The History of Maxillofacial Surgery

Elie M. Ferneini • Michael T. Goupil
Steven Halepas
Editors

The History of Maxillofacial Surgery

An Evidence-Based Journey

Springer

Editors
Elie M. Ferneini
Greater Waterbury OMS
Beau Visage Med Spa Partner
Cheshire, CT, USA

Michael T. Goupil
Division of Oral & Maxillofacial Surgery
University of Connecticut Health Center
Farmington, CT, USA

Steven Halepas
Columbia University Irving Med Center
NewYork–Presbyterian Hospital
New York, NY, USA

ISBN 978-3-030-89562-4 ISBN 978-3-030-89563-1 (eBook)
https://doi.org/10.1007/978-3-030-89563-1

This Springer imprint is published by the registered company Springer Nature Switzerland AG
The registered company address is: Gewerbestrasse 11, 6330 Cham, Switzerland

Foreword

Why write a history book, or any study of history, or of any endeavor, scientific or otherwise? Both George Santayana (1863–1952), the philosopher and author, and Winston Churchill (1874–1965), world leader and author, agreed on the maxim "those who do not remember the past are condemned to repeat it." Indeed, "the past is prologue" —Shakespeare, The Tempest.

Let us remember that all oral facial surgical specialties had their modest origins in the hands of medieval barber surgeons who extracted teeth, drained abscesses, and cauterized wounds in barns and village squares without benefit of anesthesia, asepsis, or hemostasis. Now, leave that centuries-long era of rigid dogma, profound ignorance, and superstition and fast forward to this twenty-first century of evidence-based innovative and invasive techniques and technology. This book describes the evolution in the performance of surgery and a revolution in ideas about the role of surgical specialties who operate in the orofacial region in the spectrum of healthcare.

During this author's clinical and academic career (1961–2019), OMS moved from the shadowed shallows into the bright mainstream of American surgery, despite the reefs and rocks it encountered there. This was accomplished not just through the development and importation of new techniques but also by enhanced education which placed us on a par with other surgical specialties. A bridge, albeit at times a narrow one, now unites dentistry and medicine for the well-being of patients and the continued enhancement of both professions. Surely, a basic year (or two) of general surgery education has created technically better OMS surgeons as well as expanded our knowledge and expertise in dealing with contemporary comorbidities and the emotional strains that our patients endure.

As we continue to confront the present and future frontiers of OMS, we should also seek more knowledge of the great advances of the past in order to comprehend the motives, struggles, perseverance, tenacity, and, yes, even the failures of those on whose historical shoulder we stand. Mistakes have been made even in the recent past, often resulting in a bandwagon effect, despite the present availability of evidence-based facts and lightning-fast electronic communication. By learning lessons from the past perhaps we can avoid some of the pitfalls of the present. To paraphrase

British Prime Minister Harold Macmillan (1894–1986), "the purpose of education is so that you will know when men are talking rot."

Our goals, the conquest of disease and deformity, are hardly yet accomplished, but lessons learned from the past can surely be applied to the present and the trajectory of the future. *The History of Maxillofacial Surgery* is a wonderful compilation of our professional history. It is a well-written, enlightening, and enjoyable read.

Hartford, CT, USA Morton H. Goldberg

Preface

The following introduction was drafted by the late Dr. Laskin just a few months before he passed. Dr. Laskin had a remarkable impact on the field of oral and maxillofacial surgery. The editors would like to thank him for his dedication to our specialty and for the generation of surgeons he trained. While he was unable to see the final version of the book, we find it only fitting we share his thoughts on the "History of Maxillofacial Surgery."

Maxillofacial surgery has a unique scope that is rooted in both medicine and dentistry. Therefore, to describe its complete history in a single publication would not allow for sufficient discussion of the most important aspects. To avoid this problem, the editors of this book have chosen to focus on those aspects that they consider to be of greatest significance.

The 23 chapters have been divided into 3 sections: an overview of the early history of maxillofacial surgery, a discussion of the conventional procedures within its scope, and the history of the more advanced procedures and techniques such as management of cleft lip and palate, surgery for craniosynostosis, temporomandibular joint surgery, distraction osteogenesis, and cosmetic surgery.

To provide the most detailed and accurate information, the various chapters are multi-authored and multi-specialty based. Moreover, in all surgical areas, the discussions are evidence based. Accompanying the text are numerous illustrations, figures, diagrams, and tables.

The editors are to be complimented for their unique approach to this complex story. This book should not only be of interest to the different surgical professionals who practice varying aspects of maxillofacial surgery but also to those practitioners who refer patients for such procedures.

Richmond, VA, USA — Daniel M. Laskin

Contents

Contributors

Samina H. Aziz The Wardlaw Hartridge School, Edison, NJ, USA

Shahid R. Aziz, DMD, MD, FACS, FRCSEd Department of Oral and Maxillofacial Surgery, Rutgers School of Dental Medicine, Newark, NJ, USA

Vernon Burke, DMD, MD, FACS High Desert Oral & Facial Surgery, El Paso, TX, USA

Eric R. Carlson, DMD, MD, EdM, FACS Department of Oral and Maxillofacial Surgery, University of Tennessee Medical Center, Knoxville, TN, USA

Charles Castiglione, MD, MBA, FACS Division of Plastic Surgery, Hartford Hospital and Connecticut Children's Medical Center/University of Connecticut, Hartford, CT, USA

Joy X. Chen, DMD, MD Will Surgical Arts, Rockville, MD, USA

Andrew Deek, DDS, MD Department of Oral and Maxillofacial Surgery, University of Tennessee Medical Center, Knoxville, TN, USA

Preston Dekker, DDS Department of Oral & Maxillofacial Surgery, University of Illinois at Chicago, Chicago, IL, USA

Brett H. Diamond, MD Department of Radiation Oncology, Tufts University School of Medicine, Boston, MA, USA

Sidney B. Eisig, DDS, FACS Oral and Maxillofacial Surgery, Columbia University Irving Medical Center, New York, NY, USA

Edward Ellis III, DDS, MS, FACS Department of Oral and Maxillofacial Surgery, UT Health San Antonio, San Antonio, TX, USA

Andrew R. Emery, DMD, MD Oral and Maxillofacial Surgery, Massachusetts General Hospital, Harvard School of Dental Medicine, Boston, MA, USA

M. Alejandro Fajardo, MD Department of General Surgery, School of Medicine, University of Connecticut, Farmington, CT, USA

Justin Fazzolari, DMD Oral and Maxillofacial Surgery, Columbia University Irving Medical Center, New York, NY, USA

Bridget Ferguson, DDS Oral and Maxillofacial Surgery, Columbia University Irving Medical Center, New York, NY, USA

Elie M. Ferneini, DMD, MD, MHS, MBA, FACS, FACD Division of Oral and Maxillofacial Surgery, University of Connecticut, Farmington, CT, USA

Beau Visage Med Spa and Greater Waterbury OMS, Cheshire, CT, USA

Department of Surgery, Frank H Netter MD School of Medicine, Quinnipiac University, North Haven, CT, USA

Michael S. Forman, DMD, MD Division of Oral and Maxillofacial Surgery, NewYork-Presbyterian/Columbia University Irving Medical Center, New York, NY, USA

Joel M. Friedman, DDS, FACD, FICD, FPFA Division of Oral and Maxillofacial Surgery, NewYork-Presbyterian/Columbia University Irving Medical Center, New York, NY, USA

Morton H. Goldberg, DMD, MD Division of Oral and Maxillofacial Surgery, University of Connecticut, Farmington, CT, USA

Michael T. Goupil, DDS, MEd, MBA, FACD Division of Oral and Maxillofacial Surgery, University of Connecticut, Farmington, CT, USA

Consultant in Oral and Maxillofacial Surgery, Carmel, IN, USA

Eric J. Granquist, DMD, MD Department of Oral and Maxillofacial Surgery, Hospital of the University of Pennsylvania, Philadelphia, PA, USA

Steven Halepas, DMD, MD, FACD Division of Oral and Maxillofacial Surgery, NewYork-Presbyterian/Columbia University Irving Medical Center, New York, NY, USA

Gabriel M. Hayek, DMD, MD Division of Oral and Maxillofacial Surgery, University of Connecticut, Farmington, CT, USA

Carlos R. Hernandez, DDS Department of Oral and Maxillofacial Surgery, UT Health San Antonio, San Antonio, TX, USA

Kathryn E. Huber, MD, PhD Department of Radiation Oncology, Tufts University School of Medicine, Boston, MA, USA

Christopher Hughes, MD, MPH Division of Plastic Surgery, Hartford Hospital and Connecticut Children's Medical Center/University of Connecticut, Hartford, CT, USA

Leonard B. Kaban, DMD, MD, FACS Oral and Maxillofacial Surgery, Massachusetts General Hospital, Harvard School of Dental Medicine, Boston, MA, USA

Alia Koch, DDS, MD, FACS Division of Oral and Maxillofacial Surgery, NewYork-Presbyterian/Columbia University Irving Medical Center, New York, NY, USA

Kenneth Kufta, DMD, MD Department of Oral and Maxillofacial Surgery, Hospital of the University of Pennsylvania, Philadelphia, PA, USA

Jessica S. Lee, DDS, MD, MA Private Practice, Northeast Facial & Oral Surgery Specialists, Florham Park, NJ, USA

Kenneth MacCormac, DMD Division of Oral and Maxillofacial Surgery, University of Connecticut, Farmington, CT, USA

John A. McNulty, PhD Loyola University Chicago, Stritch School of Medicine, Maywood, IL, USA

Margaret A. McNulty, PhD Department of Anatomy, Cell Biology and Physiology, Indiana University School of Medicine, Indianapolis, IN, USA

Christopher S. Midtling, DDS, MD Department of Oral & Maxillofacial Surgery, University of North Carolina, Chapel Hill, NC, USA

University of North Carolina, Chapel Hill, NC, USA

Michael Miloro, DMD, MD, FACS Department of Oral & Maxillofacial Surgery, University of Illinois at Chicago, Chicago, IL, USA

Keyur Naik, DDS, MD Department of Oral and Maxillofacial Surgery, New York University Langone Medical Center/Bellevue Hospital Center, New York, NY, USA

Christine E. Niekrash, DMD, MDentSc Frank H Netter MD School of Medicine, Quinnipiac University, North Haven, CT, USA

Benjamin Palla, DMD, MD Department of Oral & Maxillofacial Surgery, University of Illinois at Chicago, Chicago, IL, USA

Daniel E. Perez, DDS, MS, FACS Department of Oral and Maxillofacial Surgery, UT Health San Antonio, San Antonio, TX, USA

Michael Perrino, DDS, MD Riverside Oral Surgery, River Edge, NJ, USA

Peter D. Quinn, DMD, MD Department of Oral and Maxillofacial Surgery, Hospital of the University of Pennsylvania, Philadelphia, PA, USA

Utkarsh C. Shukla, MD Department of Radiation Oncology, Tufts University School of Medicine, Boston, MA, USA

Dani Stanbouly, BS College of Dental Medicine, Columbia University, New York, NY, USA

Mark H. Sueyoshi, MD Department of Radiation Oncology, Tufts University School of Medicine, Boston, MA, USA

Pasquale G. Tolomeo, DDS, MD Tulsa Surgical Arts, Tulsa, OK, USA

Derek J. Tow, DMD, MD Division of Oral and Maxillofacial Surgery, University of Connecticut, Farmington, CT, USA

Scott H. Troob, MD Department of Otolaryngology-Head & Neck Surgery, NewYork-Presbyterian/Columbia University Irving Medical Center, New York, NY, USA

Timothy A. Turvey, DDS, FACS Department of Oral & Maxillofacial Surgery, University of North Carolina, Chapel Hill, NC, USA

University of North Carolina, Chapel Hill, NC, USA

Brian M. Will, DDS Division of Oral and Maxillofacial Surgery, NewYork-Presbyterian/Columbia University Irving Medical Center, New York, NY, USA

Elizabeth M. Will, MD Department of Obstetrics & Gynecology, New York University Langone Medical Center/Bellevue Hospital Center, New York, NY, USA

Michael J. Will, DDS, MD, FACS Will Surgical Arts, Urbana, MD, USA

Jason W. Yu, DMD, MD Section of Oral & Maxillofacial Surgery, UCLA School of Dentistry, Los Angeles, CA, USA

Part I
Early History

Saint Apollonia: Patron Saint of Dentistry

Christine E. Niekrash

1 Introduction

The exquisite pain of a toothache has afflicted humanity since ancient times. An archaic Sumerian clay tablet written in approximately 5000 BCE describes dental pain. Toothaches are mentioned frequently throughout literature worldwide. The famous French barber-surgeon Ambroise Pare, writing in the 1500s CE, stated, "Toothache is, of all others, the most atrocious pain that can torment a man, followed by death."

Dental pain appears in several of Shakespeare's plays (*Othello*, *Cymbeline*, *Much Ado about Nothing*). The famous Scottish poet Robert Burns wrote his "Address to the Toothache" following his tormented bout with dental pain in 1786. For millennia, people searched for relief from this debilitating pain, with many resorting to crude methods of tooth extraction, pain relief, magic, and prayer.

For 1700 years, Christians around the world have implored Saint Apollonia (Fig. 1) to extinguish their dental pain and to prevent it. For example, Cervantes wrote in his epic work *Don Quixote* (published in 1615 CE): "'Be in no pain then,' replied the bachelor, 'but go home, in Heaven's name, and get something warm for breakfast, and on your way repeat the prayer of Saint Apollonia – if you know it.' 'Bless me!' replied the housekeeper, 'the prayer of Saint Apollonia, say you? That might do something if my master's distemper laid in his gums, but alas! It is all in

Some tortures are physical, And some are mental, But the one that is both is dental. — Ogden Nash

C. E. Niekrash (✉)
Frank H Netter MD School of Medicine, Quinnipiac University, North Haven, CT, USA
e-mail: Christine.Niekrash@quinnipiac.edu

E. M. Ferneini et al. (eds.), *The History of Maxillofacial Surgery*,
https://doi.org/10.1007/978-3-030-89563-1_1

Fig. 1 Saint Apollonia. Attributed to Piero della Francesca c. 1455–1460. (Courtesy National Gallery of Art, Washington, D.C. Reprinted without alteration)

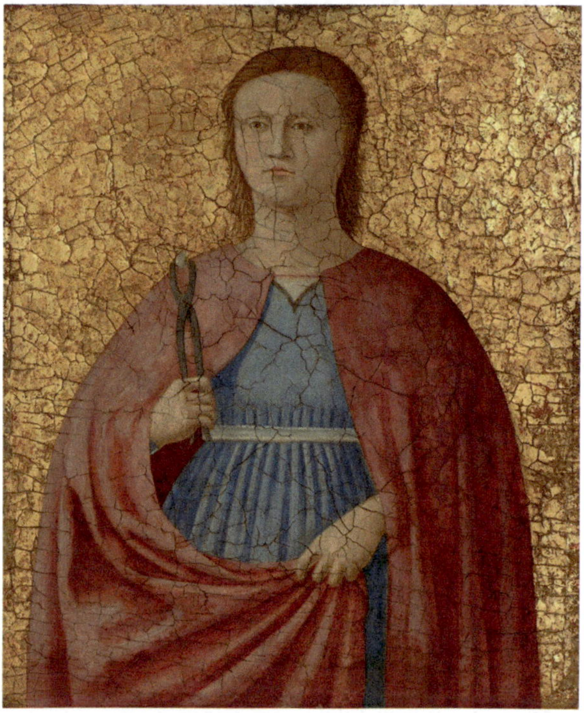

his brains.'" In 1557 CE, Francisco Martinez wrote the following prayer in his book on dentistry published in Valladolid, Spain, one of many prayers to her:

> "Illustrious virgin martyr, Apollonia,
> Pray to the Lord for us
> Lest our offenses and sins we be punished
> By diseases of the teeth."

Her life and legend are described below.

2 Egypt 249 CE, the First Written Description of Saint Apollonia

Alexandria is a port city on the Mediterranean Sea in northern Egypt, famous in the past for its vast ancient library, its lighthouse, and the large pagan Temple of Serapis. In the year 249 CE, it was a site of considerable turbulence and social unrest. The city was controlled by the Roman Empire which was then in the middle of its Imperial Crisis (235–284 CE), a period when various generals fought for control of the empire. This era witnessed the rise and collapse of over 20 emperors and the splintering of the huge empire. Widespread public discord resulted from the lack of a clear policy for succession of the emperors which incited civil wars, inflation and economic depression, the increased need for a larger army to provide protection of the extensive empire against invading tribes, and the arrival of the plague.

In addition, burgeoning tensions and social strife arose between the increasing number of Christians in the Roman Empire and those members of the polytheistic pagan majority. In Alexandria in the mid-third-century CE, rioting and mob violence were common. From 244 to 249 CE, many Christians fled from Alexandria during the rule of Roman Emperor Philip the Arabian (Marcus Julius Philippus (reigned Feb 244–Sept 249)).

Celebrations were held in 248 CE to commemorate the millennium of the founding of Rome (set at 753 BCE). During the festivities, a Roman poet is said to have foreseen catastrophe caused by the Christians. As a result, a heathen mob inflicted "bloody outrages on the Christians whom the authorities made no effort to protect" (Kirsch 1907).

Saint Dionysius (then the Christian bishop of Alexandria), writing to Bishop Fabius of Antioch, describes a specific incidence of pagan mob violence that tortured several Christian individuals after the mob was incited by this poet. Saint Dionysius wrote, "And the prophet and poet of evil to this city, whoever he was, was beforehand in moving and exciting the heathen crowds against us, rekindling their zeal for the national superstitions. So, they being aroused by him and availing themselves of all lawful authority for their unholy doings, conceived that the only piety, the proper worship of their gods was this—to thirst for our blood." In the letter, he continues to describe the polytheistic mobs torturing several Christians. He continues, "Thereupon they all with one consent made a rush on the houses of the believers, and, falling each upon those whom they recognized as neighbours, plundered, harried and despoiled them, setting aside the more valuable of their possessions and casting out into the streets and burning the cheaper things and such as were made of wood, till they produced the appearance of a city devastated by the enemy. But the brethren gave way and submitted and accepted the plundering of their possessions with joy…" (Feltoe 1918).

Saint Dionysius documents, "Another notable case was that of the aged virgin Apollonia, whom they seized and knocked out all her teeth, striking her on the jaws: then they made a pyre before the city and threatened to burn her alive, if she would not join them in uttering blasphemies. But she asked for a brief respite, and being let go, suddenly leapt into the fire and was devoured by the flames." There are variations and embellishments of this story, some stating that she made the sign of the cross when forced to worship the pagan idol, causing the statue of the Roman god to explode. In fact, Apollonia most likely was an older Christian Deaconess from a Greek family living in Alexandria. However, all versions of her life agree in reporting that her teeth were shattered and violently extracted to torture her before she died because she would not renounce her faith. She is recognized as a Christian martyr and was canonized about 50 years later, becoming Saint Apollonia.

3 The Legend

With the passage of time, St. Apollonia's story became romanticized and embellished. She evolved to become younger, more beautiful, and even more virtuous. According to the developing legend, Apollonia's father was a magistrate and her parents were opulent, loving, and happy. Their only regret was their inability to have children. Their frequent prayers to the pagan gods were unanswered. However, three Christian pilgrims visited their home and presented the story and teachings of Christ to the magistrate's wife. The woman then prayed to the Virgin Mary and Christ. Through this request, she subsequently gave birth to a daughter, Apollonia.

Jacobus de Voragine wrote a chapter on Saint Apollonia in 1260 in his treatise "The Golden Legend: Readings on the Saints," one of the most widely read medieval documents (de Voragine 1993). He describes her excruciating dental torture and ultimate martyrdom in the fire. He concludes, "Oh, great and wondrous struggle of this virgin, who by the grace of a compassionate God, went to the fire so as not to be burned and was burned so as not to be consumed, as if neither fire nor torture could touch her! There would have been safety in freedom, but no glory for one who avoided the fight." He continues, "The merit of this virgin, so gloriously and blessedly triumphant, excels and shines out among martyrs."

During the 1500s, the legend of Saint Apollonia was explained in the "Rappresentazione di Santa Apollonia Vergine e Martire" (Eramo et al. 2017), a stage production from Florence, Italy, that involved approximately 20 performing actors and a still undiscovered musical score. This production corresponds with six paintings of St. Apollonia by mannerist painter Francesco Granacci (Florence, 1469–1543) currently housed in the Accademia Gallery of Florence that illustrate the key points of the Sacra Rappresentazione.

This religious drama, similar to the passion plays of Germany, further embellishes the legend of Saint Apollonia. In this version, her father is King Tarsus. She is raised as a pagan, but her interest in Christianity remains sparked by her mother's story of the role of the Virgin Mary in her birth. Apollonia is then converted to Christianity by a hermit (Leonine, disciple of Saint Anthony) who baptizes her. Ecstatic, she returns to Alexandria to preach and to convert the people, which angers her father the king.

The production script describes that her father, furious with his daughter's response, sentences punishment for Apollonia by declaring,

"Take her and break her teeth
With pain as much as raw and strong
So that she experiences harsher torments
To make her error clear
And to set an example for rebels"

After she endures these tortures, Apollonia declares that even without teeth, she can still speak well and continue to convert the people, and she refuses to worship the idols. The emperor then orders her decapitation and a "cloud takes Saint Apollonia's soul and picks it up to Heaven."

4 The Patroness of Dentistry and the Healer of Dental Pain

Christian patron saints are named to act as protectors or intermediaries between humans and God and to intercede on the behalf of individuals who pray to them. Often, the saint becomes the patron saint to protect against pain or affliction in the particular part of the body that reflected their martyrdom. Because Apollonia had been tortured by the destruction and extraction of her teeth, she became the patron saint for those who suffered from toothaches and later by extension for those who alleviate this pain, the profession of dentistry. In the Middle Ages, dental ailments were prevalent and treated by a variety of procedures including bloodletting, leeching, blistering of the skin, laxatives, cupping, placing garlic cloves in the ear, and destroying the dental nerves by cautery using a red-hot iron or strong acid (Walsh 1897). The last resort solution was a brutal tooth extraction by barber-surgeons, blacksmiths, or tooth-drawers at a monastery or a fair, all without anesthesia. On certain days on the top of Capitoline Hill at the top of Araceli's marble staircase in Rome, Franciscan friars would extract teeth (Kelley 1919). Home remedies, elixirs, amulets, or magic spells offered minimal or no relief (please see Chap. 3: Barber-Surgeons). During the medieval period, physicians first advised those experiencing dental pain to pray to Saint Apollonia for divine intercession and relief. Journeyman tooth-drawers typically wore pointed hats bearing the insignia of Saint Apollonia, patron saint of toothache sufferers, and a necklace of extracted human teeth (Wynbrandt 1998). In 1508 in Holland, Utrecht Brevier first mentions Saint Apollonia as patroness of those who suffer from toothache. Churches and chapels, statues, and paintings were created and dedicated in her honor.

Her feast day is celebrated on February 9 of each year by the Roman Catholic Church, Alexandrian Church, Eastern Orthodox Church, and Coptic Church.

5 Relics

Within Christianity, relics are all or part of the mortal remains or objects associated with a holy figure. (Harper and Hallam 1995). Christians have been venerating relics since the days of the Roman Catacombs (200–900 CE). Barbara Drake Boehm explains the importance of relics in Christianity, writing "Relics were more than mementos. The New Testament refers to the healing power of objects that were touched by Christ or his apostles. The body of the saint provided a spiritual link between life and death, between man and God: 'Because of the grace remaining in the martyr, they were an inestimable treasure for the holy congregation of the faithful.' Fueled by the Christian belief in the afterlife and resurrection, in the power of the soul, and in the role of saints as advocates for humankind in heaven, the veneration of relics in the Middle Ages came to rival the sacraments in the daily life of the medieval church" (Boehm 2000).

In addition, and if possible, saints' graves and churches housing relics were visited to attain divine intervention (pilgrimages). But the actual graves could be difficult to visit if they were located outside the city walls or far away. As a result, the saint's remains were exhumed and transported all over medieval Europe, usually in pieces, and the relics were stored in churches and by royalty and the wealthy.

Christian relics reached their peak during the Middle Ages, but fraud often occurred. King Philip II of Spain who reigned in Spain from 1556 to 1598, according to Carlos Fuentes in *The Buried Mirror* (Fuentes 1992), "…surrounding himself with such an avalanche of saintly relics. His agents searched far and wide to bring him the skulls, shinbones, and withered hands of saints and martyrs, the relics of Christ's thorns and the True Cross, which he worshiped more than gold and silver. In fact, Philip managed to amass all 290 holy teeth from the mouth of Saint Apollonia, the patroness of toothache. The relic deposit at El Escorial must looked like Citizen Kane's warehouse at Xanadu."

In 1543, church authorities ruled that every relic should have a special seal (autentica), but the veracity of relics is difficult or impossible to ascertain. Reliquaries (often very elaborate works of art) display and protect relics. They are often carried in procession on the saint's feast day and other holy days. This still occurs to commemorate Saint Apollonia in various locations around the world, such as the Church of St. Brice in the Belgian city of Tournai.

Relics of Saint Apollonia were collected and displayed across Europe. According to Kelley (Kelley 1919), her head was housed in the ancient Basilica of Santa Maria in Trastevere in Rome, her arms in Basilica di San Lorenzo in Rome, and part of her jaw in San Basilio also in Rome. Currently, in Rome, there is a Piazza Saint Apollonia. Other Saint Apollonia relics have been attributed to a Jesuit church at Antwerp, St. Augustine's at Brussels, a Jesuit church at Mechlin (Belgium), St. Cross at Liege (Belgium), and several churches in Cologne (Walsh 1897). Some of these churches have closed or distributed their ancient relics, and records are difficult to verify.

An elaborate reliquary in the Cathedral in Porto, Portugal, displays a purported tooth of Saint Apollonia (Fig. 2). Her alleged upper right first premolar with cervical caries is displayed in the cathedral treasury of Rab (Croatia) (Skrobonja et al. 2009).

Saint Apollonia relics also exist in the United States. Examples include St. Mary's College in St. Marys, Kansas, the Shrine of All Saints at Saint Martha of Bethany Church in Morton Grove, Illinois (personal correspondence with Father Dennis), and the Church of St. Joan of Arc, Powell, Ohio (relics of St. Apollonia are under the main altar with three other saint relics).

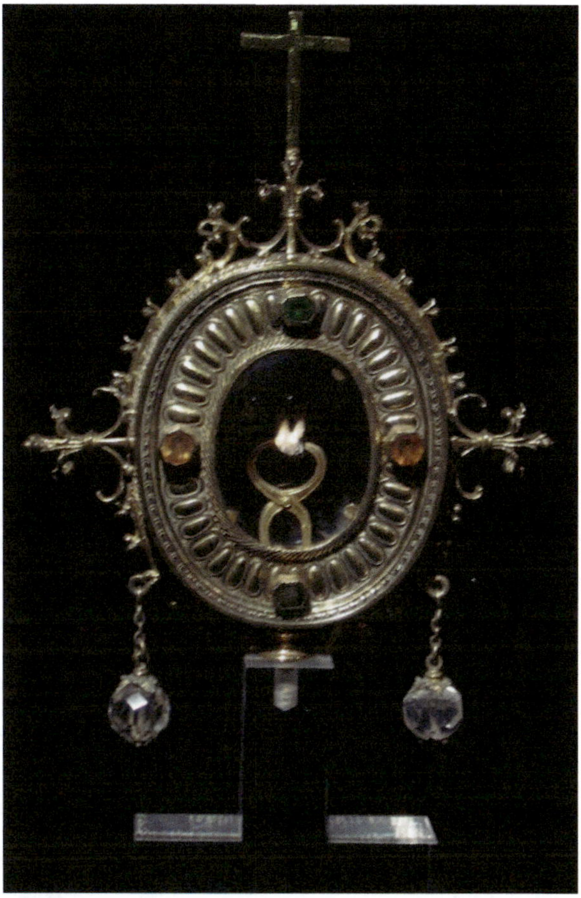

Fig. 2 Reliquary allegedly contains tooth of Saint Apollonia, Cathedral of Porto, Portugal. (Wiki Commons Image, reproduced without alteration)

6 St. Apollonia Commemorations: Statues, Churches, Plazas, Paintings, Stained Glass Windows

Saint Apollonia is usually depicted as young and beautiful and with the same identifying symbols. She is most often holding forceps which frequently hold a tooth. She is depicted with a crown (halo) or palm frond symbolizing martyrdom. Some images include the pyre. Ancient art often displayed Saint Apollonia with a golden tooth hanging from her necklace.

Germany houses many small chapels of Saint Apollonia (Aachen, Stein, etc.) Lisbon, Portugal, named its train station Apollonia. England is home to more than 50 works commemorating her (Beal 1996), including chapels, stained glass, paintings, and statues. Her image forms the side support of the coat of arms of the British Dental Association. Belgium, Sweden, and the Netherlands also host many images and commemorations of Saint Apollonia.

In the United States, Chicago houses a stained glass window depicting Saint Apollonia in the Loyola University Madonna Della Strada Chapel (Fig. 3).

A statue of Saint Apollonia by Vincenzo Luccardi stands at the entrance of the Leon Levy Library (Dental Medicine) in the University of Pennsylvania. She is portrayed with a bandage around her jaw. The Boston Guild of Saint Apollonia, founded in April 1920, performed charitable work among parochial school children in the Boston area.

Paintings of Saint Apollonia appear in prominent museum collections such as the Louvre, the National Gallery of Art, the Philadelphia Museum of Art, the Royal Dental Institute of Stockholm, Sweden, and in a host of churches, chapels, and smaller museums. Recently (1984), Andy Warhol created a series of silk screen paintings of Saint Apollonia.

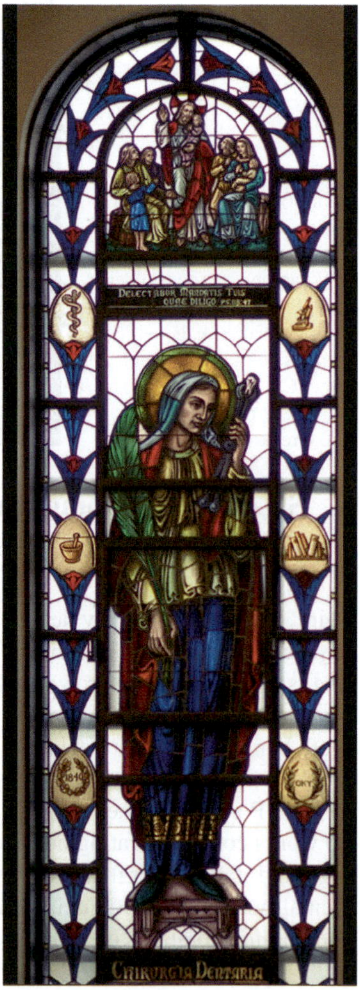

Fig. 3 Photographer: Mark Beane, "Madonna della Strada Chapel – St. Apollonia of Alexandria Window," *Loyola University Chicago Digital Special Collections*, accessed July 23, 2020, http://www.lib.luc.edu/specialcollections/items/show/164. Reproduced without alterations

Commemorations of Saint Apollonia are numerous, ancient and contemporary, and in a variety of forms. To this day, in early February (to commemorate Saint Apollonia's February 9 feast day), special pancakes called Geutelingen are baked in the Belgian town of Elst. It is believed that chewing this special pancake will offer protection from toothaches.

Summary This chapter describes what is known about the life of Saint Apollonia, a Christian martyr who was tortured by the violent extraction and destruction of her teeth in 249 CE. She has been named the patron saint of those suffering from toothache and for those who alleviate that pain, the dental profession. This chapter describes the evolution of her depictions and commemorations and the location of various relics and works of art honoring her. Saint Apollonia is usually portrayed holding a forceps displaying a tooth or wearing a necklace with a dangling golden tooth. Her feast day is celebrated every February 9.

References

Beal JF. Representations of Saint Apollonia in British Churches. Dental Hist. 1996;30:3–19.

Boehm BD. Relics and Reliquaries in Medieval Christianity. In: Heilbrunn timeline of art history. New York: The Metropolitan Museum of Art; 2000. http://www.metmuseum.org/toah/hd/relc/hd_relc.htm (originally published October 2001, last revised April 2011).

de Voragine J. The golden legend: readings on the Saints (c.1260). Translated by Ryan, W. Princeton: Princeton University Press; 1993.

Eramo S, Natali A, Bravi M, Cella D, Milia E. A "Sacra Rappresentazione" of Saint Apollonia's martyrdom. J Hist Dent. 2017;65(2):63–72.

Feltoe CL. (translator from the Greek) Saint Dionysius of Alexandria: letters and treatises (36). London. The Macmillan Company; 1918. Translations of Christian Literature. Series I. Greek Texts.

Fuentes C. The buried mirror: reflections on Spain and the New World. Boston: Houghton Mifflin Company; 1992. p. 164.

Harper J, Hallam E. Secrets of the middle ages. New York: Kenecky and Kenecky; 1995.

Kelley H. Saint Apollonia-the patron saint of dentistry. J National Dent Assoc. 1919;6(5):400–12.

Kirsch J. St. Apollonia. The Catholic Encyclopedia. Vol. 1. New York: Robert Appleton Company; 1907. http://www.newadvent.org/cathen/01617c.htm.

Skrobonja A, Rotschild V, Culina T. Saint Apollonia's Tooth – A Relic in the Cathedral Treasury of Rab (Croatia). Br Dent J. 2009;207:499–50.

Walsh W. Curiosities of popular customs and of rites, ceremonies, observances and miscellaneous antiquities. Philadelphia: Lippincott; 1897.

Wynbrandt J. The excruciating history of dentistry: toothsome tales and oral oddities from Babylon to Braces. New York: St. Martin's Griffin; 1998.

Anatomists: The Basis of Surgery

Margaret A. McNulty and John A. McNulty

1 Introduction

Surgery has been a part of dentistry and medicine since the beginning of civilization with archeological evidence showing that as far back as 12,000 years ago, people were subjected to drilling holes in the cranium (trepanation) supposedly to relieve intracranial pressure or other neurological complaints (Gross 2012). Skeletal remains in this same period had incisors with excavated pits (Oxilia et al. 2017), while skeletal material dating to about 200 BCE included dental fillings comprising a bronze wire inserted into the tooth canal (Yeomans 2019). Clearly, some knowledge of anatomy was valuable to these early surgeons, but it was not until Claudius Galen (129–199 CE) formally introduced anatomy and physiology in ancient Greece as the disciplines comprising the foundation of dentistry and medicine.

This chapter highlights some of the historical hallmarks of anatomy, touching on a few anatomical facts and anecdotes which are not typically covered elsewhere and which we hope the reader will find interesting. For instance, it includes information on the history of the sphenoid bone because it provides a specific example of how anatomy has influenced dentistry and medicine over the years. Why the sphenoid bone? Not only is it highly relevant to dentistry because it transmits important nerves to the maxilla and mandible, but it has long mystified anatomists because of its complexity and its obscure location at the base of the skull. Other sections of the chapter review the evolution of modern anatomical imaging, as well as the history

M. A. McNulty (✉)
Department of Anatomy, Cell Biology and Physiology, Indiana University School of Medicine, Indianapolis, IN, USA
e-mail: mcnultma@iupui.edu

J. A. McNulty
Loyola University Chicago, Stritch School of Medicine, Maywood, IL, USA

E. M. Ferneini et al. (eds.), *The History of Maxillofacial Surgery*,
https://doi.org/10.1007/978-3-030-89563-1_2

of specimen acquisitions (cadavers) in anatomical education. Without the transmission of information, there can be no history. In reviewing the role of education, this chapter shares some anecdotes from more than five decades of our combined experiences as instructors of anatomy. The chapter closes with a brief history of art and anatomy. Because of their common attention to form, it has been natural that art and anatomy have been so closely aligned.

2 From Galen to Vesalius

Any recounting of the history of anatomy requires recognition of the many figures who influenced the evolution of the discipline (Malomo et al. 2006; Mavrodi et al. 2013; Ghosh and Kumar 2019). Here, we draw brief attention to two of the most notable contributors, Claudius Galen and Andreas Vesalius.

Claudius Galen of Pergamon (Fig. 1) was born into the Roman Empire in 129 CE and, at the early age of 16, began his interests in medicine, which included extended studies in Alexandria, Egypt, a well-known medical center at that time. His long career included serving as physician to several emperors until his death at age 87.

Galen's contributions to anatomy formed the foundation of medical knowledge lasting almost 1400 years. He honed many of his skills as a physician and anatomist through his treatment of gladiators wounded in the "games," treating their wounds as windows in the body, thus replacing dissections of human bodies, which were illegal at the time. Because Galen was driven by the need to visualize anatomical

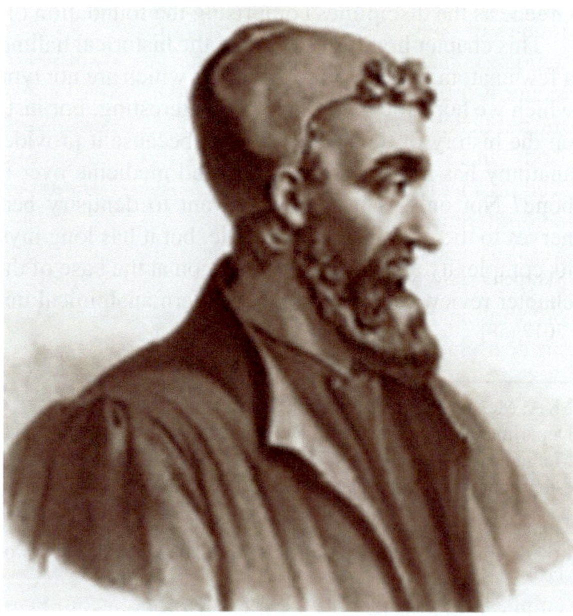

Fig. 1 Galen lithograph by Pierre Roche Vigneron. (Paris: Lith de Gregoire et Deneux, ca. 1865)

structures through dissection, many of his observations were based on animal models, including Barbary apes. Among his most notable anatomical observations were correct descriptions of seven of the 12 cranial nerves, the four valves of the heart, the arterial/venous system, and functions of spinal nerves, especially the role of the phrenic nerve in controlling contraction of the diaphragm (Malomo et al. 2006).

Galen was a prolific author completing several hundred publications, many of which served as medical handbooks that formed the basis of medical education in medieval universities once they were translated into Latin. These writings promoted the discoveries of earlier physicians such as Hippocrates and Herophilus, but only where they agreed with his observations. However, Galen's works began to lose favor when, by the mid-sixteenth century, the Flemish physician, Andreas Vesalius, emphasized that Galen's anatomical descriptions were principally from animals rather than humans and contained numerous errors. Nevertheless, Galen still is rightly recognized for his role in contributing to the rise of modern science and the experimental method.

Galen's publication (circa 180 CE) describing the skull bones is of particular note because it was probably the earliest work known that included human material. Most importantly to the subject of this chapter, he described the anatomy of the sphenoid bone for the first time as "the bone which resembles a wedge (sphen hence sphenoid) between the vault of the skull and the upper jaw" (Singer 1952). His description goes on to include the sutures running along the temples meeting with the coronal suture and descending to the palate to form a boundary with the upper jaw. References to the winglike pterygoid plates were made.

As did Galen, Andreas Vesalius began his training in medicine and anatomy at the early age of 18 in 1532 at the University of Paris, during which time he developed his skills in human dissection by venturing outside the walls of Paris to the mound of Mounfacon where the decomposing bodies of executed criminals were deposited (Mavrodi et al. 2013). He quickly rose in statue for his knowledge of anatomy, giving lectures at the university using human material and culminating in the publication of his book *De humani corporis fabrica* (On the Fabric of the Human Body) in 1543 (Ghosh and Kumar 2019). As discussed below, this book revolutionized the medical world and replaced the Galenistic views of anatomy as the preeminent reference because it provided more accurate descriptions of the human body. Vesalius paid a high professional price and was roundly criticized for his corrections of Galen's writings (Malomo et al. 2006). He left the university, abandoned any preparations of future studies, and lived out his remaining years as a physician until his death in 1564.

3 The Sphenoid Bone

"Gentlemen, damn the sphenoid bone!" This quote attributed to Oliver Wendell Holmes Sr. in his lecture to the Harvard medical class in the 1800s (Tubbs 2016) emphasized dramatically the mystery and anatomical intricacies of this bone. It is worth briefly noting that women were not admitted to medical school at that time, though as Dean of Harvard Medical School, he worked to reform the admission process to eventually include women (Tubbs et al. 2012).

The sphenoid bone contributes extensively to forming the base of the skull and in this position articulates with a large number of other bones including the frontal, parietal, ethmoid, zygomatic, temporal, occipital, palatine, and vomer bones and through these articulations connects the neurocranium with the facial bones (Jamil and Callahan 2020). Its complex anatomy is due in part to its embryological origin from both mesodermal and neural crest derivatives. The principal components include the body with the sella turcica housing the pituitary gland, the lesser wing that transmits four cranial nerves to the orbit, the greater wings that contribute to the calvarium, and the two pterygoid processes that serve as attachments for important muscles of mastication. The greater wing contains the foramen rotundum transmitting the maxillary nerve to the upper jaw and the foramen ovale for the mandibular nerve innervating the lower jaw and tongue. The overall shape of the bone reminded early anatomists of a bird or a bat with its body, wings, and legs (pterygoid processes).

The long history of the sphenoid bone was recently reviewed by Costea et al. (Costea et al. 2018). Highlights of this review pointed out the contributions of Vesalius (1555 CE), who referred to the bone as the cuneiform bone with "extraordinary varied form" contributing to its designation as a "polymorphous" bone. Vesalius presented all of the anatomy of the sphenoid bone up to that time (Fig. 2) and corrected many of the errors in the anatomical descriptions of the bone,

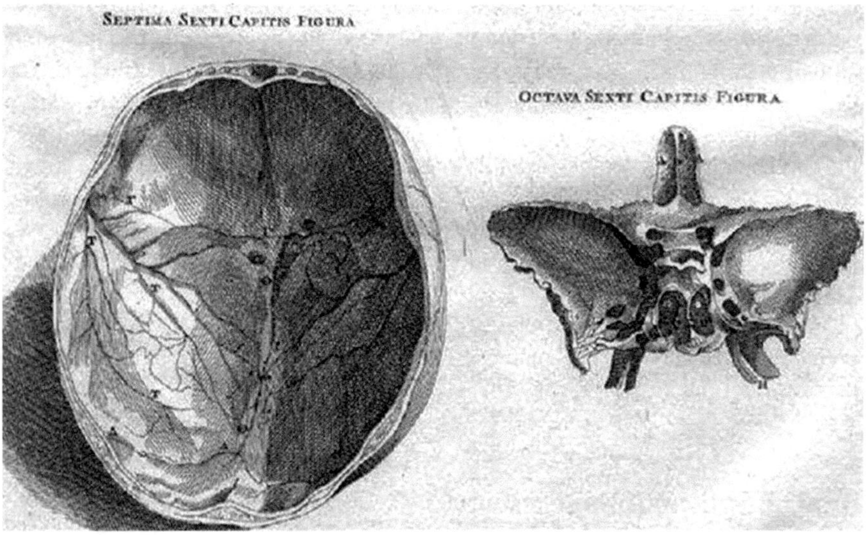

Fig. 2 Drawings of the cranium and sphenoid bone, taken from Andreas Vesalius' *De corporis humani fabrica*, 1543

including those of Galen. Most importantly, Vesalius detailed all of the foramina and structures (nerves, arteries, veins) passing through each foramen. This anatomical detail greatly expanded the importance of anatomy to medicine and surgery because, as pointed out above, the cranial nerve innervation to the upper and lower jaws pass through these foramina. More recent innovations have produced 360-degree interactive models allowing easier understanding of the complexity of the bone and its foramina as well as surrounding structures (Jacquesson et al. 2017).

Medical issues specifically involving the sphenoid bone are not common, but in 1895, there was a remarkable account of severe caries in the sphenoid bone of a physician (Day 1895). The disease progressed over a period of several months, and its severity can be gleaned from the following description: "an area of diseased bone 2 cm. in length by 1 cm. in breadth could be seen and it was evident that the body of the sphenoid and basilar process of the occipital bone were disintegrating." On postmortem examination, "The entire body of the sphenoid and basilar process of the occipital bone were riddled with sinuses, exposing the external surface of the dura and leaving it as the only protection and support of that part of the base of the brain resting on the clivus blumenbachii. The pterygoid processes and ascending rami of the palatine bones were carious and loose. The vomer was entirely gone, as also the perpendicular plate of the ethmoid." It was clearly a desperate situation.

4 Modern Anatomical Imaging

The foundation of dental surgery is based upon proper imaging of the anatomy, and therefore, radiology plays an integral role in the history of dental surgery. Dental imaging begins with the discovery of X-rays, a type of electromagnetic radiation characterized by short wavelengths, by Wilhelm Conrad Röntgen, a professor of physics at the University of Würzburg in Germany, in 1895. He discovered these new rays, which he deemed "X-rays," after noticing light near a glass vacuum (Crookes) tube during one of his experiments. After his discovery of X-rays, Röntgen was able to persuade his wife, Anna Bertha Röntgen, to place her hand on a photographic plate, thus creating the first radiographic image of a human subject. From there, it is unclear who made the first dental radiograph. Several individuals in Germany, England, and the United States were using X-rays to take images of teeth in early 1896, shortly after Röntgen's discovery (Campbell 1995). However, Friedrich Otto Walkhoff has been credited as taking the first dental radiograph, of his own teeth, by holding an ordinary photographic glass plate during the 25-minute exposure (Riaud 2014) (Fig. 3). Dr. C. Edmund Kells was likely the first dentist in the United States to take intraoral X-rays in a living patient by developing a film holder that would allow the patient to swallow during the process, which required at least 15 minutes' exposure time (Langland et al. 1972). In the early 1900s, dental radiography increased in popularity, and German and American companies began manufacturing dental X-ray machines.

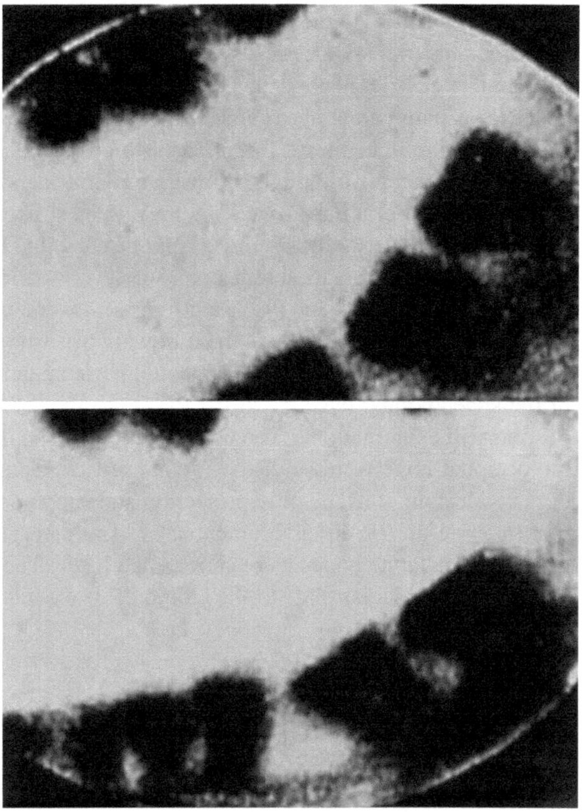

Fig. 3 The first dental X-ray image depicting the teeth of Otto Walkhoff (1896)

Unfortunately, these early X-rays were crude and not useful, and the dangers of X-rays were soon realized by early radiology pioneers and those who volunteered early on to serve as subjects. These subjects experienced radiodermatitis and ultimately radiation-induced carcinomas following repeated exposure to the damaging X-rays. Indeed, Dr. Kells himself suffered from extensive lesions on his hands that refused to heal, ultimately resulting in 35 surgeries culminating in the amputation of his entire left arm at the shoulder in 1926 (Langland et al. 1972). It was not long before the correlation was made between the development of adverse health effects secondary to X-ray exposure, though it was unclear to these individuals as to whether the dangers came from exposure to the X-rays themselves or by the action of the current passing outside of the tube (Kells 1899). However, further refinement in the technique led to safer applications in the dental field. William Herbert Rollins, a practicing dentist, was responsible for many techniques and devices that reduced X-ray exposures. In 1896, he began to investigate the properties of X-rays, mostly focused toward dental applications (Kathren and William 1964). In 1901, he published a paper that correlated lesions on his hands to repeated and prolonged X-ray exposure; he subsequently suggested other dentists and medical professionals properly protect themselves, for example, by using glasses lined with lead and enclosing the X-ray tube in a leaded box (Rollins 1901). However, his warnings were not heeded until years later, and thusly, he ultimately became known as the "Father of Radiation Protection."

In the succeeding years, incorporation of radiological principles in the dental field was assisted by several technical developments that made the technology safer and more efficient for dental uses. In the mid-1920s, film replaced glass plates for visualizing radiographic images. By 1925, the radiograph had become part of the foundation of the practice of dentistry, and it was deemed necessary for diagnosing and treating diseases and issues related to the teeth and jaws (Mooney 1925). H. R. Raper introduced his new "bitewing" technique in 1926 and subsequently published the details of his technique in a textbook (Raper 1926), which was widely accepted at the time by those in the field as a large step in dental preventative medicine (R H N. 1927), as it allowed visualization of the occlusal surfaces of the teeth. Extraoral panoramic radiography was developed in 1949 by Yrjo V. Paatero, and launched dental radiography forward, as it allowed for an unobstructed, two-dimensional image of the entire mouth (Hallikainen 1996). However, it was not until the 1960s when commercial panoramic radiology units were manufactured in Europe and the United States and were readily available to those practicing in the field.

The technology that resulted in digital radiography known today was developed beginning in the late 1970s with digital subtraction angiography (Korner et al. 2007). Numerous other technological advances have resulted in digital radiography becoming increasingly available, even in remote hospitals and practices. These advancements have made the process of obtaining oral radiographs far more efficient and resulted in less radiation exposure for the patient and practitioner. Digital radiography was first introduced into the dental field in 1987 by Dr. Francois Mugnon with his RadioVisioGraphy system (Frommer and Stabulas-Savage 2011), and the first digital dental panoramic unit was built by W. Doss McDavid at the University of Texas Health Sciences Center in San Antonio. Shortly after, in 1995, digital panoramic X-ray systems were available on the market.

More advanced radiological imaging techniques used to accurately assess anatomical structures, such as computed tomography (CT) and magnetic resonance imaging (MRI), have been increasingly integrated in dental practice. Originally developed in 1967 by Sir Godfrey Hounsfield, CT scans were initially extremely time-consuming, thus limiting their dental applications. Technological advances in the imaging technique have significantly decreased scanning time and made the imaging modality far more suitable for dentistry. Some applications include identifying bony pathologies and assessing paranasal sinuses and the bony components of the temporomandibular joint (Parks 2000). However, CT has not been widely utilized in dental practice due to the high radiation dosage, cost associated with the procedure, the lack of access to scanners, and experience required to adequately interpret images, which is knowledge often not readily found in practicing dentists (Kumar et al. 2015). Cone beam CT (CBCT), first introduced in the 1990s, allows for accurate, 3D imaging of hard tissue structures using only a single rotation where patient movement is not required and can negate the concerns associated with traditional CT in dental practice, resulting in improved diagnoses and patient safety (Howerton and Mora 2007). The applications of CBCT in dental surgery include identifying the exact anatomical location of pathologies such as tumors or bone lesions, assessing impacted and supernumerary teeth, evaluating severity of osteonecrosis of the jaw, and evaluating paranasal sinuses (Fig. 4), among other applications, and are more widely utilized in oral surgery compared to traditional CT imaging.

In the history of radiological imaging, MRI is a relative latecomer to the field. While the research in physics that led to the development of MRI dates back to 1938, it was not until the 1970s that it was demonstrated to be possible to use nuclear MR to create an image (Lauterbur 1973). Compared to the other radiological imaging modalities that utilize ionizing radiation, MRI has a promising future in dentistry. The ability of the technique to distinguish between various soft tissues makes it an ideal imaging technique to diagnose temporomandibular joint dysfunction (TMD) and dental implant planning (Niraj et al. 2016). MRI techniques are also being used for a variety of other conditions that benefit from identifying the exact anatomical location and extent of disease, including early bone changes secondary to tumor formation and fractures (Niraj et al. 2016).

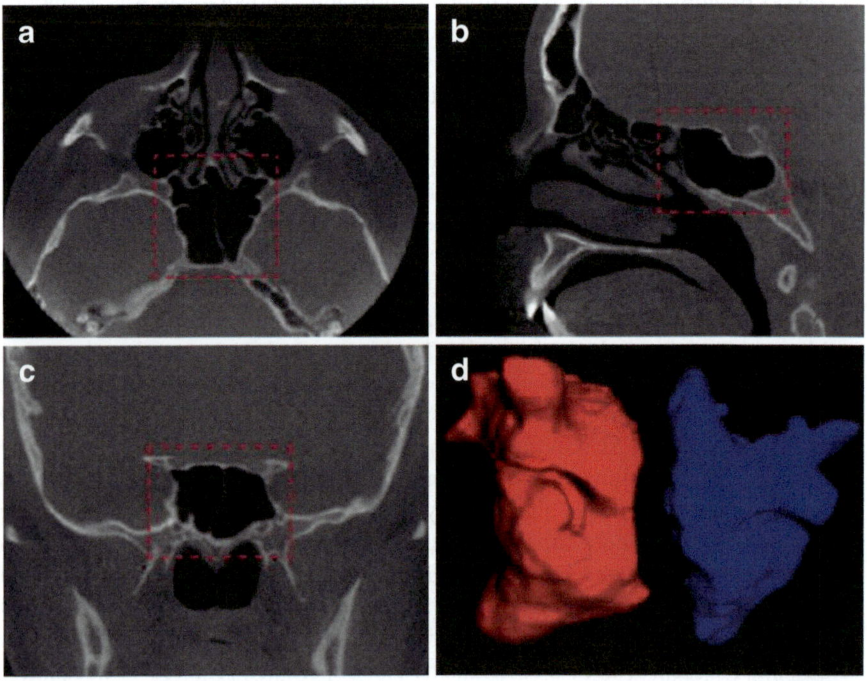

Fig. 4 Three-dimensional reconstruction of the sphenoid sinus using CBCT. (**a**) axial view, (**b**) sagittal view, (**c**) coronal view, (**d**) final volumetric reconstruction (Nejaim et al. 2019)

5 A Brief History of Cadaver Acquisition for Education

The study of anatomy is an active science involving dissection of the human body to discover its parts, hence a need for human material, which provided a tumultuous history of its own affected by cultural mores, religious constraints, and superstitions. Leonardo da Vinci in the late fifteenth century was among the first to incorporate dissections to accomplish his detailed renditions of the human body. His dissections of human corpses were mostly from hospitals in Florence, Milan, and Rome, and they led to a better understanding of the physiology and the mechanics of joint movements. Vesalius followed shortly thereafter, and in contrast to da Vinci, who had many eclectic interests, he was much more focused on the surgical and anatomical specialties. Vesalius was a strong proponent of dissection as a teaching tool and relied for the most part on executed criminals for his studies. One such dissection of a felon (Jacob Karrer) from Switzerland prepared by Vesalius in 1543 resulted in a well-preserved and the oldest surviving skeletal preparation displayed in the Anatomisches Museum at the University of Basel.

This reliance on executed criminals for anatomical studies has persisted since the sixteenth century. Siegfried Zitzelsperger, an anatomist who trained in Germany in the early 1930s, recounted as a young student waiting for completion of an execution before he and his colleagues rushed in to quickly remove the spleen from the deceased to perfuse it with latex to make a case of the circulatory system (personal comm.). More recently, the Visible Human Project (VHP) (2019) compiled a large data set of cryosectioned, cross-sectional images from a male and a female. The male donor was Joseph Paul Jernigan, a 38-year-old Texas murderer who was executed by lethal injection. The VHP was funded by the National Institutes of Health Library of Medicine to increase the availability of high-resolution electronic images correlated with both MRI and CT images. The anatomical axial images were collected from the removal of cryosections at 4 mm intervals for the male and 0.33 mm intervals for the female. The completed data sets have been widely licensed for use in noncommercial and commercial applications for education and research.

The use of executed criminals for dissection was legitimized in the Murder Act of 1751 by the Parliament of Great Britain (Mitchell et al. 2011). It was intended to prevent acts of murder if potential offenders knew that they would be dissected following execution. The act also provided a supply of bodies to the Royal College of Surgeons for this purpose. While executions of convicts provided a source of cadavers for study, it was not terribly reliable and did not provide sufficient numbers of cadavers as dental and medical education programs grew in number. In order to make up this supply gap, rather gruesome activities sprang up including murder of the homeless and grave robbing. One notorious episode occurred in Scotland in the early 1800s where two Irishmen murdered 16 unsuspecting people under different conditions and sold their bodies to a member of the Royal College of Surgeons of Edinburgh who taught anatomy and advertised demonstrations using fresh anatomical subjects for each lecture. The crime of murder for the purpose of selling bodies for dissection became known as "burking," named after one of the offenders,

William Burke (Harris 1920). A direct consequence of this "burking" incident was the passage of the British Anatomy Act of 1832, which rescinded the Murder Act and enhanced the availability of human bodies from physicians legally responsible for patients who had died in hospitals and other facilities and who had not been claimed by relatives in over 48 hours.

If murder or legal acquisition of human bodies was not an option, then stealing bodies which had already been buried became an alternative. Over time, an important distinction has arisen between "grave robbers" and "body snatchers." The former includes those who rob burial sites for profit (including archeological sites). The latter are those individuals interested only in the deceased, usually for sale to medical schools or other professionals to dissect. One example occurred in the 1850s in Illinois. According to the account published in the Joliet Herald News (1997), three physicians in the area required a body to dissect to resolve some unanswered anatomical questions. A young medical student (Keeny), the brother-in-law of one of the physicians, volunteered to recover the body of an elderly woman recently interred. Keeny delivered, the physicians dissected, but Keeny lost his nerve when returning the body to the grave and left it in a quarry covered with stones and snow not to be discovered until the spring thaw. The newspaper account included courtroom dramas involving false accusations and a local play recounting the affair, but the story ended without resolving the fate of Keeny and the three physicians.

Today, cadavers for anatomical teaching and research are obtained legally through donor programs that rely on the altruism of the general public to donate their remains upon their death. In most cases, individual medical schools have their own programs to support their needs. In other cases, several universities consolidate resources such as the Anatomical Gifts Association in Illinois, which collects and distributes donors to seven medical schools in the greater Chicago area. Government regulations strictly control the distribution and use of any human remains.

6 Anatomy Through Art and Atlases

The human body as the subject of art is a constant from the earliest cave drawings with the prevailing link between art and anatomy (other than the human form) being reliance on the visual sense. As the artist lends perspective through a painting, the anatomist reveals relations of structures through dissection. This anthropocentric nature of art and anatomy is highlighted by the dependence of anatomical study on artists' abilities to capture and render complicated anatomical elements in a three-dimensional perspective. Examples of these artistic accomplishments are abundant (Mavrodi et al. 2013).

In 1490 AD, Leonardo da Vinci (1452–1519), an accepted genius for his contributions in mathematics, chemistry, mechanics, and art, sketched a drawing of the proportions of the human body he made from measurements of models in Milan, Italy. The drawing represents accurate proportions of the human body within a square and a circle. It is referred to as "Vitruvian Man" (Fig. 5) because it was based on descriptions of the Roman architect Vitruvius. It combines mathematics (proportions) and art as only Leonard da Vinci could do, which qualified it as an important message we have sent into space many times on formal embroidered patches worn by NASA astronauts. One design includes an astronaut in a space-walk suit in the same position depicted in the "Vitruvian Man" and is worn on the right shoulder of US space suits engaged in extravehicular activity space walks. The "Vitruvian Man" was also featured on patches worn by NASA's Expedition 37 crew that traveled to the International Space Station in 2013.

One of the more famous paintings combining art and anatomy was "The Anatomy Lesson of Dr. Nicolaes Tulp" by Rembrandt (1632) (Fig. 6). The painting depicts Dr. Nicolaes Tulp, who was Doctor of Medicine and Praelector Anatomiae to the Amsterdam Guild of Surgeons, demonstrating a dissection of the forearm to other members of the guild. Such demonstrations were common in medical centers across Europe, and though they originally were for educational purposes, they evolved to

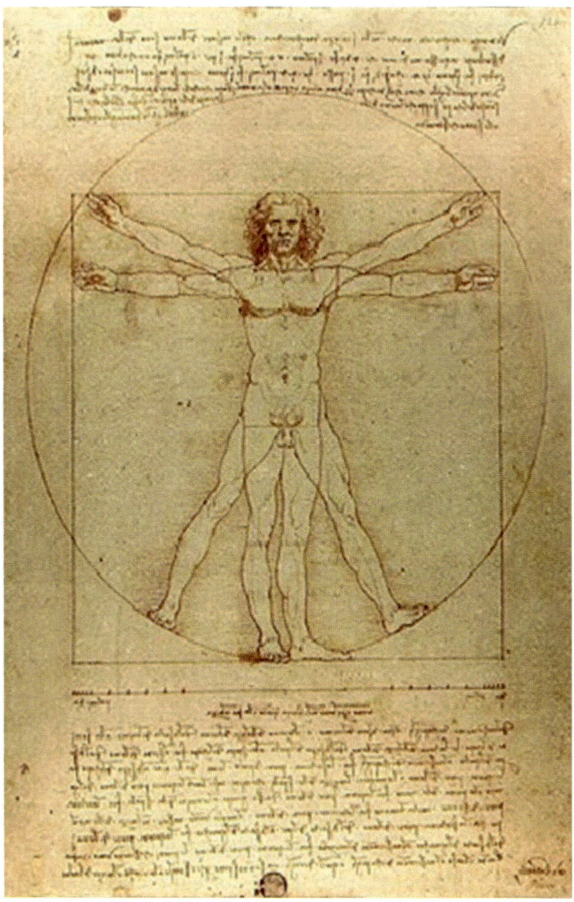

Fig. 5 Vitruvian Man by Leonardo da Vinci

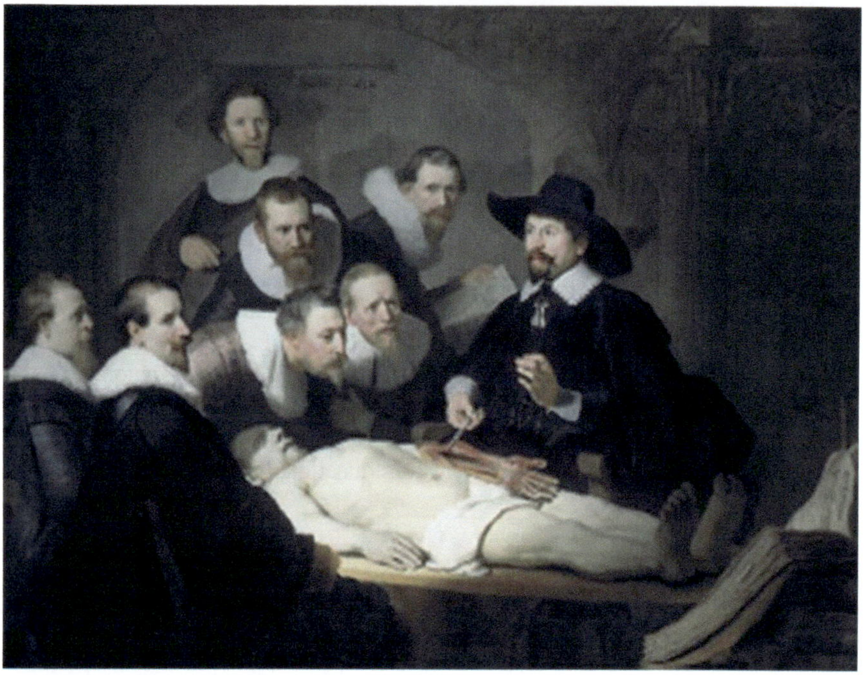

Fig. 6 "The Anatomy Lesson of Dr. Nicolaes Tulp" by Rembrandt (1632)

become more public events where local residents would pay an entry fee to the anatomy theater where they viewed skeletal material when there was no cadaver dissection.

Over the years, anatomists have questioned whether Rembrandt erred in his depiction of the muscles shown dissected in the left forearm, specifically whether the extensor or the flexor muscles are represented. The suggestion of an error was based primarily on anatomic atlas drawings, especially on the origin of the muscles that Dr. Tulp is holding in his forceps. These muscles appear to originate from the lateral epicondyle of the humerus. However, if he painted the flexor (anterior) aspect of the forearm as suggested by the position of the thumb, those flexor muscles originate from the other side of the humerus, the medial epicondyle. One compelling argument that the dissection represents the flexor forearm muscles is the clarity with which the tendons of the superficial flexors of the digits divide to allow passage of the tendons of the deep flexors are painted on the distal digits. In order to address this question of whether or not the painting was in error, Ijpma et al. undertook a detailed dissection of a male cadaver's flexor forearm photographed at different stages of the dissection (FF et al. 2006). They reported that Rembrandt's depiction of Dr. Tulp's dissection could be reasonably reproduced by selectively cutting and displacing specific forearm muscles supporting the notion that Rembrandt did not err in his painting. Though it must be pointed out that even if he had erred, it would not have distracted from the historical blending of art and anatomy.

The relationship between art and anatomy transformed into drawings to help supplement the dissection and especially in those cases where dissection was not possible to substitute with detail as lifelike as possible. The period of the fifteenth to the seventeenth century was a time of rapid development of visual aids important to the furtherance of the anatomical sciences. Leonard da Vinci (1452–1519) set the stage with his drawings of the skeletal system (Fig. 7), muscular system, the heart and vascular system, and sex organs along with other internal organs.

Soon after, Andreas Vesalius (1514–1564) compiled what can be considered the first comprehensive atlas of anatomy, *De Humani Corporis Fabrica* ("On the Fabric of the Human Body"). The Fabrica comprised a series of books on the skeletal system, muscular system, nervous system, vascular system, brain, and heart and was most likely the large book depicted in Rembrandt's painting, "The Anatomy Lesson of Dr. Nicolas Tulp." The following 300 years saw further refinements in the anatomical publications combining text and drawings including authors very familiar to anatomists such as Morgagni and Charles Bell (Bell's palsy).

What can be considered a second milestone in the evolution of atlases and textbooks in anatomy was the work of Henry Gray (1827–1861) who published in 1858 the legendary book "Anatomy, Descriptive and Surgical" otherwise known as "Gray's Anatomy." This book has become the central authority of human anatomy and is a common fixture on anatomists' bookshelves. As a member of the Royal College of Surgeons and as the book's title implied, Henry Gray had as his main

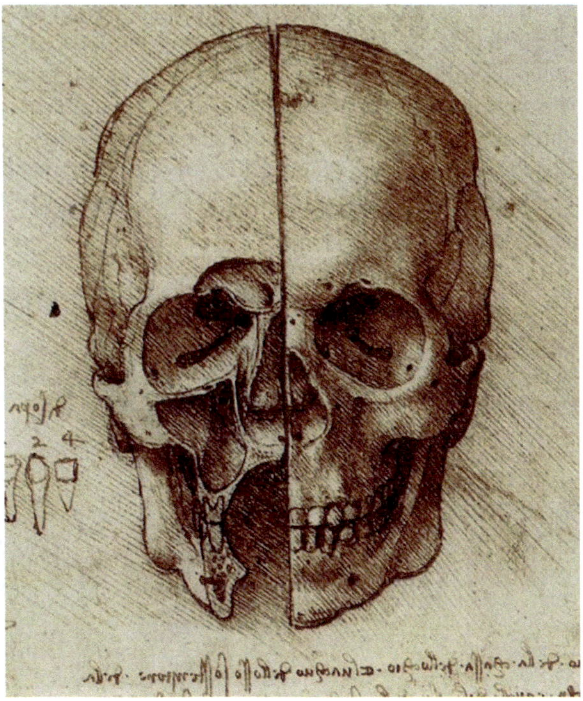

Fig. 7 "The skull" by Leonardo Da Vinci, 1489

objective to improve the skills of surgeons through the application of detailed anatomical knowledge. The book was the culmination of years of personal, methodical dissections, and its success was greatly enhanced by the illustrations made by Henry Carter, a demonstrator working with Gray. Carter's illustrations were direct and nomenclature added for ease of reference with the text, a style that has persisted to the present. It was another century before the next milestone in anatomical atlases arrived with the publication of Frank Netter's "Atlas of Human Anatomy" in 1989. Netter's training as a physician and an illustrator combined to produce color illustrations that were rich in detail and lifelike rendition. His atlas is a staple of medical education and, along with "Gray's Anatomy," has found a place on most bookshelves of anatomists and surgeons.

As the Internet and computer technology expanded in the twenty-first century, it allowed individual anatomists to become publishers and to produce their own anatomical "atlas" and either publish to the wider audience or keep them solely for in-house use within their own courses. Paramount to this process was the ease with which dissections could be photographed and distributed to fulfill any need essentially on the fly. The extension of multimedia to include videos allowed dynamic, dimensional anatomical presentations that static illustrations can never duplicate. Combined with the technological advancements in radiological imaging, including the ease of obtaining CT and MRI scans of living individuals, it has never been easier to obtain high-resolution images of anatomical structures. Combine the ease of obtaining images with the ease for anyone to create a website, and the result is a large variety of Internet-based resources created by anatomists and institutions around the world. These technological and specifically imaging advancements are of particular use to surgeons who rely on detailed knowledge of head and neck anatomy, which has been previously difficult to comprehend due to its complexity. It is now possible to create detailed digital anatomical resources that can incorporate soft tissue and osseous structures into three-dimensional images that can be manipulated by the learner, such as the structures surrounding and passing through the complex sphenoid bone (Nowinski and Thaung 2018) (Fig. 8). There are many

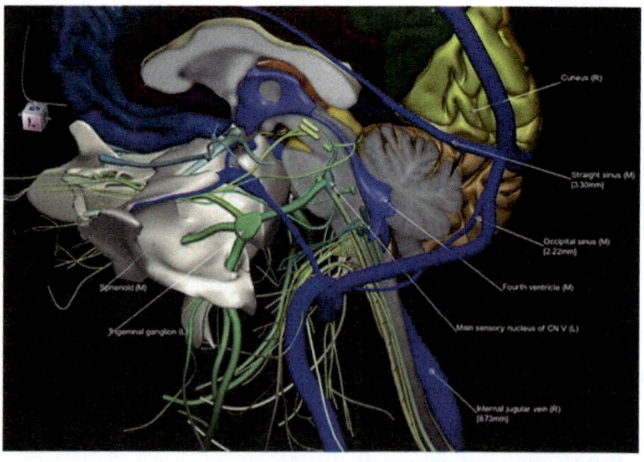

Fig. 8 A 3D reconstruction of MRI and high-resolution CT scans of the sphenoid bone with surrounding neurovasculature, taken from a normal male (Nowinski and Thaung 2018)

digital resources that are also freely available to the general public, creating an opportunity for the anatomy of the human body to be freely explored by those both within the medical fields and the general public. These resources are not limited to only digital; 3D printing of anatomical structures, including pathologies from actual patients, allows clinicians to perform simulated surgeries on these printed structures to determine the best course of surgical action, which has not been previously possible preoperatively (Lin et al. 2018).

With the continued development of artificial intelligence algorithms and virtual reality, it is easy to imagine how future anatomists and surgeons will experience anatomical and surgical education in the comfort of their chair. And indeed, this has already become a reality for most students and instructors of anatomy as a direct result of the COVID-19 pandemic. Research conducted prior to the shift to entirely virtual instruction indicated that learning supplemented with these novel digital resources improved short-term learning of anatomy compared those who only learned via dissection-based methods (Wilson et al. 2019). While research is still ongoing as to the ultimate impacts of COVID-19 online anatomy instruction for professional medical and dental students, it is increasingly apparent that these novel digital technologies are primarily useful as a *supplement* to anatomy instruction and will not be able to replace in-person dissection of human cadavers (Singal et al. 2020; Iwanaga et al. 2021).

7 Summary

The knowledge of anatomy is the building block that all surgical principles rely on. Our species understanding of anatomy and physiology is the foundation of medicine. With the advancement of medical imaging and computer technology, the future of studying human anatomy will continue to evolve dramatically.

References

1850S ANATOMY LESSON. Herald News, The (Joliet, IL). 1997 July 06;Sect. A (1).
Campbell DJ. A brief history of dental radiography. N Z Dent J. 1995;91(406):127–33.
Costea C, Turliuc S, Cucu A, Dumitrescu G, Carauleanu A, Buzduga C, et al. The "polymorphous" history of a polymorphous skull bone: the sphenoid. Anat Sci Int. 2018;93(1):14–22.
Day EW. Report of a CASE of caries of the sphenoid bone. JAMA. 1895;25(21):890.
Frommer HH, Stabulas-Savage JJ. Radiology for the dental professional. 9th ed. Missouri: Mosby Elsevier; 2011.
Ghosh SK, Kumar A. The rich heritage of anatomical texts during renaissance and thereafter: a lead up to Henry Gray's masterpiece. Anat Cell Biol. 2019;52(4):357–68.
Gross CG. A hole in the head: more tales in the history of neuroscience. The MIT Press; 2012.
Hallikainen D. History of panoramic radiography. Acta Radiol. 1996;37(3 Pt 2):441–5.
Harris DF. History of the events which led to the passing of the British Anatomy Act, A.D. 1832. Can Med Assoc J. 1920;10(3):283–4.

Howerton WB, Mora MA. Use of cone beam computed tomography in dentistry. Gen Dent. 2007;55(1):54–7; quiz 58, 79.

IJpma FF, van de Graaf RC, Nicolai JP, Meek MF. The anatomy lesson of Dr. Nicolaes Tulp by Rembrandt (1632): a comparison of the painting with a dissected left forearm of a Dutch male cadaver. J Hand Surg Am. 2006;31(6):882–91.

Iwanaga J, Loukas M, Dumont AS, Tubbs RS. A review of anatomy education during and after the COVID-19 pandemic: revisiting traditional and modern methods to achieve future innovation. Clin Anat. 2021;34(1):108–14.

Jacquesson T, Mertens P, Berhouma M, Jouanneau E, Simon E. The 360 photography: a new anatomical insight of the sphenoid bone. Interest for anatomy teaching and skull base surgery. Surg Radiol Anat. 2017;39(1):17–22.

Jamil RT, Callahan AL. Anatomy, sphenoid bone. In: StatPearls. Treasure Island: StatPearls Publishing LLC; 2020.

Kathren RL, William H. Rollins (1852-1929): X-ray protection pioneer. J Hist Med Allied Sci. 1964;19:287–94.

Kells CE. Roentgen Rays. Dental Cosmos. 1899;41(10):1014.

Korner M, Weber CH, Wirth S, Pfeifer KJ, Reiser MF, Treitl M. Advances in digital radiography: physical principles and system overview. Radiographics. 2007;27(3):675–86.

Kumar M, Shanavas M, Sidappa A, Kiran M. Cone beam computed tomography – know its secrets. J Int Oral Health. 2015;7(2):64–8.

Langland OE, Fortier AP, Kells CE. Oral Surg Oral Med Oral Pathol. 1972;34(4):680.

Lauterbur PC. Image formation by induced local interactions: examples employing nuclear magnetic resonance. Nature. 1973;242:190.

Lin J, Zhou Z, Guan J, Zhu Y, Liu Y, Yang Z, et al. Using three-dimensional printing to create individualized cranial nerve models for skull base tumor surgery. World Neurosurg. 2018;120:e142–52.

Malomo A, Idowu O, Osuagwu F. Lessons from history: human anatomy, from the origin to the renaissance. Int J Morphol. 2006;24(1):99.

Mavrodi A, Paraskevas G, Kitsoulis P. The history and the art of anatomy: a source of inspiration even nowadays. Ital J Anat Embryol. 2013;118(3):267–76.

Mitchell PD, Boston C, Chamberlain AT, Chaplin S, Chauhan V, Evans J, et al. The study of anatomy in England from 1700 to the early 20th century. J Anat. 2011;219(2):91–9.

Mooney BR. The importance of the dental surgeon in medicine and the value of radiography in dental practice. Can Med Assoc J. 1925;15(12):1245–7.

Nejaim Y, Farias Gomes A, Valadares CV, Costa ED, Peroni LV, Groppo FC, et al. Evaluation of volume of the sphenoid sinus according to sex, facial type, skeletal class, and presence of a septum: a cone-beam computed tomographic study. Br J Oral Maxillofac Surg. 2019;57(4):336–40.

Niraj LK, Patthi B, Singla A, Gupta R, Ali I, Dhama K, et al. MRI in dentistry- a future towards radiation free imaging - systematic review. J Clin Diagn Res. 2016;10(10):ZE14–9.

Nowinski WL, Thaung TSL. A 3D stereotactic atlas of the adult human skull base. Brain Inform. 2018;5(2):1.

Oxilia G, Fiorillo F, Boschin F, Boaretto E, Apicella SA, Matteucci C, et al. The dawn of dentistry in the late upper paleolithic: an early case of pathological intervention at Riparo Fredian. Am J Phys Anthropol. 2017;163(3):446–61.

Parks ET. Computed tomography applications for dentistry. Dent Clin N Am. 2000;44(2):371–94.

R H N. Clinical preventative dentistry. Radiol. 1927;9(6):534.

Raper HR. Clinical preventative dentistry: based on a new type of X-ray examination. Rochester: Ritter Dental Manufacturing Company, Inc.; 1926.

Riaud X. First dental radiograph (1896). Dent Hist. 2014;59(2):87–8.

Rollins W. X-light kills. Boston Med Surg J. 1901;144(7):173.

Singal A, Bansal A, Chaudhary P, Singh H, Patra A. Anatomy education of medical and dental students during COVID-19 pandemic: a reality check. Surg Radiol Anat. 2020.

Singer C. Galen's elementary course on bones. Proc R Soc Med. 1952;45(11):767–76.
That National Library of Medicine's Visible Human Project [Internet].: National Library of Medicine; 2019 [updated July 08; cited December 14, 2020]. Available from: https://www.nlm.nih.gov/research/visible/visible_human.html.
Tubbs RS. Gentlemen, damn the sphenoid bone! Clin Anat. 2016;29(1):1.
Tubbs RS, Shoja MM, Loukas M, Carmichael SW. Oliver Wendell Holmes, Sr. (1809-1894): physician, jurist, poet, inventor, pioneer, and anatomist. Clin Anat. 2012;25(8):992–7.
Wilson AB, Brown KM, Misch J, Miller CH, Klein BA, Taylor MA, et al. Breaking with tradition: a scoping meta-analysis analyzing the effects of student-centered learning and computer-aided instruction on student performance in anatomy. Anat Sci Educ. 2019;12(1):61–73.
Yeomans S. Medicine in the Ancient World. 2019 December 28. https://www.biblicalarchaeology.org/daily/ancient-cultures/daily-life-and-practice/medicine-in-the-ancient-world/.

The Barber-Surgeons

Michael T. Goupil

1 Introduction

The barber-surgeons were the primary surgical healthcare providers from the eleventh to the seventeenth centuries in Europe. As barbers, they were experienced in the use of sharp instruments and thus well adapted to fill the void that physicians were unable to perform. Their procedures ranged from cutting hair to bloodletting, tooth removal, and setting bones (Fig. 1).

2 Origins

Barber-surgeons came into existence around 1000 CE. They were considered the medical and grooming experts of Europe (Hue 2017). The separation of surgery from traditional medicine dates back to the early Hippocratic Oaths that cautioned physicians from practicing surgery due to their lack of knowledge (Thamer 2015).

The origin of barber-surgeons is attributed to a number of edicts proclaimed by the popes in the twelfth century. One of the functions of the religious prior to these edicts was to provide for both the spiritual and physical health of their followers. Pope Innocent II issued edicts against the study and practice of medicine through the Council of Clermont (1130), Council of Rheims (1131), and Lateran Council (1139). The interpretation of the edicts in general prevented monks from conducting procedures that led to bleeding. This prohibition was reinforced with the edicts of Pope Alexander III through the Councils of Montpellier (1162) and Tours (1163).

M. T. Goupil (✉)
Division of Oral and Maxillofacial Surgery, University of Connecticut, Farmington, CT, USA

Consultant in Oral and Maxillofacial Surgery, Carmel, IN, USA

E. M. Ferneini et al. (eds.), *The History of Maxillofacial Surgery*,
https://doi.org/10.1007/978-3-030-89563-1_3

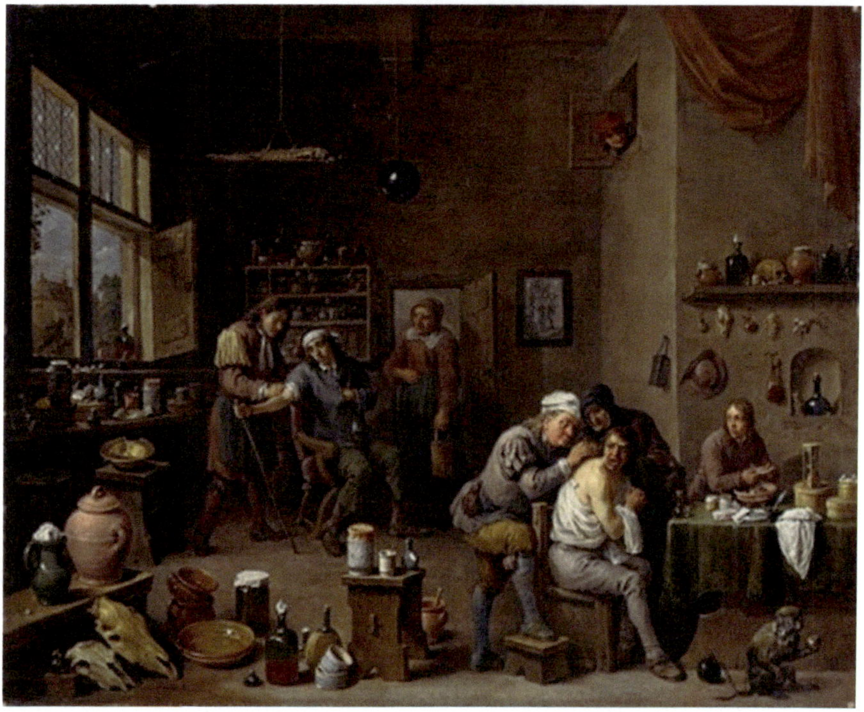

Fig. 1 "The Surgeon" by David Teniers the Younger, 1670s. (Reproduced without alteration, public domain image)

Initially, the edicts prohibited higher clergy from the study and teaching of medicine, but the later edicts extended to lower monks and eventually forbade all bleeding and cutting (Amundsen 1978).

Barbers were already part of monastic societies as monks had specific grooming needs for their required tonsures. As barbers were well versed in the use of razors and scissors, it was only natural for the monks to teach the barbers the surgical techniques they were no longer permitted to perform (Amundsen 1978; Hue 2017).

The Black Plague in the fourteenth and fifteenth centuries led to the demise of many of the university-trained physicians. This led to an ever-increasing need for barber-surgeons and their expanded surgical role.

3 Scope of Practice

Two of the most common procedures performed by barber-surgeons were the drawing of teeth (see Chap. 9, Evolution of Tooth Removal) and bloodletting which was based on Greek and Roman medical practice (Fig. 2). One of the continued beliefs in the Middle Ages, for the cause of disease, was an imbalance of the four

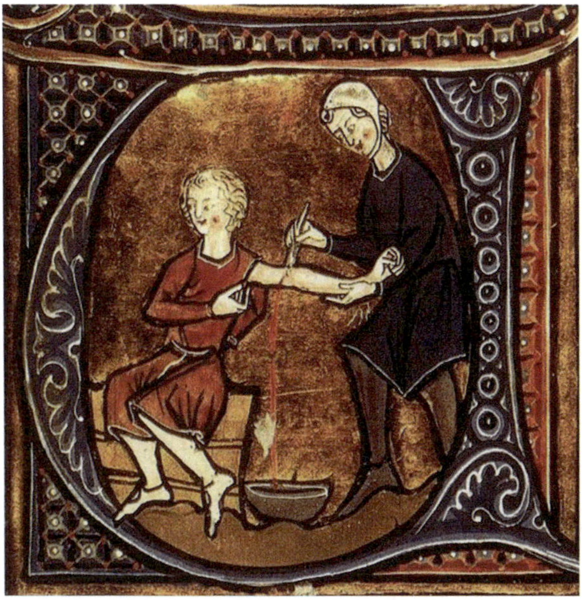

Fig. 2 The ancient art of bloodletting. Reproduced without alteration, public domain image

humors – sanguine, choleric, melancholic, and phlegmatic. A common practice in diagnosing an hormonal imbalance was to examine the urine for color, consistency, and taste (The Gory History of Barber Surgeons 2019). Once the diagnosis was made, the patient underwent bloodletting, by cutting one of the veins, to reestablish a balance in the humors.

War was a popular pastime in the Middle Ages, and this led to an expansion of the barber-surgeons scope of practice. The craft of barber-surgeons was limited to basic trauma, stabilization of broken bones, sword and knife wounds, and now the new injuries associated with gunpowder (Schneider 2020). Broken bones were set, limbs were amputated, and bleeding was stopped. The one benefit of armed conflict is the development and expansion of surgical procedures. As monasteries took on a larger role as hospitals, barber-surgeons provided bone setting and limb amputation in the surrounding community.

4 European Medical Education

The first secular European medical school was established in Italy at Salerno. Subsequently, medical schools were established at Montpelier, Bologna, Paris, Oxford, and Cambridge (Bagwell 2005). Surgery was considered part of the medical education system in Italy, and thus, barber-surgeons did not play a prominent role there as opposed to France and England.

In France, medical education was provided on three levels. Physicians were at the top of the healthcare pyramid. They received their education at universities and were licensed by the university. In the thirteenth century, physicians were required to take an oath not to perform surgery. Second in hierarchy were the surgeons of the long robe. They studied medicine for two years and surgery for two years before entering the surgeon's guild as Master Surgeons. The hallmark of the physicians' and surgeons' education was their instruction was conducted in Latin and Greek. At the hierarchy bottom were the barber-surgeons or the surgeons of the short robe. Lacking the ability to read, write, or speak Latin or Greek, they had no formal medical education. The barber-surgeons learned their craft through an apprenticeship usually lasting at least 5 years before they were eligible to be examined and obtain the designation of Master Barber-Surgeon (Garant 2013).

The Guild of Barbers was formed in Paris in 1210. The distinction between the long robe and the short robe was based on education (Ring 1985). The long robe indicates a university education, whereas the short robe designates an apprenticeship supervised by a guild. By royal decree in the fourteenth century, surgeons of the short robe were prohibited from performing surgery until passing an examination given by the surgeons of the long robe (Wynbrandt 1998).

5 Notable Barber-Surgeons

Ambroise Paré (see Chap. 4, The Three Pillars of Surgery) became the greatest surgeon of the sixteenth century, and because of his advances in surgery gained through his military experiences and extensive writings, he is often called the Father of Modern Surgery (Fig. 3).

He was born in 1510 in northwest France. Paré's father, elder brother, and brother-in-law were all barber-surgeons. He moved to Paris for his apprenticeship and eventually became a wound dresser at the Hôtel-Dieu de Paris, the oldest hospital in Paris. He eventually passed his examination for the rank of Master Barber-Surgeon in 1536.

He spent the next 30 years in the military where he developed new techniques for the treatment of gunshot wounds. He drew significant criticism from physicians and surgeons of the long robe as his writings were in the French vernacular as opposed to the traditional Latin of the medical profession.

Because of his reputation as a compassionate and innovative practitioner, he became the barber-surgeon to four French Kings – Henri II, Francois II, Charles IX, and Henri III. Paré also had an extensive dental practice, stabilizing jaw fractures with gold wire and replanting avulsed teeth (Garant 2013; Ring 1985; Swartz 2015).

Richard le Barbour became the first Master of the Barbers in London in 1308. He was responsible for the supervision of all barbers in the city of London. Based on monthly inspections, he was to ensure that barbers were not "keeping brothels or acting in an unseemly way" (Sprague 2008).

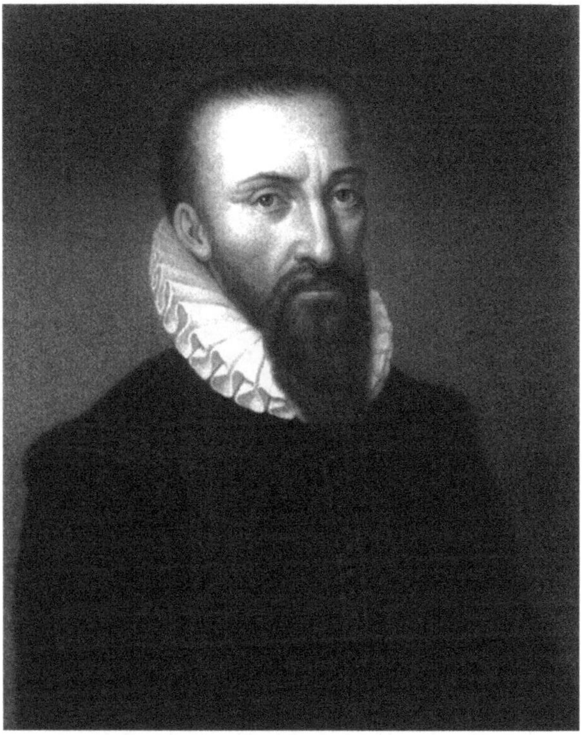

Fig. 3 Portrait of Ambroise Paré (1510–1590) by William Holl. Reproduced without alteration, public domain image

Barber-surgeons were the first healthcare professionals to focus on providing medical care to soldiers in both war and peace time. Hinsikinus was the first barber-surgeon referenced in Finland. He was hired to prepare medicine and care for the wounded from 1324 to 1326. Finland gained its independence in 1917 and no longer felt that there was a need to provide barber-surgeons for the military (Kuronen and Heikkinen 2019).

Jan van Riebeeck (1618–1677) was inducted into the Guild of Barber-Surgeons in Amsterdam in 1634 where he served a 4-year apprenticeship. He was the first founder of the Colony of Good Hope which is now known at the Republic of South Africa (Bird 1965).

6 The London Barber-Surgeons' Guild

Guilds and companies were originally established for social and religious interaction. The trade guilds were responsible for apprenticeships and the regulation of their specific trades.

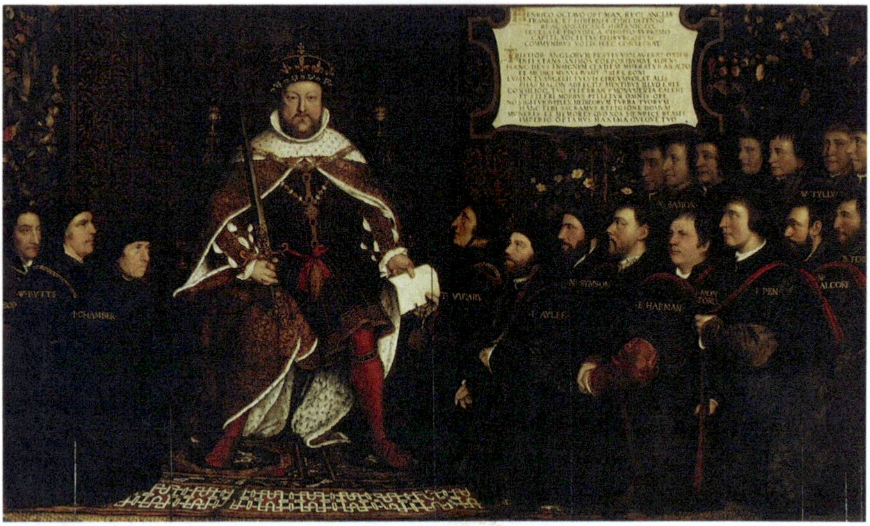

Fig. 4 Henry VIII and the Barber-Surgeons, by Hans Holbein the Younger; The Worshipful Company of Barbers

The Worshipful Company of Barbers has been in existence for over 700 years. This first reference to this guild was in the early twelfth century and probably was founded earlier than that. As noted above, Richard le Barbour was the first Master Barber. The first surgeon was admitted to the company in 1312.

A surgeons' guild was established in London in 1435, and they claimed the right to regulate the practice of surgery, thus competing with the barbers. In 1462, King Edward IV granted the barbers its first royal charter to regulate practice of surgery. This act was commemorated in a painting by Holbein (Fig. 4).

In 1540, an Act of Parliament established the Company of Barbers and Surgeons of London and established their respective roles. Surgeons could no longer cut hair, and barbers could no longer perform surgery, but both groups could continue to draw teeth.

In 1745, the surgeons left the company and formed the Royal College of Surgeons of England. In 1919, the relationship between the surgeons and barbers was reestablished, and surgeons are now regularly admitted to the company. The company has returned to the original intent of the guild system for social and charitable activities (Dobson 1974; The Worshipful Company of Surgeons (Dobson and Walker 1979).

7 Barber Pole

Because the majority of people were unable to read, businesses and professionals used signage to indicate the services that they provided. The well-known red and white barber pole indicated the services of the barber-surgeon. The red on the pole

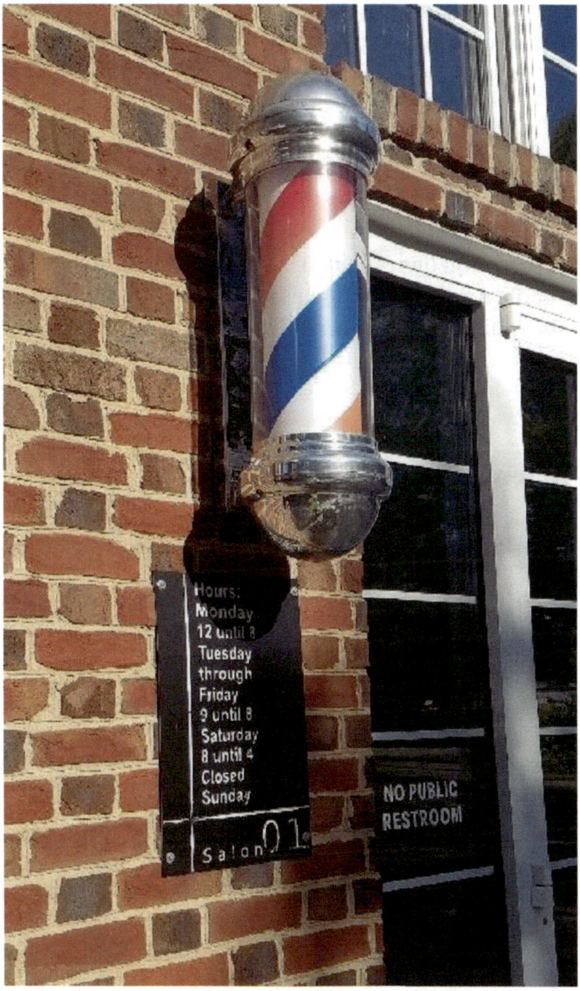
Hours:
Monday
Tuesday
through
Friday
9 until 8
Saturday
8 until 4
Closed
Sunday
Salon01
NO PUBLIC
RESTROOM

Fig. 5 Modern-day barber pole

represented the blood from the primary service of bloodletting, and the white on the pole symbolized bandages. The blue stripe represents the "blue pole" that was displayed outside of the offices of surgeons (Wynbrandt 1998). Even though barbers no longer provide surgical services, many barber shops have retained this universal symbol (Fig. 5).

8 End of an Era

The need for formal medical education as part of a surgeon's training had been recognized. In 1743, Louis XV, the King of France, prohibited any barber or wig maker from performing surgery (The Gory History of Barber Surgeons 2019), while in

London in 1745, the surgeons separated from the barbers to form their own professional society. The extraction of teeth could still be accomplished by either surgeons or barbers.

9 Summary

Barber-surgeons provided a significant role in the delivery of healthcare during the Middle Ages and the Renaissance. The innovations and writings of barber-surgeons like Ambroise Paré during this period helped develop and shape the field of surgery as known it today.

References

Amundsen DW. Medieval canon law on medical and surgical practice by the clergy. Bull Hist Med. 1978;52(1):22–4.
Bagwell CE. "Respectful image" revenge of the barber surgeon. Ann Surg. 2005;241(6):872–8.
Bird RV. Personalities and pages form dental history in South Africa. J D.A.S.A., Sept:266–268; 1965.
Dobson J. Barber into surgeons. Ann R Coll Surg. 1974;54:84–91.
Dobson J, Walker M. Barbers and barber surgeons of London. Oxford: Blackwell Scientific Publications; 1979.
Garant RG. The long climb. Hanover Park: Quintessence, Publishing Co, Inc; 2013.
Hue DL. The history of the barber surgeon. https:/barbersurgeonsguildcom/a/dispatch/author/Daniel-lee-hue/. 2017.
Kuronen J, Heikkinen J. Barber-surgeons in military surgery and occupational health in Finland, 1324-1944. Mil Med. 2019;184(1/2):14–21.
Ring ME. Dentistry an illustrated history. St Louis: CV Mosby, Inc; 1985.
Schneider D. The invention of surgery. New York: Pegasus Books; 2020.
Sprague C. In: Burn I, editor. Introduction in notable barber surgeons. London: Farrand Press; 2008.
Swartz SI. The anatomist, the barber-surgeon, and the king: how the accidental death of Henry II of France changed the world. New York: Humanity Books; 2015.
Thamer S. Bloody history of barber surgeons https:/Mdrynyu.Org/Fall-2015-Bloody-History-Of-Surgeons/.
The Gory History of Barber Surgeons: Medieval Medicine Gone Mad. Ancient origins: reconstructing the story of humanity's past. Ancientorigins.net. 2019.
The Worshipful Company of Surgeons. Barberscompany.org.
Wynbrandt J. The excruciating history of dentistry. New York: St Martin's Press; 1998.

The Three Pillars of Surgery

Morton H. Goldberg

1 Introduction

The triad of hemostasis, anesthesia, and asepsis is the three pillared foundation of the contemporary glory and wonder that is twenty-first-century surgery and all of its specialties and subspecialties. Without prevention and control of bleeding, pain management, and infection control, one would never have progressed from the not-so-distant era of screaming, restrained patients undergoing burning cautery control of hemorrhage, or facing death from deep or generalized infections. More simply put, a three-legged stool has little value if one or more of its struts is absent or inadequate.

The solution and management of these fundamental surgical problems can be attributed to many physicians and surgeons throughout history. But because of their keen observation skills, appreciation of medical history, common sense, and courage to go against the established norms, even in the face of intense criticism, three names rise to the surface – Paré, Wells, and Lister.

2 Hemostasis – Ambroise Paré

Ambrose Paré (1510–1590) was born in Bourg-Hersnet near Laval, France (Fig. 1). Little is known of his early life. His father has been described as a cabinet maker, but tradition describes him as the valet de chambre and barber to the Sieur de Voul (Hernigou 2013a). Paré's older brother and his brother-in-law were both barber-surgeons, and thus, it is not surprising that Paré followed in the family tradition and was apprenticed as a barber-surgeon (Ellis and Abdella 2019a). Because of his

M. H. Goldberg (✉)
Division of Oral and Maxillofacial Surgery, University of Connecticut, Farmington, CT, USA

E. M. Ferneini et al. (eds.), *The History of Maxillofacial Surgery*,
https://doi.org/10.1007/978-3-030-89563-1_4

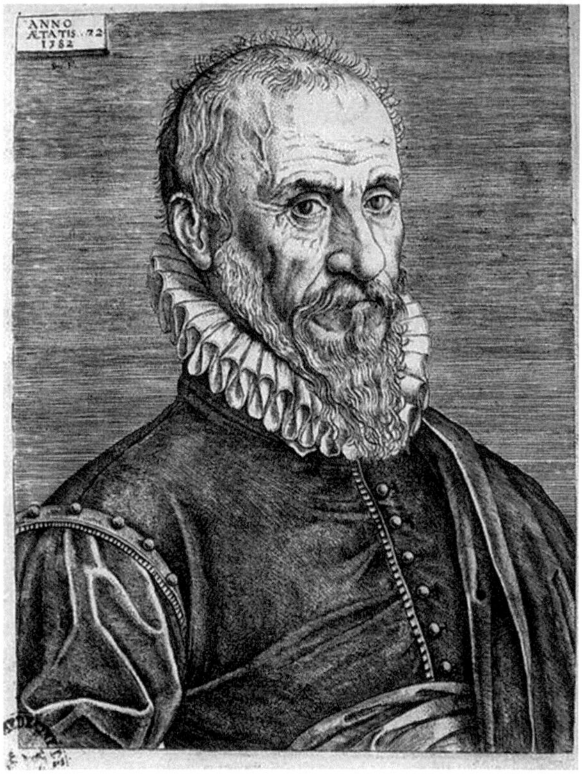

Fig. 1 Portrait of Ambroise Paré, 1582. Reproduced without alteration, public domain image

interest in surgery, Paré, at the age of 22, went to the Hôtel Dieu (Sherzoi 1999) which was the oldest hospital in Paris where he continued to study as a barber-surgeon treating the sick and poor. Fortunately for Paré, the Hôtel Dieu had recently become associated with the University of Paris, and as a barber-surgeon, he was able to attend lectures in anatomy and surgery at the medical school (Bracker 2008; Markatos et al. 2018). Additionally, he was able to receive hands-on experience from the attending surgeons.

Because of a lack of finances, Paré was unable to pay for his examination as a master barber-surgeon at the end of his apprenticeship. Instead, at the age of 26, he started his career as a military surgeon (Ellis and Abdella 2019a). He served his first of 17 military campaigns (Goyal and Williams 2010) at the Siege of Turin (1536–1537) where he made his first major contribution to military surgery. The traditional method of treating battlefield wounds was boiling oil. Paré was a compassionate practitioner, and the pain induced by this treatment caused him a great deal of stress. Because of the inflicted pain and now a shortage of oil, Paré sought an alternate treatment method. He formulated a salve composed of egg yolk, oil of rose, and turpentine, a method that had been used by the Romans a thousand years earlier (Bishop 1995a; Ring 1985a). The next morning, he noted that the wounds treated by boiling oil were showing signs of infection as opposed to those treated with his salve. Paré published this technique in 1545 *The Method of Treating Wounds by Arquebus and Other Firearms.* Not only had Paré broken with the traditional Galenic medical practice, but he also published his work in the French vernacular as opposed to the accepted medical writing if Latin (Bracker 2008; Ring 1985b.).

Wounds on those numerous battlefields were created by early forms of the matchlock musket (arquebus) as well as by arrows, lances, and swords. Those who suffered deep wounds of the abdomen, chest, or cranium were left to their inevitable fate, but combatants with limb or facial wounds might survive if the initial hemorrhage could be controlled. The traditional method of wound hemostasis had been, for centuries, burning by red-hot iron cautery or by pouring boiling oil into the wound. Some of the battlefield barber-surgeons of that era boiled puppies in the oil, convinced that this contributed to controlling blood loss.

Paré, the Father of Modern Surgery, had learned the use of cautery at the Hôtel Dieu in Paris, but he recognized that the burned tissue frequently became infected, necessitating amputation which led to further blood loss and the need for more cauterization. Amputation was one of the most common surgical procedures performed in the sixteenth century (Baskett 2004). His contemporaries, however, believed that many wound infections were the result of "gunpowder poisoning." The technique of suturing for lacerations or cutaneous surgery had been utilized for centuries in China and the Arab world. Paré reasoned that suturing could be applied to large deep wounds in lieu of cautery or hot oil and puppies. Hence, his innovative and often lifesaving development of the suture ligature. In order to clamp a bleeding vessel prior to tying in with a ligature, he modified the "bec de corbin" (crow's beak) which is considered to be the precursor of the modern hemostat (Hollingsham 2008a). Though suturing of wounds had been advocated by Hippocrates, Galen, Celsus, and Avicenna, Paré was the first to put his technique to a practical use when performing an amputation (Markatos et al. 2018; Hernigou 2013b). His first attempt was at the Siege of Danville in 1552 (Ellis and Abdella 2019a; Shah 1992), later publishing the technique in his classic *Treatise on Surgery (Dix livres de la chirurgie)* in 1564 (Fig. 2).

While also developing innovative dressings and sliding skin flaps to close defects created by injury or excision, Paré's fame spread, ultimately resulting in him becoming court surgeon to the infamous French queen, Catherine de Medici, having served as court surgeon to five French kings. His discoveries and procedures were accomplished despite centuries old entrenched surgical dogma, but he prevailed. He had erected the first of the three pillars of successful modern surgery, hemostasis.

Perhaps William Halsted, the "father of American Surgery," had Paré in mind when, 300 years later, he taught his oft-repeated maxim "treat tissue gently and it will reward you by healing quickly." One of Halsted's fellow surgeons at John Hopkins built further on Parés' concepts and perfected hemostatic clamps: thank you, Dr. Howard Kelly!

Today, every day, surgeons clamp, ligate, and suture in ORs, and ERs, and offices while stabilizing facial fractures, removing third molars, performing bone grafting and osteotomies, placing implants, and excising soft and hard tissue lesions. To the benefit of patients, society now has blood banks, vessel repair, catheter-placed

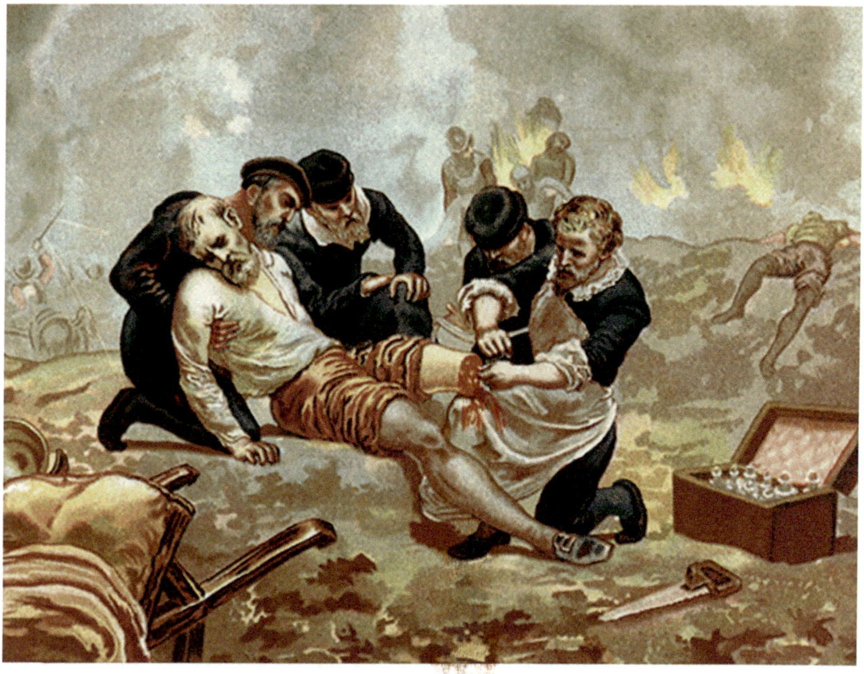

Fig. 2 Ambroise Paré performing a leg amputation of a wounded soldier in the field of battle (illustration for "La Ciencia Y Sus Hombres" by Louis Figuier; D Jaime Seix, 1876)

hemostatic emboli, pinpoint electrocautery, and collagen plugs. Over four centuries later, humanity owes a considerable debt to Ambrose Paré.

Five things are proper to the duties of a churgian. To take away that which is superfluous. To restore to those places, such things as are displaced. To separate those things which are joyned together. To join those which are separated. To supply the defects of nature. (from "THE EPISTLE DEDICTORIE TO HENRY THE THIRD, THE MOST CHRISTIAN KING OF FRANCE AND POLAND" 8 FEBRUARY ANNO DOMINI 1579, PARIS).

Ambroise Paré' possessed all the attributes of a great surgeon – manual skill, experience, judgment, courage, and compassion. He was a very humble man as evidenced by his most often recognized quote found on the base of his statue in level – "Je le pansy, Dieu le guérit" (I dressed him, God healed him) (Bishop 1995b).

3 Anesthesia – Horace Wells

Horace Well was born on January 21, 1815, in Hartford, Vermont (Fig. 3). The son of prosperous farmers, he was educated in New Hampshire and Massachusetts (Gordon 2000). At the age of 19, he moved to Boston for a 2-year apprenticeship in

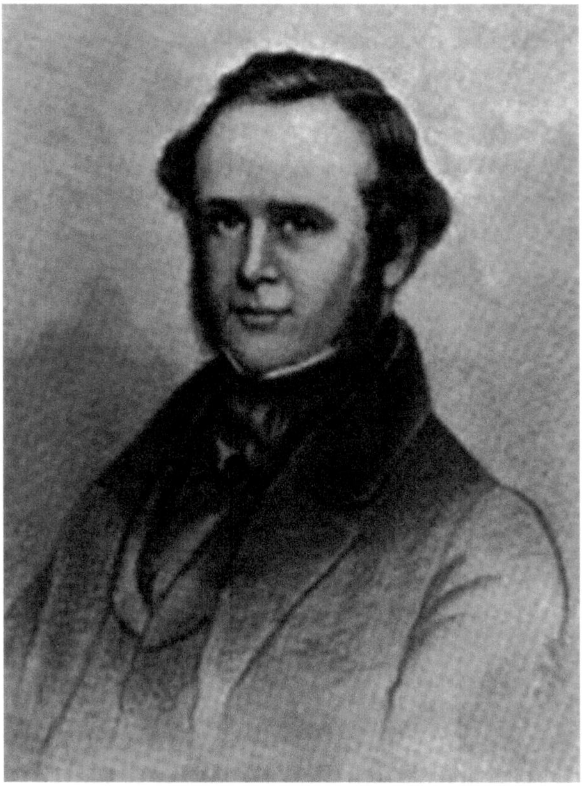

Fig. 3 Dr. Horace Wells 1815–1848. (Reproduced without alteration, public domain image)

dentistry. Upon completing his apprenticeship, Wells then moved to Hartford, Connecticut, where he started a lucrative dental practice (Jacobson 1995).

Fast forward to December 11, 1844, in Hartford, Connecticut, a 29-year-old dentist reluctantly agreed to accompany his wife to a theater where Gordon Quincy Colton, an itinerant showman and "medicine man," was performing. Colton administered nitrous oxide, contained in a leather bag, to volunteers from the audience who, while "analgesialized," unwittingly stumbled and tripped across the stage to the delight of the locals. One of the participants, Samuel A. Cooley, an apothecary clerk, struck his leg against a chair but did not cry out nor, when questioned afterward by Wells, did he recall the injury (Haridas 2013).

"Chance favors the prepared mind." Put otherwise, keen observation and rational deduction often lead to profound revelations and discoveries. That young dentist, Horace Wells, having observed, then reasoned that the nitrous oxide must have obtunded that man's pain, a glorious feat never before accomplished, except by large doses of laudanum (opium).

The following day in his office, Wells wittingly and willingly underwent extraction of one of his own teeth, with nitrous oxide as the successful anesthetic. In attendance were his practice partner William Morton and the wielder of the forceps,

John Riggs (Haridas 2013). It was certainly one of the greatest advances, perhaps the greatest gift to mankind, in the history of surgery.

The widely held tradition is a subsequent attempt by Wells to anesthetize a patient during a longer procedure – excision of a mass – in the amphitheater of the Massachusetts General Hospital (MGH) failed. That patient's screams did not shock the jaded assembled black, frocked-coated surgeons who then collectively stamped their feet and shouted "humbug, humbug," a mid-nineteenth-century term for deceptive behavior.

There is no primary evidence for this tradition. More likely, a medical student had a tooth extracted with nitrous oxide in a public hall on Washington St. in Boston. The failure of the procedure in front of medical colleagues indeed is true. Wells attributed the failure of achieving pain-free surgery was due to removing the nitrous oxide bag too soon. When the medical student who was having his tooth extracted was questioned, he stated that he had not felt any pain (Jacobson 1995; Haridas 2013).

Two years later, Morton successfully demonstrated the use of ether at the MGH. This news was rapidly transmitted, overcoming brief initial doubts. In England, its demonstration was greeted not with "humbug" but with the accolade "this is no Yankee dodge" (lie).

Disappointed by his failure to receive credit for his discovery of anesthesia, Wells left Hartford, his family, and his practice for New York, where he wandered the streets, certainly depressed, perhaps psychotic and was arrested for assault. He was imprisoned in the Tombs, the ancient, infamous, and aptly named Manhattan prison. There on January 24, 1848, at age 33, he committed suicide with a razor (Haridas 2013). In the early 1960s when I was an OMFS resident at Bellevue Hospital in New York City, my fellow residents and I frequently treated patients on the locked prison ward, those sent, shackled, from the still extant Tombs.

Perhaps Wells was predestined for greatness. Surely, his gift to mankind ended millennia of unbearable pain, but his postdiscovery life was a tragedy, although not quite a Sophoclean Greek Tragedy. His ultimate fate may have been predetermined by his own flaws and fragility, the outcome perhaps predictable, even if not by a Delphian Oracle or a Cassandra.

Morton has been described by many historians as an inflexible, narcissistic, antisocial, financial con man who had hoped (but failed) to gain great profit from ether. He died in 1868. Riggs later investigated and published the first accurate description of periodontal disease, known for many decades thereafter by the eponym Riggs' disease.

The debate continues about who really discovered general anesthesia – Long, Wells, Morton, Jacobson, or others. Sir Humphrey Davy discovered nitrous oxide in 1798 and felt that it had the potential to be used to alleviate surgical pain, but it was Wells that conceived of its application according to a letter written by Riggs (Menczer and Jacobson 1992). Long claimed to have performed surgery in 1842 but failed to publish his work until after the success of Wells and Morton. Although ether had been used earlier than nitrous oxide, nitrous oxide has proven more effective because of its low risk and analgesic properties and continues to be used today.

Three days after the death of Wells, the Societé Mēdicale Française "recognized Dr. Horace Wells as the first person to discover and successfully apply vapors or gases for painless operations" (López-Valverde et al. 2011). Furthermore, in 1864, the American Dental Association passed a resolution "to Horace Wells of Hartford, Connecticut belongs the credit and honor of the introduction of anesthesia in the United States" (Ring 1985c). The debate should be over.

A bronze plaque on the outside wall of an office building close to the old State Capitol in Hartford commemorates the site of Wells' office and the monumental first-anesthetized surgery. In a park adjacent to the present capitol building, a true monument, a statue of Horace, stands appropriately on a pedestal (pillar). His grave, the plaque, and the statue are preserved by the Horace Wells Club, a 40-member group of dentists who meets annually, early in December, at a black-tie dinner to pay homage to Wells.

4 Asepsis – Joseph Lister

The development of surgery ground to a halt and could go no further until the problem of surgical infection could be resolved. Surgeons knew how the body worked, they could control blood loss, and they even could put a patient to sleep while they operated (Hollingsham 2008b).

The third pillar which supports our twenty-first-century surgical edifice is asepsis, the prevention and therapy of surgical infection. Of this triad of hemostasis, anesthesia, and asepsis, only the last of these remain a persistent and controversial issue, i.e., the overuse and abuse of antibiotics. The incision and drainage (I&D) is probably the oldest surgical procedure performed many millennia ago by tribal shamans or witch doctors using sharp sticks or splinters of flint. Our more contemporary predecessors, barber-surgeons, may have utilized metal lancets, but the cause of infection remained a mystery shrouded in superstition.

In 1674 in Delf, Holland, while utilizing a primitive microscope (lenses, mirrors, candles), Antoine Van Leuwenhoek discovered microbes. This 42-year-old linen draper and amateur naturalist was shocked to find "tiny moving animals" observed in a drop of saliva and food debris which he had scraped from his teeth! It was a great revelation to the very early and quite small scientific community of his era, but its relationship to disease and infection could not even be theorized after 15 centuries of (Greco-Roman) Galen's fixed ingrained dogma which taught that illness was caused by an imbalance of blood, phlegm, and bile. Like his contemporaries of the seventeenth-century Enlightenment (Descartes, Spinoza, Locke, and Newton), Van Leuwenhoek had opened and expanded man's comprehension of the universe: Galileo had done so with a telescope, Van Leuwenhoek with a microscope.

Centuries earlier, physicians of the Arab world were far more advanced than their Middle Ages European contemporaries. Notable was Moses Maimonides, the twelfth-century physician, astronomer, theologian, and philosopher: "You must accept the truth from whatever source it comes." He observed and reasoned that the frequency of infection might be diminished if physicians and surgeons were to wash their hands before examining or treating patients. Even if his discoveries and writings, in Arabic and Hebrew, had reached Europe, it is highly unlikely that they would have been accepted.

Nor later was the clinical experiment of Ignaz Semmelweis, a Hungarian obstetrician practicing (1848) at the Allegmeines Krankenhaus in Vienna. Appalled by the high (22%) death rate from childbirth puerperal fever, he observed and reasoned that something other than "airborne miasmas" might be the cause, perhaps from the hands of medical students who were on call to assist at childbirth, often coming directly from fresh autopsies of cadavers who frequently had expired from that era's most common cause of death: infections. He instructed the students to wash their hands prior to examining the mothers or delivering their babies, and the infection rate fell to 1%. Unfortunately, Semmelweis's work was not translated into English until 1941 (Ellis and Abdella 2019b).

His fellow obstetricians refused to accept the obvious conclusion from his successful clinical trials. Because of age-old rigid dogma, jealous professionalism, and the unpopularity of Hungarians in Vienna in 1848 – the "year of revolutions" in Europe – Semmelweis was committed to an asylum, though later released. Ironically, he died as the result of an infection of a cut sustained while performing an autopsy.

In one of medicine's most unlikely coincidences, the conquest of puerperal fever occurred simultaneously in Boston, Massachusetts. Physician Oliver Wendell Holmes Sr., also a poet and writer ("a moment's insight is sometimes worth a life's experience"), discovered and published his handwashing experience preventing "childbed fever," which was accepted by his peers and was widely distributed.

Although Louis Pasteur ("chance favors the prepared mind") and Robert Koch (four postulates) in the mid-late nineteenth century had proven, beyond any doubt, that microbes were the causative agents of infection, the Germ Theory was only hesitantly accepted. Even the great Virchow, originator of the concept of cells and cellular pathology, rejected the theory because he was "sure" that the etiology of infection came from within cells rather than from invading microorganisms. He was unwilling to challenge his own new "truths."

In 1867, British surgeon Joseph Lister introduced the concept of sterile surgery by utilizing a dilute solution of carbolic acid to disinfect traumatized tissue or prior to surgical incision, as well as for cleaning surgical instruments. He had observed that carbolic acid was being used to control the odor from sewage, and he reasoned that the chemical would be safe because it had no apparent deleterious effects on livestock.

Joseph Lister was born in Upton, Essex, England, of Quaker parents (Fig. 4). His father was a wine merchant and the inventor of a microscope that did not distort color ("achromatic" microscope) (Brand 2010). Lister came by his interest in research and science as a child. Because of his Quaker religion, Lister was unable to attend either Oxford or Cambridge. He attended the University College of London, entering the undergraduate curriculum at age 16 in 1844 and graduating from the medical school in 1851 (Schneider 2020a).

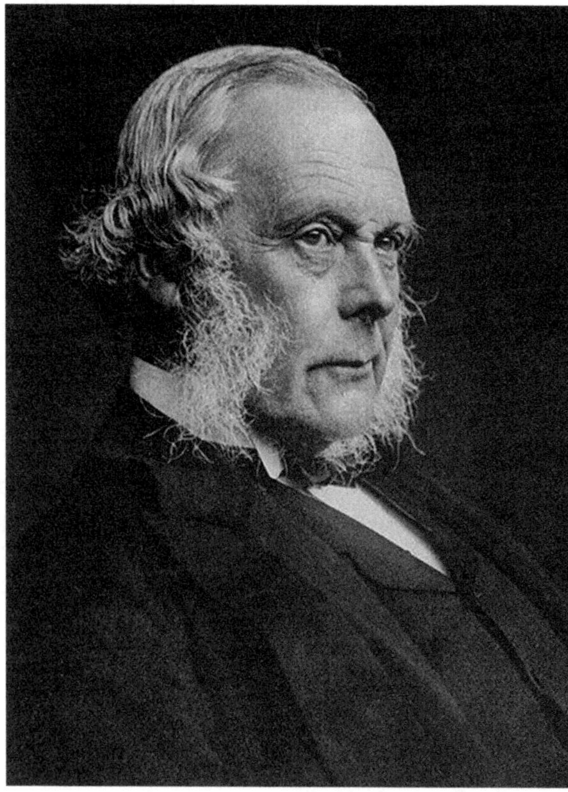

Fig. 4 Joseph Lister at age 69, taken during the meeting of the British Medical Association in Liverpool, 1896. (Reproduced without alteration, public domain image)

For centuries, compound fractures of the limbs had been treated by early amputation to avoid osteomyelitis and death from sepsis. Lister's first use of his dogma defying revolutionary idea (1865) was on 11-year-old James Greenlees who sustained a compound fracture of the leg. The normal progression of open fractures was infection, amputation, further infection, and then death. Lister applied frequent dressings soaked in carbolic acid: no infection, no necrosis, no osteomyelitis, no sepsis, and no death! After 6 weeks of immobilization, James was discharged, intact, and aseptic (Hollingsham 2008c; Fitzharris 2017).

After successfully treating 9 of 11 compound fractures, Lister published his work in 1867. This was at a time when the death rate from amputation was 25–60%, the more common course of an open fracture (Bishop 1995c). Lister's techniques were put to the test by the Germans in the Franco-Prussian War (July 1870–May 1871). The end result was that "for the first time in warfare history, fewer men died of infection than from the trauma itself" (Schneider 2020b).

However, the concept of aseptic surgery was much slower to gain acceptance by surgeons than had been the introduction of general anesthesia almost a quarter of a century earlier. In the United States, one of the staunchest advocates of Lister's innovative antisepsis was William Halsted who had returned (1880) from surgical training in the great hospitals and Krankenhausen of Europe. Initially at Bellevue

Hospital in NY City and later at the John Hopkins Hospital in Baltimore, Maryland, he developed techniques for hernia repair and mastectomy while also performing the first mandibular nerve block, utilizing cocaine (procaine was not synthesized until 1905). He also formalized the pyramidal residency training program, a great educational leap forward from the traditional pay-as-you-learn (observe) surgical apprenticeships. He also introduced rubber (sterile) gloves – to protect the hands of his scrub nurse from the carbolic acid. He later married her.

During the 1880s, Halsted traveled from New York to Albany to treat a middle-aged woman who was dying of acute, severe cholecystitis, complicated, no doubt, by dehydration and electrolyte imbalance – an unknown entity in that era. On her kitchen table, using open-drop ether (Morton), antisepsis (Lister), and ligation of blood vessels (Paré), he performed the first surgical removal of gallstones and drainage of the gallbladder. His mother survived!

Certainly, a history of the great advances in surgical infection control must include Alexander Fleming and his chance discovery of penicillin (1928), the "wonder drug," thus creating the antibiotic era, now including multiple generations of cephalosporins, quinolones, macrolides, and aminoglycosides, while penicillin begat ampicillin, which begat amoxicillin, which begat Augmentin, etc. Unfortunately, his momentous history-changing observation of fungal growth on an agar plate languished in an obscure journal of laboratory bacteriology until first used clinically – in 1940, by Florey and Chain, to treat a young British policeman who was septic from an infected facial wound which had been caused by a rose-bush thorn.

Lister died in 1912. In 1883, he was created a baron by Queen Victoria, becoming the first surgeon to obtain a peerage (Ellis and Abdella 2019c). Joseph Lister revolutionized the practice of surgery by removing the almost inevitable complication of postoperative infection, introducing scientific principles to surgical investigation. He elevated the rise of surgery from a craft to a professional science (Newson 2003; Horwitz and Deupree 2012).

5 Summary

Speculatively, how many lives were lost or severely diminished during those 12 years (1928–40)? Or what if Fleming had simply discarded that contaminated petri dish rather than deducing that the penicillin fungus had destroyed its bacterial colonies? What if Lister's patients had sustained their injuries just a few years earlier: perhaps hundreds of thousands of lives and limbs might have survived the American Civil War? What if Horace Wells had not attended that performance? Indeed, what if Paul Ehrlich (1910) had discontinued his years of methodical search for a chemical cure of syphilis at compound #605 rather than progressing to #606 (Salvarsan), thus creating a new therapeutic science – chemotherapy.

The "what if" school of historical thought and speculation cannot definitively answer its own questions, but the common denominators in all of these tales of great leaps forward taken by the giants of their eras are open innovative minds, keen observation, and willingness to challenge ancient or indefensible dogma or even hostility and failure. Some achieved great fame in their lives while others succumbed without it, but they have become immortal by endowing so much to so many.

Are great historical advances and changes direct linear trajectories, or are they just chance encounters – or perhaps even providential predetermination? Is each innovator unique, or do they all stand, to some degree, on the intellectual "shoulders" of those who preceded them? How much is due simply to being at the right place at the right time? Unanswerable questions, but the solid pillars and glorious legacies remain for we who have inherited them.

References

Baskett TF. Ambroise Paré and the arrest of haemorrhage. Resuscitation. 2004;623:133–5.

Bishop WJ. The early history of surgery. New York: Barnes & Noble; 1995a. p. 79.

Bishop WJ. The early history of surgery. New York: Barnes & Noble; 1995b. p. 84.

Bishop WJ. The early history of surgery. New York: Barnes & Noble; 1995c. p. 106–7.

Bracker CB. Ambroise Paré and the birth of the gentle are of surgery. Yale J Biol Med. 2008;81(4):199–202.

Brand RA. Baron Joseph Lister, FRCS, 1827-1912. Clin Orthop Relat Res. 2010;468:2009–11.

Ellis H, Abdella S. A history of surgery. 3rd ed. Boca Raton: CRC Press; 2019b. p. 85.

Ellis H, Abdella S. A history of surgery. 3rd ed. Boca Raton: CRC Press; 2019c. p. 90.

Ellis H, Abdella SA. History of surgery. 3rd ed. Boca Raton: CRC Press; 2019a. p. 128.

Fitzharris L. The butchering art. Random House: Penguin; 2017. p. 165–6.

Gordon SH. Wells, Horace. 2000. https://doi.org/10.1093/anb/9780198606697.article1200962.

Goyal PK, Williams AH. "To illustrate and increase Chirurgie": Ambroise Paré (1510-1590). J Pediatr Surg. 2010;45:2108–14.

Haridas RP. Horace Wells' Demonstration of nitrous oxide in Boston. Anesthesiology. 2013;119:1014–22.

Hernigou P. Other aspects of Ambroise Paré's life. Int Orthop. 2013a;37:1405–12.

Hernigou P. Ambroise Paré II: Paré's contribution to amputations. Int Orthop. 2013b;37:769–72.

Hollingsham R. Blood and guts. New York: St Martin's Press; 2008a. p. 57.

Hollingsham R. Blood and guts. New York: St Martin's Press; 2008b. p. 93.

Hollingsham R. Blood and guts. New York: St Martin's Press; 2008c. p. 87–8.

Horwitz B, Deupree M. Why celebrate Joseph Lister? 2012. https://doi.org/10.1016/50140-6736(12)60245-1.

Jacobson PH. Horace Wells: discoverer of anesthesia. Anesth Prog. 1995;42:73–5.

López-Valverde A, Montero J, Albaladejo A, de Diego RG. The discovery of surgical anesthesia: discrepancies regarding its authorship. J Dent Res. 2011;90(1):31–4.

Markatos K, et al. Ambroise Paré (1510-1590) and his investigative work on the treatment of war injuries. Surg Investig. 2018;25(2):183–6.

Menczer LF, Jacobson PH. Dr. Horace Wells: The discoverer of general anesthesia. J Oral Maxillofac Surg. 1992;50:506–9.

Newson SWB. Pioneers in infection control – Joseph Lister. J Hosp Infect. 2003;55:246–53.

Ring ME. In: Harry N, editor. Dentistry an illustrated history. New York: Abrams Publishers; 1985a. p. 128.

Ring ME. In: Harry N, editor. Dentistry an illustrated history. New York: Abrams Publishers; 1985b. p. 129.

Ring ME. In: Harry N, editor. Dentistry an illustrated history. New York: Abrams Publishers; 1985c. p. 231.

Schneider D. The invention of surgery. New York: Pegasus; 2020a. p. 107.

Schneider D. The invention of surgery. New York: Pegasus; 2020b. p. 112–3.

Shah M. Premier Chiruglen du Rol: The life of Ambroise Paré (1510-1590). J R Soc Med. 1992;85:292–04.

Sherzoi M. Ambroise Pare. J Investig Surg. 1999;12:59–61.

Anesthesia

Andrew R. Emery and Leonard B. Kaban

1 Introduction

The discovery of anesthesia has been recognized as one of the most significant discoveries in the history of mankind. Massachusetts General Hospital (MGH) surgeon Henry Bigelow, the assistant surgeon at the first demonstration, claimed that anesthesia was "medicine's greatest single gift to suffering humanity" (Viets 1949). The success of inhalation anesthesia received widespread attention, interest, and rapid adoption in the practice of surgery because it was the only successful method of pain relief available for surgical patients. In the future, other routes of administration for general anesthesia and local anesthesia would also have a significant impact on pain relief. This chapter summarizes the history of general and local anesthesia and neuromuscular blockade and concludes with the concept of balanced anesthesia.

2 Inhalation Anesthetic Agents

Inhalation anesthesia is frequently what comes to mind when the origins of anesthesia are discussed. Despite a robust account of the pioneering presentation of ether in 1846 by William Morton, it is also important to consider the preceding years and scientific discoveries that set the stage for such a monumental achievement.

The earliest attempts at inhalation anesthesia date back to the middle ages when mixtures of mandrake, henbane (i.e., a source of scopolamine), and other hallucinogens were consumed (Carter 1999). Although some believe that these substances

A. R. Emery (✉) · L. B. Kaban
Oral and Maxillofacial Surgery, Massachusetts General Hospital, Harvard School of Dental Medicine, Boston, MA, USA
e-mail: aemery@partners.org

E. M. Ferneini et al. (eds.), *The History of Maxillofacial Surgery*,
https://doi.org/10.1007/978-3-030-89563-1_5

would have been most likely consumed by mouth, references made to inhaled vapors suggest that this likely represented primitive inhalation anesthesia. Despite the discovery of these hallucinogenic alkaloids, it would be centuries before true anesthesia, where patients remain immobile after a noxious stimulation, was actually discovered.

In 1275 CE, a well-known alchemist, Raymond Lully, created a solution of ethyl ether named the "sweet oil of vitriol" by mixing sulfuric acid and wine (Davison 1949). This discovery was recapitulated a few hundred years later when the collective writings of German physician Valerius Cordus, describing similar solutions, were published by Conrad Gesner in 1561 (Leake 1925a). These well-documented accounts of "sweet oil of vitriol" have led some historians to credit Cordus as the discoverer of ether. Around the same time, Paracelsus, who was a Swiss alchemist and physician, may have also discovered ethyl ether's properties. Alternatively, he found out about them from Cordus during his visits to Nuremberg and Leipzig. Paracelsus went on to describe the incapacitating and transient effects of ether on chickens but failed to realize potential surgical implications before dying in 1541 (Leake 1925a). A few years later, Italian philosopher and polymath Giambattista della Porta, also known as John Baptista Porta, contributed a collection of writings known as "Natural Magick" published in 1558. He described the ability to induce a "profound sleep" after inhaling certain vapors (Porta 1658). These historic references to inhalation anesthesia likely set the stage for what was to follow in the eighteenth and nineteenth centuries.

The next breakthrough came from Joseph Priestly, an English minister, who in 1772 heated iron filings with nitric acid producing nitrous oxide. He called this gas "dephlogisticated nitrous air." In the ensuing years, Priestly discovered other gases or "airs" including carbon dioxide (1772) named "combined fixed air," ammonia (1773) named "alkaline air," and finally sulfur dioxide (1774) named "vitriolic air" (West 2014a). Samuel Mitchell, an American physician and politician, described the anesthetic effects of nitrous oxide in 1795 (Bergman 1985). He also suggested that nitrous oxide might represent the contagion leading to all infectious disease (Riegels and Richards 2012). Mitchell's writing caught the attention of Humphry Davy, an American chemist and inventor, whose skepticism of Mitchell's contagion theory led him to investigate nitrous oxide himself (Bergman 1985). In 1798, at the invitation of Thomas Beddoes of England, Davy started working at Beddoes Pneumatic Institute, devoted to treating pulmonary tuberculosis (Leake 1925b). Davy became the first to demonstrate that gases could liquify by pressurizing them (Zimmer 2014). Davy also discovered the potential for nitrous oxide to eliminate pain during surgery in 1800, and he subsequently described his personal use of nitrous oxide for wisdom tooth pain (Riegels and Richards 2012). Davy experimented with inhaling carbon dioxide demonstrating that a 30% solution could produce narcosis associated with "a degree of giddiness and an inclination to sleep" (Riegels and Richards 2012). The change in sensation supported the hypothesis that gases had the ability to change human consciousness.

In 1805, a Japanese surgeon named Seishu Hanaoka gave an oral mixture of herbs that induced general anesthesia in a patient, allowing him to perform a successful mastectomy (Ball and Westhorpe 2011). Although not a gas, the oral elixir produced an anesthetic effect which facilitated a painless operation nearly 40 years prior to Morton's demonstration of ether. Unfortunately, this discovery was not shared with the world probably because the shogun of Japan, Tokugawa Yoshimune, would not allow its release.

In 1818, Humphry Davy's successor and English scientist, Michael Faraday, published an article describing similarities between the effects of ether and nitrous oxide (Bergman 1992). Faraday suggested that ether had recreational benefits similar to nitrous oxide. In the 1830s, recreational ether use, referred to as "ether frolics," became a popular form of social entertainment (Short 2014). Despite the sensory altering effects of these gases, it was not appreciated that they could be used for elimination of pain during surgery. With ether and nitrous oxide both under study by scientists and being used for recreational purposes, another inhaled gas, chloroform, was discovered by Frenchman Eugene Soubeiran in 1831. German scientist Justus von Liebig independently discovered chloroform in 1832 (Kyle and Shampo 1997). However, the idea to use chloroform for anesthesia would not be realized until after the demonstration of ether in 1846. In January of 1842, American medical student William Clark recorded the first use of ether to perform a dental extraction, and in March of the same year, American surgeon Crawford Williamson Long used ether to painlessly remove a tumor from the neck of his patient, James Venable (Desai et al. 2007).

On December 10, 1844, Gardner Colton, who had dropped out of medical school to put on nitrous oxide demonstrations, displayed the effects of nitrous oxide on several volunteers in Hartford, Connecticut. A practicing dentist of Hartford named Horace Wells was present for the demonstration. After observing a volunteer injure himself with little evidence of pain, Wells saw the potential for analgesia and anesthesia (Desai et al. 2007). Dental surgeons, at that time, were desperate for remedies to make tooth extractions less painful. Horace Wells then arranged for one of his own molars to be extracted the next day by John Riggs with Gardner Colton administering nitrous oxide (Desai et al. 2007; Smith and Hirsch 1991; Haridas 2013). After a few weeks of practicing with nitrous oxide on 12–15 patients, Wells traveled from Hartford, CT, to Boston, MA, in January of 1845 in hopes of demonstrating his discovery to physicians there (Haridas 2013).

As an aside, Wells initially trained as an apprentice under Nathan Cooley Keep, a revered dental surgeon in Boston, before returning to Hartford to start his practice around 1836 (Beecher and Ford 1848). There were no formal dental schools at that time. Morton, who was 4 years younger than Wells, first met Wells in Massachusetts while Wells was on a business trip and before Morton was interested in dentistry (Beecher and Ford 1848). In 1841, when Morton was 21 years old, he sought to study dentistry and went to Hartford, CT, where he learned from Wells as noted by the payment Wells documented in his day book (Archer 1944). Wells and Morton eventually partnered in Hartford, and when Wells invented a noncorrosive dental solder in 1843, they went to Boston to promote it and open another office (Beecher and Ford 1848). Their partnership dissolved in 1844, but they remained friends, and following in Wells footsteps Morton would also seek out Nathan Cooley Keep for special apprentice-style training.

Morton would eventually help connect Wells to John Collins Warren, the surgeon-in-chief at Massachusetts General Hospital (MGH), who agreed to introduce Wells to his class of Harvard Medical students after a lecture he was giving, for a demonstration of nitrous oxide (Smith and Hirsch 1991; Haridas 2013; Guralnick and Kaban 2011). Unfortunately, the nitrous was withdrawn too soon from the student volunteer who admitted to feeling pain as Wells extracted one of his teeth (Urman and Desai 2012). According to Morton, the audience "laughed and hissed," leaving Wells utterly embarrassed (Haridas 2013). This failure would eventually cause Wells to spiral into depression before taking his own life in 1848 (Guralnick and Kaban 2011).

Despite Wells' failed demonstration, Morton probably realized the potential of his attempt (Beecher and Ford 1848; Guralnick and Kaban 2011). Morton's mentor Nathan Cooley Keep, the most respected and skilled dental surgeon of the time in Boston, likely encouraged him to continue using ether, and Keep likely called upon his friend and Harvard Professor of Chemistry, Charles Thomas Jackson, for help (Guralnick and Kaban 2011; Urman and Desai 2012; Kaban and Perrott 2020). Jackson is believed to have suggested to Morton that he should use sulfuric ether instead of commercial ether (a common cleaning fluid) to produce anesthesia (Guralnick and Kaban 2011; Lopez-Valverde et al. 2011). Morton experimented with ether and tried it in animals and eventually on a patient, Ebenezer H. Frost, from whom he successfully removed a tooth on September 30, 1846 (Guralnick and Kaban 2011; Urman and Desai 2012). Morton wanted to keep the identity of the gas a secret in hopes of collecting royalties later, but MGH surgeon-in-chief Dr. John Collins Warren resisted this by delaying the initial demonstration until Morton revealed the name of the drug to him (Guralnick and Kaban 2011). Finally, on October 14, 1846, Morton was invited to MGH by Warren to demonstrate his anesthetic technique (Guralnick and Kaban 2011; LeVasseur and Desai 2012). Morton, who only had 2 days to prepare, scrambled to the last minute to finalize his conical glass inhaler with the help of local instrument maker Joseph Wightman (Viets 1949). Ultimately, he arrived late for the 10 AM demonstration but successfully anesthetized the patient, Edward Gilbert Abbott, for the ligation of the feeding vessels of a congenital vascular malformation performed by Warren (Vandam and Abbott 1984) (Fig. 1). Warren famously turned to the audience and uttered, "Gentlemen, this is no humbug" (Leake 1925b; Guralnick and Kaban 2011). However, some physicians remained skeptical of Morton's technique given the superficial nature of the operation, so Morton tried again to validate his technique by providing ether for the removal of a fatty tumor, but there were doubters once more. Morton again provided anesthesia on November 7, 1846, this time for a knee amputation performed by surgeon George Hayward, and his success left skeptics convinced. Thus, Morton's work was validated at last (Guralnick and Kaban 2011).

Morton and Jackson submitted their joint patent for "surgical insensibility by means of sulphuric ether" on November 12, 1846 (Yang et al. 2018). Eventually, Morton, Jackson, and Wells would all oppose each other in search of recognition for the roles they each respectively played in the discovery of ether anesthesia (Leake

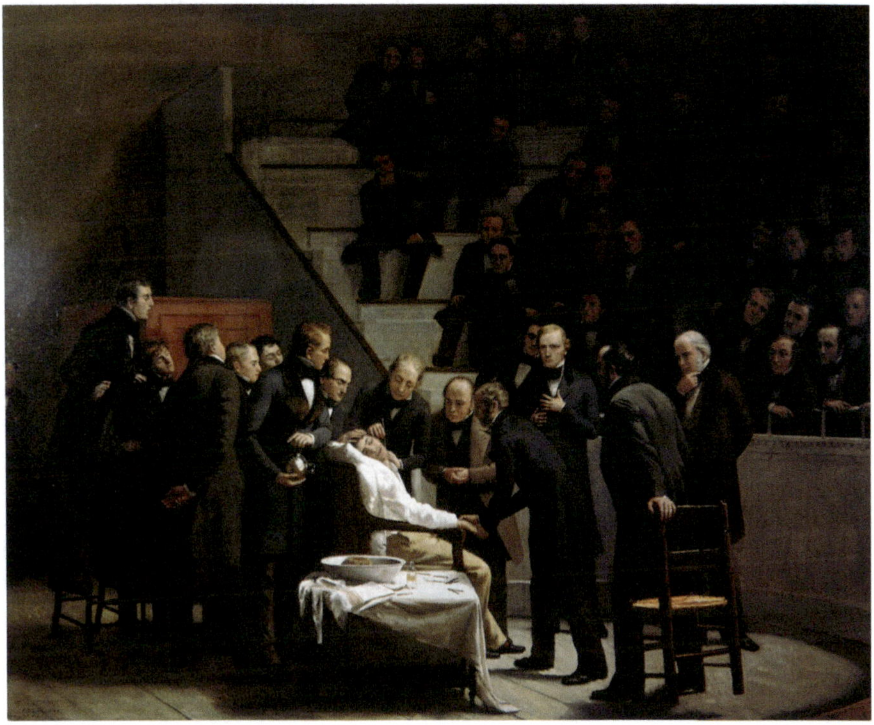

Fig. 1 Robert Cutler Hinckley oil on canvas painting from 1893 entitled The First Operation with Ether (Reprinted with permission from the Harvard Medical Library in the Francis A. Countway Library of Medicine, Boston, Massachusetts)

1925b). Years later, in 1849, Morton would appeal to Congress for a $100,000 grant for his contributions of ether anesthesia, but primary opposition from Keep, as well Jackson, would ultimately foil Morton's chances of financial remuneration (Leake 1925b; Guralnick and Kaban 2011).

On November 11, 1846, just 3 weeks after Morton's initial demonstration, ether was being used in Scotland for amputations (Viets 1949). Soon after that, Robert Liston, the preeminent surgeon in London, used ether for surgery with success and much surprise (Pieters et al. 2015). By January 19, 1847, Scottish obstetrician James Simpson became the first person to use ether for labor (Dunn 1997). On April 11, 1847, dentist Nathan Cooley Keep became the first to use ether for obstetric anesthesia in the United States. He administered ether to the wife of American poet, Henry Wadsworth Longfellow, for the delivery of their daughter Fanny in their home on Brattle Street in Cambridge, MA (Guralnick and Kaban 2011; Dunn 1997). A year later, on November 4, 1847, Simpson and colleagues experimented with various vapors in search of something less pungent for pregnant patients and came upon chloroform (Kyle and Shampo 1997). Simpson soon popularized chloroform, making it the British anesthetic of choice, while ether remained the preferred anesthetic in the United States (Kyle and Shampo 1997). John Snow, an English physician known as the father of epidemiology for his work identifying the water pump which was the source of the cholera epidemic in London, learned about these demonstrations of ether and chloroform and began studying anesthesia himself (Leake 1925b). In 1847, he described the five stages of anesthesia (Thornton 1950), and in 1853, he administered chloroform to Queen Victoria during childbirth, ending moral opposition to the relief of pain and generating greater acceptance of anesthesia use (Kyung et al. 2018).

Inhaled anesthetics would soon spread globally by the ships' captains and doctors within a year after the first demonstration, driving innovation and scientific investigation (Ellis 1976). Second-generation anesthetic gases were eventually produced including ethyl chloride (1894), ethylene gas (1923), and cyclopropane (1933) (Whalen et al. 2005). In the 1940s, due to the ongoing covert Manhattan project, attention was turned to fluorine chemistry leading to the production of fluorinated anesthetics including halothane (1951), methoxyflurane (1960), and enflurane (1963). Enflurane was then followed by isoflurane in the 1980s, which was eventually replaced by sevoflurane and desflurane in the 1990s (Wang et al. 2020). In the ensuing years, increased understanding of the mechanisms of action and metabolism of the inhaled anesthetics, patient factors, and the effects of the type of surgery being performed have guided the indications for the uses of various anesthetic gases.

3 Intubation and Inhaled Anesthesia Technology

In addition to the pharmacologic discovery of inhaled anesthetics, it is also important to consider the technological advances that kept pace and occasionally drove inhaled anesthesia innovation.

The development of techniques for surgical airways dates back as early as 3600 BCE, depicted by the healing tracheostomy wounds seen on Egyptian hieroglyphics (Rajesh and Meher 2012). In the second century CE, despite the Greek physician, Galen, describing the necessity of breathing to keep the heart beating, it was not until 1543 when Andreas Vesalius described opening the trachea of an animal to provide ventilation that interest in this subject increased (Slutsky 2015). In 1546, the first successful surgical airway on record was done by Antonio Musa Brassavola for a tonsillar obstruction; however, the term "tracheotomy" was not coined until Thomas Fienus first used it in 1649 (Rajesh and Meher 2012). A few decades later, in 1667, English scientist, philosopher, and polymath Robert Hooke demonstrated that blowing fresh air into the lungs of dogs that were not breathing was life-sustaining (West 2014b). Thus, the pure movement of the lungs was not itself essential to life, nor was it driving the movement of blood throughout the lungs or body. This realization suggested that life was sustainable with just air exchange in the lungs, whether by natural or artificial means.

In 1754, an English obstetrician named Benjamin Pugh described one of the first airway devices: an air-pipe made of tightly coiled wire for resuscitating neonates (Szmuk et al. 2008; Baskett 2000). In 1760, Buchan used an opening in the windpipe to aid in human resuscitation (Szmuk et al. 2008). Later, in 1788, Englishman Charles Kite introduced a curved metal cannula into the trachea of drowning victims to help resuscitate them (Szmuk et al. 2008).

In 1829, English physician Benjamin Guy Babington published on his "glottoscope," which consisted of a tongue depressor speculum to retract supraglottic tissues out of view and a series of mirrors used to visualize the larynx (Pieters et al. 2015). The term "laryngoscope" was adopted later by fellow colleague and physician Thomas Hodgkin, who is best known for his work on Hodgkin's disease (Pieters et al. 2015). Ultimately, the direct laryngoscope would be developed in 1910 by American physician Chevalier Jackson (Pieters et al. 2015).

In 1874, Jacob M. Heiberg, a surgeon from Norway, described the jaw thrust maneuver for opening up airways (Matioc 2016). In 1876, Alfred Woillez developed a manual ventilator, which was later replaced by the iron lung (Slutsky 2015). Eventually in 1885, using high-pressure oxygen cylinders with high-pressure nitrous oxide, the SS White Company patented the first anesthesia machine (Bause 2009). In 1893, Austrian physician Victor Eisenmenger described using an inflatable cuff around an endotracheal tube paving the way for the designs used today for endotracheal intubation (Gillespie 1946). In 1967, English physician Ian Calder performed the first fiber-optic bronchoscopy (Pieters et al. 2015), and in 2001, Canadian surgeon John Pacey invented the first commercially available video laryngoscopes known as the GlideScope (Pieters et al. 2015).

In addition to technical advances, in 1895, Harvey Cushing and Amory Codman, both Harvard medical students, first proposed the idea of keeping an anesthesia record, which included information such as the pulse, respiratory rate, depth of anesthesia, and amount of anesthetic given (i.e., ether) (Fisher et al. 1994), which remains standard practice today.

4 Parenteral Anesthesia

Some of the most important and frequently used anesthetics today are those intravenously administered. While the separate historical timelines of inhalation, local, and parenteral anesthesia can be thought of as parallel themes at times unfolding simultaneously, the discovery of parenteral anesthesia arguably started earlier than the rest.

It seems most appropriate to start the story of parenteral anesthesia with the establishment of intravenous access. The earliest record of intravenous access for medication administration appears to date back to 1656 when the English architect Christopher Wren performed a cutdown to access the leg vein of a dog. Wren delivered ale via a goose quill as the needle and animal bladders as the syringe (Dorrington and Poole 2013; Dagnino 2009), leaving the dog transiently senseless before later regaining full consciousness and surviving. Johann D. Major, a German graduate of Padua University, tried this technique on humans in 1662 (Barsoum and Kleeman 2002; Foster 2005), but the resulting mortality paralyzed the scientific advancement of this technique for another 200 years until Adam Neuner developed a syringe in 1827 while studying cataract surgery (Blake 1960). From 1827 onward, the concentrated efforts of many individuals on improving syringe and needle design were paramount to the future of both local and parenteral anesthesia.

4.1 Opioids

General anesthesia has been defined as a state in which a patient is rendered amnestic, unconscious, immobile, and free of pain (Dodds 1999). Although inhalation anesthetics produce rapid unconsciousness with rapid recovery, opioids in high enough doses can also produce similar anesthetic effects, but often with a longer recovery period. Opioids are effective because of their strong analgesic effects, which blunt the pain inflicted by surgical incision, dissection, and manipulation, thereby reducing the reflex stress response to pain which results in withdrawal from the stimulus, tachycardia, and hypertension. As a result, opioids are powerful anesthetics or anesthetic adjuncts depending on their dose and the circumstances of their use.

Opium is a substance derived from the poppy plant and well known since 3000 BCE in Mesopotamia (Brownstein 1993; The History of Opiates | Michael's House Treatment Center 2020). After thousands of years, morphine was extracted from opium by Friedrich Sertürner in 1806 (Schmitz 1985). A few years later in 1832, codeine was identified as an impurity associated with morphine and isolated for use as an analgesic drug (Eddy et al. 1968). In 1898, heroin (known as diacetylmorphine) was commercialized by the Bayer company (Leverkusen, Germany), also involved in the discovery of aspirin around the same time (Sneader 1998). Heroin was initially marketed as a cough suppressant with a presumed lower risk of addiction compared to morphine. However, a decade later, concerns for addiction and drug dependence would begin challenging the drug's acceptance. Heroin was banned in the United States in 1924 (Sneader 1998).

In 1921, hydromorphone was discovered in Germany and found its way into clinical medicine by 1926 (Murray and Hagen 2005). In 1939, meperidine was synthesized (Batterman and Himmelsbach 1943) about the same time that the long-acting opioid, methadone, was synthesized (Fishman et al. 2002). In 1960, fentanyl was synthesized for the first time, and the synthesis of other fentanyl-like medications followed: sufentanil, alfentanil, and remifentanil (Stanley 2014). Each of these medications were integrated into the practice of anesthesia providing the analgesia component of the balanced anesthesia strategy.

5 Sedative Hypnotics and Other Intravenous Anesthetics

One of the first medications designed for intravenous use was the hypnotic medication chloral hydrate. It was synthesized by German scientist Justus von Liebig in 1832, but was not introduced into medicine until a fellow German scientist, Oskar Liebig, did so in 1869 (López-Muñoz et al. 2005).

In 1864, German chemist Adolf von Baeyer synthesized a new class of medications known as barbiturates when he created malonylurea (Cozanitis 2004). This eventually led to the synthesis of diethyl-barbituric acid in 1881 and its inauguration into clinical medicine in 1904 as the first clinically used hypnotic (López-Muñoz et al. 2005). With diethyl-barbituric acid as the parent molecule, many other iterations were spun off, including one in 1911 called phenobarbital. It was synthesized by German scientist Heinrich Horlein (López-Muñoz et al. 2005). Many other barbiturate variants were developed including butobarbital (1922), amobarbital (1923), secobarbital (1929), pentobarbital (1930), and hexobarbital (1932) (López-Muñoz et al. 2005). Thiopental was synthesized from pentobarbital by substituting the oxygen at position 2 for a sulfur group, introducing a new class of medications known as the thiobarbiturates. This class of drugs was first used clinically by Ralph Waters in 1934 (López-Muñoz et al. 2005). The addition of sulfur resolved the issue of muscle movement when the non-sulfonated precursor drug, hexobarbital, was administered.

After the Second World War, the search for shorter-acting barbiturates resulted in the discovery of methohexital (López-Muñoz et al. 2005). A distinctive property of methohexital is the excitability it produces on electroencephalograms, in contrast to the depressing effects of other barbiturates. This characteristic made it a useful agent for anesthesia during electroconvulsive therapy (Kadiyala and Kadiyala 2017).

Propofol was discovered in 1973 by Scottish veterinarian John Baird Glen (2018). Propofol has the advantage of fast onset and decreased postoperative nausea and vomiting. As a result, it has become one of the most widely used anesthetic medications, often used without inhalation anesthetics, during total intravenous anesthesia (TIVA) (White 2008). The introduction (1989) and subsequent popularity of propofol has resulted in significantly diminished barbiturate use in anesthesia.

Other medications important to parenteral anesthesia include the benzodiazepines. The first benzodiazepine, chlordiazepoxide (also known as Librium®), was discovered in 1960 by Leo Sternbach, a Polish-American chemist working at Hoffmann-La Roche pharmaceutical company (López-Muñoz et al. 2011). Additional studies aimed at simplifying the side chains of the chlordiazepoxide molecule resulted in additional benzodiazepines such as diazepam (1959), oxazepam, alprazolam, triazolam, and midazolam. These medications have been utilized in anesthesia for their amnestic, anxiolytic, and hypnotic properties (López-Muñoz et al. 2011).

Another parenteral anesthetic currently in use is ketamine. It was synthesized by Calvin Stevens, in 1962, to decrease side effects of phencyclidine (PCP) and was found to lack the cardiac or respiratory depression seen with barbiturates. However, emergence delirium, excitability, and addictive potential of this drug have restricted its use. Situations that require brief sedation, e.g., injured pediatric patients in the emergency room, remain prime opportunities to utilize ketamine effectively (Gao et al. 2016). Additionally, etomidate, a rapid-acting anesthetic, was discovered by Janssen Pharmaceuticals in 1972 (Forman 2011). It has the benefit of rapid onset, but unfortunately, it has been associated with adrenal suppression, thus relegating its use to an induction agent for rapid sequence induction (RSI).

More recently, anesthetic discovery has identified dexmedetomidine, approved by the FDA in 1999, for patients in intensive care units (Gertler et al. 2001). Its use was then broadened to include surgical patients in 2008 as it provides both sedation and decreases sympathetic output by stimulating central alpha-2 receptors (Kaur and Singh 2011).

6 Neuromuscular Blockers

In addition to unconsciousness and analgesia, general anesthesia also requires patient immobility and muscle paralysis (Dodds 1999). Although inhalation anesthetics are useful for producing unconsciousness and opioids best at reducing pain, neuromuscular blockers are superior at rendering patients immobile and paralyzing contractile tissues to facilitate surgical manipulation. This permits better conditions to perform sophisticated operations and reduces overall operating time. Therefore, neuromuscular blockers add a crucial component to the general anesthesia regimen.

Some of the earliest published accounts of parenteral anesthesia were neuromuscular blocker medications, also known as paralytics, that dated back to around 1500 CE. In 1516, Peter Martyr d'Anghera, a historian from Spain, relayed stories of those who had visited the New World overseas describing the puzzling "flying death," in reference to the poison known as curare that was used by natives (Raghavendra 2002). Wars in Europe stalled further exploration of curare's potential until 1735 when Charles de la Condamine, a French explorer, observed Ecuadorian natives shooting curare-dipped darts from their blowpipes to hunt animals (Fernie 1964). The acquisition of curare was the first step toward discovering the potential of neuromuscular blockers.

Curare was then tried in animals including rabbits, cats (Raghavendra 2002), and donkeys (Birmingham 1999), which survived due to artificial ventilation provided by bellows inserted into their airways. In 1857, curare's function as a neuromuscular junction blocker was discovered (Bowman 2006), and in 1912, German surgeon Arthur Lawen became the first to use paralytics in surgery (Czarnowski and Holmes 2007). Lawen reported that use of paralytic curarine (an extract from gourd curare) in combination with ether or chloroform produced the desired level of abdominal wall muscle relaxation unachieved by other medications (Foldes 1995). In the 1930s, curare was purified and branded under the name Intocostrin, also known as d-tubocurarine (Ball and Westhorpe 2005), and in 1942, Intocostrin was used on a patient for the first time, thus officially inaugurating neuromuscular blockade into clinical practice (Sykes 1992).

In 1946, English researcher Frederick Prescott described his frightening experience being the first human to voluntarily receive tubocurarine alone without any other anesthetic agents after which he reported being paralyzed, but sensate to pain (Prescott et al. 1946). Prescott's research also found that d-tubocurarine reduced the shock-like state that often occurred with spinal anesthesia, producing muscle relaxation like ether without prolonged postanesthetic recovery and vomiting, and it saved time as nerve blocks were time-consuming (Prescott et al. 1946).

As the pharmacology of neuromuscular blockers became more robust, so did the infrastructure that would ultimately help ventilate the paralyzed patient during surgery. Scottish physician John Dalziel in 1983 developed the first negative pressure respirator in 1838 known as the tank respirator (Kacmarek 2011). In 1911, Johann Heinrich Draeger introduced the first positive pressure ventilator known as the pulmotor (Kacmarek 2011). Paralytics and ventilators coevolved as were necessary for each to remain successful.

In the mid-twentieth century, combinations of drugs to produce anesthesia became more popular given the growing medications from which to choose. In 1946, Thomas Cecil Gray, an English anesthetist, presented this idea known as "balanced anesthesia" to the Royal Society based on 1500 patients (Shafer 2011). He described inducing anesthesia with an intravenous agent, giving curare to provide relaxation and to decrease barbiturate, and an inhaled agent for anesthesia maintenance. His thought was to combine several drugs to create a more advantageous effect and outcome, and from these descriptions, the multimodal modern anesthetic approach as we know it was born.

With the balanced anesthesia techniques now realized, scientists and clinicians turned to newer anesthetic agents and neuromuscular blockers. A depolarizing paralytic called suxamethonium, also known as succinylcholine, was introduced into clinical medicine in 1951 (Raghavendra 2002). In 1964, the non-depolarizing paralytic pancuronium was discovered (Raghavendra 2002) and essentially completely replaced curare for generating neuromuscular blockade. Following this, a number of other paralytics were discovered, notably vecuronium (1973) (McKenzie 2000), atracurium (1981) (Raghavendra 2002), mivacurium (1984) (Savarese et al. 2004), and rocuronium (1994) (Succinylcholine vs. Rocuronium: Battle of the RSI Paralytics - JEMS 2020). In addition, the Train-of-Four monitor was invented in 1972 allowing clinicians to detect the amount of neuromuscular blockade at any one time (McGrath and Hunter 2006; Ali's "train of Four" | Wood Library-Museum 2020), providing even greater control of paralysis in surgery and anesthesia. Despite the availability of glycopyrrolate and neostigmine for reversal of muscle relaxation, a new neuromuscular blocker reversal agent known as sugammadex was discovered in 2001 (Welliver et al. 2008), approved in Europe in 2008 (The Development and Regulatory History of Sugammadex in the United States - Anesthesia Patient Safety Foundation 2020) and finally in the United States in 2015 (Drug Trial Snapshot: BRIDION | FDA 2020).

As the practice of anesthesia evolves and medications become more targeted, we find the concept of balanced anesthesia more poignant than ever. Thomas Cecil Gray's concept of balanced anesthesia remains the pedagogy behind modern anesthesia and serves as the basis on which we now seek to optimize drug combinations and minimize drug side effects (Shafer 2011).

7 Parenteral and Local Anesthesia Technology

As previously mentioned, the 1820s were transformative years for local anesthesia with the arrival of the hypodermic syringe (Blake 1960). In 1827, Adam Neuner developed a syringe-like apparatus through which he was able to inject fluid into the eyes of deceased corpses to study and practice cataract surgery (Blake 1960). However, this design included a central stylet, which needed to be removed to inject fluid requiring more steps to operate (Blake 1960). Not long after, in the 1830s, French physicians were treating neuralgia in humans by pushing morphine paste down grooved trocars, functioning as rudimentary syringes (Lawrence 2002). In 1836, vascular nevi were treated by injecting an irritating chemical beneath the skin first by lancing the skin and then pushing the chemical beneath it with a blunt tip of a syringe (Blake 1960) representing yet another attempt at hypodermic injection. Eventually, in 1844, Francis Rynd of Dublin developed a hollow needle in the form of a cannula within which was a slender retractable trocar required to breach the skin, marking the first hypodermic needle (Lawrence 2002). By this syringe design, narcotic liquid followed gravity and was administered under the skin as the cannula was withdrawn—a functional but not ideal design.

In 1853, Daniel Ferguson, a surgical instrument and truss maker in London, devised a new syringe design consisting of a glass tube containing an internal plunger and piston (Blake 1960). The syringe ended in a narrow conical platinum tube with an oblique opening just proximal to the most distal trocar-like tip. Inside of that narrow platinum tube was a second slightly shorter tube, also with an oblique opening that could align with the outer one when the outer one was spun to the correct position (Blake 1960; Duce and Hernandez 1999). This design did away with the need for a removable trocar used to puncture the skin before fluid could be administered. Ferguson's design was modified by Cooper Forster, a surgeon in London, with indicators to signal when the aperture was open or closed (Blake 1960). Later in 1853, Edinburgh physician Alexander Wood further modified Ferguson's design by calibrating the barrel and creating a threaded tip on the end of the syringe for attaching a hollow needle with a beveled point (Duce and Hernandez 1999). Wood's needle that could pierce the skin without needing to lance skin or use a trocar and his syringe design, published in 1855, earned him the credit for developing the hypodermic technique. Notably, French veterinary surgeon Charles Gabriel Pravaz, who simultaneously was developing a hollow metal needle in 1853, narrowly trailed Wood for the honor of pioneering the original hypodermic syringe (Lawrence 2002). Interestingly, the term "hypodermic" was not coined until 1865 when proposed by Charles Hunter, who also garnered fame for realizing that injecting morphine locally caused systemic pain relief, in contrast to Wood who thought the effects were only local (Howard-jones 1947).

In 1867, as a component of his ongoing work on antisepsis for prevention of wound and surgical site infection, Joseph Lister described the successful use of carbolic acid for surgical wounds, which improved both mortality and morbidity (Schlich 2012; Pitt and Aubin 2012). Lister's use of carbolic acid is believed to also have extended to surgical instruments as a means to clean them (Craig 2018; Lister 1870). Later, the idea of using a pressured steam to sterilize instruments would result in the first autoclave being introduced in 1879 by Charles Chamberland, an associate of Louis Pasteur (Harvey 2011). Following this invention, in the 1880s and 1890s, Lister's assistant Ernst Tavel and Swiss physician Theodor Kocher advocated the use of pressured steam to sterilize instruments, and eventually hypodermic needles (Schlich 2012; Maclachlan 1942).

However, even 50 years later in the early 1900s, only about 1.8% of the 1039 commonly used drugs in the United States were injectable, a small market for syringe use. In 1921, after the discovery and use of insulin, there was a subsequent increase in parenterally administered drugs, making the need for a delivery system critically important (Lawrence 2002). Needles were reused at the end of the nineteenth century and the first half of the twentieth century, and despite attempts at steam sterilization, they were difficult to clean leading to complications of cellulitis with reuse (Craig 2018). Attempts to clean these needles included inserting a small wire to debride the inside followed by either passing them through an alcohol flame before inserting it, soaking the needle in carbolic solution followed by cleaning with alcohol or by boiling the needle for a few minutes in water (Hampton 1893). In 1946, the first disposable syringe, made of glass with interchangeable parts, was developed by brothers Robert Lucas and William Chance (Kantengwa 2020). In 1949, Arthur E. Smith had patented the first disposable hypodermic syringe in the United States made of glass, eliminating the need to sterilize and reuse syringes (Levy 2020). In 1955, Roehr products (Waterbury, CT) introduced the first plastic disposable hypodermic syringe (Levy 2020), which were commonly used by the 1960s (Kravetz 2005). The 1950s also brought about the introduction of many single-use items in medicine, including needles (Greene 1986). Disposable syringes and needles were also mass-produced for the polio vaccination program led by Dr. Jonas Salk, thus solidifying their utility in medicine (Levy 2020). Since the 1950s, disposable hypodermic syringes and needles have become the standard of care to administer drugs parenterally to prevent entry site and hematogenous infection.

8 Local Anesthesia

8.1 Local Anesthesia Drugs

Local anesthesia has become one of the most commonly used methods for alleviating the pain of surgical procedures and injuries. The injection of local anesthetic agents is ubiquitous in medicine, dentistry, and other areas of health care from operating rooms to outpatient clinics, private offices and in the prehospital management of injured patients.

Some of the earliest attempts at pain relief were described by Greek surgeons applying anodyne and astringent pastes to wounds during the siege of Troy around 1250 BCE (Zorab 2003a). Around 50 CE, a Greek physician named Pedanius Dioscorides, who eventually wrote a five-volume book on medicine called De Medica Materia, described mixing Memphitic stone and henbane seeds to smear onto a surgical site prior to the operation (Belfiglio 2018). This anesthetic paste is thought to have released carbonic acid producing a cold or "freezing" effect resulting in anesthesia of the operative site; this was the first topical anesthetic (Zorab 2003b; Bhimana and Bhimana 2018).

In 1539, the potential use of coca leaf as an anesthetic agent was first described by Friar Vicente de Valverde, the bishop of Cuzco (Calatayud and González 2003a). Peruvian literature suggests that coca leaves were chewed and spit into the wounds of patients to alleviate pain (Chivukula et al. 2014). The local anesthetic mechanisms of cocaine were not well understood but were clearly recognized by the way it was being used for pain relief. In 1653, the potential anesthetic properties of coca were revealed by Spanish Jesuit Bernabe Cobo in a paper describing the alleviation of a toothache by chewing coca leaves (Calatayud and González 2003b).

In 1807, Dominique Larrey, Napoleon's surgeon during the bloody and cold battle of Eylau (current day Western Russia), described the numbing effect of cold snow to produce local anesthesia and reduce the pain of amputations (Zimmer 2014). Although Larrey's tactic was rudimentary, there were few alternatives readily available as intravenous access was not yet in use. In the 1820s, with the advent of the early hypodermic syringe, the technology finally caught up to allow localized medication delivery beneath the skin for analgesic effect (Blake 1960).

In the mid-1860s, before the local anesthetic effects of cocaine had been appreciated for clinical use, British physician Benjamin Ward Richardson used ether spray to numb the skin (Leake 1925b). Later, Richardson's ether spray was changed to ethyl chloride which evaporated more rapidly and produced a faster onset of anesthesia. Ultimately, this spray technique would propel topical anesthesia forward, setting the stage for subcutaneous local anesthesia to follow.

In 1859, nearly 200 years after Cobo's paper on the numbing effects of coca leaves was published, German chemist Albert Niemann was the first to isolate pure cocaine, which he keenly noted caused numbness when placed on his own tongue (Redman 2011). Vassily von Anrep, a Russian physician also studying cocaine, described the effects of injecting cocaine into animals commenting afterward that it should be tested as a local anesthetic. Sadly, his astute recommendation was not followed, and his brilliant work went largely unnoticed (Yentis and Vlassakov 1999). Finally, in September of 1884, Carl Koller, an ophthalmology resident and roommate of Sigmund Freud who was also a resident at the Vienna General Hospital, recognized the significance of cocaine's local anesthetic potential (Goerig et al. 2012). After witnessing a colleague painlessly cut his tongue while licking cocaine off a knife, Koller appreciated the significance of the event and realized the potential of the drug. He soon tested a cocaine solution on frog corneas with demonstrable decrease in sensation (Goerig et al. 2012). This work was presented to the science community shortly thereafter and was well received. From then on, cocaine use for local anesthesia grew rapidly, which also led to the development of many regional anesthetic techniques.

On December 6, 1884, Richard John Hall and William Stewart Halsted published a report describing the first nerve block. They used 4% cocaine solution to anesthetize the inferior alveolar nerve of the mandible (Grzybowski 2008). Hall and Halstead went on to describe the techniques of regional blockade in many other parts of the body including the facial nerve, brachial plexus, and pudendal and posterior tibial nerves. In 1885, James Leonard Corning published the first report of spinal anesthesia using cocaine (Wulf 1998). The same year, Corning proposed using a tourniquet to slow the systemic absorption of local anesthesia (Giovannitti et al. 2013). It was not until 1903 that Heinrich Braun would modernize this concept by recommending the use of epinephrine as a chemical tourniquet instead (Giovannitti et al. 2013), a practice that is standard today.

However, despite cocaine's growing popularity and use, by 1891, there were 13 deaths and 200 cases of systemic intoxication, raising concern for the safety of locally injecting cocaine (Murray and f. Cocaine. 1979). Carl Ludwig Schleich developed standardized local anesthesia infiltration techniques by diluting the topical cocaine dose for use with hypodermic injection. This technique was safe and decreased cocaine mortality (Wawersik 1991). His results were presented at the 1892 Congress of the German Society for Surgery in Berlin, but his comments about infiltration anesthesia being potentially less dangerous than general anesthesia offended the surgeons in the audience. Eventually, however, the merit of his work was recognized and adopted in Germany.

The increasing mortality from the toxic effects of cocaine and its addictive nature led a movement to identify alternative substances that could be used as local anesthetics. In 1890, Eduard Ritsert, a German chemist, synthesized benzocaine (Brock and Bell 2012). Unfortunately, its poor water solubility relegated it to use mainly as a topical anesthetic. In 1903, amylocaine (Stovaine) was introduced but was soon found to irritate nerves and was promptly replaced. Procaine, better known by its brand name Novocaine, was synthesized by Alfred Einhorn in 1904. Procaine remained the main anesthetic in dentistry and medicine until tetracaine was synthesized in 1928. However, tetracaine and procaine were both esters with allergic side effects and toxicities, as compared to the more tolerable amide compound of lidocaine, discovered by Nils Lofgren and his assistant, Bengt Lundqvist, in 1948 (Giovannitti et al. 2013). Lidocaine underwent years of clinical testing before finally being introduced into practice in 1948 following FDA approval. Lidocaine's tolerability would later make it one of the most commonly used local anesthetics, even today. In 1957, Bo af Ekenstam introduced two more local anesthetics named mepivacaine and bupivacaine (Calatayud and González 2003a; Ekenstam, and af, Egner B, Pettersson G. 1957). In 1969, Nils Löfgren and Cläes Tegner synthesized prilocaine (Löfgren and Tegné 1960), and a few years later in 1972, articaine was first published in the literature by J. E. Winther (Winther and Nathalang 1972). A more recent discovery is the 2011 FDA-approved ultra-long-acting anesthetic called liposomal bupivacaine (Exparel®) (Drug Approval Package: Brand Name (Generic Name) NDA 2020). Despite a decrease in the rate of local anesthetic discovery and innovation over the last several decades, the drive to improve the effects and success of local anesthesia continues and is evolving.

9 Summary

In conclusion, the story of anesthesia is complex, with simultaneously evolving themes including inhalation, local and parenteral agents, asepsis, technology, and neuromuscular blockers. All these combine today to produce balanced anesthesia safely and appropriately for each patient. Undoubtedly, serendipity played a strong role at times in the discovery process, but history was made by also seizing the opportunities provided as demonstrated by William Morton and critical thinking of John Snow about the science at hand. These factors have driven innovation in anesthesia over the last several hundred years and solved one of humanity's greatest issues—pain during surgery.

References

af Ekenstam B, Egner B, Pettersson G. Local anaesthetics I. N-alkyl pyrrolidine and N-alkyl piperidine carboxylic acid amides. Acta Chem Scand. 1957;11(7):1183–90.

Ali's "train Of Four" | Wood Library-Museum [Internet]. [cited 2020 Dec 16]. Available from: https://www.woodlibrarymuseum.org/museum/item/787/ali's-"train-of-four".

Archer WH. Life and letters of Horace Wells discoverer of anesthesia. J Am Coll Dent. 1944;11(2):81–210.

Ball C, Westhorpe R. Muscle relaxants - Intocostrin. Anaesth Intensive Care. 2005;33(3):289.

Ball C, Westhorpe RN. The history of premedication. Anaesth Intensive Care. 2011;39(6):991.

Barsoum N, Kleeman C. Now and then, the history of parenteral fluid administration. Am J Nephrol. 2002;22(2–3):284–9.

Baskett TF. Benjamin Pugh: The air-pipe and neonatal resuscitation. Resuscitation. 2000;44(3):153–5.

Batterman RC, Himmelsbach CK. Demerol—a new synthetic analgesic: A review of its present status and comparison with morphine. J Am Med Assoc. 1943;122:222–6.

Bause GS. America's first patented series of bubble-through anesthetic vaporizers. Anesthesiology. 2009;110(1):12–21.

Beecher HK, Ford C. Some new letters of Horace Wells concerning an historic partnership. J Hist Med 1954;(January 1848):9–20.

Belfiglio V. Perioperative anesthesia in ancient Rome: 27 B.C.-A.D. 476. Neurol Neurosci Rep. 2018;1(1):1–3.

Bergman NA. Samuel Latham Mitchell (1764-1831) - a neglected American pioneer of anesthesia. J Am Med Assoc. 1985;253(5):675–8.

Bergman NA. Michael Faraday and his contribution to anesthesia. Anesthesiology. 1992;77:812–6.

Bhimana D, Bhimana V. The historical perspective of local anesthetics. Dev Anaesth Pain Manag. 2018;1(3):1–8.

Birmingham AT. Waterton and Wouralia. Br J Pharmacol. 1999;126(8):1685–90.

Blake JB. Mr. Ferguson's hypodermic syringe. J Hist Med Allied Sci. 1960;15(4):337–41.
Bowman WC. Neuromuscular block. Br J Pharmacol. 2006;147(SUPPL. 1):277–86.
Brock WJ, Bell TA. The in vitro and in vivo genotoxicity of benzocaine: a brief communication. Int J Toxicol. 2012;31(3):222–7.
Brownstein MJ. A brief history of opiates, opioid peptides, and opioid receptors. Proc Natl Acad Sci. 1993;90:5391–3.
Calatayud J, González Á. History of the development and evolution of local anesthesia since the coca leaf. Anesthesiology. 2003a;98(6):1503–8.
Calatayud J, González Á. History of the development and evolution of local anesthesia since the coca leaf. Anesthesiology [Internet] 2003b [cited 2020 May 28];98:1503–1508. Available from: www.anesthesiology.org.
Carter AJ. Dwale: an anaesthetic from old England. Br Med J. 1999;319:1623–6.
Chivukula S, Grandhi R, Friedlander RM. A brief history of early neuroanesthesia. Neurosurg Focus. 2014;36(4):1–5.
Cozanitis D. One hundred years of barbiturates and their saint. J R Soc Med. 2004;97:594–8.
Craig R. A history of syringes and needles. The University of Queensland Australia — Faculty of Medicine; 2018.
Czarnowski C, Holmes S. Curare and a Canadian connection. Can Fam Physician. 2007;53(9):1531–2.
Dagnino J. Wren, Boyle, and the origins of intravenous injections and the Royal Society of London. Anesthesiology. 2009;111(4):923–4.
Davison MHA. The discovery of ether. Anaesthesia. 1949;4(4):188–93.
Desai S, Desai MS, Pandav CS. The discovery of modern anaesthesia – Contributions of Davy, Clarke, Long, Wells and Morton. Indian J Anaesth. 2007;51(6):472–6.
Dodds C. General anaesthesia - practical recommendations and recent advances. Drugs. 1999;58(3):453–67.
Dorrington KL, Poole W. The first intravenous anaesthetic: how well was it managed and its potential realized? Br J Anaesth. 2013;110:7–12.
Drug Approval Package: Brand Name (Generic Name) NDA # [Internet]. [cited 2020 Dec 17]. Available from: https://www.accessdata.fda.gov/drugsatfda_docs/nda/2011/022496Orig1s000TOC.cfm.
Drug Trial Snapshot: BRIDION | FDA [Internet]. [cited 2020 Dec 10]. Available from: https://www.fda.gov/drugs/drug-approvals-and-databases/drug-trial-snapshot-bridion.
Duce AM, Hernandez FL. Origins of the hypodermic syringe and local anesthesia. Their influence on hernia surgery. Hernia. 1999;3:103–6.
Dunn PM. Sir James Young Simpson (1811-1870) and obstetric anaesthesia. Nature. 1997;388:F207–9.
Eddy NB, Friebel H, Hahn K-J, Halbach H. Codeine and its alternates for pain and cough relief. Ann Intern Med [Internet] 1968;38(6):673–741. Available from: http://www.ncbi.nlm.nih.gov/pubmed/18568113%0Ahttp://www.pubmedcentral.nih.gov/articlerender.fcgi?artid=PMC2424120.
Ellis RH. The introduction of ether anaesthesia to Great Britain. Anaesthesia. 1976;31:766–77.
Fernie JD. The shape of the earth. Am Sci. 1964;79(5):393–5.
Fisher JA, Bromberg IL, Eisen LB. On the design of anaesthesia record forms. Can J Anaesth. 1994;41(10):973–83.
Fishman SM, Wilsey B, Mahajan G, Molina P. Methadone reincarnated: novel clinical application with related. Pain Med. 2002;3(4):339–48.
Foldes FF. The final steps leading to the anesthetic use of muscle relaxants. Muscle Relaxants. 1995:8–12.
Forman SA. Clinical and molecular pharmacology of etomidate. Anesthesiology. 2011;114(3):695–707.
Foster R. Doctor's Review|Fear of medical mechanics [Internet]. 2005 [cited 2020 Dec 6]. Available from: http://www.doctorsreview.com/history/fear-medical-mechanics/.

Gao M, Rejaei D, Liu H. Ketamine use in current clinical practice. Acta Pharmacol Sin [Internet] 2016;37(7):865–872. Available from: https://doi.org/10.1038/aps.2016.5.
Gertler R, Brown HC, Mitchell D, Silvius E. Dexmedetomidine: a novel sedative-analgesic agent. BUMC Proc. 2001;14:13–21.
Gillespie NA. The evolution of endotracheal anaesthesia. J Hist Med Allied Sci. 1946;1(4):583–94.
Giovannitti JA, Rosenberg MB, Phero JC. Pharmacology of local anesthetics used in oral surgery. Oral Maxillofac Surg Clin North Am [Internet]. 2013;25(3):453–65. Available from:. https://doi.org/10.1016/j.coms.2013.03.003.
Glen JB. The discovery and development of propofol anesthesia | The 2018 Lasker-Debakey clinical medical research award. JAMA. 2018;320(12):1235–6.
Goerig M, Bacon D, Van Zundert A. Carl koller, cocaine, and local anesthesia: some less known and forgotten facts. Reg Anesth Pain Med. 2012;37(3):318–24.
Greene VW. Reuse of disposable medical devices: historical and current aspects. Infect Control. 1986;7(10):508–13.
Grzybowski A. Cocaine and the eye: a historical overview. Ophthalmologica. 2008;222(5):296–301.
Guralnick WC, Kaban LB. Keeping ether "En-vogue": The role of Nathan Cooley keep in the history of ether anesthesia. J Oral Maxillofac Surg [Internet] 2011;69(7):1892–1897. Available from: https://doi.org/10.1016/j.joms.2011.02.121.
Hampton IA. Nursing: its principles and practice; 1893. p. 1–484.
Haridas RP. Horace Wells' demonstration of nitrous oxide in Boston. Anesthesiology. 2013;119(5):1014–22.
Harvey J. Chamberland, Charles Edouard. In: eLS. 2011. p. 1–3.
Howard-jones N. A critical study of the origins and early development of hypodermic medication. J Hist Med Allied Sci. 1947;2(2):201–49.
Kaban LB, Perrott DH. Dual-degree Oral and Maxillofacial Surgery Training in the United States: "Back to the Future". J Oral Maxillofac Surg [Internet]. 2020;78(1):18–28. Available from: https://doi.org/10.1016/j.joms.2019.08.026.
Kacmarek RM. The mechanical ventilator: past, present, and future. Respir Care. 2011;56(8):1170–80.
Kadiyala PK, Kadiyala LD. Anaesthesia for electroconvulsive therapy: an overview with an update on its role in potentiating electroconvulsive therapy. Indian J Anaesth. 2017;61(5):373–80.
Kantengwa S. Origin of ordinary things: The syringe | The New Times | Rwanda [Internet]. The New York Times. 2020 [cited 2020 Dec 6]. Available from: https://www.newtimes.co.rw/lifestyle/origin-ordinary-things-syringe.
Kaur M, Singh P. Current role of dexmedetomidine in clinical anesthesia and intensive care. Anesth Essays Res. 2011;5(2):128–33.
Kravetz RE. Hypodermic syringe. Am J Gastroenterol. 2005;100(12):2614.
Kyle RA, Shampo MA. James Young Simpson and the introduction of chloroform anesthesia in obstetric practice. Mayo Clin Proc [Internet]. 1997;72(4):372. Available from: https://doi.org/10.4065/72.4.372.
Kyung E, Kim E, Cooper B, Desai MS. Popular literature as an educational aid for the history of anesthesia. J Anesth Hist [Internet]. 2018 [cited 2020 May 28];4(2):123–127. Available from: https://doi.org/10.1016/j.janh.2017.09.001.
Lawrence G. Tools of the trade. Lancet. 2002;359:1074.
Leake CD. Valerius Cordus and the discovery of ether. JSTOR. 1925a;7(1):14–24.
Leake CD. The historical development of surgical anesthesia. Sci Mon. 1925b;20(3):304–28.
LeVasseur R, Desai S. Ebenezer Hopkins Frost (1824 –1866): William T.G. Morton's first identified patient and why he was invited to the ether demonstration on October 16, 1846. Anesthesiology. 2012;117(2):238–42.
Levy S. The hypodermic syringe: greatest medical device of all time? [Internet]. Medical Device and Diagnostic Industry. 2014 [cited 2020 Dec 6]. Available from: https://www.mddionline.com/drug-delivery/hypodermic-syringes-greatest-medical-device-all-time.

Lister J. Further evidence regarding the effects of the antiseptic system of treatment upon the salubrity of a surgical hospital. Lancet. 1870;96:287–9.

Löfgren N, Tegnér C. Studies on local anesthetics: XX. Synthesis of some α-monoalkylamino-2.-methylpropionanilides: a new useful local anesthetic. Acta Chem Scand. 1960;14(2):486–90.

López-Muñoz F, Álamo C, García-García P. The discovery of chlordiazepoxide and the clinical introduction of benzodiazepines: half a century of anxiolytic drugs. J Anxiety Disord. 2011;25(4):554–62.

López-Muñoz F, Ucha-Udabe R, Alamo C. The history of barbiturates a century after their clinical introduction. Neuropsychiatr Dis Treat [Internet] 2005;1(4):329–343. Available from: http://www.ncbi.nlm.nih.gov/pubmed/18568113%0Ahttp://www.pubmedcentral.nih.gov/articlerender.fcgi?artid=PMC2424120.

Lopez-Valverde A, Montero J, Albaladeja A, Gomez de Diego R. The discovery of surgical anesthesia: discrepancies regarding its authorship. J Dent Res. 2011;90(1):31–4.

Maclachlan JT. Lister's antiseptic technique. Br Med J. 1942;2:466.

Matioc AA. An anesthesiologist's perspective on the history of basic airway management. Anesthesiol Clin North Am. 2016;124(2):301–11.

McGrath CD, Hunter JM. Monitoring of neuromuscular block. Continuing Education in Anaesthesia. Crit Care Pain. 2006;6(1):7–12.

McKenzie AG. Prelude to pancuronium and vecuronium. Anaesthesia. 2000;55(6):551–6.

Murray A, Hagen NA. Proceedings of the Symposium "Updates of the Clinical Pharmacology of Opioids with Special Attention to Long-Acting Drugs". J Pain Symptom Manag. 2005;29(5S):S57–66.

Murray S, f. Cocaine. Br Med J. 1979;1(6169):971–2.

Pieters BM, Eindhoven GB, Acott C, van Zundert AAJ. Pioneers of laryngoscopy: indirect, direct and video laryngoscopy. Anaesth Intensive Care. 2015;43:4–11.

Pitt D, Aubin J-M. Joseph Lister: father of modern surgery. J Can Chiropr Assoc. 2012;55(5):E8–9.

Porta JB. Printed for Thomas Young and Samuel Speed and are to be sold at the three pigeons, and at the angel in St. Paul's Church-yard. London: Natural Magick; 1658. p. 218.

Prescott F, Organe G, Rowbotham S. Tubocurarine chloride as an adjunct to anaesthesia - report on 180 cases. Lancet. 1946;248(6412):80–4.

Raghavendra T. Neuromuscular blocking drugs: discovery and development. J R Soc Med. 2002;95(7):363–7.

Rajesh O, Meher R. Historical review of tracheostomy. Internet J Otorhinolaryngol. 2012;4(2):1–4.

Redman M. Cocaine: what is the crack? A brief history of the use of Cocaine as an anesthetic. Anesthesiol Pain Med. 2011;1(2):95–7.

Riegels N, Richards MJ. Humphry Davy - his life, works, and contributions to anesthesiology. Anesthesiology. 2012;114(6):1282–8.

Savarese JJ, Belmont MR, Hashim MA, Mook RA, Boros EE, Samano V, et al. Preclinical pharmacology of GW280430A (AV430A) in the Rhesus monkey and in the cat. Anesthesiology. 2004;100:835–45.

Schlich T. Asepsis and bacteriology: a realignment of surgery and laboratory science. Med Hist. 2012;56(3):308–34.

Schmitz R. Friedrich Wilhelm Sertürner and the discovery of morphine. Pharm Hist. 1985;27(2):61–74.

Shafer SL. From d-tubocurarine to sugammadex: The contributions of T. Cecil Gray to modern anaesthetic practice. Br J Anaesth. 2011;107(1):97–102.

Short G. Ah, The staph of life! Ether frolics & gas gangrene [Internet]. Brevis Corporation. 2014 [cited 2021 Jan 3]. Available from: https://www.brevis.com/blog/tag/ether-frolics/.

Slutsky AS. History of mechanical ventilation - from Vesalius to ventilator-induced lung injury. Am J Respir Crit Care Med. 2015;191(10):1106–15.

Smith GB, Hirsch NP. Gardner Quincy Colton: Pioneer of nitrous oxide anesthesia. Anesth Analg. 1991;72(3):382–91.

Sneader W. Department of medical history The discovery of heroin. Med Hist. 1998;352:1697–9.

Stanley TH. The fentanyl story. J Pain [Internet]. 2014;15(12):1215–26. Available from:. https://doi.org/10.1016/j.jpain.2014.08.010.
Succinylcholine vs. Rocuronium: Battle of the RSI Paralytics - JEMS [Internet]. [cited 2020 Dec 10]. Available from: https://www.jems.com/patient-care/succinylcholine-vs-rocuronium-battle-of-the-rsi-paralytics/.
Sykes K. Harold Griffith Memorial lecture - The Griffith legacy. Can J Anesth. 1992;40(4):365–70.
Szmuk P, Ezri T, Evron S, Roth Y, Katz J. A brief history of tracheostomy and tracheal intubation, from the bronze age to the space age. Intensive Care Med. 2008;34(2):222–8.
The Development and Regulatory History of Sugammadex in the United States - Anesthesia Patient Safety Foundation [Internet]. [cited 2020 Dec 10]. Available from: https://www.apsf.org/article/the-development-and-regulatory-history-of-sugammadex-in-the-united-states/.
The History of Opiates | Michael's House Treatment Center [Internet]. [cited 2020 Dec 10]. Available from: https://www.michaelshouse.com/opiate-rehab/history-of-opiates/.
Thornton BYJL. John Snow, pioneer specialist-anaesthetist. Anaesthesia. 1950;5(3):129–35.
Urman RD, Desai SP. History of anesthesia for ambulatory surgery. Curr Opin Anaesthesiol. 2012;25(6):641–7.
Vandam L, Abbott JA. Edward Gilbert Abbott : enigmatic figure reprinted by permission of the New England Journal of Medicine. N Engl J Med. 1984;311:991–4.
Viets HR. The earliest printed references in newspapers and journals to the first public demonstration of ether anesthesia in 1846. J Hist Med Allied Sci. 1949;4(2):149–69.
Wang Y, Ming X-X, Zhang C-P. Fluorine-containing inhalation anesthetics: chemistry, properties, and pharmacology. Curr Med Chem. 2020;27(33):5599–652.
Wawersik J. History of anesthesia in Germany. J Clin Anesth. 1991;3(3):235–44.
Welliver M, McDonough J, Kalynych N, Redfern R. Discovery, development, and clinical application of sugammadex sodium, a selective relaxant binding agent. Drug Des Devel Ther. 2008;2:49–59.
West JB. Joseph Priestley, oxygen, and the enlightenment. Am J Physiol Lung Cell Mol Physiol. 2014a;306(2):L111–9.
West JB. Robert Hooke: early respiratory physiologist, polymath, and mechanical genius. Physiology. 2014b;29(4):222–33.
Whalen FX, Bacon DR, Smith HM. Inhaled anesthetics: an historical overview. Best Pract Res Clin Anaesthesiol. 2005;19(3):323–30.
White PF. Propofol - its role in changing the practice of anesthesia. Anesthesiology. 2008;109(6):1132–6.
Winther JE, Nathalang B. Effectivity of a new local analgesic Hoe 40 045. Eur J Oral Sci. 1972;80(4):272–8.
Wulf HFW. The centennial of spinal anesthesia. Anesthesiology. 1998;89:500–6.
Yang QH, Alston TA, Charles T. Jackson and William T.G. Morton Patented the "Ethereal Solution of Opium" of Elton Romeo Smilie. J Anesth Hist [Internet]. 2018;4(2):128–129. Available from: https://doi.org/10.1016/j.janh.2018.01.004.
Yentis SM, Vlassakov KV. Vassily von Anrep, forgotten pioneer of regional anesthesia. Anesthesiology. 1999;90:890–5.
Zimmer M. History of anaesthesia: early forms of local anaesthesia. Eur J Anaesthesiol. 2014;31(1):1–12.
Zorab J. History of anaesthesia. Anaesthesia. 2003a;58:935.
Zorab J. History of anesthesia. Anesthesia. 2003b;58:826–7.

The Legacy of Maxillofacial Surgery During the Great War

Shahid R. Aziz and Samina H. Aziz

1 Introduction

World War I, "The Great War," brought to reality a suffering, violence, and destruction that were new to the human experience. Historically, the pressure placed on the medical profession to respond to the care of the wounded during wartime has stimulated the medical sciences into new eras of advancement. It is an unfortunate truth that war often provides fuel for medical advancement. Trench warfare during World War I provided surgeons with new challenges in facial trauma management and laid the cornerstone for modern-day oral and maxillofacial surgery. The work of surgeons such as Gillies, Kazanjian, Ivy, Morestin, Valadier, and others provided the basis for facial reconstruction (Aziz 2001).

The Great War lasted from July 28, 1914, to November 11, 1918. It was a consequence of the assassination the Austro-Hungarian heir Archduke Franz Ferdinand in Sarajevo by Gavrilo Princip, a Bosnian Serb Yugoslav nationalist. The resulting Austria-Serbia conflict escalated into two competing alliances: the Triple Entente (Allied)—consisting of France, Russia, and Britain—and the Triple Alliance of Germany, Austria-Hungary, and Italy (Central Powers). After the sinking of American merchant ships by German submarines, the United States declared war on Germany on April 6, 1917. The Treaty of Versailles brought World War I to an end, signed on June 28, 1919, in Versailles, France.

As noted above, Trench warfare was a novel approach to warfare. It provided protection to the soldier for bodily injury from gunfire; however, the soldier's face

S. R. Aziz (✉)
Department of Oral and Maxillofacial Surgery, Rutgers School of Dental Medicine, Newark, NJ, USA
e-mail: AZIZSR@SDM.RUTGERS.EDU

S. H. Aziz
The Wardlaw Hartridge School, Edison, NJ, USA

E. M. Ferneini et al. (eds.), *The History of Maxillofacial Surgery*,
https://doi.org/10.1007/978-3-030-89563-1_6

was often exposed. In 1915, steel helmets were introduced, protecting to a degree from brain trauma, but the face remained bare. Further, the Great War introduced a new age of high-velocity ballistic use and injury. What resulted was a never-before-seen volume and severity of facial trauma—soft and hard tissue. It is estimated that 15% of all injuries were facial. Often, this injury rendered the soldier alive but with massive tissue loss. As a consequence, this forced the evolution and laid the foundations for modern-day facial reconstructive surgery. The reconstructive efforts could be broken into two basic efforts:

1. Frontline triage and stabilization. Typically, the soldier was stabilized, facial fractures reduced, and facial soft tissue injury treated for infection and hemorrhage. Soldiers were then transferred away from the front to more sophisticated centers. The best documented frontline efforts were by the Harvard Surgical Unit's maxillofacial team led by Dr. Varaztad Kazanjian.
2. Tertiary care centers away from the front lines where hard and soft tissue reconstructive surgery occurred. The best known of these were two:

   (a) Sidcup—led by Sir Harold Gillies
   (b) Berlin unit—led by Professor Jacques Joseph

2 Front-Line Care: Origins of the Harvard Unit

Although the US government remained officially neutral during the early years of the Great War, the American people strongly supported the cause of the Allied Powers. Sir William Osler proposed that leading American and Canadian universities should provide the Allied Forces with medical services near the fields of battle. Harvard, Johns Hopkins, Columbia, and McGill Universities arranged for medical "units" to be part of the Royal Army Medical Corps of the British Expeditionary Forces in France. On June 26, 1915, Harvard sent to England the first of 3 surgical units led by Dr. E. H. Nichols and composed of 32 surgeons, 3 dentists, and 75 nurses (the subsequent 2 units were led by Dr. David Cheever and Dr. Hugh Cabot, respectively).

When the First Harvard Unit was being formed, Dr. Nichols requested that Dr. Eugene Smith, Dean of the Harvard Dental School, select three dentists for inclusion. Smith, in turn, nominated Dr. Varaztad H. Kazanjian, who was at the time Instructor in Mechanical (Prosthetic) Dentistry and a 1905 graduate of the School, to be the Chief Dental Officer of the Dental Department of the Harvard Unit. Dr. Kazanjian readily accepted and chose as his assistants Ferdinand Brigham and Frank Cushman, both graduating seniors from Harvard Dental School. Brigham in his memoirs wrote:

> Dean Smith sensed it was the most dramatic event in the history of the school, and he intended to make the most of it. He chose Dr. Kazanjian with instinctive judgment, based on all his experience in choosing men and shaping dental events. Dr. Smith knew his man, knew that his quiet unassuming manner which has confounded many from that day to this

> into thinking that he was timid or unmethodical, cloaked a thoroughgoing ability to forge ahead, an ease of organizing, and imagination in meeting the unknown . . .. I am not aware that Dr. Smith considered any other candidate than Dr. Kazanjian. He had the interest of the school at heart. He read the future carefully (Brigham 1964).

Varaztad Kazanjian (1879-1974) was a remarkable individual. Born in what is now Eastern Turkey, of Armenian heritage, he immigrated at age 16 to the United States to avoid persecution by the Ottoman Empire. Settling in Massachusetts, he later attended Harvard Dental School, graduating in 1905, and further trained as a prosthodontist. He then served as a faculty member at the dental school. Following World War 1, Kazanjian then completed his medical degree at Boston University and returned to Harvard as a Professor of Oral Surgery and the first Professor of Plastic Surgery. He is considered to be one of the founders of modern plastic surgery, though he never forgot his roots in dentistry. (Fig. 1)

The members of the Harvard Unit had a unique status in the Royal Army. Not British subjects, they were granted temporary honorary commissions in the Royal Army Medical Corps. The British War Office assigned this unit to Number 22 General Hospital at Dannes and Camiers, France. Dannes and Camiers were two hamlets located 14 miles south of Boulogne-sur-mer. No. 22 was one of five base

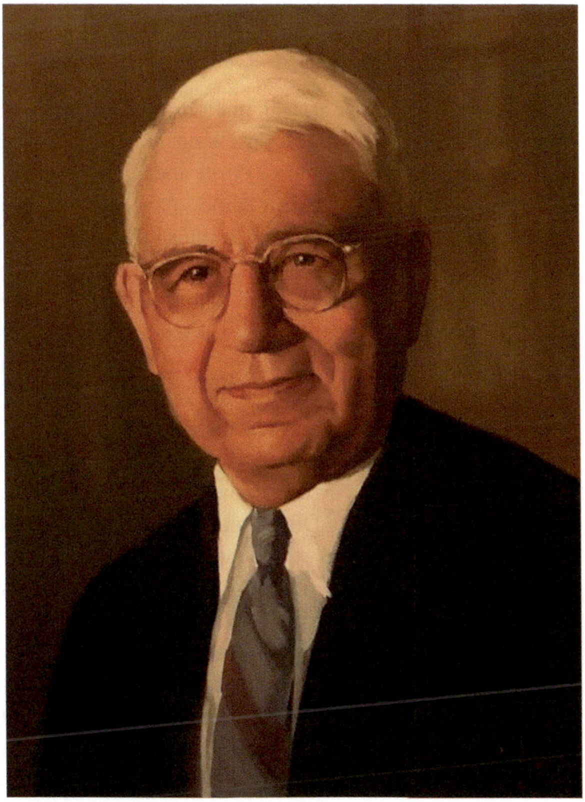

Fig. 1 Portrait of Dr. Kazanjian in foyer of the Harvard School of Dental Medicine, Boston, MA, USA. Reproduced with permission and without alterations

hospitals situated in northern France. The hospital contained 1800 beds and was equipped with surgical and medical wards and operating facilities. The professional staff was housed in waterproof tents. These military base hospitals were adjacent to the front lines of fighting and sent "surgical teams" (teams of surgeons, anesthesiologists, and nurses) to the frontline casualty-clearing stations for emergent care, for triage of the injured, and to facilitate a smooth transfer of the wounded to base hospitals.

Arriving in Dannes-Camiers, France, in July 1915, the Harvard dentists were the first to commence work. They were assigned one ward in the hospital and were kept busy with exodontia and prosthetic dentistry. Dr. Cushman later wrote in the Harvard Alumni Bulletin:

> Upon the arrival of the Unit in France, dental conditions were found to be much worse than expected. Until it became known throughout the district that fractures of the jaws were being treated by the Harvard Unit, much of the work was concerned with extraction of teeth and the making of artificial dentures. The most important phase of the work of the dental men in the Unit was, of course, the treatment of the cases of fractures of the jaws, and before the work was long underway, many cases of this sort were being brought in from the front and from other hospitals. The injuries were often very extensive, involving in addition to the jaws, other parts of the face and cranium. External wounds necessitate an entire change of procedure from the methods used in jaw fractures in civil hospitals. Owing to the drainage of Saliva through these wounds, the sepsis is widespread and persistent. Too much credit cannot be given to Dr. Kazanjian for the masterly way in which these cases are being handled (Fig. 1). Each new case requires the devising of special appliances to fit its particular needs; but this Harvard man is always found equal to every occasion (Cushman 1916).

One week after his arrival in France, Kazanjian created a plan for the Dental Department of the First Harvard Unit which consisted of two phases: (1) routine dental care for soldiers and (2) oral and maxillofacial surgery. When the 3-month term of the First Harvard Unit came to an end, the British War Office, cognizant of Kazanjian's excellent fieldwork, requested that he stay on until the end of the war or until he could train a successor. Kazanjian, while willing, was concerned about his absence from his position at the dental school. Six surgeons of the unit petitioned Harvard President Lowell to allow Kazanjian to remain. Lowell cabled an affirmative response. Kazanjian then requested that the British War Office allow his assistants to remain and to provide better facilities in which to work. The British agreed and provided Kazanjian and his unit with better space and larger wards, relocating them to General Hospital 20.

Kazanjian wrote an article in the 1917 British Medical Journal detailing the daily activities of the Dental Department of the Harvard Surgical Unit. He noted that "soldiers who have received wounds of the face and jaws have for the first time been collected in centers for treatment." Advantages of this system included a nursing staff properly trained to efficiently handle maxillofacial injuries, the development of a dental laboratory that quickly produced splints and appliances necessary for treatment, and the opportunity to maintain a "comprehensive system of records from which deductions can be made on the complications, mortality, etc...." Cases were usually admitted to the dental department 2–3 days after injury. Kazanjian divided treatment into two distinct periods: the first, or early period (usually 3–4 weeks after injury), which he considered essential for a successful outcome. During this time, soldiers usually suffered from mental shock, toxic absorption from the wounds, exhaustion secondary to blood loss, and malnutrition secondary to inflammation of the oral cavity and damage to the masticatory apparatus. Further, it was during this period that patients were at highest risk for serious complications such as hemorrhage, bronchopneumonia, and generalized sepsis. The microorganisms involved in the septicemia were thought to be streptococcal; however, no positive identification was completed. Cellulitis was observed, originating from the wound and spreading over the face and scalp and accompanied by pyrexia. Bronchopneumonia was considered the most fatal complication. Some cases occurred suddenly, others gradually. Empyema and multiple abscesses in the lung were common. The pulmonary infections seemed to originate from the inhalation of septic material from the mouth. To prevent the onset of sepsis, initial treatment involved irrigation of the mouth at 2-hour intervals during the day and night and swabbing of the soft tissues with iodine-soaked cotton. This was followed by surgical debridement of the wound under local anesthesia (Kazanjian 1917).

The second period was the convalescent period. During this time, definitive treatment of the oral and maxillofacial region was undertaken, including repair of the hard tissues by means of splints, construction of prosthetic appliances, and reconstructive operations for the repair of facial deformities. Based on his clinical experience, Kazanjian developed several basic principles for treating facial fractures: immediate immobilization of the fracture via the use of splints, reestablishment of the dental occlusion as a guide for fracture reduction, early wound care and cleansing to minimize sepsis, and the control of blood loss. Kazanjian emphasized that early immobilization of fractures was the quickest and best means for recovery, and in turn, it reduced soft tissue inflammation and the risk of infection and increased patient comfort. He noted that the primary function of splints was the fixation of bony fragments, which in turn provided support for overlying soft tissues. Nearly every splint was custom-made to suit each case. For cases of "ordinary" severity, standard splints were used to immobilize the jaw. In cases of extreme destruction of hard and soft tissues, Kazanjian found that intraoral splints were inadequate; an external support system composed of a series of vulcanite plates fitted over the forehead, and a headgear, was developed. This appliance stabilized the tissues of the mouth, nose, eyes, and neck. For extensive mandibular loss, Kazanjian created a sectional or folding artificial jaw; it acted as a framework for reconstructive operations and maintained the contour of the lower face. If the temporomandibular joint was involved in the injury, he placed a mechanical condyle to restore joint function. Before the Harvard Unit's arrival, one major flaw in the care of maxillofacial war injuries was the basic lack of dental training on the part of the military surgeon. Kazanjian noted that if a surgeon was called upon to treat a fracture of the mandible, in many instances, he approximated the segments with wires or metal plates without regard to the occlusion of the teeth, while the dentist, in attending a similar injury, almost invariably applied intermaxillary ligation or immobilization of the jaw by some form of splint attached to the teeth which brought the jaws and teeth into natural occlusion. The key to Kazanjian's success was his training as a prosthodontist.

He used dental occlusion as the guide for reduction of the fracture—a principle well known in the dental community but novel to the medical clinician. His work during the Great War with general surgeons brought to light this basic principle of fracture reduction in the medical community, bridging the "no-man's-land" between medicine and dentistry (Kazanjian 1920).

With regard to management of the soft tissues, Kazanjian wrote that "there does not appear to be much scope for primary suturing of gunshot wounds complicated by fracture of the jaw. Some advantages may follow accurate primary suture of those portions of the wound which involve the lip margins, the eyelids, the alar of the nose, portions of the external ears or the outlying tributaries of a radiating wound."[5] He advocated the use of secondary suturing to lessen the amount of scarring. Immediate cleansing and debridement to minimize sepsis were most important for facial soft tissue trauma (Fig. 2). Finally, in situations in which soft tissue reconstruction was required, Kazanjian used flap operations to cover deficiencies. He used primary and secondary suturing to reduce the region to be covered by the flaps and created an appliance to reproduce the bony tissue to serve as a framework to give a natural contour to the soft tissues of the face or neck and to prevent undue scar contraction.

During Kazanjian's 3.5 years in Dannes-Camiers, the Harvard Unit saw 3000 maxillofacial cases (Fig. 3). News of the unit's successful management of even the most complex facial injury spread throughout the Allied and German medical communities, and Kazanjian's methods soon became the standard of care for the soldier with oral and maxillofacial wounds. The British press dubbed Kazanjian the "Miracle Man of the Western Front" in honor of his surgical accomplishments. Kazanjian later wrote, "As I look back upon those busy years, it is apparent that the principles and methods evolved during World War for the treatment of maxillofacial injuries had far reaching influence on the surgical treatment of civilian injuries and

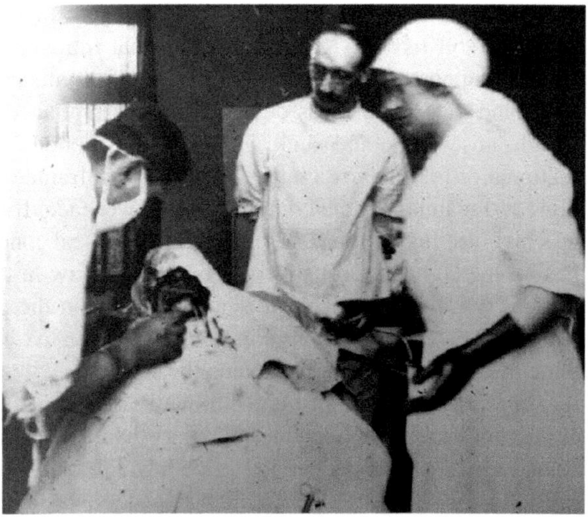

Fig. 2 Kazanjian debriding a facial wound. Courtesy Center for the History of Medicine, Francis Countway Library of Medicine, Harvard Medical School, Boston, MA, USA. Reproduced with permission and without alterations

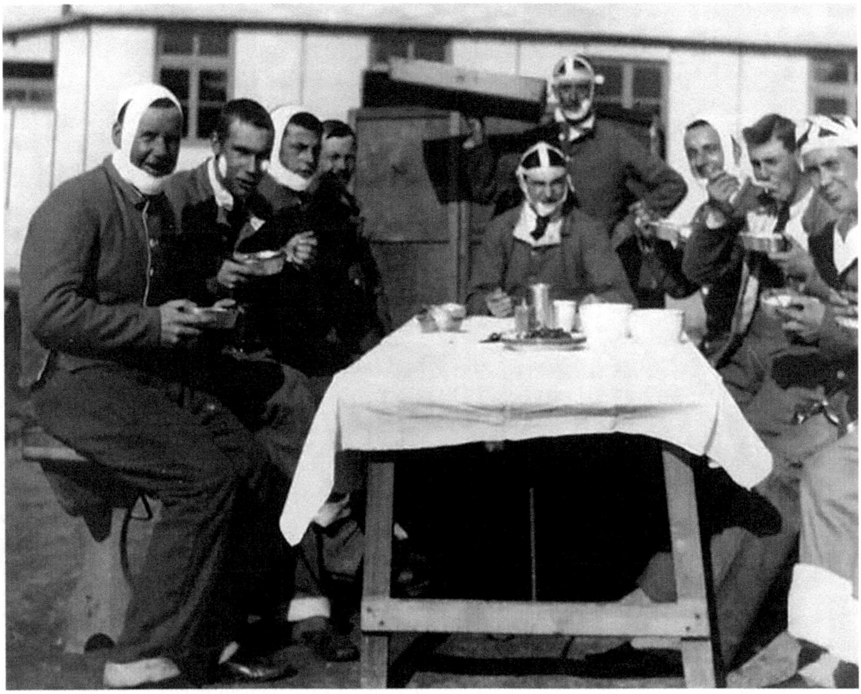

Fig. 3 Patients of Kazanjian's. Courtesy Center for the History of Medicine, Francis Countway Library of Medicine, Harvard Medical School, Boston, MA, USA. Reproduced with permission and without alterations

of acquired and congenital deformities of the face and jaw as well as other parts of the body (Converse 1919)." The Harvard Unit was retired by the British Army on January 8, 1919. Kazanjian and Hugh Cabot were both invested by King George with the "Insignia of a Companion of the Order of St. Michael and St. George" at Buckingham Palace (Fig. 4).

3 Tertiary Care—Sir Harold Delf Gillies and the Surgeons of Sidcup

As noted above, there were an unprecedented number of soldiers sustaining severe facial injury during the Great War. Many required more than stabilization—facial reconstructive surgery was necessary. These centers were reconstructing often never-before-seen facial trauma. From this brutality arose novel reconstructive techniques to meet the need. One of the landmark centers for facial reconstructive surgery was a converted estate in the English country outside of London. Later known as Queens Hospital and then Queen Mary's Hospital, this center was the brainchild

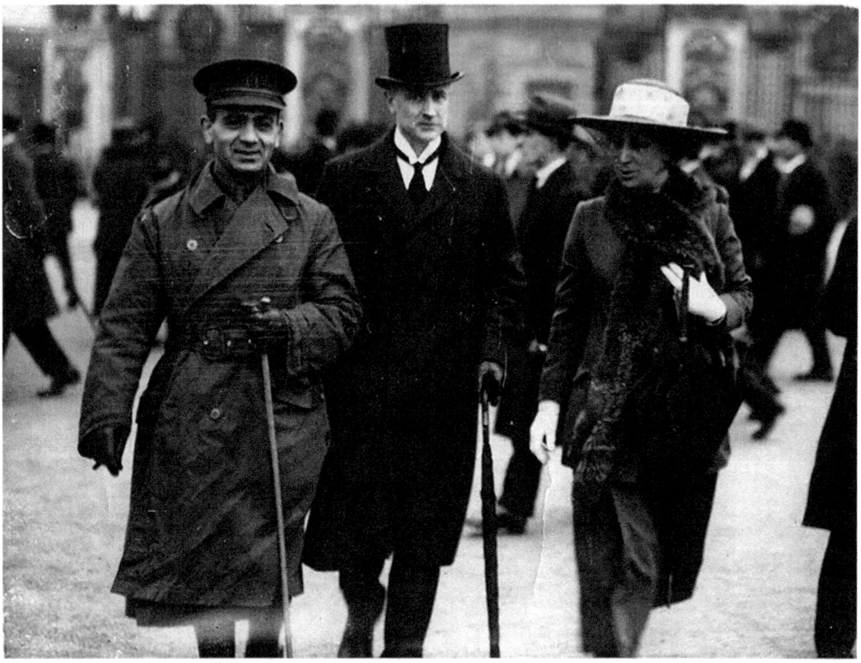

Fig. 4 Immediately after receiving his investiture outside Buckingham Palace. Courtesy Center for the History of Medicine, Francis Countway Library of Medicine, Harvard Medical School, Boston, MA, USA. Reproduced with permission and without alterations

of a British Army otolaryngologist whose work during World War I made him a world-famous plastic surgeon: Sir Harold Delf Gillies.

Gillies (1882–1960) was born in Dunedin, New Zealand. The son of a prominent family that emigrated from the Isle of Bute, Scotland, he was one of eight children. His father passed at age 4, and young Gilles then moved to Auckland. He was initially educated at Wanganui Collegiate School where he excelled as an athlete. In 1900, he was considered the premier schoolboy cricketer in all of New Zealand. Gillies then matriculated to Gonville and Caius College, the University of Cambridge, in 1901. During his time at Cambridge, he excelled in studies as well as in sports. Gillies rowed for his university as well as represented England in golf. He went on to do clinical training at St. Bartholomew's hospital in London and trained in otolaryngology under Sir Milson Rees (Bamji 2006).

In 1914 as the British war effort was developing, Gillies volunteered to serve as a British Medical Officer, working with the Red Cross (Fig. 5). In January 1915, he was sent to France where he encountered a French-American dental surgeon by the name of Charles Valadier. Valadier had established the first British jaw surgery unit at the 83rd base hospital in Wimereux. Ironically (and a nod to the historical issues oral surgeons had in hospital until the 1970s), Valadier, as a dentist, required supervision of a physician to operate, and Gilles was obliged to be said physician. Gillies assisted and observed the dentist Valadier treat mandibular trauma via bone grafting.

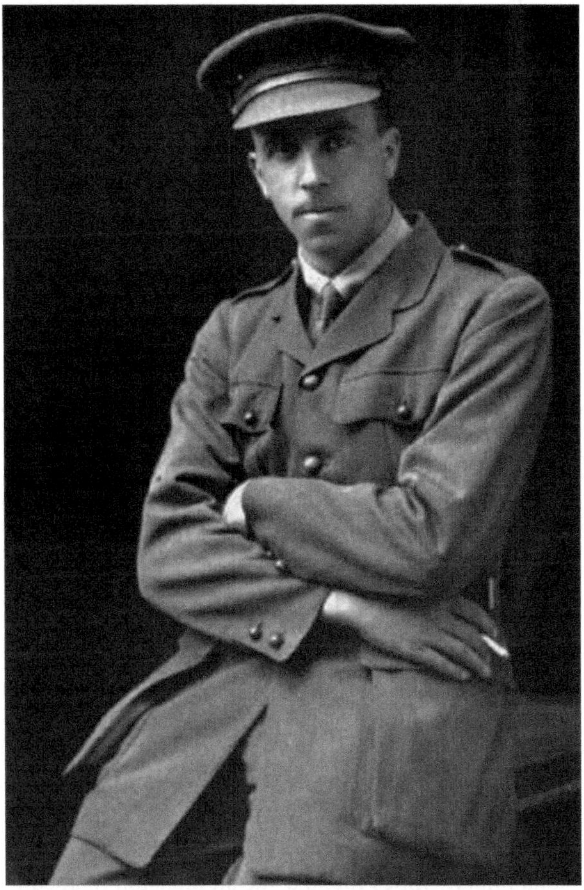

Fig. 5 Sir Harold Delf Gillies circa 1915 in British Army uniform (Meikle 2006)

Charles Valadier (1873–1931) was perhaps one of the great mystery men of his day. French-American, he was born in Paris and educated in New York. He claimed to be a graduate of what is now the Columbia University Vagelos College of Physicians and Surgeons and what is now Temple University School of Dentistry. Valadier then set up practice in New York City, though later returned to France in 1910 to be near family. He opened a dental practice in Paris and in 1914 volunteered with the British Red Cross at the outbreak of the Great War. Through his charming manner and patronization of his superior officers, Valadier was able to open his own jaw unit in Wimereux (Cruse 1987). Gillies noted that Valadier was

> a great fat man with sandy hair and a florid face, who had equipped his Rolls Royce with a dental chair, drills, and the necessary heavy metals..., with generals strapped in his chair he convinced them of the need of a plastic and jaw unit… the credit for establishing the first plastic and jaw unit must go to the remarkable linguistic talents of the smooth and genial Sir Charles Valadier (Gillies and Millard 1957).

Valadier advocated principles similar to Kazanjian—debridement and irrigation of facial injury and stabilization of the occlusion. After the war, he became a British citizen and was knighted for his efforts. Unfortunately, he developed a severe gambling problem post war and died penniless in 1931. Valadier's work inspired Gillies to pursue surgical reconstruction of the face. Gillies then traveled to Paris to spend time with the French-Creole surgeon Hippolyte Morestin.

Morestin (1869–1919) was born in Martinique, the son of a doctor. He trained as a surgeon in France. Morestin was described as a surgeon before his time—focusing on reconstruction and the aesthetic. As such, he focused from 1914 until his death in 1919 on the reconstruction of soldiers with devastating facial injury. He led a surgical unit in a military hospital in Paris—Hospital Val-de Grace. It was here that Gilles observed Morestin. Gilles later wrote:

> I stood spell bound as he removed half of a face distorted with a horrible cancer and then deftly turned a neck flap to restore not only the cheek but the side of the nose and lip in one shot... at the time it was the most thrilling thing I had ever seen. I fell in love with the work on the spot (Lalardrie 1972).

Morestin died prematurely in 1919 at the end of the Great War from influenza. While many may not know his name, he was a remarkable surgeon and Gillies's inspiration.

After Gillies's experience in France, he returned to England and petitioned the British Army's surgeon-in-chief—Arbuthnot Lane—to establish a section of the Cambridge Military Hospital, Aldershot, dedicated to the treatment of facial injuries in soldiers from the Front. From his French experience, Gillies valued the work of dentists; as such, he created a multidisciplinary unit of surgeons, dental/oral surgeons, anesthesiologists, and others. July 1916 brought the Battle of the Somme. Gillies's unit was overwhelmed with facial casualties. As such, Lane directed Gillies to establish an entire hospital, under Gillies's direction, dedicated to the repair of facial injury. Gillies found a vacant mansion (named Frognal) in Sidcup, Kent, and quickly converted it into a 1000-bed hospital which was named Queen Hospital (renamed Queen Mary's Hospital in 1928), opening in June 1917. Gillies then recruited surgeons from New Zealand, Canada, and Australia as well as the United States to set up respective units within Frognal. For the next 3 years, they treated over 5000 men. And reconstructive efforts continued from 1920 to 1929 with an estimated 8500 men treated. Gillies separated the hospital into geographic units:

1. British Unit—led by Gillies
2. Canadian Unit—led by Fulton Risdon and Carl Waldron
3. New Zealand Unit—headed by Henry Pickerill
4. Australia Unit—Henry Newland

Sidcup is long considered the place where the foundations for modern facial reconstructive surgery evolved, with Gillies its founder (Fig. 6). And while this is certainly true, Sidcup was so much more. It was a place where there was a true understanding for the need of multidisciplinary care to ensure ultimate facial reconstruction, especially the marriage between dental surgeons and medical

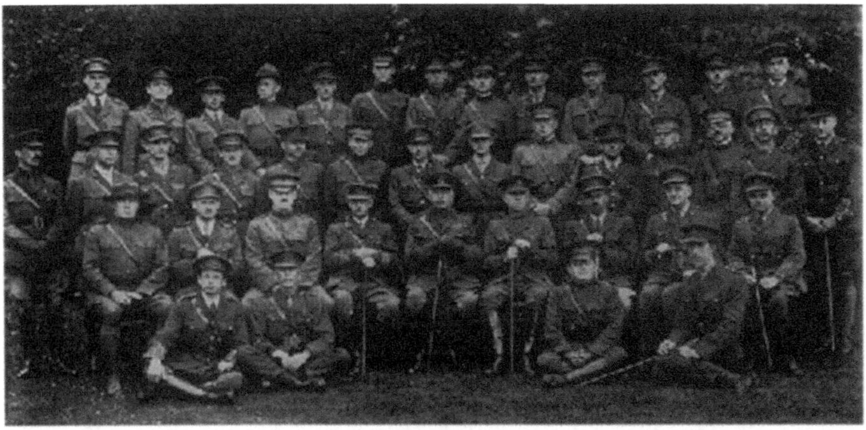

First Row.—Capt. A. Atwell, Capt. B. O. Watson, Capt. G. Johnson, Capt. C. M. Leary, Lieut. R. Waite, Capt. B. P. Lafitte, Capt. G. Seccombe Hett, Major W. J. Seruton, Capt. C. E. Aumsey, Capt. V. Macdonald, Capt. R. G. Robertson, Capt. G. M. Hick, Capt. R. F. Risdon.

Second Row.—Capt. F. Ashworth, A.D.C., Capt. J. C. Clayton, Capt. A. L. Fraser, Capt. W. Kelsey Fry, M.C., Capt. G. C. Bird, Lieut. J. I. Ogden, Capt. J. M. Turner, Capt. R. Montgomery, Capt. H. W. Brent, Lieut. H. M. Johnston, Major Roa P. McGee, Capt. J. M. Waugh, Capt. A. W. L. Campbell, Capt. B. Mendleson.

Third Row.—Major T. C. Sullivan, Major H. P. Pickerill, Major G. M. Dorrance, Lt.-Col. J. R. Colvin, H.R.H. The Duke of Connaught, Lt.-Col. H. S. Newland, D.S.O., Major H. D. Gillies, Major A. Wheeler, Major C. W. Waldron.

Fourth Row.—Capt. H. C. Malleson, Capt. H. L. Whale, Lieut. F. J. Kelly, Lieut. J. W. Edwards.

Fig. 6 Surgeons of Sidcup, June 1918 (Pickerill 1954)

"maxillofacial" surgeons. Indeed, the senior dental surgeon Kelsey Fry who worked with Gillies is said to have told Gillies on their first meeting, "I'll take the hard tissues. You take the soft."

Gillies also appreciated the need to document the work done—as such, he hired photographers, painters, and others. Of note was the surgeon turned artist Henry Tonks, who documented through drawings and painting the work done at Sidcup. The results were astonishing. The following were developed at Sidcup:

1. The tubed pedicle flap
2. Temporalis muscle transfer flap for zygomatic defects
3. Epithelial inlay flap for reconstruction of eyelids and intraoral vestibuloplasty
4. Autogenous bone grafting to the jaws as designed by oral surgeon Kelsey Fry
5. Advances in nasal reconstruction by Henry Pickerill
6. Perhaps most importantly the nasal endotracheal tube and associated forceps developed by Ivan Magill and Stanley Rowbotham

As noted earlier, much of what was being developed was in an attempt to primarily close large avulsive facial soft tissue injury. They allowed the surgeons at Sidcup to refine techniques of local and pedicled soft tissue flaps. Further, to reconstruct facial hard tissue injury, Fry and others developed techniques of bone grafting from the rib and tibia. Gillies developed a reconstructive technique known as the tubed pedicle flap. This was a myocutaneous flap. Unfortunately for Gillies, a Ukranian surgeon Vladimir Filatov independently also developed the same flap and published his technique prior to Gillies. In addition, Gillies modified Esser's epithelial inlay flap for reconstruction of eyelid injury using pedicled oral mucosa. Finally, Fry and Gillies designed an onlay flap for vestibuloplasties, using stents—a technique commonly used today.

One of the key members of Gillies multidisciplinary team was Kelsey Fry. William Kelsey Fry (1889–1963) was educated in medicine and dentistry at Guy's Hospital, receiving his medical degree in 1912 and dental qualification in 1913. It is said that Fry, while a student at Guy's, developed a love for facial and oral surgery after watching Sir Arbuthnot Lane repair a cleft palate on an infant. However, before he could start training formally in oral surgery, Fry was recruited into the British Army's medical core. Fry was dispatched to the front lines in France and was immediately wounded. He, by coincidence, convalesced at Guy's Hospital. Fry returned to France but was later posted to assist Gillies at Cambridge Hospital, later Sidcup. At Sidcup, the team of Gillies Fry and Magill dealt with facial trauma never before seen (Fig. 7). Fry utilized the methods by American field oral surgeons Kazanjian and Henry Sage Dunning (who later founded Columbia University's dental school) to stabilize facial fractures by use of external fixation and splints with Gillies's developed methods of autogenous bone grafting to mandibular defects.

Perhaps most interesting of Fry's achievements was working with anesthesiologist Ivan Magill and Stanley Rowbotham. Magill and Rowbotham championed the idea of intratracheal (endotracheal) nasal anesthesia—mainly out of necessity (Fig. 8). Prior to the Great War, anesthesia was often simply administered via mask inhalation. However, because of the degree of facial trauma, mask inhalation was

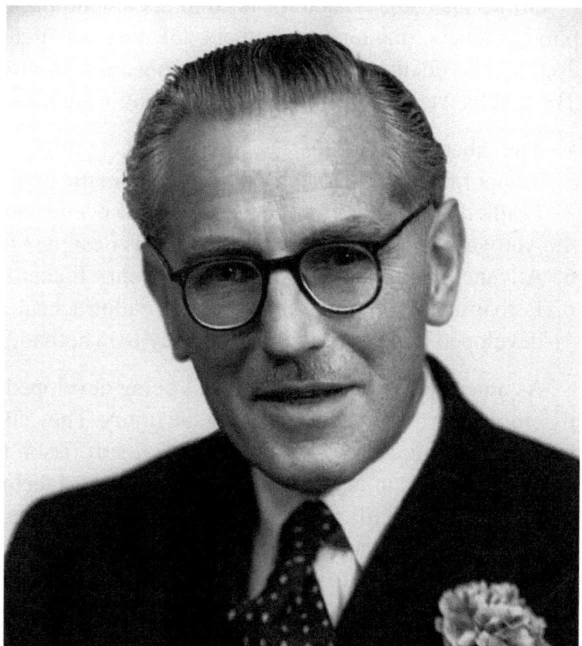

Fig. 7 Sir William Kelsey Fry. From national portrait gallery website https://www.npg.org.uk/collections/search/portrait/mw106643/Sir-William-Kelsey-Fry

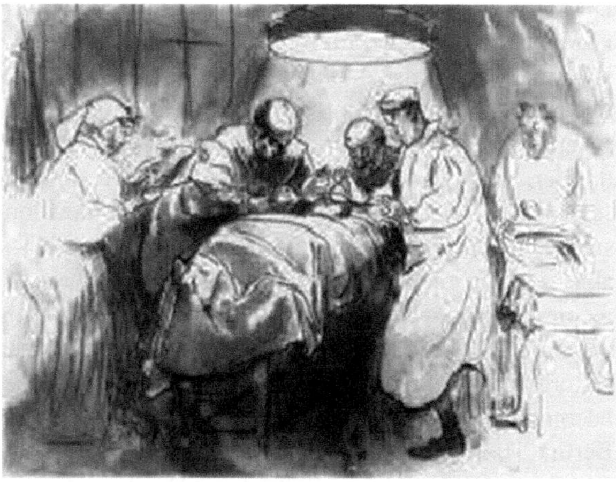

Fig. 8 Sketch by Henry Tonks of Gillies, Fry, and Magill at work in Sidcup

impossible. As such, Magill proposed using an endotracheal tube placed either through the nose, mouth, or neck out of the field of surgery. The first tube was designed by Magill and physically built by Fry in his dental laboratory in Sidcup. Needless to say, eventually, this anesthetic technique revolutionized the specialty. Fry spent his career as an academic, championed the naming and classification of the specialty of oral surgery in the United Kingdom, and ultimately helped establish the Faculty of Dentistry of the Royal College of Surgeons of England in 1947 (Anonymous 1966).

For all their efforts, Gillies and Fry (British citizens) received knighthoods, becoming Sir Harold Gillies and Sir William Kelsey Fry. Gillies went on to become known as the father of modern plastic surgery.

4 Maxillofacial Surgical Advances by the Central Powers

While the English language medical literature has detailed the exploits of Kazanjian, Gillies, and other maxillofacial surgeons of the Allied Forces, not as much has been written in English medical journals about the advances made by the German surgeons and other Central Power surgeons. However, significant and similar progress in the treatment of maxillofacial war injuries was attained by surgeons from the opposite side of the front line. In fact, some medical historians argue that many of Gillies's surgical advances were based on techniques originated by Central Power surgeons. There were two prominent centers of maxillofacial reconstructive surgery: Dusseldorf and Berlin. The prominent Central Power surgeons at these centers were Auguste Lindemann (1880–1970) (Dusseldorf), Jacques Joseph, and Johannes Esser in Berlin.

Lindemann was already a well-known facial surgeon prior to the Great War. In 1914, he founded the world's first hospital dedicated to facial surgery in

Dusseldorf—the Dusseldorf Hospital for the facially injured. During the Great War, Lindemann developed iliac crest grafting to reconstruct mandibles using wires for stabilization. He also published this work; Gillies noted that some of his reconstructive efforts were based on reading Lindemann's work. In 1916, Professor Jacques Joseph (1865–1934) was appointed to the Department of Facial Plastic Surgery at the Ear, Nose, and Throat Clinic of Charité Hospital in Berlin. Born in Prussia to a Jewish family, early in his medical career, he developed a love for facial aesthetic surgery, pioneering otoplasties and rhinoplasties. His soft tissue work was remarkable, and he meticulously documented his work. Worthy of note was Joseph's reconstruction of a Turkish soldier who had most of his midface lost to injury. Over the course of multiple soft tissue combined with dental prosthetic surgeries, Joseph restored this soldier's face (Fig. 9). After the war, Joseph focused on nasal surgery, becoming world famous in the rhinoplasty. He suddenly died in 1934 in his home in Berlin (Thomas et al. 2019).

Johannes Esser (1877–1946) was a Dutch reconstructive surgeon. Like Morestin, his landmark work in facial reconstruction is often overlooked. As a young man, Esser became the Dutch chess champion in 1903. He enrolled in medical school at the University of Leiden; his sister also attended the university's dental school. Esser managed to accompany his sister to her dental courses and thus trained simultaneously in medicine and dentistry. Following graduation, he became a country doctor but quickly found that his passion was in surgery of the face. Esser then went to Paris to study under French surgeons, including Morestin. At the start of the Great War, Esser offered his expertise to both the French and the British; neither accepted as he

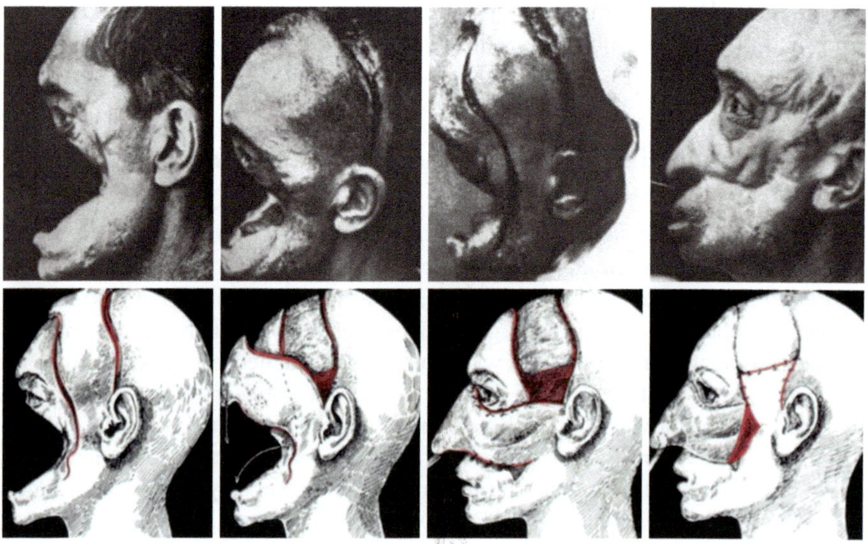

Fig. 9 Turkish lieutenant Mustafa Ipar, Joseph, Jacques. Nasenplastik und sonstige Gesichtsplastik: Nebst einem Anhang über Mammaplastik und einige weitere Operationen aus dem Gebiete der äußeren Körperplastik. Leipzig: Curt Kabitzsch, 1928–1931

was a Dutch citizen. He returned to Holland and began a facial plastic surgical practice. Esser then offered his services to the Austrian-Hungarian government, who accepted. He was posted to a hospital in the Czech Republic, where his surgical skills in facial flap surgery gained him notoriety. Esser later worked at the University of Vienna, and at the end of the war, he was given a 150-bed ward in Berlin to treat injured soldiers. From his war experience, Esser published his experience and gained significant celebrity in the European surgical community. One of his flaps, the epithelial inlay flap, was used frequently by Gillies, who called it the "Esser outlay." As World War II approached, he again offered his services to France but was once more turned down. Frustrated, Esser and his son decided to travel to the United States, hoping to establish a center for facial plastic surgery. Esser never was able to establish this center, though he did find a place in the medical community in Chicago to lecture (he was not allowed to practice medicine in the United States due to licensing restriction). Esser passed away at age 69 at his home in Chicago (Tolhurst 2015).

5 Anna Ladd and Jane Poupelet and Their Facial Masks

A synopsis of facial surgery during the Great War would not be complete without mention of two women who in their own nonsurgical way reconstructed the disfigured faces of soldiers from the front line: Anna Coleman Ladd and Jane Poupelet. Anna Ladd was born on July 15, 1878, in Bryn Mawr, Pennsylvania. She was born into a wealthy American family and grew up in Paris, France, until the age of 21. In 1900, Ladd moved to Rome to proceed in studies focused on art and sculpting. She married Maynard Ladd, a pediatric gastroenterologist.

Anna Ladd was introduced to the face masks by Lewis Hine, an English art critic. While visiting Ladd in Boston, Hine gave her an article written by British sculptor Derwent Wood. In the article, Wood explains the creation of the face masks used on soldiers who suffered from war-related disfigured faces. Due to the seriousness of the permanent facial injuries, many soldiers felt socially embarrassed—some even wished to die rather than face this agony. These masks allowed soldiers to return to a relatively normal life.

In 1917, Maynard Ladd went to France to work for the children's section of the American Red Cross. Anna Ladd of course followed him to Paris. She petitioned the American Red Cross to create a division that specialized in creating face masks. This would later become known as the Studio for Portrait Masks for Mutilated Soldiers in Paris in 1917. Ladd hired the French artist Jane Poupelet (1874–1932) as her assistant. Poupelet was born in 1874 in Dordogne, France. Prior to the war, she developed her skills in Paris. Due to the cultural and social limitations of nineteenth-century France which restricted the work of female artists, Poupelet often exhibited her work (usually female nude and farm animal sculptures) under the male pseudonym Simon de la Vergne. A patriotic French woman, she wanted to aid the injured French soldier; her meeting with Anna Coleman Ladd became the opportunity she desired.

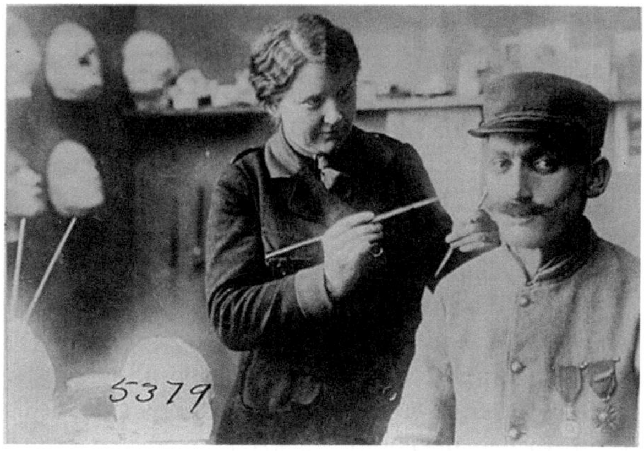

Fig. 10 Anna Coleman Ladd fitting a mask on a soldier with a mutilated face. (Library of Congress - https://www.loc.gov/pictures/resource/cph.3c37180/)

From 1917 to 1920, these women created 250 masks for soldiers. The process required several steps:

1. Moulage of disfigured soldiers' face
2. Modelling of the missing parts of the face based on pre-injury photography
3. Manufacturing a cooper prosthesis
4. Adjusting the prosthesis to the face
5. Painting the mask to appear human

Following the war, Ladd returned to Boston where she received much publicity for her work for the American Red Cross. Her masks would create new "trends" in this century by incorporating a new aspect of modernism into art and making an impact on looks in pop culture at this time. Poupelet remained in France but stopped sculpting, focusing on sketch art. Years later, they were both awarded the title of Knight of the French Legion of Honor (Room and Zacher 1982; Benmoussa et al. 2020; https://www.dailyartmagazine.com/jane-poupelet-bronze-paper-and-commitment-in-wwi/). Ladd passed away in 1939 and Poupelet in 1932 (Fig. 10).

6 Summary

Trench warfare combined with advances in ballistics created a never-before-seen number of mutilated faces requiring repair during the Great War. Ironically, horrific human conflict often leads to advances in medicine, dentistry, and surgery as a required response. The work of these surgeons made them legends as well as laid the foundation for what we as maxillofacial surgeons do today. What perhaps is most amazing is how these surgeons handled catastrophic trauma in the pre-antibiotic era.

References

Anonymous. Great teachers of surgery in the past. Sir William Kelsey Fry (1889-1963). Br J Surg. 1966;53(4):317–20.

Aziz SR. Harvard dental school and the fight for the ideals of democracy. J Oral Maxillofac Surg. 2001;59:428–33.

Bamji A. Sir Harold Gillies: Surgical Pioneer. Trauma. 2006;8:143–56.

Benmoussa N, Fanous A, Charlier P. Jane Poupelet: a woman artist devoted to the wounded soldiers from the First World War. J Stomatol Oral Maxillofac Surg. 2020;121:323–6.

Brigham F. Harvard goes to war. Harvard Dental Alumni Bull. 1964;24:100.

Converse JM. The extraordinary career of Dr Kazanjian. Plast Reconstr Surg. 1919;71:138.

Cruse WP. Auguste Charles Valadier: a Pioneer in maxillofacial surgery. Mil Med. 1987;152:7:37.

Cushman F. Work of Harvard Dental School graduates in France. Harvard Alumni Bull. 1916;28:614.

Gillies HD, Millard RD. The principles and art of plastic surgery. Boston: Little Brown; 1957. p. 6–15.

https://www.dailyartmagazine.com/jane-poupelet-bronze-paper-and-commitment-in-wwi/.

Kazanjian VH. The Department of Oral Surgery of the Harvard Surgical Unit. Br Med J. 1917;154:3.

Kazanjian VH. Observations on war surgery of the face and jaws. Dental Cosmos. 1920;62:283.

Lalardrie JP. Hippolyte Morestin 1869-1918. Br J Plast Surg. 1972;25:39–41.

Meikle MC. The evolution of plastic and maxillofacial surgery in the twentieth century: The Dunedin Connection. Surgeon. 2006;4:325–34.

Pickerill HP. The Queen's Hospital, Sidcup. Br J Plast Surg. 1954;6(4):247–9.

Room S, Zacher J. Anna Coleman Ladd: maker of masks for the facially mutilated. Plas Reconst Surg. 1982;70(1):104–11.

Thomas RL, Fries A, Hodgkinson D. Plastic surgery pioneers of the central powers in the great war. Craniomaxillofac Trauma Reconstr. 2019;12:1–7.

Tolhurst D. Pioneers in plastic surgery. Cham: Springer; 2015. p. 55–62.

Formation of Head and Neck Surgical Specialties

Gabriel M. Hayek and Michael T. Goupil

1 Introduction

The practice of surgery has a long history. The first known surgery dates back to 10,000 BCE, the New Stone Age. Skulls discovered in France in 1695 showed evidence of trephination. Considered to be the oldest surgical text, and perhaps the first book, is the Edwin Smith Papyrus (Fig. 1). These Egyptian writings date back to 1600 BCE and are believed to contain material older than that.

The first replacement of a nose, rhinoplasty, is described in the Hindu literature of the fifth century and may be considered to be the origin of otorhinolaryngology. Plastic surgery may trace its origins back to the Tsin dynasty (~266–470 BCE where a Chinese plastic surgeon treated harelip, sometimes known as cleft lip). The surgeons trained by Hippocrates were believed to treat disorders of the eyes, ears, nose, throat, and teeth. In addition, Hippocrates described immobilization methods for the treatment of jaw fractures (Bishop 1995).

The specialization in medicine can be traced back to the ancient Greek period. In 500 BCE, the Greek historian Herodotus described the specialization of Egyptian medicine: "Each physician limits himself to one area of disease. Some specialize in eyes, others in the head, teeth, the abdomen and its parts…" (Hoffman-Axthelm 1981).

Initially, head and neck surgical specialization was based on the interest and expertise of the surgeon in a regional anatomical area. Over time, specialties within these regional anatomical areas evolved, but with advances in medicine and resident

G. M. Hayek
Division of Oral and Maxillofacial Surgery, University of Connecticut, Farmington, CT, USA

M. T. Goupil (✉)
Division of Oral and Maxillofacial Surgery, University of Connecticut, Farmington, CT, USA

Consultant in Oral and Maxillofacial Surgery, Carmel, IN, USA

E. M. Ferneini et al. (eds.), *The History of Maxillofacial Surgery*,
https://doi.org/10.1007/978-3-030-89563-1_7

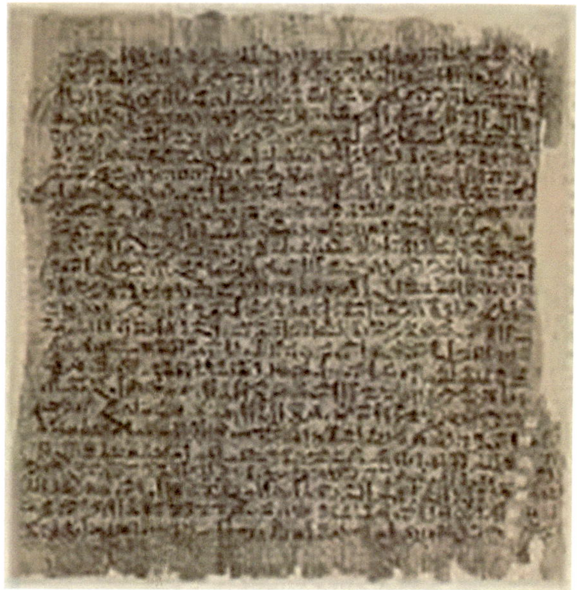

Fig. 1 Page from Edwin Smith surgical papyrus. Wellcome Library, London. (https://creativecommons.org/licenses/by/4.0/)

education, the lines of demarcation for these regional areas have blurred. This chapter will attempt to describe the evolution of the four primary surgical specialties of the facial region – otolaryngology (head and neck surgery), ophthalmology, oral and maxillofacial surgery, and plastics and reconstructive surgery.

2 Otolaryngology and Head and Neck Surgery

2.1 Birth of the Specialty

The terms otolaryngology, otorhinolaryngology, and ear, nose, and throat (ENT) surgery are the same specialty. The term used depends on geography and the target audience. The specialty developed in the early twentieth century when the separate fields of otology and laryngology were united (Weir 2000). Initially, otology was practiced by surgeons, whereas laryngology was practiced medically by clinicians.

One of the earliest physicians, the Egyptian Sekhet (~3500 BCE), appears to be the first rhinologist: "he cured the king's nostrils" (Helidonois 1993). The Edwin Smith Papyrus dating to 1600 BCE describes clinical surgery including trauma to the head and facial structures (Helidonois 1993). Similarly, the Eber's papyrus (~1500 BCE) contains a chapter on the hard of hearing including tinnitus and dizziness (Nogueira et al. 2007). The greatest in the Hindu literature for the specialty was the reconstruction of a new nose using cheek and forehead soft tissue flaps in the sixth century BC by Sushruta (Helidonois 1993).

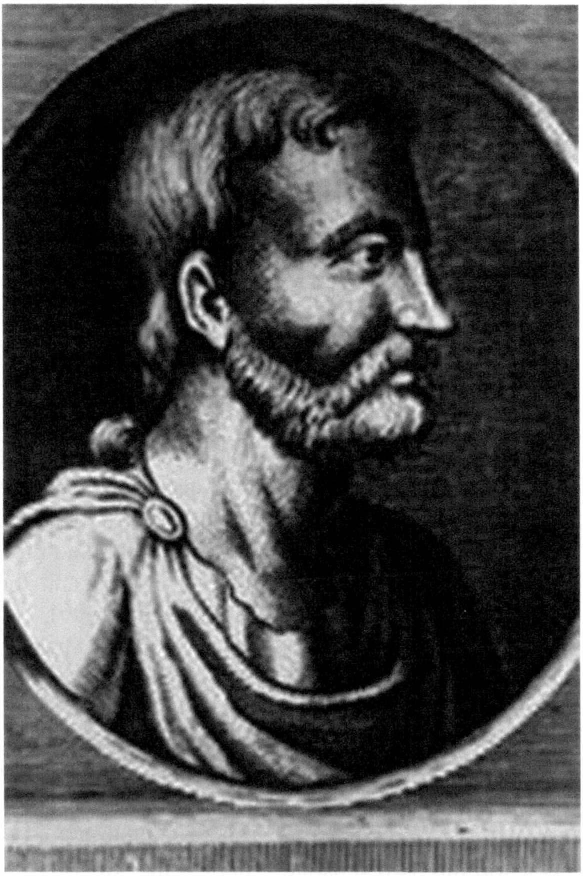

Fig. 2 Celsus, Aulus Cornelius, author (US National Library of Medicine, public domain)

The Byzantine Compiler, Paul of Aegina, among other things described the removal of tonsils using a hook and scalpel circa around 476 BCE (Helidonois 1993), though Celsus (Fig. 2), in the first century, was the first to describe a tonsillectomy using his fingers (Nogueira et al. 2007). Additionally, Celsus is often described as the first head and neck surgeon to describe the treatment of lip cancer with surgery, although this may have only been the treatment of a lacerated lip (Cantrell and Goldstein 1999).

The French surgeon Guy de Chauliac (1300–1367) contributed to the field of otology by creating the ear speculum to introduce "sunlight onto the external auditory meatus" to remove foreign bodies. He also treated quinsy by using an incision for drainage (Helidonois 1993). The father of modern otology was the physician Adam Politzer (1835–1920) who taught in Vienna. One of his students, Robert Barney (1876–1936), was the Nobel Prize winner for his work on the vestibular organ (Helidonois 1993).

The origins of laryngology are attributed to Manuel Garcia (1805–1906), a singing teacher who was able to view his own larynx with a mirror. More likely, this aspect of the specialty should be credited to Benjamin Babbington, a London physician who performed the first laryngoscopy using his "glottiscope" in 1829 (Weir 2000). One of the first larynx procedures is attributed to Alexander the Great (356–323 BCE). He saved the life of one of his soldiers by using the point of his spear to perform the first cricothyrotomy (Nogueira et al. 2007).

Significant advancements in the specialty of otolaryngology have been made throughout history by physicians, surgeons, and anatomists. This is one of the first specialties to perform procedures using local anesthesia and the first to perform surgery with microscopes and endoscopes (Nogueira et al. 2007).

2.2 *Organizations*

Medical history demonstrates that physicians that have a similar interest in a particular area form an association to share knowledge. With the development of the otoscope and the laryngoscope in the late 1850s, a number of physicians became interested in treating diseases of the ear, nose, and throat. This led to the formation of the American Otological Society in 1869 and the American Laryngological Association in 1879 (Cantrell and Goldstein 1999).

In 1896, Dr. Hal Foster, an otolaryngologist, invited colleagues to the first meeting of the Western Association of Ophthalmologists, Otologists, and Laryngologists. Noting that members were coming from all over the country, this organization became the American Academy of Ophthalmology and Otolaryngology (AAOO) in 1903. Four years later, with 434 members, it became the largest medical specialty society in America. As the academy grew larger, it became difficult to find a venue to hold the national meeting. This eventually led to a separation of the AAOO in 1979, forming two separate groups – the American Academy of Otolaryngology and the American Academy of Ophthalmology (www.aao-hns).

The name extension of head and neck was added to otolaryngology in 1978 to better define the changing scope of the specialty (Jackler and Mundry 2013). The American Academy of Otolaryngology-Head and Neck Surgery is now the largest organization in the world of specialists that treat the ear, nose, throat, and related structures (www.aao-hns).

A similar organization of ophthalmologists and otolaryngologists formed a section within the American Osteopathic Association. This became an independent organization in 1918 forming the American Osteopathic Society of Ophthalmology and Otolaryngology. This organization disbanded in 1944 and formed a coalition with the international society and is known as the Osteopathic College of Ophthalmology and Otorhinolaryngology. Like the AAO-HNS, the extension of head and neck surgery was added in 1995. They are now known as the American Osteopathic Colleges of Ophthalmology and Otolaryngology-Head and Neck Surgery (www.aocoohns.org). The main function of these organizations continues to be education, research, and adherence to high standards.

3 Ophthalmology

3.1 Birth of the Specialty

Similar to other specialties, ophthalmology has a long history dating back thousands of years. The earliest written records make note of the magical importance of the eye. This reference to the "evil eye" continues to the present day (Arrington and Marti-Ibanez 1959, p. 11). The earliest record of ocular therapeutics, including legal ramifications, "an eye for an eye," is found in the Code of Hammurabi (circa 1900 BCE) (Arrington and Marti-Ibanez 1959, p. 12, 13; Wheeler 1946).

The Indian surgeon Sushruta (800 BCE) predates Hippocrates and was considered the "father of Indian medicine." He dealt extensively with ocular anatomy and physiology. He described 76 ocular diseases. Many of his treatments were surgical in nature, and he is also considered to be the "father of cataract surgery" (Arrington and Marti-Ibanez 1959, p. 13, 14; Smith 2019). Herophilus (335 BC–280 BCE), a Greek physician, coined the term retina and gave the first description of the anatomy of the eye (Arrington and Marti-Ibanez 1959, p. 32).

Roger Bacon is credited with the use of lenses to assist old people with weak eyesight. In 1268, Bacon wrote on optics in general and specifically the use of lenses in his *Opus Magnus.* His lenses were used by placing them on the text to be read rather than worn as glasses (Wheeler 1946).

Georg Bartisch (1535–1607), a German physician considered to be the Father of Ophthalmology, started his medical education apprenticed to a barber-surgeon. He is given this title because he wrote the first textbook totally devoted to ophthalmology in 1583, *Ophthalmodouleia das ist Augendienss*, and he was the first surgeon to purposely remove an eye from a living patient. Bartisch gave the specialty its name. Bartisch's textbook was quickly followed by the first ophthalmology textbook in English, *Briefe Treatise Touching the Preservation of Eye Sight,* published by Walter Baily in 1584 (Arrington and Marti-Ibanez 1959, p. 84).

In 1803, the first formal course in ophthalmology was taught at the University of Göttingen (Tikkanen 2019). Following this in 1805, the Moorfield Eye Hospital was founded in London. This was the first institution dedicated to the practice and teaching of ophthalmology. It is home to the Institute of Ophthalmology, making it the largest eye hospital in the world (Smith 2019).

In 1851, Hermann Helmholtz published his paper describing his invention, the ophthalmoscope, making the clinical practice of ophthalmology a more exact science. The English physician Charles Babbage may actually have invented this device earlier, but unfortunately, he did not publish his work (Wheeler 1946).

3.2 Organizations

The professional organization of ophthalmology as noted above was started by the 1890s by the Kansas City ophthalmologist Hal Foster. Through his leadership, the American Academy of Ophthalmology and Otolaryngology (AAOO) was established in 1903. Due to size and logistical issues, the organization separated into two groups in 1979. The American Academy of Ophthalmology moved its headquarters to San Francisco. This academy is now the largest association of physician and surgeons dedicated to the treatment of the eye.

The American Board of Ophthalmic Examinations was formed in 1916 and, upon incorporation the following year, became the first medical specialty-certifying board in the United States (Cantrell and Goldstein 1999).

4 Oral and Maxillofacial Surgery

4.1 Birth of the Specialty

The earliest recorded history of what is now in the scope of oral and maxillofacial surgery dates to 2700 BCE Egypt, in which the Edwin Smith Papyrus details 48 cases treated by military surgeons (Laskin 2016; Tiwari et al. 2017). Among these include the treatment of mandible fractures with bandages soaked in honey and egg white, closing wounds with sutures, and the repair of broken noses. The written treatment of oral disease dates to 1200 BCE in ancient Greece. The treatments were administered in temples by priests called asclepiads who were followers of Asclepius, the Greek God of Medicine. Although these were largely herbal remedies, there is also evidence of tooth extraction.

In the fourth century BCE, Hippocrates (460–270 BCE) and Aristotle (384–322 BCE) wrote about tooth extractions (of loose teeth only) by applying substances to degrade the periodontal ligament, removing the crown, or cauterizing the pulp to stop pain, incision and drainage of abscesses, manual reduction of temporomandibular joint dislocation, and using wires across teeth to support mandible fractures.

After the fall of the Greek and Roman empires, the age of Islamic medicine would usher in the teachings of Rhazes (854–932), Albucasis (936–1013), and Avicenna (980–1037), who would detail more involving surgical procedures including the excision of oral fistulae, ranulas, epuli, frenula, thyroidectomies, and temporal artery division for the treatment of some headaches. They even recommended making incisions in the lines of skin creases, centuries before Langer would formally describe the principles of skin tension lines in 1861. Rhazes described removing teeth by loosening them with arsenic paste or the juice of boiled frogs.

The middle ages saw the separation of physicians, who formally studied medicine at universities, and surgeons, who continued to learn their trade by apprenticeship, until 1540 when the British Parliament reunited the two disciplines. The

Renaissance period would see the addition of more advanced tumor excision techniques and even gunshot wounds to the literature. Ambroise Paré (1510–1590), the Father of Surgery, treated broken jaws, excised tumors, discovered ligature to control bleeding, and improved the management of gunshot wounds by applying a mixture of egg yolk, rose water, and turpentine to the wounds, as opposed to removing bullets at all costs.

Pierre Fauchard (1678–1761), the Father of Modern Dentistry, published *The Surgeon Dentist in 1728*, a comprehensive text detailing the basic anatomy of the oral cavity and dental procedures including minor oral surgeries. Anselme Jourdain (1731–1816) would follow in 1778 with the first known oral surgery textbook, *A Treatise on the Diseases and Surgical Operations of the Mouth and Parts Adjacent*.

The name of the specialty is largely credited to James Garretson (1828–1895), whose 1869 book, *A Treatise on the Disease and Surgery of the Mouth, Jaws, and Associated Parts,* defined the scope of oral and maxillofacial surgery (Fig. 3). At this time, Garretson recommended that oral surgery be practiced by those with a medical degree only and suggested the removal of the DDS degree altogether. Most oral surgeons of the time had both degrees, though many of the biggest names – including Matthew Cryer (1840–1921), Truman Brophy (1848–1931), Thomas Gilmer (1848–1931), and Chalmers Lyons (1874–1935) – would align themselves with dental schools and strongly believed that oral surgery belonged to dentistry.

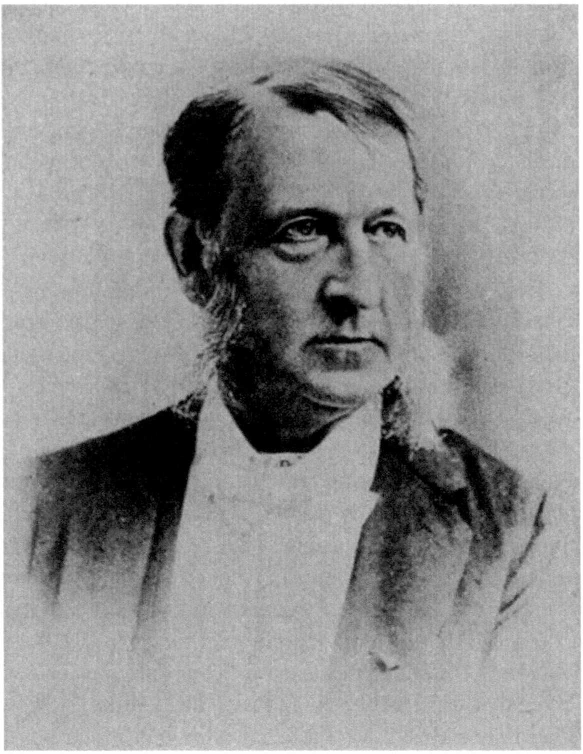

Fig. 3 Dr. James Edmund Garretson, before 1895 (History of Dental Surgery, volume 3, p. 396, public domain)

It was not until 1994 at the American Association of Oral and Maxillofacial Surgeons (AAOMS) House of Delegates meeting that the national association unanimously voted that oral and maxillofacial surgery would always remain a specialty of dentistry, and in 1997, the American Dental Association opted for a new definition of dentistry that included the full scope of the specialty (Lew 2013).

The founding of modern oral and maxillofacial surgery in North America dates to the mid-nineteenth century with the realization that deformities of the mouth and face were undertreated by the medical profession. Simon Hullihen (1810–1857), a physician with dental training from Wheeling, West Virginia, was the first to limit his professional endeavors to the face and mouth region. He would later become the first person to perform a successful mandibular osteotomy, foreshadowing the future of the field. In fact, in the last 10 years of his life, Hullihen performed 100 cleft lip and 50 cleft palate repairs, treated 100 tumors, did 200 procedures for maxillary sinus disease, and performed 85 reconstructions of the lips, nose, and mandible, a remarkable feat considering neither local nor general anesthesia yet existed.

Shortly thereafter, James Garretson would pioneer academic oral and maxillofacial surgery, introducing oral surgery as a core component of dental education at the Philadelphia Dental College, now Temple University School of Dentistry. He would become the first professor of oral surgery in the nation.

While the specialty of oral and maxillofacial surgery was being founded, America was finding itself drawn into World War I, and the two would be inextricably linked. As there was no dental corps at the time, dental officers worked closely with medical officers, treating war-ravaged facial injuries and using their dental backgrounds to help establish early principles of fracture stabilization and reconstruction with techniques for obturation, intermaxillary fixation, and prosthetic rehabilitation (Strother 2003). These techniques allowed an amazing two-thirds of wounded soldiers to return to the battlefield. These officers included prominent surgeons and founders of the modern specialty such as Robert Ivy (1881–1974), Carl Waldron (1887–1977), and Sir Kelsey Fry (1889–1963), a pioneer of British oral surgery (Lew 2013).

Before World War I, there were no formal training programs for the treatment of maxillofacial injuries; soldiers with extensive injuries often wore masks to hide their deformities (Strother 2003). The surgeon general appointed Vilray Blair (1871–1955), a general surgeon with extensive head and neck experience from Washington University in St. Louis, as the senior consultant for maxillofacial surgery. Blair named Robert Ivy, an oral surgeon from Philadelphia, as his assistant. World War I was dominated by trench warfare, resulting in an extraordinarily high percentage of wounds on the head and neck. Hospital units of "Plastic and Oral Surgery" were headed each by a team of one general surgeon and one dentist, after an intensive training course in reconstructive techniques based on the experiences of French and British surgeons including New Zealand–born Sir Harold Gillies (1882–1960) of Kent, Hippolyte Morestin (1869–1919) of Paris, and Auguste Valadier of Boulogne. These European surgeons had extensive experience in maxillofacial reconstruction already, as the United States entered the war much later. These specialized maxillofacial units had much better outcomes as they stressed immediate stabilization, early restoration of tissues and occlusion, and limited debridement. These principles of trauma would serve the specialty well in the future, as the rise of the automobile would see traumatic facial injuries become a common occurrence at home. In many regards, advancements in facial trauma continue to define the specialty today.

American oral surgery had proved its worth clinically; however, standardized formal residency training remained at large for many decades. Most residencies were 1-year clinical training programs served by part-time instructors (Lew 2013). In 1956, the 3-year training program began, in which an initial academic year was followed by 2 years of clinical training. Many of these programs, however, remained fragmented with training needing to be completed at multiple institutions. The 3-year integrated training program became standard in 1972. In 1988, the 4-year curriculum was implemented, which included a mandatory minimum of 12 months of core medical-surgical training designed to close the gaps between dental and medical education. Meanwhile, in Europe, the specialty often required a dual medical and dental background. Although a few modern oral surgeons had independently attended medical school, Walter Guralnick (1916–2017) of the Harvard/Massachusetts General Hospital program developed the dual-degree integrated residency training program in 1971 (Kaban and Perrott 2020). This included formal general surgery training, further bringing the specialty into mainstream medicine. Today, the dual-degree programs account for just under half of graduating residents. Nevertheless, controversy remains as evidenced by a review of editorials in the Journal of Oral and Maxillofacial Surgery (JOMS), and many have feared a schism in the specialty akin to many European countries who had already split into oral surgery and maxillofacial surgery (Lew 2013).

Surgeons in Germany and Austria were developing the field of corrective jaw surgery, later to be coined "orthognathic surgery." Previously, mandibular osteotomies had been described primarily for the treatment of mandibular prognathism or with transcervical approaches (Lew 2013; Bell 2018). Modern orthognathic arguably began with Hugo Obwegeser (1920–2017), the Father of European Maxillofacial Surgery, who published his intraoral bilateral sagittal split osteotomy technique in 1955 and later, in 1960, the modern LeFort I down fracture, ushering a new era of major maxillofacial surgery. In 1966, Obwegeser demonstrated his groundbreaking surgeries to a crowd of hundreds in Washington, DC. While European oral and maxillofacial surgeons were already performing dentofacial deformity correction and tumor surgery, Obwegeser would awaken the American specialty at a time when many were questioning the value of the specialty given the competition between competing specialties and a declining need for dentoalveolar surgical services.

In 1975, William Bell (1927–2016) published his landmark study on the vascularity of the maxilla, thereby demonstrating the biologic basis of orthognathic surgery. Landmark advances to treatment planning were made by Timothy Turvey and orthodontist William Proffit at the University of North Carolina at Chapel Hill, as they defined rationale and outcomes for orthognathic surgery in the 1990s. The 2000s and 2010s would see the development of virtual surgical planning, custom plates, and navigation, allowing for more precise and accurate outcomes to these complex operations (see chapter Orthognathic Surgery).

Surgery of the temporomandibular joint was long performed primarily to manage patients with ankylosis and to reconstruct mandibular form and function after ablative tumor surgery, trauma, or degenerative arthritic disease. Bruce MacIntosh of Detroit, Michigan, and Leonard Kaban of Boston, Massachusetts, had developed and clinically proven the reconstruction algorithms for costochondral rib grafts (Lew 2013). In 1963, Christenson introduced the Vitallium fossa-eminence prosthesis, and this was further improved with stock TMJ replacement devices developed by Louis Mercuri and Peter Quinn. As with many other aspects of modern surgery, computer planning now allows for custom temporomandibular joint replacements. Nonetheless, temporomandibular joint surgery developed a poor reputation with few practical uses for long-term success. The 1980s and 1990s saw the development of arthrocentesis and arthroscopy, resulting not only in minimally invasive surgical options but a much-improved understanding of articular diseases and refinement in the role of surgery.

In 1982, one of the single most influential conferences in the history of dentistry took place in Toronto, Canada. This Conference on Osseointegration in Clinical Dentistry, led by Professor Per-Ingvar Brånemark (1929–2014), would introduce modern dental implantology to North America (see chapter Dental Implants and Bone Augmentation) (Lew 2013; Block 2018). Implants were initially used for edentulous jaws but, by 1991, were being used for single tooth replacement. The field of dental implantology, however, had its origins dating back much further than this. There is evidence of implants to replace teeth as far back as Ancient Egyptian and South American civilizations. In 1938, the first long-term endosseous implant was placed by Dr. Alvin Strock (1911–1996), still in place when the patient died in 1955. Numerous iterations of the dental implant – including subperiosteal, blade endosseous, and transosteal subtypes – would follow before Brånemark's revolutionary osseointegrated titanium implant. Brånemark would begin training periodontists in the late 1980s. Before this, only oral and maxillofacial surgeons were allowed into his training courses. Implant treatment has exploded since this time with enormous technological advancements in hard and soft tissue grafting for site development, implant design, and preoperative planning.

In 1986, AAOMS sponsored a landmark conference on expanding the scope of the specialty, necessitated by the blurring of the lines of the dental specialties (Lew 2013). The potential for dental implantology to be the boon the specialty was looking for had not yet been recognized. Recommendations included enhancement in training for resident oral and maxillofacial surgeons in three distinct areas: tumor and reconstructive surgery, cleft and craniofacial surgery, and facial esthetic surgery. This has largely been met with mixed results over the last 30 years, with these disciplines being unevenly taught and performed among residency training programs and the constant legal battle to perform the full scope of the specialty being fought by organized medicine.

Among the earliest pioneers in expanded scope surgery were the tumor and reconstructive surgery fellowships with Robert Marx at Jackson Memorial Hospital, the University of Michigan led by Joseph Hellman, the University of Maryland with Robert Ord, and Legacy Emanuel Hospital in Portland, Oregon, with Dr. Bryce Potter and Eric Dierks who were dual-trained in otolaryngology (Carlson 2018). Surgeons such as R. V. Walker (1924–2011), Timothy Turvey, Douglas Sinn, Roger West, and Larry Wolford had pioneered craniofacial surgery within the specialty (Ricalde and Turvey 2018). Joseph Murray (1919–2012), a plastic surgeon at Boston Children's Hospital considered the Father of American Craniofacial Surgery, saw the need to bridge medical and dental education to achieve the full benefits of craniofacial surgery. He recruited Leonard Kaban in 1975, who is believed to be the first oral and maxillofacial surgeon to exclusively work for a children's hospital. Murray would also have a significant influence on Jeffrey Posnick, a dual-trained oral and maxillofacial and plastic and reconstructive surgeon who would develop the first full-scope craniofacial fellowship for oral and maxillofacial surgery graduates. Nonetheless, cleft lip and palate procedures have not enjoyed the same success as oncologic procedures, largely attributed to the efforts from plastic and reconstructive surgeons, who head the vast majority of the approximately 200 cleft repair teams in the United States.

Despite the difficulties, numerous fellowships have developed, which are thriving and giving new hope to what the future may hold. By 2020, there were at least 15 oncologic and reconstructive surgery fellowships and nine cleft and craniofacial surgery fellowships formally available to graduating oral and maxillofacial surgery residents (Lew 2013). The year 2011 would see the development of a formal section of oral and maxillofacial surgery within the American College of Surgeons, further recognizing the specialty's key role within the healthcare system. In 2020, the first AAOMS conference entirely dedicated to oral/head and neck oncologic and microvascular reconstructive surgery was held. By 2020, the American Board of Oral and Maxillofacial Surgery (ABOMS) was offering certificates of qualifications (CAQs) to its qualified members in these two disciplines. Cosmetic surgery of the face has also enjoyed success within the field, with over 700 AAOMS members now performing facial esthetic surgeries in their practices.

4.2 *Organizations*

The first formal residency training programs were developed at Cincinnati General Hospital in 1907 and the University of Michigan beginning in 1917. It wasn't until 1947 that the first accredited residency program in oral and maxillofacial surgery was recognized at the Pittsburgh Veterans Administration Hospital.

Dentistry's only surgical specialty would solidify its standing in 1918 with the founding of the American Association of Exodontists, when Menifee Howard (1882–1958) contacted other exodontists about the need to formally organize. At the time, its membership consisted of only 29 members (Lew 2013). One year later in 1919, the National Dental Association, now the American Dental Association (ADA), would formally recognize the specialty. In 1921, the name changed to the

American Society of Oral Surgeons and Exodontists (ASOSE), further differentiating themselves from dentists without formal specialization and more accurately reflecting the interests of the membership. In 1946, the specialty would again change its name to the American Society of Oral Surgeons (ASOS), before adopting the current nomenclature, the American Association of Oral and Maxillofacial Surgeons (AAOMS), in 1978.

5 Plastic and Reconstructive Surgery

5.1 Birth of the Specialty

The early history of plastic and reconstructive surgery as it applies to the head and neck is largely the same as oral and maxillofacial surgery. The Edwin Smith Papyrus discusses the treatment of nasal fractures via simple nasal manipulation and stabilization, closing wounds with sutures, and using raw meat to stop bleeding (Laskin 2016; Tiwari et al. 2017; Goldweyn 2008; Lawrence 2016; Singh et al. 2015; Whitaker et al. 2007). The first reconstructive surgery described dates to 600 BCE India when Sushruta described nasal reconstruction from pedicled forehead tissue. Gaspare Tagliacozzi (1545–1599) in 1597 Italy described nasal reconstruction with tissue from the forearm akin to later described tube flaps. His 1597 text *On the Surgical Restoration of Defects by Grafting* is considered the first plastic surgery book.

The historical association between oral and plastic surgery is significant. The impact of war paradoxically led to both the separation and development of the two specialties while also acting as a catalyst for cooperation and progress (Whitaker et al. 2007). After the war, surgeons focusing on post-traumatic reconstruction made their work by refining and progressing on previously never-seen-before techniques (Strother 2003). Among these included Armenian-American Varaztad Kazanjian (1879–1974) and New Zealand-born otolaryngologist Sir Harold Gillies (1882–1960), each with significant claim to the title of the Father of Modern Plastic Surgery, as well as Vilray Blair. Gillies would lay the groundwork for many craniofacial reconstructive techniques and made revolutionary discoveries in skin grafting (see chapter Surgical Flaps).

Treatment of cleft lip and palate has long been an interest in plastic and reconstructive surgery. For most of recorded history, children with congenital deformities were considered to be affected by evil spirits and often ignored or killed (Bill et al. 2006; Bhattacharya et al. 2009). The first known cleft repair was not performed until the fourth century in China on future governor-general Wei Yang-Chi. From the early fourteenth to the nineteenth century, the surgical procedure went largely unchanged, performed in cheilorrhaphy fashion, as described by Flemish surgeon Jean Yperman, with a looped suture called the sutura circumvoluta. Repair techniques finally made an advancement in 1844 when they transitioned to a cheiloplasty, as described by Joseph-François Malgaigne (1806–1865) and Germanicus Mirault (1796–1870). The modern principle of a geometric cutting procedure was first described by Werner Hagedorn (1831–1894) in 1884. This technique would be further refined by Veau (1938), LeMesurier (1949), Tennison (1952), Millard (1958), Randall (1959), and Pfeifer (1970). The first documented surgical treatment of cleft palate, meanwhile, was not until 1817, as documented by Karl Ferdinand Graefe (1787–1840). The modern concept of a morphological layered closure was first brought forth by Bernhard von Langenbeck (1810–1887) in 1861 and advanced by Victor Veau (1871–1949) in 1931.

Bone grafting was first described in the early 1600s by Dutch surgeon Job Van Meekeren (1611–1666), who attempted a cranioplasty with bone from a dog (Ricalde and Turvey 2018). The first autogenous bone graft was performed in 1821. Bone graft science began to develop with the description of creeping substitution by Barth in 1893 and a case series on bone graft healing in 1907 by Axhausen and Phemister. The modern history of craniofacial surgery starts with French oral surgeon Charles Valadier (1873–1901) who directly trained otolaryngologist Sir Harold Gillies and inspired his future work, including the first LeFort III osteotomy, though this failed after significant relapse. Afterward, Gillies reportedly told his trainees, “Never do that operation” (Wolfe 2011). Paul Tessier would awaken the world with his 1967 presentation in Rome on the successful LeFort III osteotomy, now stabilized with bone grafts, demonstrating that the quality of life for those with severe facial disfigurements could be significantly improved. Before Tessier, it was thought that the risk of infection and injury to the eyes and brain was much too high. Plastic surgeons from all over the world flocked to Paris to learn from him, as he became the Father of Craniofacial Surgery.

Cosmetic surgery of the face has been one of the most successful arenas for the plastic surgeon, although at the inception of organized plastic and reconstructive surgery, this subspecialty was looked down upon (Haiavy 2018). Cosmetic surgery has been practiced in some form since at least 2500 BCE when skin rejuvenation and hair growth techniques were documented in Egyptian papyrus texts. Elective cosmetic surgery was first discussed in the late nineteenth and early twentieth centuries with the development of general anesthesia.

The first publications in cosmetic surgery included Johann Friedrich Dieffenbach’s (1792–1847) 1845 text on rhinoplasty and Robert Talbott Ely’s (1850–1885) 1881 publication on otoplasty. Jacques Joseph (1865–1934) presented his techniques on rhinoplasty in 1898 in Berlin. Although an orthopedic surgeon by training, he is considered the father of modern rhinoplasty and is probably the first surgeon to dedicate their career to cosmetic surgery (see chapter Facial Cosmetic Surgery).

Today, the most common cosmetic procedure is injectables (see chapter Minimally Invasive Cosmetic Procedures). The first noted history of fillers was in the 1890s with the use of paraffin injections. The original use was for testicular enlargement after tuberculosis infection. The decades leading to today have been filled with debate on whether cosmetic surgery belongs to plastic surgery or should be its own discipline. In 1985, the American Academy of Cosmetic Surgery (AACS) was founded by combining multiple previous organizations and was headed by the Father of American Cosmetic Surgery, Richard Webster. Dr. Webster, of Brookline, Massachusetts, completed his formal training with Dr. Kazanjian in Boston. He would eventually limit his practice to cosmetic surgery and was the principal negotiator in the amalgamation of the various cosmetic surgery organizations as he believed that plastic surgery did not equate to cosmetic surgery and that all knowledge must be shared. The pure number and types of cosmetic surgery procedures have exploded over the last half a century. Cosmetic surgery is now practiced by members of all head and neck specialties, and fellowships dedicated to cosmetic surgery continue to grow in number.

The culmination of plastic and reconstructive surgery of the head and neck was achieved in 2005 with the first successful partial face transplantation in Amiens, France (Rifkin et al. 2018). As it often does, history repeated itself with the fields of plastic and reconstructive surgery and oral and maxillofacial surgery intertwined to complete this most complex of operations. A new era of reconstructive surgery had arrived, offering new possibilities for the repair of severe disfigurements. By April 2006, the first complete facial transplantation was completed in Xi'an, the capital of Shaanxi province in China. Approximately 50 partial and complete face transplants have now been performed worldwide as advances in allograft design, computerized planning, surgical technique, and postoperative revision are helping to push the boundaries.

5.2 *Organizations*

Kazanjian, an American dentist so instrumental in the war that he was known as the "Miracle Man of the Western Front," returned to Boston as professor of oral surgery (Strother 2003). Oral surgery, however, at the time, was just beginning its own history. Kazanjian would return to medical school and by 1941 was named the first professor of plastic surgery at Harvard University. St. Louis native Vilray Blair returned from the war to establish a multidisciplinary team at Walter Reed Hospital in Washington, DC, dedicated to the reconstruction of head and neck war injuries. He was instrumental to the creation of plastic surgery as a separate specialty and would eventually become the first non-oral surgeon elected to the American Association of Plastic Surgeons and later a founder of the American Board of Plastic Surgery in 1938. His assistant Robert Ivy who was dual-trained in medicine and dentistry would form the first multidisciplinary team for the treatment of cleft lip and palate in North America. He would remain active in professional organizations of both plastic and oral surgery throughout his career.

From war to peacetime, the field flourished by applying techniques to own not just an anatomical area, like the other head and neck specialties, but to become experts in reconstructive techniques throughout the body (Poswillo 1977). Although the earliest idea for a society of plastic surgeons appears to be brought forth in 1914 by William Shearer of Nebraska, the society known at the time as the American

Association of Oral Surgeons (AAOS) was not formed until 1921 (Goldweyn 2008; Lawrence 2016; Singh et al. 2015; Whitaker et al. 2007). Young surgeons returning from World War I realized that the "unknown and impossible" reconstructive surgeries they were performing were not part of any known specialty.

The AAOS was formally organized by Truman Brophy (1848–1928), Henry Sage Dunning (1880–1957), and Frederick Morehead. Membership was limited to those with both medical and dental degrees; even Vilray Blair with his single medical degree was allowed only associate membership. In 1923, the dual-degree requirement was dropped, though membership remained exclusive, and it would take years before the society changed its name to the American Association of Oral and Plastic Surgeons. In 1942, the society adopted its current name – American Association of Plastic Surgeons.

Meanwhile, in 1931, Jacques Malinac, shunned by the American Association of Oral Surgeons, and based on the idea by Gustave Aufricht of New York City, founded the Society of Plastic and Reconstructive Surgery for all those "engaged in the ethical practice of reconstructive surgery." The name changed to the American Society of Plastic and Reconstructive Surgeons in 1944, and the field of plastic surgery remains with two major societies today.

6 Summary

The foundations of today's head and neck specialties stem from the earliest practice of medicine in India, Asia, Greece, and Rome. Significant contributions have been made by the likes of the anatomists Vesalius and De Vinci. Innovations and substantial contributions have been made by countless physicians from around the world throughout the ages. There are too many of these figures to mention in this short chapter.

The head and neck surgical specialties are primarily based on regional anatomy with significant overlap. Surgeons of similar interests have banded together into specialty organizations. These specialty organizations have similar goals: provide a forum for the exchange of ideas, education for current and future providers, research to improve diagnostics and treatments within the specialty, and the setting of high ethical standards to protect the interests of the patients they serve.

References

Arrington GE, Marti-Ibanez F. A history of ophthalmology. 1st ed. New York: MD Publications; 1959.

Bell RB. A history of orthognathic surgery in North America. J Oral Maxillofac Surg. 2018;76:2466–81.

Bhattacharya S, Khanna V, Kohli R. Cleft lip: the historical perspective. Indian J Plast Surg. 2009;42(Suppl):S4–8.

Bill J, Proff P, Bayerlein T, Weingaertner J, Fanghanel J. Treatment of patients with cleft lip, alveolus, and palate - a short outline of history and current interdisciplinary treatment approaches. J Cranio-Maxillofac Surg. 2006;34:17–21.

Bishop WJ. The early history of surgery. New York: Barnes and Noble; 1995. pages 20, 38, 41, and 50.

Block M. Dental implants: the last 100 years. J Oral Maxillofac Surg. 2018;76:11–26.

Cantrell RW, Goldstein JC. The American Board of Otolaryngology, 1924-1999. Arch Otolaryngol Head Neck Surg. 1999;125(10):1071–9.

Carlson E. Oral/head and neck oncologic and reconstructive surgery: the creation of a subspecialty in oral and maxillofacial surgery. J Oral Maxillofac Surg. 2018;76:237–47.

Goldweyn R. The early history of plastic and reconstructive surgery. Plast Reconstr Surg. 2008;121(4):1489–98.

Haiavy J. Cosmetic surgery history of the specialty: the importance of AACS fellowships and the Webster legacy. Am J Cosmetic Surg. 2018;35(2):64–73.

Helidonois ES. The history of otolaryngology from ancient to modern times. Am J Otolaryngol. 1993;14(6):382–3.

Hoffman-Axthelm W. History of dentistry. Chicago: Quintessence Publishing Co. Inc; 1981. p. 19.

Jackler RK, Mundry A. Otolaryngology: "It's all Greek to me". 2013. https://doi.org/10.1177/0194599813514366.

Kaban L, Perrott D. Dual-degree Oral and Maxillofacial Surgery Training in the United States: "Back to the Future". J Oral Maxillofac Surg. 2020;78:18–28.

Laskin D. Oral and maxillofacial surgery: the mystery behind the history. J Oral Maxillofac Surg Med Pathol. 2016;28:101–4.

Lawrence WT. The American Association of Plastic Surgeons recent history, with a review of the past. Plast Reconstr Surg. 2016;138(1):288–96.

Lew D. A historical overview of AAOMS. American Association of Oral and Maxillofacial Surgeons; 2013.

Nogueira JF Jr, et al. A brief history of otorhinolaryngology: otology, laryngology and rhinology. Braz J Otorhinolaryngol. 2007;73(5):693–703.

Poswillo D. The relationship between oral and plastic surgery. Br J Plast Surg. 1977;30:74–80.

Ricalde P, Turvey T. History of craniofacial surgery in the United States: the role of the oral and maxillofacial surgeon. J Oral Maxillofac Surg. 2018;76:1842–6.

Rifkin W, David J, Plana N, Kantar R, Diaz-Siso JR, Gelb B, Ceradini D, Rodriguez E. Achievements and challenges in facial transplantation. Ann Surg. 2018;268(2):260–70.

Singh M, Noone RB, Afolabi H, Caterson E. A tribute to the founding figures of the American board of plastic surgery. Plast Reconstr Surg. 2015;135(6):1047–54.

Smith Y. History of ophthalmology. 2019. https://www.news-medical/health/History-of-Ophthalmology.aspx.

Strother E. Maxillofacial surgery in World War I: the role of the dentists and surgeons. J Oral Maxillofac Surg. 2003;61:943–50.

Tikkanen A. Ophthalmology, Encyclopedia Britannica. 2019. https://britannica.com/sciemce/ophthalmology.

Tiwari R, Pendyala C, Gurukarthik G, Bhattacharjee A. History of oral and maxillofacial surgery - a review. J Dental Med Sci. 2017;16(3):99–102.

Weir N. Otorhinolaryngology. Postgrad Med J. 2000;76:65–9.

Wheeler JR. History of ophthalmology through the ages. Br J Ophthalmol. 1946;30(5):264–75.

Whitaker I, Karoo R, Spyrou G, Fenton O. The birth of plastic surgery: the story of nasal reconstruction from the Edwin Smith papyrus to the twenty-first century. Plast Reconstr Surg. 2007;120(1):327–36.

Wolfe SA. A man from Heric: The life and world of Paul Tessier, MD, father of craniofacial surgery, vol. 1. S. A. Wolfe; 2011. p. 79.

www.aao-hns.

www.aocoohns.org.

Part II
Conventional Procedures

Head and Neck Infections

Justin Fazzolari, Bridget Ferguson, and Sidney B. Eisig

1 Prehistory

To understand the history of maxillofacial infections, we will begin by examining their impact on humans over time. Early human experience with maxillofacial infections may not have mirrored our own modern experiences. Fortunately for us, the fossil record is incredibly useful for this purpose, and abundant, well-preserved skulls from various eras and geographic locations tell a story of how these infections played out.

Teeth number among the hardest tissues in the human body. Furthermore, they tend to remain embedded in alveolar bone long after a person's death. The fossil record unsurprisingly offers a measure of an individual's dental health and snapshot of chronic or acute maxillofacial infections present at the time of death.

The earliest record of periapical abscesses dates back to two million years BCE, found in an individual from our own genus, *Homo*. In this individual, abscesses originating directly from the apices of multiple incisors point toward the presence of significant odontogenic infection rather than systemic osteolytic disease. It has been suggested that the severity, number, and unhealed state of the infections may indicate they contributed to the individual's death (Towle and Irish 2019).

While definitive evidence for maxillofacial infections in our most ancient ancestors certainly exists, it is important to note the relative scarcity of dental pathology in the oldest fossils. Caries rates as low as 3% have been noted in populations of early hominids (Grine et al. 1990). Rates of caries varied across time and location even within a single species, suggesting behavior and dietary habits played a key

J. Fazzolari · B. Ferguson · S. B. Eisig (✉)
Oral and Maxillofacial Surgery, Columbia University Irving Medical Center, New York, NY, USA
e-mail: Jf3252@cumc.columbia.edu; Bf2310@cumc.columbia.edu; Sbe2002@cumc.columbia.edu

E. M. Ferneini et al. (eds.), *The History of Maxillofacial Surgery*,
https://doi.org/10.1007/978-3-030-89563-1_8

role in rates of odontogenic infection (Nicklisch et al. 2016). There is one thing all our predecessors have in common, however: significantly lower caries rates than modern humans.

A look at our closest surviving relatives, apes, reveals a different cause for most maxillofacial infections: severe attrition and trauma leading to tooth fractures and pulp exposures (Legge 2012). This is borne out by examining fossils from humans just prior to the agricultural revolution, wherein high rates of attrition are thought to have obliterated carious lesions as they formed, lessening their impact (Lieverse et al. 2007).

Additionally, pulpal exposure by gradual attrition was less likely to lead to the severe periapical abscesses that we are accustomed to seeing today. It has been posited that the "abscesses" recorded in many of our ancestors' maxillae and mandibles may actually represent more benign lesions: "Such periapical granulomata and apical periodontal cysts, with far less serious implications for the health of the individuals. Individuals with multiple periapical cavities … were not, therefore, necessarily ill" (Dias and Tayles 1997).

The most significant historical development in terms of maxillofacial infections is undeniably the agricultural revolution. Changes in our diet and food preparation techniques ushered in previously unseen levels of dental decay and associated infections (Eshed et al. 2006). Modern humans, in fact, appear to suffer from the highest rates of dental caries compared to all populations throughout history. Caries has eclipsed attrition and trauma as the #1 cause of odontogenic infections, which have implications for detection, diagnosis, and management (Stránská 2013).

This transition from high rates of attrition to low rates of caries in prehistory to the high caries rates of modernity sets the stage for our modern understanding of odontogenic infection and head and neck infections. This understanding has been characterized by severe, fulminant infectious illness from caries-induced abscesses, with acute loss of bone and potentially lethal spread into various deep spaces of the head and neck. The shift toward this mechanism of disease would dictate both our understanding of maxillofacial infections and our treatment of them over the course of history.

2 Treatment of Infection in Antiquity

Introduction: Throughout most of human history, limited medical knowledge meant that few effective treatments were available to those suffering from disease. As nomadic hunter-gatherers began to develop permanent, agriculture-based settlements, technology advanced and written language began to emerge. Before long, the origins of medical and surgical treatment started to take hold in increasingly specialized societies. Many of the advances and beliefs that were written down survive to today, providing a glimpse into the knowledge base and treatments of ancient peoples.

Ancient Egypt: Some of the earliest known writings pertaining to the treatment of maxillofacial infections can be traced back to ancient Egypt, a civilization at its peak from approximately 3000 BCE–1000 BCE. Our knowledge of the ancient Egyptians is sourced from translations of original medical accounts from papyrus, wood carvings, and inscriptions on tombs and monuments (Figs. 1 and 2). Much of this information is quite specific and rich in detail, with formal titles for medical professionals such as surgeons and dentists referenced in original texts (Forshaw 2009).

Despite a plethora of information about ancient Egyptian medical practices, evidence is sorely lacking to support the surgical treatment of maxillofacial infections or even simple tooth extractions. Some scholars go so far as to "strongly reject" that dental surgery or abscess drainage was routinely performed (Blomstedt 2013). No instruments for dentoalveolar surgery have ever been discovered (Forshaw 2009) (unlike for many other cultures), and human remains consistently demonstrate periodontally involved teeth that could easily have been extracted but were not (Miller and Fields 2009).

Instead, it appears that treatment of odontogenic infections mainly involved applying pastes and masticatories directly to the painful site—treatment of a medical rather than surgical nature (Guerini 1909). Some of these treatments may have had mild analgesic effects, but the actual efficacy of these medicaments is highly dubious. A number of complex recipes have survived until modern times, seen above. Despite being so advanced for an early culture, it appears very little was done for maxillofacial infections in ancient Egypt, with maxillofacial surgery a rarity.

Greece and Rome: Following the relative decline of Egyptian power, ancient Greek culture rose to prominence in the Mediterranean and began making its own contributions to medical and surgical understanding. A number of influential Greek physicians laid the groundwork for the expansion of formal medical education and training in prosperous regions.

Surviving texts indicate that the Greeks respected ancient Egyptian medicine, although it is difficult to determine precisely which Greek practices derived from Egyptian methods. Greek medicine originated with a heavy focus on mysticism, which oftentimes implicated divine intervention in sickness and in health. This framework evolved over time into more rational, cause-and-effect style reasoning,

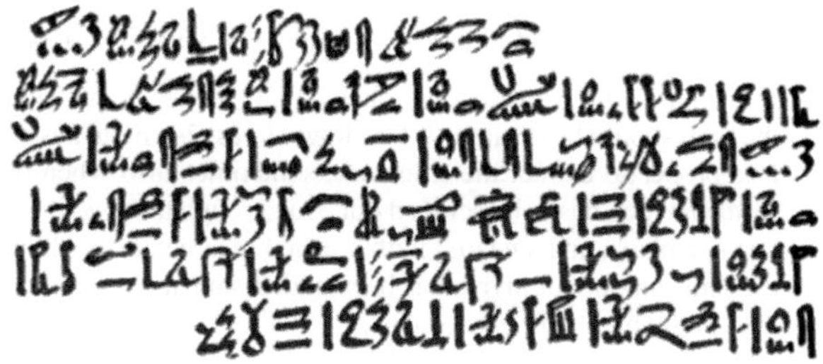

Fig. 1 Egyptian hieroglyphs on papyrus detailing a recipe for medical treatment of odontogenic infection (Guerini 1909)

Fig. 2 English translation of Egyptian recipe for medication to treat odontogenic infection (Guerini 1909)

"Cow's milk	Part 1
Fresh dates	" 1
Uah corn	" 1

To be left stand and then to be masticated nine times."

This is the second receipt:

"Anest-plant	Part 1
Dough	" 1
Green lead	" 1
Sebests[2]	" 1
Cake	" 1
Dâm-plant	" 1
Fennel seeds	" 1
Olive oil	" 1
Water	" 1

To be used like the preceding one."

even if this was dominated by beliefs about balances and imbalances of "humors" we consider erroneous today. Roman medicine largely carried on and advanced the medical theory of Greece, so we will discuss these two cultures together.

The Greeks and Romans, like the peoples before them, placed a heavy emphasis on the application of medicaments in the forms of pastes, poultices, and masticatories with regard to the oral and maxillofacial region. One of the most significant departures from previous eras, however, is the emergence of surgery as a legitimate treatment option.

The work of Aulus Celsus (n.d.-a, n.d.-b), a Roman encyclopedist in the first century, represents one of the most complete primary sources of medical knowledge in Roman times. Entire paragraphs dedicated to the medical and surgical treatment of maxillofacial infections can be found in his compilation *De Medicina.* These passages demonstrate the understanding in Rome that proper treatment may require both medical and surgical interventions. We will quote three of these segments at length:

> In the mouth too some conditions are treated by surgery. In the first place, teeth sometimes become loose, either from weakness of the roots, or from disease drying up the gums. In either case the cautery should be applied so as to touch the gums lightly without pressure. The gums so cauterized are smeared with honey and swilled with honey wine. When the ulcerations have begun to clean, dry medicaments, acting as repressants, are dusted on. But if a tooth gives pain and it is decided to extract it because medicaments afford no relief, the tooth should be scraped round in order that the gum may become separated from it; then the tooth is to be shaken. This is to be done until it is quite moveable: for it is very dangerous to extract a tooth that is tight, and sometimes the jaw is dislocated. With the upper teeth there is even greater danger, for the temples or eyes may be concussed. Then the tooth is to be extracted, by hand, if possible, failing that with the forceps. (Celsus n.d.-a)

> But a hot poultice made of flour and a fig is then to be put on until pus is formed there: then the gum should be cut into. A free flow of pus also indicates a fragment of bone; so then too it is proper to extract the fragment; sometimes also when the bone is injured a fistula is formed which has to be scraped out. But a rough tooth is to be scraped in the part which has become black, and smeared with crushed rose-petals to which a fourth part of ox-galls and the same amount of myrrh has been added; and at frequent intervals undiluted wine is to be held in the mouth. (Celsus n.d.-a)

> Should suppuration show itself, it will be necessary to use the above mentioned steam for a longer period; to keep in the mouth hot mulse, in which some figs have been cooked, and to lance the tumor before it is perfectly ripe, so that the pus may not, by remaining too long in the diseased part, injure the bone. But if the tumor be of great size, it will be more advisable to remove it entirely, so that the tooth remain free on both sides. After the pus has been extracted, if the wound be a small one, it is sufficient to keep hot water in the mouth, and to use externally fomentations of steam, as mentioned above; if it be large, it will be fitting to use the decoction of lentils and the same remedies with which all other ulcers of the mouth are cured. It also happens, sometimes, that from an ulcer of the gums—whether it follow a parulis or not—one may have for a long period a discharge of pus, on account of a broken or rotten tooth, or else on account of a disease of the bone; in this case there very often exists a fistula. Then the latter must be opened, the tooth extracted, and if any bony fragment exist, this should be removed; and if there be anything else diseased, this should be scraped away. Afterward, the same remedies which have been indicated for the other ulcers of the mouth must be used. (Guerini 1909)

The above passages help illuminate the contemporary knowledge of odontogenic infection by the time of ancient Rome. Celsus documents a sophisticated understanding of the relationship between dental decay and infections. By this time, it was widely accepted that a decayed or fractured tooth could lead to abscess development in the jawbones, which should then be treated by incision and drainage of the abscess, removal of the offending tooth, curettage of the site, and removal of bony sequestra—hallmarks of treatment which are still practiced today.

The earliest known specialized instruments for maxillofacial surgery can be traced to this era. Archaeological digs and surviving medical texts from the era showcase instruments recognizable to surgeons today. These instruments, shown below (Figs. 3 and 4), include bone levers, bone forceps, osteotomes, scalpels,

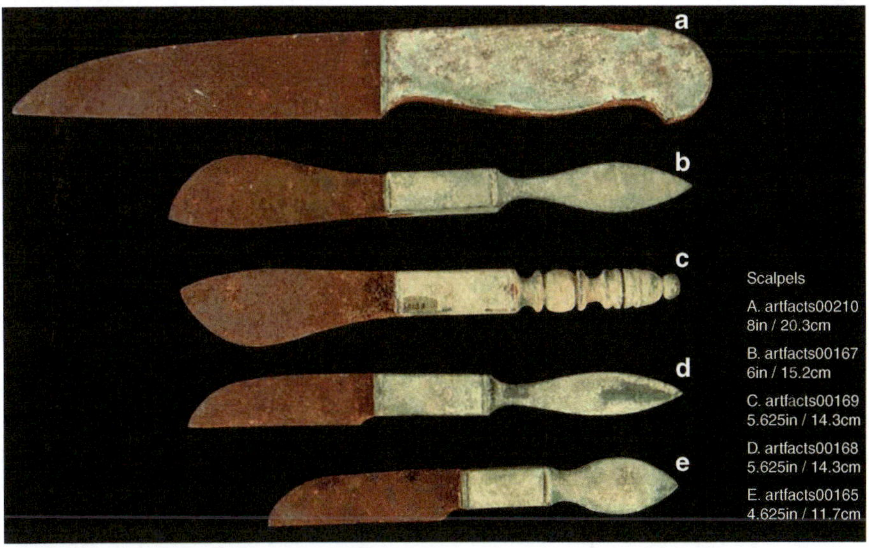

Fig. 3 Scalpels from ancient Rome in the first century CE. (Courtesy of Historical Collections & Services, Claude Moore Health Sciences Library, University of Virginia)

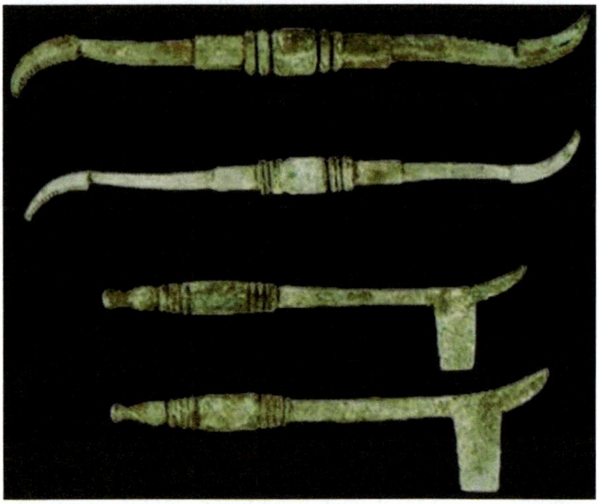

Fig. 4 Bone levers, also used to extract teeth, from ancient Rome in the first century CE. (Courtesy of Historical Collections & Services, Claude Moore Health Sciences Library, University of Virginia)

cauteries, and curettes—all necessary tools in an armamentarium for maxillofacial surgery. There is also mention of bone files, rasps, and tooth elevators from Galen, a Roman physician in the second century.

Taken together, these records make it abundantly clear that maxillofacial surgery had considerably advanced by the time of the late Roman Empire. It is important, however, to balance this knowledge with the reality that surgery was still a dangerous and unpredictable affair. It often represented the last resort for an affliction that would not resolve on its own. We will leave the Romans with this: "The ancients regarded tooth extraction as an operation to be avoided wherever possible. Caelius Aurelianus says death had followed in some cases, and that in the temple of Apollo at Delos there hung a tooth forceps of lead as a reminder for operators to exert little force in tooth extraction" (Milne 1907).

Islamic Medicine: After the fall of Rome, progress in the medical field stagnated across much of Europe. Meanwhile, Islamic scholars were hard at work preserving, translating, and advancing many of the medical practices that came before it (Campbell 2013). In many ways, Arab cultures picked up where the ancient Greeks and Romans left off. Their approach to the provision of medical care—in dedicated, academically oriented hospitals rather than the ad hoc practice settings of the past—allowed for both the centralization and institutionalization of medical care and surgery. These hospitals gave Islamic physicians centers to practice medicine, learn from others, and pass knowledge and skills to their trainees (Pormann and Savage-Smith 2007).

While medical care as a whole advanced in Islamic society, physicians of the time were still hesitant to engage in surgery due to the significant risks involved and low success rates. Even procedures with favorable success rates in Greek and Roman literature were not necessarily embraced by Islamic doctors (Pormann and Savage-Smith 2007). When surgical procedures were performed, however, practitioners were known to engage in antisepsis, a practice not widespread in previous eras, and proper hygiene was emphasized in medical settings. Islamic surgeons pioneered the use of catgut sutures to close wounds, laying the groundwork for the various types gut-style sutures we use today (Amr and Tbakhi 2007).

Despite these advances, maxillofacial surgery was not particularly changed, and many erroneous notions persisted. As late as the eighteenth century, "tooth worms" (Fig. 5) were blamed for dental problems and associated infections. Some emphasis was made on dental hygiene, which may have helped prevent infections (Boss 1993), but the treatment of maxillofacial infections once they developed was substantially unchanged.

Medieval Europe: For several centuries after the fall of Rome, medicine in Europe made minimal advances. Literacy declined and populations de-urbanized, leading to a significant decrease in learning and knowledge transfer (Riché 1976). Roman medical practices continued in southeastern Europe as part of the Byzantine Empire, although language differences (Latin vs. Greek) kept Western Europe more or less in the dark (Stahl 1962).

Despite these troubles, organized society began to coalesce again around 1000 CE in Western Europe, and with it, a revival in learning. Universities began to

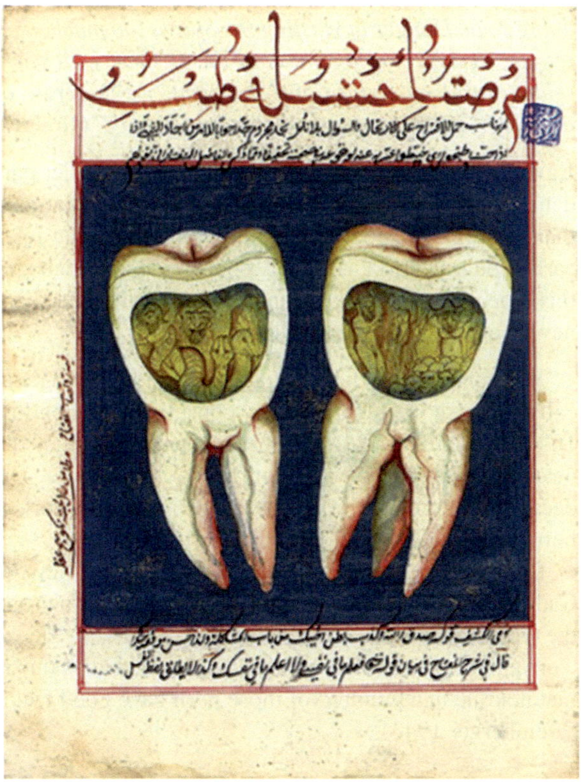

Fig. 5 Eighteenth-century hand-illustrated page from Ottoman dental book depicting tooth worms

emerge, and eventually, the translation of Greek, Latin, and Islamic texts renewed interest in medicine (Hunt 1992). Within these universities, formal dissections and autopsies were practiced like never before, greatly advancing knowledge of surgical anatomy (Bylebyl 1979).

Treatment of oral and maxillofacial conditions do not appear to have been significantly improved from previous practices discussed. The usual erroneous beliefs prevailed (tooth worms, humours, etc.), while treatment often relied on herbal remedies of dubious efficacy. Tooth extractions were performed generally by laypeople or barber-surgeons.

Notably, rates of dental caries appear to have been relatively low in medieval populations. Modern studies of medieval archaeological samples generally estimate the prevalence of caries to have been below 20% (Moore and Corbett 1971, 1973, 1975). Numerous factors are likely to cause for this, including a diet high in vegetables and low in refined carbohydrates (DeWitte and Bekvalac 2010). It is reasonable to infer from these low caries rates that severe odontogenic infections were not encountered with great frequency during this period in time.

Although not specific to the maxillofacial region, the experience of the bubonic plague is worth briefly discussing as it appears to have emboldened physicians of the time to more frequently surgically intervene in cases of frank infection: "*We do not wait for the Suppuration of a Buboe until it breaks of itself, when the Pain and other Symptoms continue very severe without Remission; besides, there would in doing so be Danger of wasting the Spirits too much, and letting the morbifick Matter retreat, besides the Smalness of the Orifice, which when they open themselves, is seldom large enough to give due Vent; we therefore open them by Incision, or to prevent Mortification, by a potential Cautery*" (Hodges and Quincy 1720).

Early Modern Period: As we remarked in earlier paragraphs, archaeological evidence indicates significantly lower rates of dental caries across historical periods than we are accustomed to today. This all began to change, however, during the early modern period, generally considered to have begun in the early 1600s. Around this time, dietary habits began to change as refined sugar became available at a scale never before experienced (Clarke 1999).

With changes in diet, dental caries and odontogenic infections began to drastically increase in prevalence. By consulting the London Bills of Mortality from the 1600s, we can see that "teeth" were consistently listed among the leading causes of death (Hull 1964; Weinberger 1948). Meanwhile, Dutch artists began depicting decayed dentition on most individuals in their artwork as the sugar-refining industry boomed around Amsterdam (Clarke 1999).

Dental infections were commonplace in the New World as well (Clarke 1999). Cadwallader Colden, a colonial New York governor and physician, remarked about the typical appearance of a young boy of the era: "He is pale of complexion, has bad teeth and often troubled with the toothache but as this is endemial to the country so that not one in a hundred of those born have good teeth or are free from toothache" (Weinberger 1948).

Unfortunately for those suffering from maxillofacial infections at the time, understanding of the disease process was incomplete and still tied to the faulty notion of "internal humours" (Guerini 1909). Treatments were similarly archaic. Cupping, cautery, medicaments, and bloodletting remained the mainstay of medical treatment of maxillofacial infection (Guerini 1909).

By the early 1700s, surgical literature began to more consistently endorse interventions such as incisions and drainage of odontogenic abscesses: "the opening in time of abscesses of the gums and of the palate even before they be completely matured, in order to prevent the suppurative process from extending and damaging the bone below" (Mauquest de la Motte 1732). Surgeons also demonstrated an understanding that bone loss is frequently involved in maxillofacial infections, a key step in understanding the disease process overall.

Pierre Fauchard's book *Le Chirurgien Dentiste* was among the first modern publications of scientific dentistry which documented the development, progression, and treatment of odontogenic infections:

> The patient was suffering with a large abscess on the right side of the lower jaw, accompanied by such great swelling of the cheek that it was impossible to open the mouth wide enough to examine the teeth. [The surgeon] Juton proposed opening the abscess immediately, but the patient would not consent. The following day he was sent for in great haste. The gathering had changed its seat, making its way between the skin and muscles of the neck, where it now formed so huge a tumefaction that the patient was in danger of being suffocated. The abscess was now immediately opened, but the swelling of the face still persisted; it was therefore only after a month had elapsed that it was possible to extract the root of the last molar, which had been the original cause of the whole malady. The surgeon observed that the liquid injected into the fistulous opening in the neck issued from the alveolus of the last molar. After the extraction of the root a prompt recovery was effected. (Spielman 2007)

German dentist Philip Pfaff arrived at a similar conclusion and stated forcefully in his textbook *Treatise on the Teeth of the Human Body and Their Diseases:* "Gingival abscesses as well as fistulae of the maxillary region almost always owe their origin to decayed teeth, and can, therefore, in general, not be cured except by the extraction of these teeth"(Guerini 1909).

Foundations of Modern Understanding: By the nineteenth century, scientific and technological advances began to accelerate at a rate never before seen. Many of the advances in knowledge around this time laid the most fundamental groundwork for our modern understanding of infectious disease. Perhaps most influential of these to our discussion is the widespread acceptance of "germ theory"—the idea that microscopic organisms could invade human tissue, causing disease. Germ theory overthrew the long-held "miasma" theory which gave credit to foul air spreading disease (Last 2007).

WD Miller, a dual-degree American dentist, was a leader in the application of germ theory to the mouth, characterizing and classifying numerous microbes he cultured from maxillofacial infections. Miller was a strong proponent of the theory that dental caries were directly related to the by-products of bacterial colonization.

He posited in 1891 that “the human mouth, as gathering-place and incubator of diverse pathogenic germs, performs a significant role in the production of varied disorders of the body.” He characterized odontogenic infections as follows:

> Alveolar abscess is an infectious disease, primarily of local character, but frequently, or usually, accompanied by general symptoms of varying intensity, and sometimes attended by complications of most serious nature. Severe cases of alveolar abscess, particularly in weak persons, not unfrequently present symptoms of an alarming nature. The extensive oedema, general debility, fever, chills, forcibly suggest the thought of general infection, which, it must be admitted, is always possible where large masses of pus accumulate about the point of the root. General blood-poisoning (septicaemia), with speedily fatal termination, has been seen to result from accumulations of infectious material about the roots of tooth. (Miller 1891)

Miller goes on to describe common and serious complications from odontogenic infections and mandibular fractures, including osteomyelitis, mediastinitis, and Ludwig’s angina. He describes a dangerous route of spread familiar to us today as progressing “through the floor of the mouth and retrotonsillar tissue into the mediastinum, producing pleuritis, pericarditis, etc., with purulent exudations.” He considered it highly probable based on the evidence available at the time that maxillofacial infections are “the result of the invasion of micro-organisms through slight wounds, ulcerations, or other breaks in the continuity of the mucous membrane, or by way of diseased teeth, or of the tonsils, or of the ducts of the sublingual and submaxillary glands”(Miller 1891).

Indeed, the most remarkable development of the late nineteenth century is the shift in the understanding of how maxillofacial infections arise. Rather than viewing each type of infection as its own discrete entity, with varying and often superstitious associated treatments and causes, scientists of the time rightly began to view them simply as differing manifestations of the same broad phenomenon, the same overarching theme: invasion of body tissue by microorganisms (Miller 1891).

So central to our understanding of maxillofacial infections, this idea became that scientists like WD Miller dedicated their careers to meticulously observe and document the properties of the microorganisms found in each case they encountered. Although much remained to be learned, patterns began to emerge and names similar to those used today began to be assigned to various species: *Bacillus dentalis viridans, Streptococcus septopyaemicus, , Actinomyces*etc.

Around the turn of the twentieth century, a more advanced understanding of infectious disease was becoming widespread in medical literature. By examining contemporary research into Ludwig’s angina in particular, we are able to glean considerable insight into the ideas of the time with regard to what was considered “acute septic infection of the throat and neck.” In a 1906 *Annals of Surgery* article, Dr. Gwilym G. Davis lays out several points which must be known to adequately understand the pathology of a disease:

> (1) what is the germ or germs that start the infection; (2) how do they gain access to the tissues; (3) what tissues are attacked; (4) how the infection progresses; (5) how it influences the parts locally and, finally, (6) how it affects the system generally. (Davis III 1906)

In the same article, Davis makes clear that oftentimes, one bacterial species predominates but that mixed infections are also common. The thoroughly modern understanding of maxillofacial infections was thus outlined: "When the teeth are the starting point the inflammation involves the periosteum of the lower jaw and thence invades all the surrounding tissues… No matter how it commences, it spreads along the connective tissues by direct continuity. It is not transmitted by the lymphatics" (Davis III 1906). With regard to Ludwig's angina in particular, he demonstrates an understanding that edema is the main issue with pus forming secondarily.

By this time, odontogenic sources had been identified as the most common cause of Ludwig's angina. Despite this, dentists were loath to treat it properly for fears of liability. As explained by Davis, "dentists will neither extract the offending tooth, nor open the abscess, nor attempt any operative means of relief for fear they should be held accountable for subsequent results." This is considered a mistake, as Davis states, "I am firmly convinced that the disease in its early stage is a purely local affection whose extension can be promptly cut short by fearless surgical treatment… In edema of the epiglottis and larynx, ice and inhalations (spray) of cocaine and adrenaline may be of service, but tracheotomy should not be deferred too long" (Davis III 1906). Prior to antibiotics, surgeons of the time had only a short to window to intervene before infection overwhelmed.

The above advanced understanding of Ludwig's angina should be contrasted with Ludwig's own explanations, only 60 years earlier: "Therapy was decided upon after consideration of the season of the year, epidemic-like character of the illness… and was chiefly as follows: local and general blood-letting, softening poultices and cataplasms, external and internal use of mercurial, relief of spasm by the remote application of sinapisms and vesicants; cathartics, diuretics and diaphoretics according to momentary requirements; in the later stages of the disease, local irritants according to the degree of the mortification process, and internal medications for the typhus process, directed particularly to the head and chest organs" (Burke 1939). Mentions are made of the dangerous effects of letting patients "catch cold," an idea now understood to be unrelated to the development of infection.

Advances in the understanding of infectious processes were in no way limited to treatment of acute septic maxillofacial infections. Similarly in trauma cases, it became understood that the retention of teeth in fracture lines allowed oral bacteria unimpeded access to internal tissue. In cases of osteomyelitis, complete excision of necrotic bone was emphasized to remove foci of infection. In just a short time, germ theory revolutionized our understanding of infectious disease and appropriate treatments.

Asepsis: In studying germ theory, pioneering lab scientists like Louis Pasteur understood that surgical and lab instruments could harbor microbes of their own, thereby causing contamination of any environment into which they are introduced. Pasteur subsequently demonstrated the effectiveness of heat sterilization in preventing the spread and replication of microbes (Ligon 2002). It might be expected that the same principles would naturally carry over to surgical procedures, but the adoption of antiseptic or aseptic techniques by surgeons was uneven and significantly delayed from its adoption in labs. When physician Ignaz Semmelweis advocated for the careful washing of hands to reduce hospital infections, his findings were initially met with disdain and fierce resistance (Semmelweis 1983).

One of the early proponents of aseptic technique, Joseph Lister, published his first article with the use of carbolic acid antisepsis in *The Lancet* in 1867 (Lister 1867a). Lister was a strong proponent of asepsis, and over time, other surgeons began following similar techniques. Not all surgeons agreed that germ theory was necessarily to blame for postsurgical infections, but they could not argue with the published and reproducible results from adhering to aseptic technique—higher surgical success rates and fewer complications (Lister 1867b).

By the 1890s, papers were being published in medical literature regarding the use of antiseptics and disinfectants specifically in dental surgery (Miller 1891). The antiseptics detailed had differing uses—some for the application to instruments, some to be applied directly to surgical sites, and still others for use as mouth rinses (Gish 1888). The use of such antimicrobial substances both improved the safety of surgical interventions in head and neck infection cases and simultaneously reduced the incidence of infections secondary to other maxillofacial surgeries. Gradually, more and more surgeons came on board with the practice of aseptic technique. These ideas eventually formed the basis for practices we follow today in surgically treating maxillofacial infections—the use of sterile instruments, chlorhexidine rinses, and povidone-iodine preps, among others.

The Antibiotic Era: In the late nineteenth century, scientists around the world began noting the inhibitory effects on bacterial growth exhibited by the presence of certain types of mold. In 1928, so the story goes, Alexander Fleming discovered the substance penicillin (Tan and Tatsumura 2015). Chemists succeeded in purifying penicillin, and the drug saw widespread use as the first highly effective systemic antibiotic in the 1940s (Mestrovic 2010).

These developments which revolutionized the treatment of infectious diseases unsurprisingly had major impacts on the treatment of maxillofacial infections. As early as 1947, Dr. Kurt Thoma, an American oral and maxillofacial surgeon, began addressing these changes: "In some instances, these new agents are so effective that surgical interference is eliminated, while in others they make possible earlier surgical measures with greater safety to the patient and a more rapid convalescence. In most instances, however, the use of antibiotics combined with carefully planned and adequate surgery gives the best results" (Thoma 1947).

Wound cultures took on even greater importance as the identification of causative microbes could now directly influence treatment. Thoma encouraged a "thorough bacteriologic study" of all cases and advised physicians to avoid contamination of culture samples from other microbes present in the mouth (Thoma 1947).

We also begin to see at this time the balancing act of when to consider conservative treatment with antibiotics versus an urgent tooth extraction. Timely initiation of antibiotic treatment was found to be adequate for some limited types of cases, but for many others, it was clear that a timely extraction remained necessary to definitively cure the condition. In any case, the use of antibiotics was found to greatly improve the safety profile of necessary surgical interventions such as extractions and incision and drainage (I&D) procedures. As remains the case today, however, Thoma noted, "Many patients do not present themselves for treatment early enough, however, and require elimination of accumulated pus and excision of dead bone" (Thoma 1947).

The promise of antibiotics was so great that surgeons of the time began to experiment with different methods of drug delivery. Systemic administration of penicillin had already been found to have significant effects on bacterial infection, even with low circulating concentrations in the blood. Surgeons surmised that higher local concentrations may be beneficial when applied directly to infected sites. To achieve this, rubber catheters were frequently left in difficult-to-treat infections such as osteomyelitis to allow antibiotics to be "instilled" directly into the site (Thoma 1947; Coe 1951).

By the middle of the twentieth century, surgeons were advocating for supportive care regimens similar to what is used in hospitals today (Thoma 1947). Foremost, antibiotics were recommended to be continued until all signs of infection abated. Proper nutrition, fluid management, and oral hygiene were seen as crucial to recovery and the prevention of secondary infection. Even the penicillin-based drugs most commonly used to treat odontogenic infection today are direct descendants of the drugs pioneered at this time.

Unsurprisingly, not all practices remain prevalent—Dr. Thoma advocated that "repeated blood transfusions greatly aid in improving the general condition of dental patients afflicted with chronic suppuration and help to overcome the infection," a treatment modality unthinkable today.

Diagnostic X-Ray Imaging: For most of human history, physicians had limited tools at their disposal for diagnosing infections: the symptoms reported by the patient and the physical signs observed upon examination. This would all change after William Roentgen used his first X-ray in 1895. In less than 30 years from its first use, X-ray imaging was widely used in dentistry, and radiography became a compulsory component of professional education (Read 1925).

The plain radiographs (Fig. 6) available for most of the century were incredibly useful to dentists and physicians looking to localize the source of an infection in the maxillofacial region. The jawbones lend themselves well to diagnostic imaging as regions of resorbed bone associated with odontogenic infection are readily visible. With the ability to accurately diagnose sources of odontogenic infection, treatment could be targeted to the involved teeth while sparing vital ones.

Encouraged by the successful and widespread adoption of diagnostic X-ray imaging, researchers in the early 1900s experimented with additional applications of the novel technology. Undesirable effects of ionizing radiation well known to us today—skin burns, hair loss, etc.—were noted relatively early into its adoption. The same process that damaged our cells, however, also appeared to damage the cells of microbial invaders. Before long, doctors were directly irradiating infected tissue to

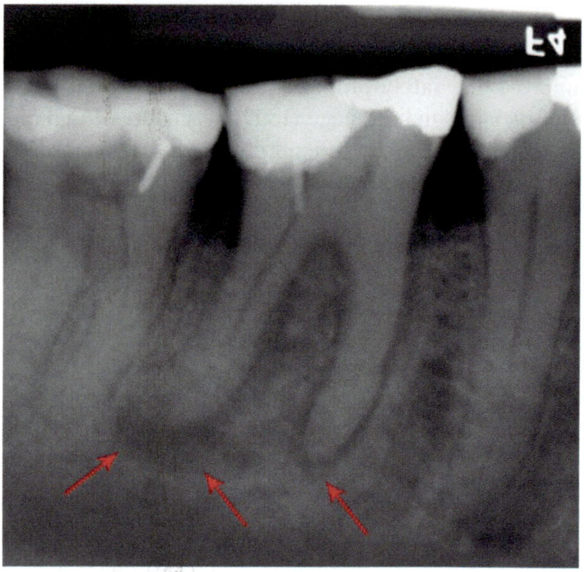

Fig. 6 Two-dimensional radiographic view of posterior tooth with periapical abscesses. (Coronation Dental Specialty Group, CC BY-SA 3.0 https://creativecommons.org/licenses/by-sa/3.0, via Wikimedia Commons)

neutralize infection and promote healing (van Dijk et al. 2020). The mechanism was suggested to be a combination of direct effects on bacterial populations and host immune alterations that enhanced phagocytosis (Calabrese 2013).

The medical community of the time generally accepted that X-ray irradiation could serve as an effective adjunct to surgery and sometimes a superior alternative. As late as the 1940s, cases of cellulitis secondary to maxillofacial surgery are reported in the literature as being treated with ionizing radiation in conjunction with antibiotic therapy. Despite being an apparently effective treatment for soft tissue infections, the use of X-rays began to fall out of favor as more serious side effects started to come to light—in particular, associations with salivary gland neoplasms (Schneider et al. 1998). The availability of a wider range of more effective antibiotics over time effectively rendered the technology obsolete.

In the 1980s, the availability of CT (computed tomography) imaging further expanded the capabilities of radiography in treating head and neck infections. For the first time, doctors could visualize "slices" of the imaged region, allowing a three-dimensional analysis of exactly where infections lay. The contributions from this technology were summed up as follows in a 1985 article in The Laryngoscope:

> The influence of CT scanning on therapy of masticator space infections and tumors is profound… CT determines the need for surgery in infections by differentiating cellulitis from abscess formation. When abscess formation is present, CT defines the best surgical approach and positioning of drains. It can demonstrate osteomyelitis and unsuspected abscesses. Postoperatively, CT can determine the presence of undrained abscesses. (Doxey et al. 1985)

This notion was corroborated by many surgeons of the time, including a 1982 article by *Flood* et al. which praised CT scanning for its utility in localizing infection and planning surgical approaches to odontogenic infections with orbital involvement (Flood et al. 1982).

Development of Contemporary Evidence-Based Care: As the medical literature matured and high-quality studies were conducted with greater frequency, we began to amass greater knowledge of the safest and most effective ways to manage maxillofacial infections. This fund of knowledge allowed practitioners of the mid- to late twentieth century to refine practices and recommend effective treatments while abandoning less favorable options.

For example, in the early 1900s, chlorophyll garnered some degree of notoriety as a potential game-changing treatment for maxillofacial infections due to apparently favorable results in initial studies (Gruskin 1940). As more studies emerged, however, the efficacy of this treatment came into question, with more rigorous analyses showing little to no benefit. Coupled with the availability of efficacious antibiotic alternatives, chlorophyll faded from use to the point that few practicing surgeons would consider its use today.

Similarly, the "instillation" of antibiotic solutions directly into wounds previously discussed became less prevalent as doubts over its effectiveness and concerns about costs and antibiotic resistance emerged. Several studies through the early twenty-first century claimed no benefit for bacterial killing with the irrigation of wounds with combination antibiotic solution (Goswami et al. 2019). Evidence against this practice mounted to the point that international researchers, including those at the 2018 International Consensus Meeting on Musculoskeletal Infection, voted strongly against the use of polymyxin-bacitracin in wound irrigation solutions (Dyrda 2018).

On the other hand, concrete evidence of efficacy in medical literature has allowed better practices to disseminate throughout the community more uniformly. One such example is the use of antibiotic prophylaxis to prevent infections related to maxillofacial surgery. Preventing an infection is undoubtedly preferable to treating one, although this must be weighed against potential complications from antibiotic treatment. Currently, literature supports perioperative antibiotics in the case of open trauma surgery (ORIF) and orthognathic surgery, but not routine dental extractions (Zallen and Curry 1975; Kreutzer et al. 2014).

Once an infection has developed, there still exists some debate on when surgical intervention is warranted. Recent reviews such as a 2017 study in *Oral and Maxillofacial Surgery Clinics* have suggested a less aggressive approach to treating infections may be reasonable, given the availability of highly effective broad-spectrum antibiotics. The authors recommend limiting surgical incision and drainage to "spaces that have identifiable purulent collections" and argue that cellulitis may be managed medically so long as the source of infection is removed (Taub et al. 2017).

Furthermore, consensus in the medical literature can confirm the utility of established practices and support their continued use. Recent studies have demonstrated that the combination of clinical examination with contrast CT imaging is significantly more effective than either option on its own (Miller et al. 1999).

As new technologies emerge and established practices are scrutinized, we can expect the treatment of maxillofacial infections to continue to evolve. Today's sterile and highly controlled operating rooms are a far cry from our barber-surgeon roots. Antibiotics and radiographic technologies now provide surgeons with improved tools to quickly combat head and neck infections and avoid morbidity and mortality.

References

Amr SS, Tbakhi. Abu Al Qasim Al Zahrawi (Albucasis): pioneer of modern surgery. Ann Saudi Med. 2007;27(3):220–1. https://doi.org/10.5144/0256-4947.2007.220.

Blomstedt P. Dental surgery in ancient Egypt. J Hist Dent. 2013;61:129–42.

Boss G. The miswāk, an aspect of dental care in Islam. Med Hist. 1993;37:68–79.

Burke J. Angina Ludovici, a translation, together with a biography of Wilhelm Frederick von Ludwig. Bull Hist Med. 1939;7:1115–26.

Bylebyl JJ. The School of Padua: humanistic medicine in the 16th century. Health, Medicine and Mortality in the Sixteenth Century; 1979.

Calabrese EJ. X-ray treatment of carbuncles and furuncles (boils): a historical assessment. Hum Exp Toxicol. 2013;32(8):817–27. https://doi.org/10.1177/0960327112467046. PMID: 23821639. Accessed 1 Dec 2020.

Campbell D. Arabian medicine and its influence on the middle ages. Routledge; 2013. p. 2–20. ISBN 978-1-317-83312-3.

Celsus A. On medicine, Book VII. n.d.-a. URL https://penelope.uchicago.edu/Thayer/E/Roman/Texts/Celsus/7*.html. Accessed 20 Oct 2020.

Celsus A. On medicine, Book VI. n.d.-b. URL https://penelope.uchicago.edu/Thayer/E/Roman/Texts/Celsus/6*.html. Accessed 15 Oct 2020.

Clarke JH. Toothaches and death. J Hist Dent. 1999;47(1):11–3.

Coe RP. Instillation of streptomycin into the pericardial sac in tuberculous pericarditis. Br Med J. 1951;1(4696):18–9. https://doi.org/10.1136/bmj.1.4696.18. PMID: 14792080; PMCID: PMC2068143.

Davis GG III. Acute septic infection of the throat and neck; Ludwig's angina. Ann Surg. 1906;44(2):175–92. https://doi.org/10.1097/00000658-190608000-00003.

DeWitte SN, Bekvalac J. Oral health and frailty in the medieval English cemetery of St. Mary Graces. Am J Phys Anthropol. 2010;142:341–54. https://doi.org/10.1002/ajpa.21228.

Dias G, Tayles N. 'Abscess cavity'—a misnomer. Int J Osteoarchaeol. 1997;7:548–54. https://doi.org/10.1002/(SICI)1099-1212(199709/10)7:5<548::AID-OA369>3.0.CO;2-I.

Doxey GP, Harnsberger HR, Hardin CW, Davis RK. The masticator space: the influence of ct scanning on therapy. Laryngoscope. 1985;95:1444–7. https://doi.org/10.1288/00005537-198512000-00002. Accessed 1 Dec 2020.

Dyrda L. Orthopedic joint infection prevention: key takeaways from the 2018 international consensus meeting on musculoskeletal infection. 2018. https://www.beckersspine.com/orthopedic/item/42091-orthopedic-joint-infection-prevention-key-takeaways-from-the-2018-international-consensus-meeting-on-musculoskeletal-infection.html?tmpl=component&print=1. Accessed 1 Dec 2020.

Eshed V, Gopher A, Hershkovitz I. Tooth wear and dental pathology at the advent of agriculture: new evidence from the Levant. Am J Phys Anthropol. 2006;130:145–59. https://doi.org/10.1002/ajpa.20362.

Flood TP, Braude LS, Jampol LM, Herzog S. Computed tomography in the management of orbital infections associated with dental disease. Br J Ophthalmol. 1982;66:269–74.

Forshaw RJ. The practice of dentistry in ancient Egypt. Br Dent J. 2009;206:481–6. https://doi.org/10.1038/sj.bdj.2009.355.

Gish JL. Oral antisepsis. Dental Regr. 1888;42(7):327–32.

Goswami K, Cho J, Foltz C, Manrique J, Tan T, Fillingham Y, Higuera C, Valle CD, Parvizi J. Polymyxin and bacitracin in the irrigation solution provide no benefit for bacterial killing in vitro. J Bone Joint Surg. 2019;101:1689–97. https://doi.org/10.2106/JBJS.18.01362.

Grine FE, Gwinnett AJ, Oaks JH. Early hominid dental pathology: interproximal caries in 1.5 million-year-old Paranthropus robustus from Swartkrans. Arch Oral Biol. 1990;35:381–6. https://doi.org/10.1016/0003-9969(90)90185-D

Gruskin B. Chlorophyll—its therapeutic place in acute and suppurative disease: preliminary report of clinical use and rationale. Am J Surg. 1940;49:49–55. https://doi.org/10.1016/S0002-9610(40)90685-7.

Guerini V. A history of dentistry from the most ancient times until the end of the eighteenth century. Lea & Febiger; 1909.

Hodges N, Quincy J. Loimologia: or, an historical account of the plague in London in 1665 with precautionary directions against the like contagion. Oxford; 1720.

Hull CW. Economic writings of Sir William Petty, Vol. II in Reprints of Economic Classics. New York: August M. Kelly, Bookseller; 1964.

Hunt T. The medieval surgery. Boydell & Brewer; 1992.

Kreutzer K, Storck K, Weitz J. Current evidence regarding prophylactic antibiotics in head and neck and maxillofacial surgery. Biomed Res Int. 2014;2014:879437. https://doi.org/10.1155/2014/879437.

Last JM, editor. "miasma theory". A dictionary of public health. Westminster College, Pennsylvania: Oxford University Press; 2007.

Legge SS. Dentoalveolar abscess variation among three groups of chimpanzees (Pan troglodytes schweinfurthii, Pan troglodytes troglodytes, and Pan paniscus). Int J Paleopathol. 2012;2:1–9. https://doi.org/10.1016/j.ijpp.2012.06.002.

Lieverse AR, Link DW, Bazaliiskiy VI, Goriunova OI, Weber AW. Dental health indicators of hunter–gatherer adaptation and cultural change in Siberia's Cis-Baikal. Am J Phys Anthropol. 2007;134:323–39. https://doi.org/10.1002/ajpa.20672.

Ligon BL. Biography: Louis Pasteur: a controversial figure in a debate on scientific ethics. Semin Pediatr Infect Dis. 2002;13(2):134–41.

Lister J. On the antiseptic principle in the practice of surgery. Lancet. 1867a;90(2299):353–6. ISSN 0140-6736, https://doi.org/10.1016/S0140-6736(02)51827-4.

Lister J. On a new method of treating compound fracture, abscess, etc., with observations on the conditions of suppuration. Lancet. 1867b:336–9.

Mauquest de la Motte G. Traité complet de chirurgie: contenant des observations & des reflexions sur toutes les maladies chirurgicales & surla maniere de les traiter. France: chez Clousier; 1732.

Mestrovic T. Penicillin production. Medical News. Published May 13, 2010. https://www.news-medical.net/health/Penicillin-Production.aspx. Accessed 18 May 2021.

Miller WD. The human mouth as a focus of infection. Lancet. 1891;138:340–2. https://doi.org/10.1016/S0140-6736(02)01387-9.

Miller J, Fields M. An appraisal of the skulls and dentition of ancient Egyptians, highlighting the pathology and speculating on the influence of diet and environment. BAR International Series 1794 Archaeopress, Oxford, UK 2008; 143 pp ISBN 13: 978 1 407302829. Int J Osteoarchaeol. 2009;19:443–5. https://doi.org/10.1002/oa.1092.

Miller WD, Furst IM, Sàndor GK, Keller MA. A prospective, blinded comparison of clinical examination and computed tomography in deep neck infections. Laryngoscope. 1999;109:1873–9. https://doi.org/10.1097/00005537-199911000-00029.

Milne JS. Surgical instruments in Greek and Roman Times. Oxford; 1907.

Moore WJ, Corbett ME. The distribution of dental caries in ancient British populations. 1. Anglo-saxon period. Caries Res. 1971;5(2):151–68.

Moore WJ, Corbett E. The distribution of dental caries in ancient British populations. II. Iron Age, Romano-British and Mediaeval periods. Caries Res. 1973;7(2):139–53.

Moore WJ, Corbett ME. Distribution of dental caries in ancient British populations. III. The 17th century. Caries Res. 1975;9(2):163–75.

Nicklisch N, Ganslmeier R, Siebert A, Friederich S, Meller H, Alt KW. Holes in teeth – dental caries in Neolithic and early bronze age populations in central Germany. Ann Anat. 2016;203:90–9. https://doi.org/10.1016/j.aanat.2015.02.001

Pormann PE, Savage-Smith E. Medieval Islamic medicine. Edinburgh University Press; 2007. ISBN 978-0-7486-2066-1.

Read C. Dental focal infection and its diagnosis by X-rays *paper read before the southern medical society, 26th February, 1925. Glasgow Med J. 1925;103:356–62.

Riché P. Education and culture in the Barbarian West: from the Jeremy Marcelino II. Columbia: University of South Carolina Press; 1976. p. 100–29.

Schneider AB, et al. Salivary gland tumors after childhood radiation treatment for benign conditions of the head and neck: dose-response relationships. Radiat Res. 1998;149(6):625–30. JSTOR, www.jstor.org/stable/3579909. Accessed 14 Oct 2020.

Semmelweis I. Etiology, concept and prophylaxis of childbed fever (trans: Codell CK). University of Wisconsin Press; 1983. ISBN 0-299-09364-6.

Spielman AI. The birth of the most important 18th century dental text: Pierre Fauchard's Le chirurgien dentist. J Dent Res. 2007;86(10):922–6.

Stahl W. Roman science. Madison: Univ. of Wisconsin Pr; 1962. p. 120–33.

Stránská P. Možnosti hodnocení dentální patologie na archeologickém kostrovém materiálu: prevalence zubního kazu od pravěku po novověk [Evaluation of the dental pathology in archaeological skeletal material: prevalence of dental caries since prehistory to modern age]. Cas Lek Cesk. 2013;152(4):196–205.

Tan SY, Tatsumura Y. Alexander Fleming (1881-1955): discoverer of penicillin. Singap Med J. 2015;56(7):366–7. https://doi.org/10.11622/smedj.2015105

Taub D, Yampolsky A, Diecidue R, Gold L. Controversies in the management of oral and maxillofacial infections. Oral Maxillofac Surg Clin North Am. 2017;29:465–73. https://doi.org/10.1016/j.coms.2017.06.004.

Thoma KH. Odontogenic infections of the jaws and associated soft tissues and their treatment with the aid of antibiotics. Surg Clin North Am. 1947;27:1321–9. https://doi.org/10.1016/S0039-6109(16)32263-0.

Towle I, Irish JD. Dental abscesses on the maxilla of a two million-year-old early Homo specimen. bioRxiv. 2019:595595. https://doi.org/10.1101/595595.

van Dijk B, Lemans JVC, Hoogendoorn RM, et al. Treating infections with ionizing radiation: a historical perspective and emerging techniques. Antimicrob Resist Infect Control. 2020;9:121.

Weinberger BW. An introduction to the history of dentistry in America, vol. II. St. Louis: Mosby; 1948.

Zallen RD, Curry JT. A study of antibiotic usage in compound mandibular fractures. J Oral Surg. 1975;33:431–4.

Evolution of Tooth Removal

Michael T. Goupil and Vernon Burke

1 Introduction

The removal of teeth is most likely one of the earliest surgical procedures performed. Probably, the first tooth was removed from a blow to the face, either accidently or as part of an interpersonal altercation. It is speculated that the first purposeful removal of a tooth was accomplished with the "the ancient healer using a hickory stick and stone mallet" (Bremner 1954, p. 341).

Over time, the removal of teeth became a specialized niche within medicine. Specific instruments were developed, but the primary tooth removal instrument, the forceps, has not changed dramatically since ancient times.

The removal of teeth, including impacted third molars, continues to be one of the most common surgical procedures performed today. Oral surgeons over the recent past have established the indications, classification systems, risk-benefit analysis, and surgical methods employed by the vast majority of oral and maxillofacial surgeons worldwide.

M. T. Goupil (✉)
Division of Oral and Maxillofacial Surgery, University of Connecticut, Farmington, CT, USA

Consultant in Oral and Maxillofacial Surgery, Carmel, IN, USA

V. Burke
High Desert Oral & Facial Surgery, El Paso, TX, USA

E. M. Ferneini et al. (eds.), *The History of Maxillofacial Surgery*,
https://doi.org/10.1007/978-3-030-89563-1_9

2 Ancient History

2.1 Prehistory Humans

The intentional removal of teeth dates to the Stone Age and most likely makes it one of the first surgical procedures performed by humankind. There is evidence that one or more incisors were intentionally removed in the late Stone Age (prior to 10,000 BCE). Evidence from both Asia and North Africa indicate that these teeth were not removed for pathological purposes but more likely to represent a significant social event such as the onset of puberty and social maturation (De Groote and Humphrey 2016; Willman et al. 2016). Most likely, these surgical procedures were performed by an ancient healer using a hickory stick and a stone mallet (Wynbrandt 1998, p. 5; Bremner 1954, p. 341) (Fig. 1).

The course diet of the Stone Age people, where the food was mixed with sand and gravel, would lead to severe tooth abrasion. The result of this abrasion would be severe pain and pulp necrosis. It is quite likely that this pain would lead to tooth removal. Our Neolithic ancestors may have used the finger and thumb to remove teeth (Anonymous 1914, p. 10).

With a change to a farming culture, more than 12,000 years ago, an increase in caries was noted. There is evidence that there was tool-assisted manipulation to the tooth in an attempt to remove the necrotic or infected pulp (Oxilia et al. 2015, 2017). The use of a flint drill was used to treat caries in the Neolithic period (Coppa et al. 2006).

2.2 Eastern and Egyptian Era

There were traces of "one who treats teeth" found at the Step Pyramid of King Djoser (Hoffmann-Axthelm 1981b). At that time, Hesy-Rei was considered to be the first dentist and dates back to 2500–2600 BCE (Leek 1967). Since dental disease was considered to be caused by spirits, treatment usually consisted of incantations,

Fig. 1 Stone Age mallet. (Image of the public domain)

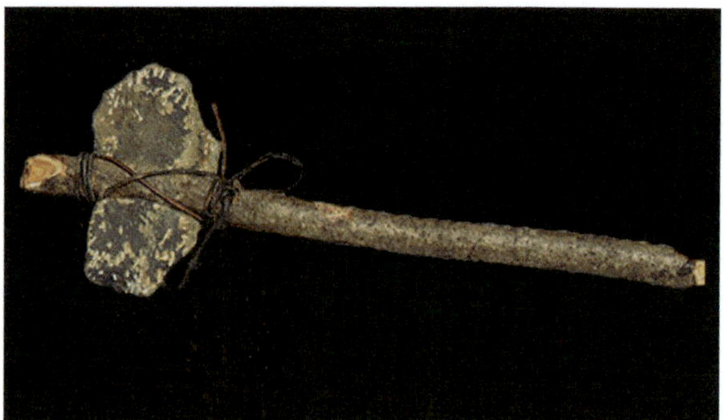

magic spells, and prayers (Wynbrandt 1998, p. 11). Most of the dental treatment was restricted to pharmaceutical preparations which did little to alleviate the widespread and painful dental disease (Forshaw 2009).

The often-quoted Ebers Papyrus, written around 1550 BCE, is among the oldest written works on medicine and is believed to contain material dating back to 3700 BCE. Although this papyrus does contain entries on surgical procedures as well as the treatment of teeth, there is no mention of dental operations including the extraction of teeth. Because there is an absence of evidence for surgical procedures on teeth, the assumption has been made that dental extractions did not occur (Guerini 1909, p. 25). This papyrus contains 11 dental treatments and consists of plasters, mouthwashes, masticatories, and incantations (Wynbrandt 1998, p. 12).

The Edwin Smith Papyrus dates from the same area and is considered to be the oldest known surgical treatise, and it contains descriptions for the treatment of jaw fractures. As dental forceps are found on stella and wall carvings, and Egyptians suffered a variety of dental diseases, the assumption is that dental extractions did occur during this era (Ring 1985, p. 35). In Additionally, Sir Marc Armand Ruffer stated, "it is difficult to believe that extractions were not practiced at this time, but the evidence is nil" (Leek 1967).

Rhazes (Abdu Bakr Muhammad ibn Zakariyyā al-Rāzī, 854–925 CE), a Persian physician, described an interesting way of extracting a tooth – "extraction, a last resort, is aided by first applying loosening agents such as arsenic paste or the juices of a boiled frog" (Ring 1985, p. 35).

Albucasis (Abū al-Qāsim Khalaf ibn al-'Abbās al-Zahrāwī al Ansari, 936–1013 CE), an Arab physician and surgeon, described a variety of dental instruments and techniques to remove fractured teeth. He gave us one of the fundamental precepts for performing extractions – "it is necessary first to ascertain which is the aching tooth, as very often the pain deceives the patient, so that he may indicate as to the very seat of the pain another tooth which is perfectly sound, and desires it to be extracted; after a while, naturally, the pain does not cease…" (Garant 2013). Like the Roman physician, Celsus, he also advocated filling the crown of a decayed tooth before extraction to minimize the crushing of the crown during the extraction procedure (Ring 1985, p. 35).

The Chinese and Japanese cultures are both known for the non-instrument, finger method of extracting teeth. In fact, practitioners in Japan were taught to extract teeth by removing pegs pounded into a wooden board simply by using their fingers (Bremner 1954, p. 341).

2.3 Greek and Roman Era

During the twelfth century BCE, the Greek physician and god of medicine Æsculapius was recognized as the inventor of purgatives and the extraction of teeth (Anonymous 1914, p. 21; Hussain and Kahn 2014). The model for the extraction

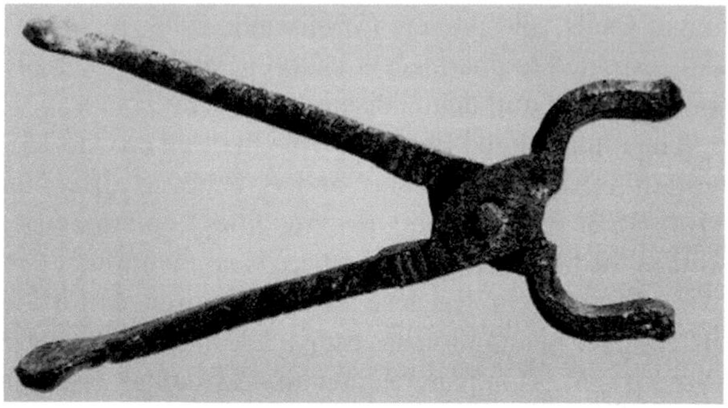

Fig. 2 Lead odontogagon found in the temple of Apollo. (Image of the public domain (Guerini 1909, p. 46))

forceps, the odontogagon (Fig. 2), was a pincer made of lead that was found in the temple of Apollo and predates the temple of Æsculapius (Guerini 1909, p. 45).

Hippocrates and Aristotle wrote about dentistry including the extraction of teeth in 500–300 BCE. Hippocrates's description for extracting a tooth using the plumberous odontogagon is said to be the first described dental operation (Ring 1985, p. 19).

Aristotle (384–322 BCE) described the application of the forceps (odontogagon) in a passage from *Mechanics*. "It is formed by two levers…By means of this; it is much easier to move the tooth, it is then easier to extract it with the hand than with the instrument" (Wynbrandt 1998, p. 19, 20).

Like the Greeks, the Roman also performed dental extractions using the dentiduceum which was based on the Greek odontogagon. In the first century, a Roman dental patient could choose between a physician specializing in dentistry, a barber-surgeon, or a tooth-drawer to perform a dental extraction (Ring 1985, p. 41).

Aulus Cornelius Celsus (25 BCE–50 CE), a Roman encyclopedist, described in his book series, *De Medicina*, tooth removal using a variety of botanicals to cause a tooth to fall out. Celsus advocated packing the decayed cavity of the tooth with lint or lead to prevent fracture of the tooth crown during extraction (Wynbrandt 1998, p. 21). He further described the classical method for tooth removal used today – "the gum must be detached all around, and then the tooth is shaken until it is loosened" (Bremner 1954, p. 53).

This was further refined by Paul of Ægina, a seventh-century Roman physician: "the extraction is begun by detaching the gum all around it as far as the alveolar bone, then the tooth is seized with the forceps, shaken loose, and drawn out" (Guerini 1909, p. 86).

2.4 *Practitioners*

The earliest "professional" recognized practitioners to extract teeth were university-trained physicians as evidenced by Hippocrates, Aristotle, Rhazes, and Albucasis. Eventually, the physicians took a more of a hands-off approach to care and delegated the extraction of teeth to barber-surgeons.

The barber-surgeons were apprenticed trained for around five years. Their existence dates back to 1000 CE. Most physicians in Western Europe at that time were members of the clergy. The papal edicts of the twelfth century prohibited members of the clergy from letting blood, and thus, the barber-surgeons took on a greater role in the extraction of teeth. Physicians that had also trained in surgery continued to extract teeth (see Chap. 3 - Barber-Surgeons).

One of the foremost recognized barber-surgeons was Ambroise Paré (1510–1590). He underwent his apprenticeship in Paris and honed his skills as a military surgeon. He was a prolific writer and inventor and made significant contributions to both medicine and dentistry. His texts, *Complete Works* and *Dix livres de la chirurgie,* contain illustrations of many of the dental instruments that he designed to extract teeth (Guerini 1909, p. 18).

The third option that patients had for dental extractions was the tooth-drawer or tooth-puller. These "practitioners" had little, if any, training. They were popular at fairs as a type of entertainment. Their one skill was speed. Due to the lack of anesthesia, having an extraction was painful and the faster the better. The downside of these rapid procedures was the potential for life-threatening complications, but by that time, the tooth-puller had moved on to the next town (Ring 1985, p. 128, 132).

3 Early Instruments

The odontogagon, as noted above, is considered to be the prototype of the dental forceps, and the basic design has not changed significantly to this day.

Giovanni d'Arcoli (1412–1484) described a number of tooth extraction instruments in his commentary on the work of Arculanus. His invention of the "dental pelican" was used into the eighteenth century for pulling teeth. Arcoli also advocated the use of cautery to stop bleeding, a technique still practiced today (Fig. 3) (Zampetti and Riva 2020).

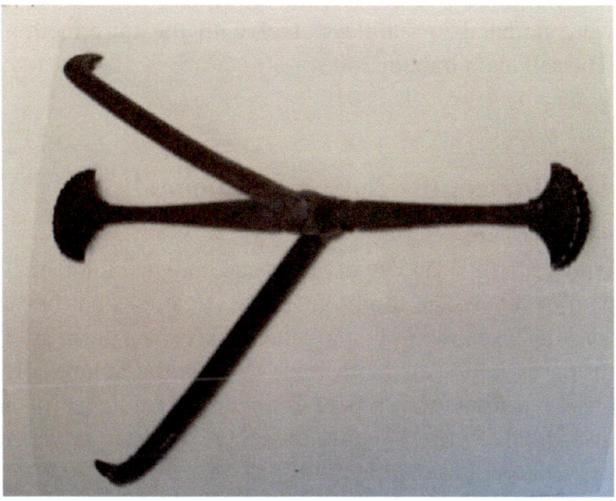

Fig. 3 Pelican c.1650 (Bennion 1986)

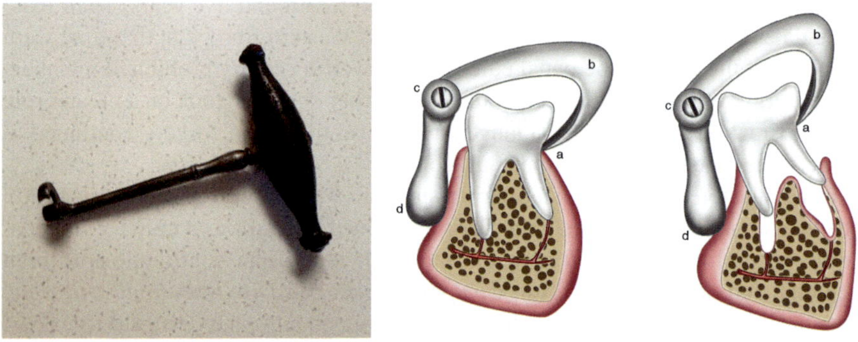

Fig. 4 Tooth key circa 1890 (courtesy of author MTG) and method of use (Hoffmann-Axthelm 1981a)

Walther Hermann Ryff (1500–1548), a German surgeon, was a prolific writer. One of his texts contained a number of woodblock prints portraying dental instruments, including forceps and elevators, that were in use at that time (Guerini 1909, p. 166).

Pierre Fauchard (1678–1761), a French physician, is considered to be the "Father of Modern Dentistry." He gave specific instructions on the use of tooth extraction instruments. He described separating the gum from the tooth, as previously advocated by Celsus, loosening the tooth with an elevator, and placing the claw of the pelican as far down on the root as possible. After loosening the tooth by "shaking" it, next is completing the procedure with elevators, pincers, and fingers (Atkinson 2002).

The tooth key dates back to circa 1740 and was based on a typical door key of the period (Fig. 4). The bolster was placed against the tooth, and the hinged claw was placed around the crown. The tooth was then removed by rapidly twisting the key like turning a key in a lock (Kravetz 2003).

Albucasis provided the first drawings of extraction elevators in 1122. Elevators in the eighteenth and seventeenth century had handles made of ivory or wood; they were updated to stainless steel with the introduction of sterilization procedures (Bussell and Graham 2008).

4 Nineteenth-Century Pioneers

For over a thousand years, little had changed in the methodology for the removal of painful teeth. The tooth-pullers were sought out because their reputation for performing an extraction rapidly meant less pain during the procedure. A major advance in the evolution of tooth removal was the control of pain. Horace Wells, a keen observer, noted that a person under the influence of nitrous oxide appeared to be insensible to pain. He tested his theory by having one of his own teeth extracted in December 1844 (Clark 1999).

The anesthetic properties of cocaine were first described by the Spanish Jesuit Bernabé Cobi (1582–1657) as treatment for toothache. But it was William Halsted and Richard Hall that developed the technique of nerve block in 1885 that revolutionized the practice of odontology (López-Valverde et al. 2011). One of the problems of the use of cocaine is its addictive properties. The German chemist Alfred Einhorn overcame this addiction problem when he synthesized the aminoester, procaine. He patented this local anesthetic under the trade name of "Novocain," which became the primary dental local anesthetic until it was supplanted by lidocaine and mepivacaine in the twentieth century (Sheikh and Dua 2020). The removal of teeth could now be conducted in a safe and comfortable environment.

The removal of teeth using forceps had remained relatively unchanged since the twelfth-century odontogagon found in the Temple of Apollo. In 1826, Cyrus Fay, an American dentist practicing in London, developed a new set of forceps. He designed forceps that adapted to the cervical portion of the various human teeth (Bussell and Graham 2008). Modern extraction techniques were further refined with the introduction of the anatomical forceps designed, in 1840, by Tomes, an English dentist. These were a set of instruments adaptable to the various shapes of individual teeth (Rounds and Rounds 1953, p. 23).

The title of Father of Oral Surgery has been attributed to Simon P. Hullihen (1810–1857). Although perhaps more known for his jaw surgeries, Hullihen also contributed to the evolution of tooth removal with his innovations in equipment design. He also made dental extractions a part of his practice as noted in his article "Odontalgia: Observations on Toothache" printed in the American Journal of Dental Science (Hullihen 1839; Armbrecht 1937).

5 Twentieth-Century Notables

The twentieth century was led off by the first text totally dedicated to the removal of teeth, *Exodontia*, published in 1913, by George B. Winter. At that time, he coined the terms "exodontia" and "exodontist." In 1926, Winter published the definitive text on the removal of a single tooth, the *Impacted Third Molar*, which provided one of the commonly used classification systems still in use today (Rounds and Rounds 1953, p. 25).

The other well-known impacted third molar classification system currently in use is the Pell and Gregory Classification System. This method was published in the Dental Digest in 1933. Though other classification systems have been developed over the past few decades, the Winter's and Pell and Gregory Classification Systems remain and are known worldwide (Pell and Gregory 1933).

For many centuries, teeth were removed primarily for the relief of pain and infection. Most techniques for tooth removal were still fraught with traumatic injuries during the surgery. As indications for the removal of teeth changed, a less traumatic means for tooth extraction was required. The use of the mallet and chisel was described by Boyd Gardner, in 1911, for the removal of normally placed as well as mispositioned and impacted teeth. Gardner felt this technique was safe and effective even in the hands of less experienced operators. The use of a mallet and chisel allowed the removal of a tooth in its entirety with a minimal amount of trauma (Gardner 1921).

The increase in the removal of impacted third molar teeth furthered necessitated a safe and predictable surgical technique. Although the dental drill has a long history, many of the earliest surgical techniques were based on the use of the mallet and chisel. In Pell and Gregory's 1933 paper, they described the use of a chisel to split the impacted third molar into several pieces depending on the angulation of the tooth (Pell and Gregory 1933). This technique saw a resurgence during the Covid-19 era with the current concern about aerosolization caused by high-speed rotary instruments. It is a useful technique to know for those practitioners providing care in remote third world areas where resources are very limited.

Another method for impacted third molar removal using a chisel is the split bone technique popularized in England. This method was introduced and taught by Sir William Kelsey Fry and subsequently published by Terrence Ward in 1956. This technique involves the removal of the mandibular lingual plate to deliver the impacted tooth (Ward 1956).

Most oral surgeons utilize high-speed rotary instruments for the removal of bone and the sectioning of teeth. One of the early proponents for the use of the dental drill for removal of impacted teeth was Wilton Cogswell. His book *Dental Oral* Surgery was published in 1932. In it, he described sectioning teeth into multiple pieces based on the position of the impacted teeth when only a belt-driven engine and steel burs were available (Nassimbene 2011). Cogswell's descriptions of tooth sectioning techniques still apply today. Through his extensive international lecturing and live training with the use of over 200 wax models he had created, he influenced later generations of surgeons in the techniques used by most surgeons today to extract teeth. This includes our lead author (MTG), who subsequently taught this technique like many others to their trainees.

Surgical techniques have been refined but are essentially the same as advocated by Pell and Gregory and Cogswell. Improvements in radiographic imaging has allowed improved assessment and risk/complication predictions. The techniques and instrumentation have become more refined especially with the current goal of replacing teeth with dental implants and the need to preserve bone.

6 Summary

The extraction of teeth is most likely the earliest surgical procedure performed by humankind dating back to the Stone Age. Although performed primarily for the relief of pain, extractions also contributed to aesthetics and cultural norms. Many of the current surgical instruments utilized today have a fundamental design dating back thousands of years. Prominent physicians and dentists over the years have refined the indications and techniques for the removal of teeth. This includes the removal of impacted teeth including third molars. A review of history should always be conducted before declaring something is "new."

References

Anonymous. The dental art in ancient times, American Medical Association lecture memoranda. London: Burrough's Wellcome and Co.; 1914.

Armbrecht EC. Hullihen, the Oral Surgeon. Int J Orthod Oral Surg. 1937;23(5):511–4.

Atkinson H. Some early dental extraction instruments including the pelican, bird or axe? Aust Dent J. 2002;47(2):90–3.

Bennion E. Antique dental instruments. 1st ed. New York: Harper & Row; 1986. p. 32.

Bremner M. The story of dentistry. 3rd ed. Brooklyn: Dental Items of Interest Publishing Co.; 1954.

Bussell M, Graham R. The history of commonly used dental elevators. Br Dent J. 2008;205(9):506–8.

Clark JH. Toothache and death. J Hist Dent. 1999;47(1):11–3.

Coppa A, et al. Early Neolithic tradition of dentistry. Nature. 2006;440(6):755.

De Groote I, Humphrey L. Characteristic evulsion in the later stone age Maghreb: age, sex, and effects in mastication. Quat Int. 2016;413:50–61.

Forshaw R. The practice of dentistry in ancient Egypt. Br Dent J. 2009;206(9):481–6.

Garant P. The long climb: from barber-surgeons to doctors of; dental surgery. 1st ed. Hanover Park: Quintessence Publishing Co.; 2013. p. 17–8.

Gardner BS. The use of the chisel and mallet in the extraction of teeth. Int J Orthod Oral Surg. 1921;7(3):145–51.

Guerini V. History of dentistry from the most ancient times until the end of the eighteenth century. 1st ed. Philadelphia: Lea & Febiger; 1909.

Hoffmann-Axthelm W. History of dentistry. 1st ed. Chicago: Quintessence Publishing Co; 1981a. p. 327.

Hoffmann-Axthelm W. History of dentistry (trans: Koehler). Chicago: Quintessence Publishing Co; 1981b. p. 21.

Hullihen SP. Odontalgia: observations on tooth-ache. Am J Dent Sci. 1839;1(5):105–11.

Hussain A, Kahn FA. History of dentistry. Arch Med Health Sci. 2014;2(1):106–10.

Kravetz R. A look back: tooth key. Am J Gastroenterol. 2003;98(11):2561–2.

Leek F. The practice of dentistry in ancient Egypt. J Egypt Archaeol. 1967;54:51–8.

López-Valverde A, De Vicente J, Cutando A. The surgeons Halsted and Hall, cocaine and the discovery of the dental anesthesia by nerve block. Br Dent J. 2011;211(10):485–7.

Nassimbene L. History of oral surgery in Colorado. 1st ed. Colorado Springs: Mountain Express Printing; 2011. p. 45.

Oxilia G, et al. Earliest evidence of dental caries manipulation in the late upper Palaeolithic. Sci Rep. 2015;5(1):1–10. https://doi.org/10.1038/sre12150.

Oxilia G, et al. The dawn of dentistry in the late upper Paleolithic: an early case of pathological intervention at Riparo Fredian. Am J Phys Anthropol. 2017;163:446–61.

Pell GJ, Gregory GT. Impacted third molars: classification and modified technique for removal. Dent Dig. 1933;39(9):325–38.

Ring M. Dentistry an illustrated history. 1st ed. St. Louis: C V Mosby; 1985.

Rounds FW, Rounds CE. Principles and techniques of exodontia. 1st ed. St Louis: CV Mosby; 1953.

Sheikh NK, Dua A. Procaine [updated 2020 Oct 11]. In: StatPearls [Internet]. Treasure Island: StarPearls Publishing; 2020. Available from: https://www.ncbi.nlm.nih.gov/books/NBK551666/.

Ward TG. The split bone technique for the removal of lower third molars. Br Dent J. 1956;101:297–304.
Willman J, Shackelford L, Demeter F. Incisor ablation among the late upper Paleolithic people of Tam Hanh (Northern Laos): social identity, mortuary practice, and oral health. Am J Phys Anthropol. 2016;160:519–28.
Wynbrandt J. The excruciating history of dentistry. 1st ed. New York: St. Martin's Press; 1998.
Zampetti P, Riva M. Giovani of Arcoli. Br Dent J. 2020;228(4):227.

Dental Implants and Bone Augmentation

Steven Halepas, Kenneth MacCormac, and Elie M. Ferneini

1 Introduction

Humans have waged a long battle against edentulism. Ancient history is poorly documented in the scientific literature. A simple Google search supplies tales of the earliest evidence of tooth replacement that is suspected to begin in 2000 BCE when bamboo was carved into peg teeth and used as replacement in edentulous sites (López-Píriz et al. 2019). A millennium later, a copper peg was hammered into the upper jaw of an Egyptian king (Smith 2019). It is unknown, however, whether the tooth was replaced during life or postmortem. In 500 BCE, Hippocrates wrote about using artificial teeth bonded with gold or silk. Archaeological excavations in France have uncovered a Celtic grave with a fake tooth composed of iron that is believed to have originated from approximately 300 BCE (Smith 2019). Archeologists have found many ancient civilizations with evidence of such tooth replacements made from ivory, metals, and the teeth of other animals. Most scholars believe that these replacements occurred postmortem as these implants would have likely had early

S. Halepas (✉)
Division of Oral and Maxillofacial Surgery, NewYork-Presbyterian/Columbia University Irving Medical Center, New York, NY, USA
e-mail: sh3808@cumc.columbia.edu

K. MacCormac
Division of Oral and Maxillofacial Surgery, University of Connecticut, Farmington, CT, USA

E. M. Ferneini
Division of Oral and Maxillofacial Surgery, University of Connecticut, Farmington, CT, USA

Beau Visage Med Spa and Greater Waterbury OMS, Cheshire, CT, USA

Department of Surgery, Frank H Netter MD School of Medicine, Quinnipiac University, North Haven, CT, USA

E. M. Ferneini et al. (eds.), *The History of Maxillofacial Surgery*,
https://doi.org/10.1007/978-3-030-89563-1_10

failure. In the first century CE, Aulus Cornelius Celsus mentioned the possibility of replacing missing teeth with cadaver teeth. The collections of the Peabody Museum of Archaeology and Ethnology at Harvard University include a Mayan mandible dated to the seventh to eighth CE in which three shell pieces were used as lower incisor replacements (Pasqualini and Pasqualini 2009; Bobbio 1972).

The earliest evidence of attempted bone repair with a foreign material comes from the Neolithic period between 10,000 and 4500 BCE. The skull of an ancient Peruvian tribal chief was discovered with a large frontal bone defect that was repaired with an implanted hammered gold plate (Pryor et al. 2009). While this may seem quite primitive by modern standards, the Neolithic period is known widely for the development of metallurgy and directly preceded the Bronze and Iron ages, so this approach would have represented the absolute forefront of medical technology (Lubbock 1865).

Jumping forward to 2000 BCE, we see the first example of a xenograft from the ancient Khurtis people that inhabited modern Armenia. The anthropologist A. Jagharian, former head of operative surgery at the Erivan Medical Institute in Armenia, discovered two skulls with evidence of attempted grafting not far from Lake Sevan (Pryor et al. 2009). One of the skulls showed a 7 mm traumatic injury repaired with a single piece of animal bone. We can tell several millennia later that the patient survived this procedure for several years afterward because the cranium demonstrated signs of regrowth surrounding the grafted material (Pryor et al. 2009). The second skull discovered by Jagharian demonstrated a similar repair of a smaller 2.5 mm defect caused by a sharpened instrument (Pryor et al. 2009). Unfortunately, these finds predate reliable archival documentation by several thousand years. Therefore, it is impossible to get a sense of whether these procedures were commonplace or one-off experiments. Thankfully, much of the early history of dental implants has been described elsewhere in the literature. The authors implore you to explore the wonderful work of Ugo Pasqualini and Marco Pasqualini entitled "Treatise of Dental Implant Dentistry: The Italian Tribute to Modern Implantology (Pasqualini and Pasqualini 2009)." As an entire textbook can and has been devoted to this subject, the authors herein will attempt to highlight some of the monumental work that allowed for the development of modern implantology.

Several centuries after the collapse of the Mayan civilization, many scholars during the European Renaissance advocated for the splinting of lost teeth to adjacent teeth using wire or thread. Pierre Fauchard, considered to be one of the founders of dentistry, reported several cases of replantation and transplantation of teeth (Pasqualini and Pasqualini 2009). The idea of replantation of natural teeth occurred through the 1700s, until 1806 when Giuseppangelo Fonzi invented the first porcelain tooth (Anonymous 1968). Maggiolo then introduced the use of gold in the shape of tooth roots, stating that it added stability when stabilizing to adjacent teeth (Maggiolo 1809; Tanunja 2018). The use of metals for implantation into extraction sockets became widespread during the nineteenth century. It is believed that in the 1840s, Chapin Harris and Horace Hayden, founders of the Baltimore College of

Dental Surgery, attempted implants with lead-coated platinum posts into artificial sockets. Others in the United States tried different metals including lead, gold, silver, platinum, and nickel (Pasqualini and Pasqualini 2009).

2 Implants in the Early Twentieth Century

The central focus of this chapter is the beginning of the twentieth century, during which procedures that resemble the modern implant began to emerge. Advancements in implantology during this period primarily occurred through two avenues. The first was new understanding in dental and osseous materials, and the second was biomechanical principles and the refinement of the implant shape. In 1913, Greenfield developed an endosseous hollow-cylinder basket shape implant made of iridium and gold soldering as artificial roots (Greenfield 2008; Block 2018a). He presented the stepwise use of drills increasing diameters that is still practiced today. These implants were used as a single tooth replacement. In the 1930s, Drs. Alvin and Moses Strock were researching the Vitallium® orthopedic screw fixtures used in hips. They used this metal to place a series of implants for teeth in animals and humans at Harvard. Vitallium is a cobalt-chrome-molybdenum alloy (originally manufactured by Howmedica Osteonics Corporation, now Stryker, Mathway, NJ) that was fabricated into a threaded design and placed as an immediate implant. In 1938, Adams developed and patented a submergible threaded cylindrical implant with a smooth gingival portion and healing abutment. The prosthetic used was a ball-hitch design for an overdenture (Burch 1997). Many new designs were fabricated at this time, many of which mirrored the typical wood screw with a helical thread pattern. Implants were typically a solid screw or hollow basket design composed of different alloy materials that result in a fibrous implant interface (Linkow 1966).

Prior to the hypothesis of osseointegration, implants used a fibrous-osseous integration system, which at the time was believed to be the ideal circumstance for stability of the prosthesis. It was not until the concept of osseointegration or direct integration of the bone to the metal that changed this fundamental thinking. In 1924, Zierold researched the reaction of different metals in dogs (Zierold 1924). Some of his observations were "gold, aluminum, and stellite were readily tolerated by bone and tended to be encapsulated with fibrous tissue; they were inert materials, unaffected by the living cells and body fluids; (2) silver and lead were slightly less tolerable to bone, but they easily underwent corrosion, and created a greater connective tissue response; (3) zinc corroded easily and caused a slight connective tissue reaction; (4) copper caused definite stimulation of bone, although it underwent slow corrosion; (5) steel and iron definitely inhibited bone regeneration and steel readily underwent corrosion (Rudy et al. 2008)." The search of the perfect biocompatible material continued. In 1940, the concept of osseointegration, specifically titanium, was first described by Bothe et al. in Great Britain (Bothe et al. 1940; Jokstad 2017).

Later, a researcher in the United States reaffirmed this proposition stating, "since titanium adheres to bone, it may prove to be an ideal metal for prosthesis (Leventhal 1951)." In the same year, Dahl invented the subperiosteal implant design (Linkow and Dorfman 1991).

Linkow reported on the blade implant in 1968 (Linkow 1966). Prior to this, vertical post-type implants with spiral shafts, vents, and pins were primarily used as anchors for prosthetic support. Linkow noted difficulties with knife-edge ridges in terms of placement and resorption. This observation led to the idea of thin blades of larger anterior-posterior length rather than diameter. These were preformed after raising full-thickness flaps, exposing all the bone. High-speed drills were used to create channels, and the blades were tapped into the final position. Blade implants were used with some initial success. Linkow stated the blade implants formed a fibro-osseous integration that he believed was like the periodontal ligament of teeth from a histological perspective (Linkow and Rinaldi 1987).

In the mid-1970s, trans-osseous implants were used for overdentures in the anterior mandible. Kent et al. reported on the use of a mandibular staple bone plate to support a dental prosthesis through an extraoral incision in the submental parasymphysis region from the late 1970s. The plate was made from a titanium alloy (6% aluminum and 4% vanadium). They reported promising results in terms of stability in 160 patients. Bosker and van Dijk subsequently reported on 368 patients who underwent the procedure, 43 had reversible complications, and 1 had unilateral hypesthesia (Bosker and van Dijk 1989). The disadvantages to this approach were the extraoral incision, the need for general anesthesia, and less than ideal gingival implant interface.

In 1978, the National Institutes of Health (NIH) held a Dental Implant Consensus Conference in Boston, Massachusetts, with the Harvard Tooth Implant-Transplant Research Unit at the School of Dental Medicine (Anonymous 1978). At this point, thousands of patients had been treated with dental implants for years. While many had been successful, many others had early failures and complications. The American Dental Association (ADA) had developed an implant registry to establish uniform case reports. The Food and Drug Administration (FDA) had begun to implement standards, classifications, and limitations on medical devices including implants. The panel described success as "functional service for five years in 75% of the cases." The subject criteria for success included "adequate function, absence of discomfort, improved aesthetics, and improved emotional and psychological attitude." The conference reported statistics on subperiosteal, transosteal, blade, and staple implants (Fig. 1). Ultimately, the conference identified the need for clinical trials to determine the best protocols for dental implants.

Professor George Zarb in Toronto, Canada, recognized the need for the continued clinical research expressed in the 1978 NIH conference. Notably, titanium was not even mentioned at this 1978 conference. In 1982, the first Toronto Osseointegration Conference was held. It was the first opportunity for the most prominent prosthodontic and oral and maxillofacial surgery community in North America to come and learn from the most prominent dental implant researchers in the world at the time (Jokstad 2008). Among them was Dr. Brånemark and his research team.

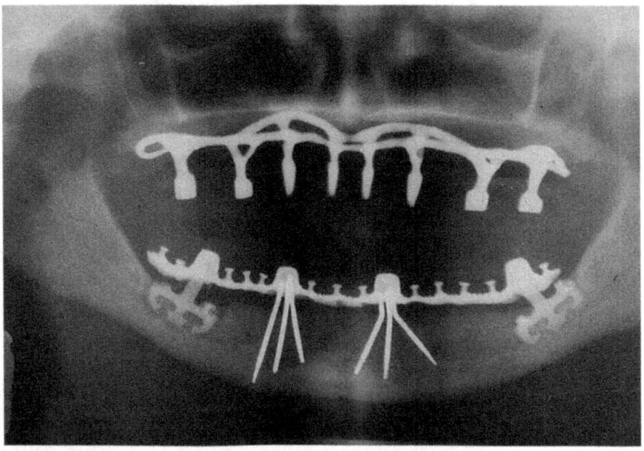

Fig. 1 The X-ray controlling from 1976 to 1977 shows a subperiosteal implant (according to Cherchéve) in the maxilla. Two implant tripods (according to Pruin) in the lower canine region and two stabilized blade implants (according to Heinrich) in the molar region. (Image from Wikimedia commons. Public domain image. Reproduced without alterations. https://commons.wikimedia.org/w/index.php?search=blade+implants&title=Special:Search&go=Go&ns0=1&ns6=1&ns12=1&ns14=1&ns100=1&ns106=1#/media/File:Panoramic_radiograph_of_historic_dental_implants.jpg. This image is licensed under the Creative Commons Attribution-Share Alike 3.0 Unported license. https://creativecommons.org/licenses/by-sa/3.0/deed.en. CC BY-SA 3.0)

3 Brånemark and the Foundations of Modern Implantology

The development of the dental implant relied heavily on the progression of various businesses throughout the second half of the twentieth century. Many different companies played important roles. While it would be too time-consuming to discuss the history of every business in the industry, we would be remiss not to include the contributions of Straumann and Nobel BioCare due to the contributions of Drs. Brånemark and Straumann. Reinhard Straumann founded the research institute Dr. Ing R. Straumann AG in Waldenburg, Germany, in 1954. In 1981, Professor Brånemark and the Swedish company Bofors cofounded Nobelpharma which later became Nobel Biocare in 1996.

It was not until 1982 that Per-Ingvar Brånemark, MD, PhD, introduced the titanium osseointegration implant to North America (Fig. 2). Professor Brånemark was a physician and anatomist in Sweden who discovered the concept of osseointegration in 1952 while studying blood flow in rabbit bone. He placed a titanium-housed optical component to a rabbit's leg which allowed him to study the bones microcirculation (Fig. 3) (Brånemark 1983). After the completion of the study, he found he was unable to remove the device. He noted that titanium components can bond irreversibly with bone. This resulted in a pivotal movement in his team's work, which quickly identified the value of titanium in this context.

Brånemark was not the first to propose that titanium was a suitable biomaterial for implantation in bone. Biological researchers in dentistry and medicine, including Beder, Ploger, Emneus, and Stenram, were some of Professor Brånemark's

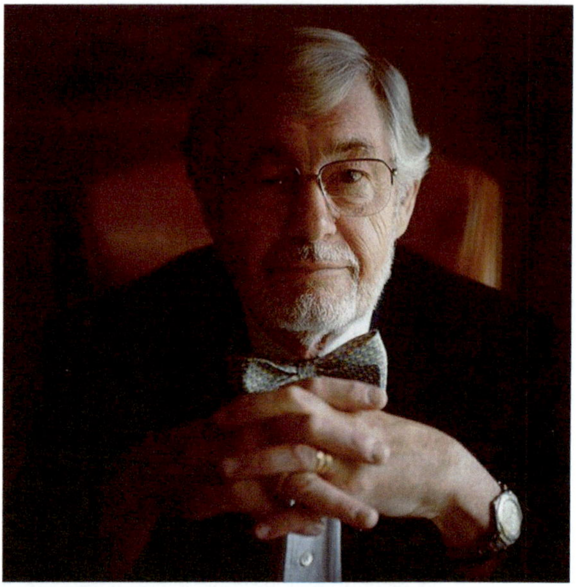

Fig. 2 Photograph of Professor Brånemark in June 2013. (Image from Wikimedia commons. Public domain image. Reproduced without alterations. https://commons.wikimedia.org/wiki/File:Branemark_headshot2. This image is licensed under the Creative Commons Attribution-Share Alike 3.0 Unported license. https://creativecommons.org/licenses/by-sa/3.0/deed.en. CC BY-SA 3.0)

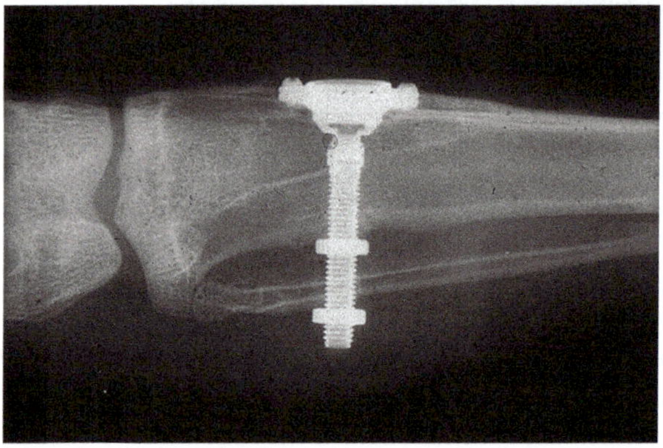

Fig. 3 Radiograph of Per-Ingvar Brånemark's rabbit specimen, showing a titanium optic chamber fixed to the rabbit's tibia and fibula. (Image from Wikimedia commons. Public domain image. Reproduced without alterations. https://upload.wikimedia.org/wikipedia/commons/4/47/Branemark%27s_initial_radiograph.jpg. This image is licensed under the Creative Commons Attribution-Share Alike 3.0 Unported license. https://creativecommons.org/licenses/by-sa/3.0/deed.en. CC BY-SA 3.0)

early mentors who demonstrated that bone tolerated implanted titanium well (Emneus and Stenram 1960; Beder and Ploger 1959). "A simple search for titanium on PubMed generates some 350 papers published before December 31, 1970 (Jokstad 2017)." But while his background was in orthopedics and anatomy, he saw the immense opportunity in dental implants. His group extracted teeth in dogs and replaced them by screw-shaped titanium implants. The implants were allowed to heal under a mucoperiosteal flap. Fixed prosthesis was connected after 3 to 4 months without loading. Radiological and histological analyses of the anchoring tissues showed integration at 10 years (Brånemark 1983). In 1977, Brånemark et al. reported on the osseointegration system for clinical jaw reconstruction using titanium-based implants (Brånemark et al. 1977). In 1983, they published a 5- to 9-year success rate of 3000 osteointegrated implants inserted into edentulous jaws of 400 consecutive patients in Gothenburg, Sweden (Brånemark et al. 1983). Two revelations were noted at this time. The first is the concept of osseointegration between the implant and the bone. The second was the establishment of a biological seal around the abutments penetrating the soft tissue, thus decreasing the inflammatory reaction. In 1974, Straumann engineered the first titanium hollow cylinder implant (Sutter et al. 1983). In 1997, NobelReplace released the first tapered dental implant designs, a design that better mimics tooth root morphology.

Brånemark quickly understood the issue with successive bone loss over time as well as the issue of inadequate bone for implant placement. In 1984, he and his colleagues reported on osseointegrated implants penetrating the maxillary sinus. They first conducted an experimental study in dogs and later a clinical study in humans. A total of 139 implants were placed that pierced the sinus or nasal cavity in 101 patients. At 5- to 10-year follow-up, the success rate was 70% in sinus-penetrating implants and 72% in nasal bone/mucosa implants (Brånemark et al. 1984). In 1988, Smalley et al. with the aid of Brånemark published on osseointegrated titanium implants in the maxilla, zygomatic, frontal, and occipital bones for maxillofacial protraction in *Macaca nemestrina* monkeys (Smalley et al. 1988). While this was monumental in the world of orthodontics in terms of eliciting skeletal changes, it was also the foundation for zygomatic implants in dental rehabilitation in the atrophic maxilla. The 1990s saw the use of maxillofacial implants for various reconstructions of the skeletal complex after trauma or ablative therapy.

Many important advancements occurred in the 1990s that allowed for further work with zygomatic implants. In 1995, Brånemark et al. described 156 edentulous patients who were fully rehabilitated by fixed prosthesis with either four or six titanium implants. After 3–4 months in the mandible and 5–8 months in the maxilla, abutments were placed, and prostheses were fabricated. This landmark study was the cornerstone for modern full-arch dental rehabilitation concepts we use today (Brånemark et al. 1995). Two years later, Tarnow et al. reported on immediate loading of threaded implants in 10 patients. Of 69 implants that were loaded, 67 integrated. Six patients were treated with Nobel Biocare implants, one with ITI Bonefit, two with Astra Tech TiOblast implants, and one with 3i implants (Tarnow et al. 1997). This was groundbreaking evidence as up until this point, Adell and Brånemark had maintained that a prerequisite for successful osseointegration was a non-loaded environment. The ITI® (International Team for Implantology by Straumann) released the SLA (sandblasted, large grit, acid-etched) surface implant in June 1998, increasing our understanding of osseointegration and implant success (Scacchi et al. 2000).

In the search for a suitable esthetic fixed prostheses supported by dental implants, Fortin et al. described the Marius bridge in 2002 (Fortin et al. 2002). The Marius bridge was named after the first patient treated with this prosthesis. The implants were placed between 1991 and 1994, and the bridge restorations were placed in patients between 1993 and 1995 and followed for a period of 5 years. The process required utilization of the concept of anterior-posterior spread, a fundamental principle in 2020. The authors noted that moderate to severely resorbed maxilla often have too thin of bone to allow vertical placement of implants, specifically in the posterior region. The authors used tilted implants to overcome this obstacle. It is a principle that will be carried forward over the next two decades. The "All-on-Four" concept was first learned in 1998 with Maló, Rangert, and Nobre in collaboration with Nobel Biocare. In 2003, Maló et al. described in the literature the use of the "All-on-Four" immediate function with the Brånemark System for complete edentulous maxillae with a 1-year follow-up in 32 patients. They used both straight and angulated (17° and 30°) implants with Brånemark System multiunit abutments. Immediate provisional complete arch acrylic prostheses were delivered the day of the surgery, and a final prosthetic was delivered at 12 months postoperatively (Maló et al. 2003).

Armed with information about immediate loading and anterior-posterior spread, tremendous advancements in zygomatic implants for dental rehabilitation were possible. Prior to this, implants in the maxillofacial complex were targeted for reconstruction of the skeletal structure rather than dental function. In 2000, Tamura et al. published a case report of zygomatic implants following subtotal maxillectomy with fabrication of a maxillary prosthesis (Tamura et al. 2000). In 2004, Brånemark et al. published on 52 zygomatic fixtures for the atrophic maxilla with an overall prosthetic rehabilitation rate of 96% after at least 5 years of function (Brånemark et al. 2004). Two years later, Anlgren et al. reported on 25 successful zygomatic implants placed from 199 to 2001, with an 11- to 49-month follow-up (Ahlgren et al. 2006). That same year, Bedrossian et al. described the immediate function with the zygomatic implants in 14 patients (28 bilateral zygomatic implants and 55 premaxillary implants) that supported an immediate fixed provisional prosthesis (Bedrossian et al. 2006).

The desire for flapless surgery and immediate loading accelerated the development of computer-aided treatment planning and fabrication of surgical stents and prosthesis. In 2005, NobelGuide was released by Nobel Biocare as one of the first guided surgery systems (Marchack 2005). In 2007, Bedrossian published a report on the use of NobelGuide for a computer-guided, implant-supported complete maxillary rehabilitation (Bedrossian 2007).

4 Bone Augmentation

The modern era of bone grafting began in the mid-seventeenth century with a Dutch surgeon named Job Van Meekeren. In 1668, Van Meekeren performed the first heterologous grafting procedure on an injured soldier (de Boer 1988). He used a fragment of dog bone to repair a skull puncture wound, and the procedure was successful overall (de Boer 1988). However, in the eyes of the Christian church at that time, the implantation of nonhuman tissues was considered blasphemous and resulted in the excommunication of the soldier from the church. After enduring the unfortunate consequences of excommunication from the permanent institution of the church, the soldier returned to Van Meekeren to have the dog bone fragment removed so he could be readmitted to the church. Unfortunately for the soldier, upon reentering the site of the graft, Van Meekeren discovered that the fragment had completely incorporated into the surrounding tissues (de Boer 1988).

In the late seventeenth and early eighteenth centuries, orthopedic surgeons began to focus their research efforts on the microscopic structure of bone aided by advances in microscope technology. The earliest of descriptions of the microscopic anatomy of bone came from Antonie van Leeuwenhoek. In 1674, van Leeuwenhoek published the first description of the canal-based structure of cancellous bone and also began to define the terms "implant," "resorption," and "bone callus" (de Boer 1988). This foundational work opened the door for later research advances in bone physiology and grafting. The discoveries and descriptions provided by van Leeuwenhoek's publications started an era of intense debate over the origins of osteogenic potential in bone. In 1739, Henri-Louis Duhamel performed an animal experiment in which he implanted silver wires beneath the periosteum and allowed the surgical wound to heal for several weeks before reentering the site (Hernigou 2015). When he observed the wires several weeks later, he discovered that they had become buried in bone (Hernigou 2015). Duhamel used these experimental results and repeated the experiments of some of his predecessors to validate his assertion that the periosteum had osteogenic potential (Hernigou 2015).

Duhamel's publications were met with mixed reception by his contemporaries. His biggest opponent, Albrecht Von Haller, believed instead that the periosteum was merely a support system for the blood vessels and that exudation from blood vessels was the true cause of osteogenesis (Hernigou 2015). In 1763, Von Haller published his book *Experimentorum de Ossium Formatione* in which he elaborated on the idea that blood vessels carried the mineral elements required for osteogenesis and therefore were the major source of osteogenic potential. At the time, this was an extremely controversial notion. The feud between the two men, who represented the two leading theories of the era, became notorious enough that it came to be known as "Duhamel-Haller Controversy" (Hernigou 2015). Unfortunately, neither of the two men would live to see the dispute settled. Jean Pierre Marie Flourens went a long way in settling this controversy when he conclusively showed in his 1842 publication that periosteum was osteogenic and was the chief agent in healing and repair of bone defects (Hernigou 2015).

Surgeons did not stand idle awaiting the resolution of academic conflicts and chose to forge ahead with experimental procedures. In 1820, the German surgeon Phillips Von Walters described the first use of a bone autograph (Henkel et al. 2013). Walters successfully repaired trepanation holes – created during a procedure to relieve intracranial pressure – with pieces of bone harvested from other sites on the patient's skull (Henkel et al. 2013).

Advances in both bone biology and bone grafting technology in the mid-nineteenth century were dominated by Louis Léopold Ollier. Ollier was a French surgeon who began his career as a botanist and closely studied the microscopic organization of tree bark, which perhaps sparked his eventual interest in periosteum (Donati et al. 2007). In 1858, Ollier took the first scientific experimental approach to solve the riddle of osteogenesis. Despite a lack of sterile surgical technique or modern histological tools, Ollier made several discoveries and is credited with the first use of the term "bone graft" in an 1861 publication (Donati et al. 2007). He determined that transplanted bone and periosteum survived and became osteogenic if given the proper conditions. In a textbook published in 1867, Ollier noted that periosteum-coated grafts were best for transplanting and further stated that the contents of the haversian canals and the endosteum were also osteogenic (Hernigou 2015).

These assertions were considered and incorporated into cutting-edge subperiosteal and subcapsular surgical excision techniques, which became the standard of care in the treatment of bony malunion secondary to traumatic fracture (Hernigou 2015). At this time, malunion was commonly treated with large resections or even amputations. Therefore, the subperiosteal resection technique offered another means to achieve bone healing and avoid amputation. These contributions earned Ollier the Great Prize for Surgery established by Napoleon III. Despite being widely considered an authority in the field by his colleagues and contemporaries, Ollier's publications were not without dissenters (Donati et al. 2007). In the late 1800s, Arthur Barth, a German surgeon, began publishing the findings of his own experiments in which he directly refuted the claim that the graft survived past the first few days of implantation. Barth asserted that the implanted material underwent gradual necrotic change (Henkel et al. 2013). He used rabbit and dog models to show that dead graft material was resorbed and replaced by native tissues (Henkel et al. 2013). This difference of opinions was one of the innumerable scientific feuds that would not be resolved until after the time of both Ollier and Barth.

Around 1885, Ollier began to revisit some of his earlier experiments in xenografting. With the emergence of sterile surgical technique in the mid-1860s, he was curious to see if new sterilization protocols would improve the outcomes of some of his earlier failures (Hernigou 2015). Grafts were found to experience less morbidity when the recipient [rabbit or cat] was from a higher species and the donor [chicken] was a member of a less advanced species (Hernigou 2015). Ollier was also able to successfully graft from one mammal to another; however, he noted that over time, the graft material would disappear. He further noted that there was no guarantee of a graft taking in a human recipient unless the donor material had come from a very closely related species, such as monkeys, and even in that case, the graft only provided transient benefit (Hernigou 2015). With this in mind, Ollier concluded that homographs and autographs were the most reliable options to repair bony defects with the limitation of technology.

Despite focused research efforts from Ollier and his contemporaries, use of non-autologous grafts in human patients were seriously considered until late in the nineteenth century. The reason is not exactly clear; perhaps there were some religious or moral concerns stemming from the experience of Van Meekeren a few centuries earlier. In 1880, the Scottish surgeon William Macewen pushed the field into the modern era when he published his case report from 1879, in which tibial bone from one child infected with rickets was grafted into the heavily deformed humerus of another child that had been resected secondary to osteomyelitis (Hernigou 2015). This represented the first successful documented bone allograft in a human. The achievement effectively opened up a new field in bone surgery. In the years that followed this initial success, Macewen would earn further recognition by being the first surgeon to repair a mandibular defect with bone harvested from the ribs (de Boer 1988).

Abel M. Phelps was another important contributor to the early development of bone grafting technology. In 1891, he published a landmark case report of a young man with ununited leg fractures who has undergone several previous surgeries with minimal success. Phelps was initially reluctant to continue attempting surgical repair; however, sensing the desperation of the patient's parents to avoid amputation, he agreed to try one last-resort measure (Hernigou 2015). Phelps transplanted a portion of bone from the foreleg of a dog into the leg of his patient. Both donor and host were left attached to each other for 2 weeks to maintain circulation to the graft. Phelps believed that leaving the vascular supply of the graft intact would initiate the growth of new bone in the boy's limb (Hernigou 2015). About 15 days after the graft, the patients were separated, and Phelps noted that the boy's bone graft had become irregularly covered in new bone. Both patients had a brief convalescence after the operation (Hernigou 2015). Phelps claimed no specific references when asked how he planned and designed the procedure. Instead, he said that "observation in my studies during the past two years convinced me that circulation between two opposite species could be established with safety" (Hernigou 2015). While the procedure was ultimately a failure, it still represents a landmark in the overall field as it was the first example of a vascularized flap used in a human patient. Abel Phelps' meticulous documentation of his procedure, observations, and insightful commentary on possible reasons for his failure allowed even his unsuccessful work to become a stepping stone and invaluable training resource for the surgeons and researchers that would follow.

The early twentieth century saw a new group of researchers such as Putti, Phemister, and Albee rise to the forefront of bone grafting research and publication. In 1912, Vittorio Putti, an Italian orthopedic surgeon, published a review of the state-of-the-art research in the field of bone grafting and biology at the time. He reviewed the work of previous authors, his contemporaries, and combined this information with his own personal clinical experience and observations to elucidate some generalized clinical indications for the use of bone grafts (Donati et al. 2007). Putti also proposed a bone-lengthening technique, which is now called distraction osteogenesis, and suggested novel uses of bone grafts such as grafting growth-plate cartilage into adult patients (Donati et al. 2007). This report represented a unification and clarification of many emerging principles of the era and formed the foundation of much of the progress to follow.

In 1914, Dallas Burton Phemister performed several experiments in dogs to further investigate osteogenesis. Earlier works had heavily debated the osteogenic potential of the graft itself. There was ongoing disagreement about whether grafts integrated via osteogenesis or if the existing donor tissue was responsible for integration (Donati et al. 2007). Phemister took a big step in introducing the modern concept of bone resorption when he described a phenomenon he called "creeping substitution" (Donati et al. 2007). He went further to say that the amount of time a graft needed to complete its resorption was anywhere from 3 to 12 months depending on the size, thickness, and location of the graft (Donati et al. 2007). He explained how the proximity of the endosteum and periosteum to adequate blood supply would allow those tissues to survive, while the relative lack of circulation of the deeper portions of the graft would cause cellular necrosis and resorption of the inorganic portion of the cellular matrix (Hernigou 2015). Phemister's 1914 publication would become one of the most frequently cited English works in the field. This authoritative publication was followed by an almost equally important work from FH Albee. Albee published his "Rules for Using Bone Grafts" in 1915 which described data from his own surgeries on various autologous bone harvesting sites such as the iliac crest, trochanter, tibia, metatarsal, olecranon, fibula, and cranium (Albee 1923).

By the mid-1940s, autologous and homologous bone grafting had become widely used procedures. Alberto Inclan published an article in the Journal of Bone and Joint Surgery in 1942 in which he presented the outcomes of a large number of his cases and discussed the common issues of the current technology (Inclan 1942). At that time, medical science was beginning to understand the immunological challenges related to homologous grafts. Inclan discussed that a homologous graft between two living patients of the same blood group was possible, albeit inconvenient at times. He and his colleagues began to hint at the modern concept of storing bone material for future use (Donati et al. 2007). In his 1942 publication, Inclan began to outline a storage protocol for bone grafts. He wrote that grafts should be kept immersed in the donor or host's blood within a sterile glass container in a refrigerated environment between 2 and 5 °C (Donati et al. 2007). While the implementation of the modern bone bank would have to wait for improved refrigeration technology, the idea of uncoupling the harvesting and use of bone grafts was revolutionary for the time (Donati et al. 2007).

While many of the brightest and most influential minds of the scientific community were trying to define the best way to perform bone grafts using human tissues, an equally dedicated group was beginning to research alternative materials to replace bone. As early as 1892, Dressman was exploring the use of calcium sulfate (plaster of Paris) for the repair of large bony defects (Donati et al. 2007). In his 1912 publication, Putti also commented on the use of ivory as a possible bone substitute when harvesting adequate material from the donor or the host was not possible (Donati et al. 2007). However, many early bone substitutes at this time led to the same unfortunate outcome: infection, graft rejection, and, ultimately, failure of the procedure. Medical science would need to make several key advances before materials could be designed to avoid some of the pitfalls of their earlier predecessors.

Calcium orthophosphates were discovered and described as early as the 1770s. However, the use of materials such as hydroxyapatite (HA) in bone grafting studies only began to gain momentum in the 1950s (Kattimani et al. 2016). HA has properties that make it nonreactive with the adjacent living tissues. For that reason, it remains one of the more popular materials that accounts for a large quantity of the regenerative graft materials available today (Kattimani et al. 2016). HA-based grafting materials were truly revolutionary for the field of bone grafting overall. These materials gave rise to what would later be called the first generation of biomaterials (Hench and Thompson 2010). Professor Bill Bonfield, a medical materials researcher at Cambridge University, was one of the pioneers whose research efforts led to the widespread incorporation of bioactivity as a consideration in the design of new materials and allowed the acceleration of the field from the 1960s forward (Hench and Thompson 2010). During the 1960s and 1970s, the primary goal in the development of new grafting materials was to diminish the biological response to the foreign body (Hench and Thompson 2010). This was achieved by eliminating release of toxic by-products. These materials are called "bioinert" as they create no response in the surrounding tissues (Hench and Thompson 2010).

Despite the success of the first generation of biomaterials and the improvements they provided in the lives of millions of patients, Bonfield recognized the need for an improved generation of biomaterials. The 1980s saw the rise of the second-generation biomaterials, such as Hapex, a material trademarked by Bonfield's research laboratory (Hench and Thompson 2010). Second-generation biomaterials were designed to incorporate the concept of bioactivity, which aimed not only to closely mirror the architecture of native tissues and their mechanical properties but also to create a beneficial response in the tissues surrounding the graft (Hench and Thompson 2010). These innovative materials were composed of polymeric matrices of polyethylene with HA particles dispersed throughout. Bonfield continued designing and discovering new biomaterials, such as Si-substituted HA, which is still considered a successful bone grafting material (Hench and Thompson 2010). By the mid-1980s, bioactive bone grafting had reached clinical use in a variety of orthopedic and dental applications, largely thanks to the research and commercialization efforts of the Bonfield laboratory.

Second-generation biomaterials explored the utility of bioactivity and materials that were reliably and predictably resorbed by the host. These advances converged in the third generation of biomaterials starting in the 2000s (Hench and Thompson 2010). Now, resorbable polymer systems are being modified on the molecular level to elicit specific interactions with cellular integrins and thereby encouraging cellular differentiation and extracellular matrix production and organization (Hench and Thompson 2010). These materials generally fit into one of two categories: bioactive glass or hierarchical porous foams that activate genes in neighboring tissues and stimulate regeneration of living tissues (Hench and Thompson 2010).

The future of bone grafting materials is likely to be governed by two competing schools of thought. In one camp, there are materials designed for in situ tissue regeneration, and in the other, there is tissue engineering. The emerging field of tissue engineering aims to seed progenitor cells on molecularly modified scaffolds outside the body to allow the cells to become differentiated and mimic native tissues. Engineered tissues are then implanted to replace diseased or damaged tissues.

By contrast, in situ tissue regeneration materials aim to achieve the same result by implanting a material initially that will encourage the local tissue to regenerate or repair itself. The addition of these concepts to improving knowledge of immunology and endocrinology will lead to the emergence of new materials with multifaceted effects on regeneration and repair of local tissues.

5 Guided Bone Regeneration

Guided bone regeneration (GBR) procedures are dental surgical procedures which use a membrane to guide the growth of bone and gingival tissues in areas that may be lacking tissue for a variety of reasons. At present time, GBR is the intersection of bone grafting technology with clinical dentistry. The rising popularity of dental implants has driven interest in both the preservation and creation of bone as means of developing sites for later prostheses. In 1976, Dr. Tony Melcher began defining the basic principles and theories of GBR for use in dental applications (Melcher 1976). One of Melcher's largest contributions was his recognition of the importance of using implantable barriers to exclude unwanted cell lineages from prematurely colonizing graft material (Melcher 1976). The positive results of Melcher's studies up to the 1980s and their application to periodontics sparked interest in the study of rebuilding larger alveolar bone defects with guided bone regeneration. GBR was first attempted by Dahlin et al. in 1988 on rats. They found that if the bone was protected and kept away from adjacent tissues, via a membrane, there was improved ingrowth of bone-forming cells into a bony defect; this was confirmed in a study by Kostopoulos and Karring in 1994 (Kostopoulos and Karring 1994). Recent systematic review has shown that the outcomes following GTR are highly variable, both between and within studies, meaning that clinicians must still take great care in case selection to ensure the best possible outcomes (Needleman et al. 2006).

6 Sinus Lifts

The maxillary sinuses sometimes are in the way of placing maxillary posterior implants. The development of both dental implants and bone augmentation materials has allowed this procedure to develop and evolve. The first lateral window or direct sinus-lift procedure is credited to Dr. Hilt Tatum in 1973. Dr. Tatum graduated from the Emory University Dental School in 1957. He performed the first sinus graft in 1975 at Lee County Hospital in Opelika, Alabama. This was followed by successful placement of two implants. As many are aware, the sinus membrane is quite thin and easily damaged. Early on, the sinus elevation was done using inflatable catheters. Eventually, instruments were fabricated to better handle this delicate tissue. Dr. Tatum was presenting his findings at the American Academy of Implant

Dentistry in the late 1970s, and Dr. Philip Boyne was in attendance. Dr. Boyne and his colleague Dr. James would advance this technique and publish their methods in 1980 (Tatum Jr. 1986; Boyne and James 1980). Dr. Robert Summers is believed to have described first the internal/indirect sinus lift for sinuses that needed to be lifted less than 4 mm. This technique is accomplished by preforming the osteotomies with drills just shy of the sinus floor and using osteotomes to tap up the sinus floor leaving the membrane intact. Bone particulate graft is then placed to keep the sinus elevated, and the dental implants can be placed (Summers 1998). The lateral window for direct sinus lift is an invasive approach and may be falling out of favor. Dr. Block published a technique in 2019 describing a crestal window approach for direct sinus elevation with successful outcomes (Block 2018b). While sinus lift will likely always have some indications, with the use of smaller implants, this technique could become less utilized.

7 The Twenty-First Century

Recently, there has been a renewed interest in the use of platelet-rich plasma (PRP) and platelet-rich fibrin (PRF). Marx first described the use of PRP and PRF in the dental field in 1998, where he reported positive healing of the alveolar bone with its use (Marx et al. 1998). PRP is a concentration of platelet and plasma proteins derived from whole blood that is placed in a centrifuge to remove the red blood cells. PRP is believed to work via the degranulation of the alpha granules in platelets which contain several growth factors (Scully et al. 2018). PRP contains a variety of growth factors/cytokines such as transforming growth factor beta (TGF -beta), platelet-derived growth factor (PDGF), insulin-like growth factor (IGF), and epidermal growth factor (EGF).

A study performed using 72 dental implants in nine beagles dogs attempted to analyze the bone remodeling using PRP and PRF. After 3-month follow-up, the authors concluded that there was no increase in primary or secondary implant stability, but they did see a biological improvement in the peri-implant bone volume and structural integration (Huang et al. 2019). Although clinical effects have yet to be established, a biological effect is being consistently observed. In one in vitro study, in which roughened titanium dental implants were treated with PRP, the authors found that the number of cells observed around the implant at day 5 was double that of the non-PRP-coated implant (Lee et al. 2016). Research into the use of such biologics to increase osseointegration and soft tissue healing will likely continue over the next several decades. A randomized, split mouth design was conducted for eight patients who needed bilateral widening of keratinized mucosa around dental implants in the mandible. On one side of the mouth, a free gingival graft was placed, while on the other, a PRF membrane was placed. The mean amount of keratinized mucosa at the implant at the PRF-only site was 3.3 mm ± 0.9 and 3.8 mm ± 1.0 at the free gingival graft site (Temmerman et al. 2018). Now that integration of the implants is well established, the interest in dental implants have pivoted to longevity and precision. Soft tissue appears to be a key component in implant longevity and late failure.

One of the greatest advancements so far of the early twenty-first century was not so much in the dental materials but in treatment planning. Much of this is due to better data collection primarily from computer-aided technology such as cone beam computed tomography (CBCT), intraoral scanners, and treatment planning software allowing virtual planning and milling of surgical guides. The twentieth century had emphasis on getting stability and integration of the implant. The twenty-first century has been about placing the implants in the ideal location to allow for optimal dental prosthetic rehabilitation. When CBCTs first became available, radiographic stents with fiducial markers are needed to be used with the planning software that made its utilization cumbersome and required significant time by the provider. With the advancement of scanners and software, fiducial markers are no longer needed. Many companies have created user-friendly planning software to design implant treatment plans and seamlessly use 3D printing technology to make surgical stents. The use of a well-designed surgical stent results in less than 2 mm crestal and apical deviation and less than 5-degree angulation error (Block 2018a; Luebbers et al. 2008; Nijmeh et al. 2005; Ewers et al. 2005).

Dynamic navigation has become common practice in the operating room, especially in cancer ablative surgery, and in surgery with difficult access. Dynamic navigation uses the data from CT scans and optical sensors to track in live time where the surgeon's instruments are in relation to the patient's anatomical structures on the computer, allowing for more precision in operative technique. Dynamic navigation has found its way into the world of dental implants with companies such as X-Nav Technologies®. These systems have many advantages including more precision with smaller flap designs given the improved accuracy even with less surgical access.

8 Future Direction

The twentieth century revealed that titanium appears to be the metal most biocompatible with bone. The first two decades of the twenty-first century has seen refinement of titanium to increase success rates as well as escalate accuracy of placement and restorations. Sandblasting, acid etching, and other techniques to cause roughened surfaces of the titanium have allowed more successful bone-implant interfaces (Wennerberg et al. 2018). Companies like Straumann and Nobel Biocare are continuing to refine their implant systems. In 2020, it is well established that long-term implant survival relies on adjacent healthy soft tissue. Nobel Biocare has released the TiUltra, which has advanced the field from focusing strictly on the bone-implant interface to also incorporate the soft tissue-implant interface (Karl and Albrektsson 2017).

The future of tooth replacement is likely not in the world of implantology but in regeneration. While full summarization of the current knowledge of tooth regeneration is outside the scope of this chapter, the authors felt it was appropriate to address the path that tooth replacement will likely take. Through the understanding of odontogenesis, tooth regeneration can be divided into scaffold-based and scaffold-free models (Bhanja and D'Souza 2016). In 2002, Young et al. used a poly L-lactide-co-glycolide scaffold using third molar tooth buds of pigs and were able to grow mineralized tooth structures in immunodeficient rat hosts (Young et al. 2002). This scaffolding work continues by many researchers including Duailibi, Honda, and Young with promising results (Young et al. 2005; Honda et al. 2005; Duailibi et al. 2004). The major drawback of the scaffold technique is the developed teeth are often very small and the size and shape are difficult to control. In 2004, Ohazama et al. developed a primordial tooth by recombination technique with a scaffold-free design that successfully developed normal histology (Ohazama et al. 2004). Nakao et al. in 2007 developed a novel 3D organ culture method in which they regenerated a tooth germ in a renal capsule and later transplanted to the jaw (Nakao et al. 2007). In 2009, Ikeda et al. used a similar 3D organ method and transplanted tooth germ into the first upper molar region of mice. The tooth demonstrated correct structure, including enamel, dentin, cementum, pulp, and periodontal ligament space, but the tooth was smaller than the natural teeth (Ikeda et al. 2009). Many challenges still exist in tooth regeneration, the first being an appropriate cell source and the second induction of odontogenic potency. Human urine-induced pluripotent stem cells (iPSCs) have been shown to possess odontogenic competence in the right microenvironment, but there is still a need for identification of a "tooth inducer (Li et al. 2019)." Whether it be full tooth regeneration or cell-biased repair, the future of tooth replacement is likely not in the world of biomaterials but in molecular and cell biology.

9 Summary

The search for the optimal way to replace missing teeth is still at large. The search for the best biomaterial and shape for dental implants consumed much of the twentieth century. Early metals allowed for fibrous-osseous stability, but it was not until the understanding of osseointegration with titanium that dental implants became a mainstay treatment. Work on bone grafting substances to regenerate bone has allowed providers to place dental implants in atrophic mandibles. The first two decades of the twenty-first century have seen refinement of titanium to increase success rates, as well as increased accuracy of placement and restorations using technological advances such as cone beam computed tomography (CBCT) and intraoral scanners. Treatment planning software has further advanced accuracy through virtual planning and milling of surgical guides and the creation of dynamic navigation. While dental implants have come a long way, the future of tooth replacement likely resides not in the world of biomaterials but in molecular and cell biology.

References

Ahlgren F, Størksen K, Tornes K. A study of 25 zygomatic dental implants with 11 to 49 months' follow-up after loading. Int J Oral Maxillofac Implants. 2006;21:421.

Albee FH. Fundamentals in bone transplantation: experiences in three thousand bone graft operations. J Am Med Assoc. 1923;81:1429.

Anonymous. [In honor of Giuseppangelo Fonzi, inventor and maker of the 1st porcelain teeth in 1806]. Dent Cadmos. 1968;36:1185.

Anonymous. Dental implants: benefit and risks. In: Online NCS, editor. Dental implant consensus conference. Boston; 1978. p. 13.

Beder OW, Ploger WJ. Intraoral titanium implants. Oral Surg Oral Med Oral Pathol. 1959;12:787.

Bedrossian E. Laboratory and prosthetic considerations in computer-guided surgery and immediate loading. J Oral Maxillofac Surg. 2007;65:47.

Bedrossian E, Rangert B, Stumpel L, Indresano T. Immediate function with the zygomatic implant: a graftless solution for the patient with mild to advanced atrophy of the maxilla. Int J Oral Maxillofac Implants. 2006;21:937.

Bhanja A, D'Souza DS. Mapping the milestones in tooth regeneration: current trends and future research. Med J Armed Forces India. 2016;72:S24.

Block MS. Dental implants: the last 100 years. J Oral Maxillofac Surg. 2018a;76:11.

Block MS. The Crestal window approach for sinus floor grafting with delayed implant placement: a preliminary report. J Oral Maxillofac Surg. 2018b;76:2319.

Bobbio A. The first endosseous alloplastic implant in the history of man. Bull Hist Dent. 1972;20:1.

Bosker H, van Dijk L. The transmandibular implant: a 12-year follow-up study. J Oral Maxillofac Surg. 1989;47:442.

Bothe S, Beaton R, Davenport H. Reaction of bone to multiple metallic implants. Surg Gynecol Obstet. 1940;71:592.

Boyne PJ, James RA. Grafting of the maxillary sinus floor with autogenous marrow and bone. J Oral Surg. 1980;38:613.

Brånemark PI. Osseointegration and its experimental background. J Prosthet Dent. 1983;50:399.

Brånemark PI, Hansson BO, Adell R, Breine U, Lindström J, Hallén O, Ohman A. Osseointegrated implants in the treatment of the edentulous jaw. Experience from a 10-year period. Scand J Plast Reconstr Surg Suppl. 1977;16:1.

Brånemark PI, Adell R, Albrektsson T, Lekholm U, Lundkvist S, Rockler B. Osseointegrated titanium fixtures in the treatment of edentulousness. Biomaterials. 1983;4:25.

Brånemark PI, Adell R, Albrektsson T, Lekholm U, Lindström J, Rockler B. An experimental and clinical study of osseointegrated implants penetrating the nasal cavity and maxillary sinus. J Oral Maxillofac Surg. 1984;42:497.

Brånemark PI, Svensson B, van Steenberghe D. Ten-year survival rates of fixed prostheses on four or six implants ad modum Brånemark in full edentulism. Clin Oral Implants Res. 1995;6:227.

Brånemark PI, Gröndahl K, Ohrnell LO, Nilsson P, Petruson B, Svensson B, Engstrand P, Nannmark U. Zygoma fixture in the management of advanced atrophy of the maxilla: technique and long-term results. Scand J Plast Reconstr Surg Hand Surg. 2004;38:70.

Burch RH. Dr. Pinkney Adams – a dentist before his time. Ark Dent. 1997;68:14.

de Boer HH. The history of bone grafts. Clin Orthop Relat Res. 1988;226:292.

Donati D, Zolezzi C, Tomba P, Viganò A. Bone grafting: historical and conceptual review, starting with an old manuscript by Vittorio putti. Acta Orthop. 2007;78:19.
Duailibi MT, Duailibi SE, Young CS, Bartlett JD, Vacanti JP, Yelick PC. Bioengineered teeth from cultured rat tooth bud cells. J Dent Res. 2004;83:523.
Emneus H, Stenram U. Reaction of tissues to alloys used in osteosynthesis. Experimental, histological examination of reaction of soft tissues in animals. Acta Orthop Scand. 1960;29:315.
Ewers R, Schicho K, Undt G, Wanschitz F, Truppe M, Seemann R, Wagner A. Basic research and 12 years of clinical experience in computer-assisted navigation technology: a review. Int J Oral Maxillofac Surg. 2005;34:1.
Fortin Y, Sullivan RM, Rangert BR. The Marius implant bridge: surgical and prosthetic rehabilitation for the completely edentulous upper jaw with moderate to severe resorption: a 5-year retrospective clinical study. Clin Implant Dent Relat Res. 2002;4:69.
Greenfield EJ. Implantation of artificial crown and bridge abutments. 1913. Compend Contin Educ Dent. 2008;29:232.
Hench LL, Thompson I. Twenty-first century challenges for biomaterials. J R Soc Interface. 2010;7:S379.
Henkel J, Woodruff MA, Epari DR, Steck R, Glatt V, Dickinson IC, Choong PF, Schuetz MA, Hutmacher DW. Bone regeneration based on tissue engineering conceptions - a 21st century perspective. Bone Res. 2013;1:216.
Hernigou P. Bone transplantation and tissue engineering. Part II: bone graft and osteogenesis in the seventeenth, eighteenth and nineteenth centuries (Duhamel, Haller, Ollier and MacEwen). Int Orthop. 2015;39:193.
Honda MJ, Sumita Y, Kagami H, Ueda M. Histological and immunohistochemical studies of tissue engineered odontogenesis. Arch Histol Cytol. 2005;68:89.
Huang Y, Li Z, Van Dessel J, Salmon B, Huang B, Lambrichts I, Politis C, Jacobs R. Effect of platelet-rich plasma on peri-implant trabecular bone volume and architecture: a preclinical micro-CT study in beagle dogs. Clin Oral Implants Res. 2019;30(12):1190–9.
Ikeda E, Morita R, Nakao K, Ishida K, Nakamura T, Takano-Yamamoto T, Ogawa M, Mizuno M, Kasugai S, Tsuji T. Fully functional bioengineered tooth replacement as an organ replacement therapy. Proc Natl Acad Sci. 2009;106:13475.
Inclan A. The use of preserved bone graft in orthopaedic surgery. JBJS. 1942;24:81–96.
Jokstad A. The Toronto Osseointegration conference revisited. Osseointegration; 2008.
Jokstad A. Why did Professor Per-Ingvar Brånemark never receive the Nobel Prize in Medicine? Clin Exp Dent Res. 2017;3:79.
Karl M, Albrektsson T. Clinical performance of dental implants with a moderately rough (TiUnite) surface: a meta-analysis of prospective clinical studies. Int J Oral Maxillofac Implants. 2017;32:717.
Kattimani VS, Kondaka S, Lingamaneni KP. Hydroxyapatite–past, present, and future in bone regeneration. Bone Tissue Regen Insights. 2016;7:BTRI.S36138.
Kostopoulos L, Karring T. Augmentation of the rat mandible using guided tissue regeneration. Clin Oral Implants Res. 1994;5:75.
Lee JH, Nam J, Nam KW, Kim HJ, Yoo JJ. Pre-treatment of titanium alloy with platelet-rich plasma enhances human osteoblast responses. Tissue Eng Regen Med. 2016;13:335.
Leventhal GS. Titanium, a metal for surgery. J Bone Joint Surg Am. 1951;33-a:473.
Li L, Tang Q, Wang A, Chen Y. Regrowing a tooth: in vitro and in vivo approaches. Curr Opin Cell Biol. 2019;61:126.
Linkow LI. Clinical evalusation of the various designed endosseous implants. J Oral Implant Transplant Surg. 1966;12:35.
Linkow LI, Dorfman JD. Implantology in dentistry. A brief historical perspective. N Y State Dent J. 1991;57:31.
Linkow LI, Rinaldi AW. The significance of "fibro-osseous integration" and "osseointegration" in endosseous dental implants. Int J Oral Implantol. 1987;4:41.

López-Píriz R, Cabal B, Goyos-Ball L, Fernández A, Bartolomé JF, Moya JS, Torrecillas R. Current state-of-the-art and future perspectives of the three main modern implant-dentistry concerns: aesthetic requirements, mechanical properties, and peri-implantitis prevention. J Biomed Mater Res A. 2019;107:1466.

Lubbock J. Pre-historic times: as illustrated by ancient remains, and the manners and customs of modern savages. London: Edinburgh, Williams and Norgate; 1865.

Luebbers H-T, Messmer P, Obwegeser JA, Zwahlen RA, Kikinis R, Graetz KW, Matthews F. Comparison of different registration methods for surgical navigation in cranio-maxillofacial surgery. J Cranio-Maxillofac Surg. 2008;36:109.

Maggiolo J. Manuel de l'art dentaire (Manual of dentalart). Nancy, France: C Le Seure; 1809.

Maló P, Rangert B, Nobre M. "All-on-Four" immediate-function concept with Brånemark System implants for completely edentulous mandibles: a retrospective clinical study. Clin Implant Dent Relat Res. 2003;5(Suppl 1):2.

Marchack CB. An immediately loaded CAD/CAM-guided definitive prosthesis: a clinical report. J Prosthet Dent. 2005;93:8.

Marx RE, Carlson ER, Eichstaedt RM, Schimmele SR, Strauss JE, Georgeff KR. Platelet-rich plasma: growth factor enhancement for bone grafts. Oral Surg Oral Med Oral Pathol Oral Radiol Endod. 1998;85:638.

Melcher AH. On the repair potential of periodontal tissues. J Periodontol. 1976;47:256.

Nakao K, Morita R, Saji Y, Ishida K, Tomita Y, Ogawa M, Saitoh M, Tomooka Y, Tsuji T. The development of a bioengineered organ germ method. Nat Methods. 2007;4:227.

Needleman IG, Worthington HV, Giedrys-Leeper E, Tucker RJ. Guided tissue regeneration for periodontal infra-bony defects. Cochrane Database Syst Rev. 2006;(2):CD001724.

Nijmeh AD, Goodger NM, Hawkes D, Edwards PJ, McGurk M. Image-guided navigation in oral and maxillofacial surgery. Br J Oral Maxillofac Surg. 2005;43:294.

Ohazama A, Modino SAC, Miletich I, Sharpe PT. Stem-cell-based tissue engineering of murine teeth. J Dent Res. 2004;83:518.

Pasqualini U, Pasqualini ME. Treatise of implant dentistry: the Italian tribute to modern implantology. Carimate: Ariesdue; 2009. © Copyright 2009 Azienda Pubblica di Servizi alla Persona "Suor Agnese".

Pryor LS, Gage E, Langevin CJ, Herrera F, Breithaupt AD, Gordon CR, Afifi AM, Zins JE, Meltzer H, Gosman A, Cohen SR, Holmes R. Review of bone substitutes. Craniomaxillofac Trauma Reconstr. 2009;2:151.

Rudy RJ, Levi PA, Bonacci FJ, Weisgold AS, Engler-Hamm D. Intraosseous anchorage of dental prostheses: an early 20th century contribution. Compend Contin Educ Dent. 2008;29:220.

Scacchi M, Merz BR, Schär AR. The development of the ITI dental implant system. Part 2: 1998–2000: steps into the next millennium. Clin Oral Implants Res. 2000;11(Suppl 1):22.

Scully D, Naseem KM, Matsakas A. Platelet biology in regenerative medicine of skeletal muscle. Acta Physiol (Oxf). 2018;223:e13071.

Smalley WM, Shapiro PA, Hohl TH, Kokich VG, Brånemark PI. Osseointegrated titanium implants for maxillofacial protraction in monkeys. Am J Orthod Dentofac Orthop. 1988;94:285.

Smith Y. History of dental implants. 2019.

Summers RB. Sinus floor elevation with osteotomes. J Esthet Dent. 1998;10:164.

Sutter F, Schroeder A, Straumann F. Engineering and design aspects of the I.T.I. hollow-basket implants. J Oral Implantol. 1983;10:535.

Tamura H, Sasaki K, Watahiki R. Primary insertion of implants in the zygomatic bone following subtotal maxillectomy. Bull Tokyo Dent Coll. 2000;41:21.

Tanunja. A complete review of Dental Implant Materials. Int J Recent Scientific Res. 2018;9:29665.

Tarnow DP, Emtiaz S, Classi A. Immediate loading of threaded implants at stage 1 surgery in edentulous arches: ten consecutive case reports with 1- to 5-year data. Int J Oral Maxillofac Implants. 1997;12:319.

Tatum H Jr. Maxillary and sinus implant reconstructions. Dent Clin N Am. 1986;30:207.

Temmerman A, Cleeren GJ, Castro AB, Teughels W, Quirynen M. L-PRF for increasing the width of keratinized mucosa around implants: a split-mouth, randomized, controlled pilot clinical trial. J Periodontal Res. 2018;53:793.

Wennerberg A, Albrektsson T, Chrcanovic B. Long-term clinical outcome of implants with different surface modifications. Eur J Oral Implantol. 2018;11(Suppl 1):S123.

Young CS, Terada S, Vacanti JP, Honda M, Bartlett JD, Yelick PC. Tissue engineering of complex tooth structures on biodegradable polymer scaffolds. J Dent Res. 2002;81:695.

Young C, Abukawa H, Asrican R, Ravens M, Troulis M, Kaban L, Vacanti J, Yelick PC. Tissue-engineered hybrid tooth and bone. Tissue Eng. 2005;11:1599.

Zierold AA. Reaction of bone to various metals. Arch Surg. 1924;9:365.

Midface Trauma

Michael S. Forman, Joy X. Chen, Joel M. Friedman, and Shahid R. Aziz

1 Introduction

The earliest known text to reference the management of facial trauma is the *Edwin Smith Papyrus*, a scroll of trauma cases from ancient Egypt, dating back to at least 1700 BCE and postulated to reference texts as late as 3000 BCE (van Middendorp et al. 2010; Breasted 1930). The series of cases outlining surgical traumas described multiple cases of facial fractures. Maxillofacial trauma cases in the text include various facial lacerations, head injuries, and fractures of the nasal bone, maxilla, zygoma, and mandible. Some of these early cases will be described in the relevant sections of this chapter.

The midface serves a critical function in not only facial appearance but also by providing vertical strength to the head through its many buttresses. Adequate repair of midface fractures restores much of what makes up an individual's self-image and enables one to speak, eat, and function appropriately. Given its importance, it is no surprise that early writings focus on repairs of midface injuries.

Outside of the papyrus, one of earliest, well-documented descriptions of the management of facial fractures can also be traced to Hippocrates (460–375 BCE). His translated work reads "If the teeth at the point of injury are displaced or loosened, when the bone is adjusted fasten them to one another…preferably with gold

M. S. Forman (✉) · J. M. Friedman
Division of Oral and Maxillofacial Surgery, NewYork-Presbyterian/Columbia University Irving Medical Center, New York, NY, USA
e-mail: Mf3097@cumc.columbia.edu

J. X. Chen
Will Surgical Arts, Rockville, MD, USA

S. R. Aziz
Department of Oral and Maxillofacial Surgery, Rutgers School of Dental Medicine, Newark, NJ, USA

E. M. Ferneini et al. (eds.), *The History of Maxillofacial Surgery*,
https://doi.org/10.1007/978-3-030-89563-1_11

wire, but, lacking that, with linen thread, till consolidation takes place" (Dingman and Natvig 1964). Medical historians believe that based on how casually he describes this technique, that the method of using wire or bandages to stabilize facial fractures had been around for quite some time prior to Hippocrates' writings.

Most well-documented "modern" principles and techniques developed for the treatment of midface trauma date back to the early twentieth century (Table 1). Commonly, many advances in medicine or surgery occurred through wars, where horrific injuries and crude conditions consequently led to clinical innovations and breakthroughs. Unfortunately, it was the midface that was exposed and a major

Table 1 A timeline of important breakthroughs related to the management of maxillofacial trauma

1823	Von Graefe describes an apparatus to immobilize a fracture of the upper jaw with a metal bar fixed to the premolars and tied to a headband.
1840	Baudens uses circumferential wiring to immobilize an oblique fracture of mandible.
1844	Strohmeyer describes the reduction of depressed zygoma fractures using a 1-prong hook.
1847	Buck is credited with applying wire sutures directly to fractured bones for stabilization.
1866	Gunning reports on treatment of fracture of the lower jaw by interdental splints.
1880s	Open reduction and internal fixation with metal plates.
1885	Roentgen develops radiographic imaging.
1898	Use of frontal sinus ablation for frontal sinus disease.
1901	Introduction of the Le Fort classification system of midface trauma.
1921	Lynch describes the frontoethmoidectomy procedure.
1936	Anderson develops external appliance and pin fixation for the management of edentulous mandible fractures.
1938	Konrad Zuse develops the first electromechanical binary programmable computer.
1942	Penicillin (discovered by Alexander Fleming in 1928) is first used to treat infection.
1942	Adams introduces the technique of internal craniofacial suspension of the midface and direct wiring of zygomatic fractures.
1942	John Atanasoff and Clifford Berry complete development of the first digital computer.
1943	Transantral reduction of late fractures of the orbit with fat.
1944	Converse and Smith describe a surgical approach for repairing orbital fractures, autogenous bone grafts, and early surgery.
1955	Bergara and Itoiz describe the use of the frontal sinus osteoplastic flap.
1958	Goodale and Montgomery describe the ablative frontal sinus procedure.
1960s	Luhr and Perren et al. introduce Vitallium compression plates.
1964	Mustardé and Dingman and Natvig describe open repair and transnasal wiring to address the medial canthal tendon.
1970	May et al. report on the importance of nasofrontal ducts.
1970s	Introduction of rigid fixation concepts and absolute immobility.
1972	Hounsfield develops the first clinical CT procedure.
1972	Michelet and Festal introduce osteosynthesis with miniplates.
1977	Claussen et al. report on computed tomography and craniofacial injuries.
1978	Donald and Bernstein describe the first cranialization procedure.
1978	Champy et al. introduce the monocortical miniplate tension band technique.

Table 1 (continued)

1983	Gentry et al. describe facial buttresses based on high-resolution CT analysis.
1985	Stanley and Nowack and later Gruss et al. report on reconstruction of facial buttresses in the management of complex facial trauma.
1985	Gruss et al. and others describe the role of primary bone grafting in NOE fractures.
1985	Ewers and Härle report on bioabsorbable plates and screws in the management of maxillofacial trauma.
1986	Levine et al. report on stratification of the management of frontal sinus fractures based on injury.
1991	Markowitz et al. introduce a NOE classification system based on the medial canthal tendon.
1991	Putterman advocates CT findings for stratification of surgery.
1993	Hosemann et al. describe endoscopy and observation in the management of nasofrontal ducts and NOE fractures.
1994	Gleason et al. combine 3D computer-reconstructed neuro-images with a novel video registration technique for virtual reality-based, image-guided neurosurgery.
1997	Saunders et al. report on the use of the endoscope for orbital floor fractures.
2013	Weathers et al. describe the conservative shift in frontal sinus fracture management.

Louis and Morlandt (2018)
Abbreviations: *3D* 3-dimensional, *CT* computed tomographic, *NOE* naso-orbito-ethmoid

victim of trench warfare—where more protection was naturally provided to the trunk and limbs. Thus many of the pioneers in plastic, oral, and maxillofacial surgery with both medical and dental backgrounds were able to publish based on their experiences in the Great War, World War II, or the Balkan war. Original surgical pioneers such as Harold Delf Gillies, Varaztad Kazanjian, and Robert Ivy all faced unchartered circumstances with terribly wounded soldiers during World War I. In part, the formal field of plastic surgery emerged after the world wars with Harold Gillies serving as the founder and first president of the British Association of Plastic Surgery in 1946.

During the Great War, many multidisciplinary teams emerged to take care of facial injuries since most doctors were not accustomed to treating the injuries that presented from missiles, explosions, and bullets. As mentioned, Harold Gillies, a New Zealand native, became widely recognized as one of the founders of facial and plastic surgery. Much of this occurred at the Queen's Hospital at Sidcup, Kent, United Kingdom. To demonstrate the multiple collaborations that occurred, in many of Gillies' writings, he credits a dentist with whom he worked closely with for inspiration, Charles Valadier. Valadier was a dentist originally born in Paris, but raised in America. He volunteered via the British Red Cross Society to help out in the war in 1914. Gillies wrote, "The credit for establishing the first Plastic and Jaw Unit, which so facilitated the later progress of plastic surgery, must go to…Charles Valadier" (McAuley 1974). Historically speaking, it is described that much of the facial surgery done during the wars were completed by a multidisciplinary team of providers working together. Gillies met Valadier when he volunteered for the Red Cross in 1915 (Simpson and David 2004).

It was Valadier in 1917 who was one of the first to outline the principles for the management of facial trauma through his wartime experiences (Valadier and Whale 1917). He described a few key principles: (1) All remaining teeth should be preserved to provide support for interdental splints. He keenly notes that the secret to effective repair was to obtain proper occlusion of teeth. Interestingly, he commented an English soldier's mouth was difficult to treat because their teeth were generally "poor in quality and few in number" (Valadier and Whale 1917). (2) Wounds should be closed as soon as possible. He sharply noticed that lacerated tissues retracted and subsequently made closure difficult to impossible. At the same time he commented that closure can also lead to scar formation and trismus and that tissue stents will be required to maintain volume as the tissue contracts. (3) Ultimately, for the management of facial bone fractures, he used a series of interdental positioning stents to stabilize midface and jaw fractures with the addition of wire or suture fixation. He fabricated a stent for each individual patient and each unique fracture pattern. The goal was always the same—to stabilize and immobilize the segments of the bone across the fracture lines. At times he utilized extraoral devices to help manipulate the segments to their appropriate positions. A combination of tooth-borne fixation devices and wiring allowed him to treat the plethora or midface trauma injuries he encountered.

Lastly, for wound care and to prevent infection following stabilization of the midface and closure of the soft tissues, he placed a drain into the wound. He developed an apparatus nicknamed by wartime patients, as the "Fire Engine" (Valadier and Whale 1917). It was a device he travelled through the wards with, irrigating wounds under pressure with boiled water to keep his surgical sites clean.

Most of the novel principles described during World War I and by Charles Valadier are still in practice today and have led to incredible achievements in maxillofacial surgery since that time. More information regarding their experiences during the war can be found in the dedicated chapter on this topic. However, it is important to understand the impact of the wars as a key period for advancing oral and facial surgery. Dental professionals and, in particular, oral and maxillofacial surgeons have always played a critical role in the management of these injuries. In this chapter we will review the earliest documented procedures our research revealed related to the maxilla, zygoma, and nasal bones. Remarkably, many guiding principles have not changed significantly over the past 1000 or more years compared to present-day standard of care.

Fortunately, several important advances in the management of maxillofacial trauma in the last 40 years have resulted in improved outcomes. These include the development of high-resolution computed tomography (CT), rigid fixation techniques, improved biomaterials, soft tissue resuspension, and primary bone grafting. Further advances in outcomes have occurred with the use of virtual surgical planning, endoscopic techniques, and surgical navigation.

2 Imaging

One of the most important advancements in medicine is the advent of modern imaging techniques. Since the first use of radiographic imaging by Wilhelm Conrad Roentgen in 1895, no significant changes in medical imaging occurred until the advent of the computer. The computer allowed for more sophisticated imaging techniques with greater diagnostic capability. In 1972, an engineer named Godfrey Hounsfield performed groundbreaking research that led to the development of the first clinical computer tomography (CT) scanner. He shared the Nobel Prize in Medicine and Physiology in 1979 with Allen Gormack, a physicist, for the development of computer tomography (Seeram 1994). In 1977, Claussen et al. reported the first use of computed tomography in diagnosing craniofacial injuries which allowed for unprecedented visualization and analysis of the complex anatomy associated with craniomaxillofacial surgery (Claussen et al. 1977).

With advancements in CT technology, the modern clinician can evaluate craniofacial injuries and fracture patterns in great detail via individual cuts or 3D-rendered reconstructions. Three-dimensional imaging paved the way for the development of guided surgical navigation, virtual surgical planning, and patient-specific implants.

3 The Maxilla, Rene Le Fort, and Le Fort I, II, and III Fractures

One of the earliest treatment methods for fractures of the maxilla dates back to 1832, when Karl Ferdinand von Graefe, a German surgeon, introduced an apparatus for the treatment of maxillary fractures (Dingman and Natvig 1964). The device utilized extra-skeletal fixation via use of a circumferential fronto-occipital band of metals as an anchor with two adjustable vertical supports. The vertical supports housed curved hooks to fit over the patient's teeth for stabilization. This ultimately immobilized the maxilla, using anterior teeth as a point of fixation to the forehead, providing extra-skeletal fixation. Interestingly, similar methods utilized this creative device well into the mid- twentieth century. In 1887, an American, Thomas Gilmer, is credited with the development of intermaxillary fixation (IMF) via wiring and described its use for the management of complex jaw fractures (Gilmer 1904). Fractures of the maxilla are rarely encountered alone, but often in conjunction with other facial bone fractures. Thus, while principles of maxillary fractures will be introduced and explained here, relevant principles will be further expanded upon in other sections of this chapter.

In 1901, Rene Le Fort, a French surgeon, completed a series of cadaveric experiments that led to perhaps the most widely used and known fracture classification system in effect today. No midface history chapter would be complete without a brief review of these novel and infamous experiments. He set to evaluate the manner in which fractures propagated throughout the midface and questioned midface contiguity with the skull base. He tested three main conditions: (1) *the point of application of the force*, (2) *the direction of the wounding agents*, and (3) *the position of the head during the trauma* (Tessier, 1972a). Le Fort utilized a variety of different methods such as "administering a very violent blow with a wooden club" or "violently projecting the skull against the autopsy table" (Tessier 1972a). He deliberately applied an array of forces to specific areas of the face (e.g., nose, malar bone, or alveolus) with the head stationary, dangling off the autopsy table or being propelled itself. Through his findings, he described "great lines of weakness" which later contributed to what we now call a Le Fort I, II, or III fracture.

The first great weak line—which he described as the protection barrier of the cranial cavity—is the nasal septum and vomer. A second great weak line "circumscribes the whole middle part of the face, in which the malar bones are not involved" which we understand today as a Le Fort II.

He observed that the maxilla, despite its anatomical connections to the skull base, is physiologically independent from it (Tessier 1972a). He discovered there are bony columns in place above the alveolar arch that are able to distribute the natural vertical forces from the lower jaw over a very broad cranial area. Laterally this includes the malar bones which distribute the forces into large areas of the maxilla and skull base. He also identified certain weak points in this area which caused facial bones to break in a manner preserving forces distributed to the brain. He noticed that trauma involving the malar bones can cause the separation of the face from the skull (Le Fort III). When describing this weak line, he wrote "this line passes through the nasal bones…The upper part is very resistant. When it yields, the cribriform plate of the ethmoid bone yields also. From the nasal bones the fracture line runs toward the orbit" (Tessier 1972b).

Finally, he described a third weak line which cuts across the face—starting from the lower part of the pyriform aperture; crossing the canine fossa, below the malar bone; and meeting the second line (which ultimately rises posterior to cross the pterygomaxillary fissure and cut the pterygoid process). This of course referred to the most common type of fracture, a Le Fort I. These imaginative and ferocious studies aid surgeons to this day in understanding the anatomy of common facial fracture patterns.

The treatment principles of maxillary fractures and the described Le Fort I, II, or III fractures are all based on the re-establishment of functional dental occlusion and fragment immobilization. These principles were demonstrated with the extra-skeletal facial devices employed in the 1800s. Generally, the main methods developed to accomplish these primary objectives were intermaxillary fixation (IMF) and either internal or external fixation. The first was considered a closed treatment option commonly achieved with Erich arch bars, or an equivalent method, to re-establish occlusion and provide stabilization of the fractured segments. The pressure of the mandible against the maxilla both reduces the fracture and stabilizes it in place (Dingman and Natvig 1964). This principle is well understood today for the management of the same fractures.

The alternatives to intraoral fixation alone were a form of external or internal fixation as modern hardware did not get introduced until the 1970s. We will spend some time reviewing the principles of such treatments here, which are germane to the other sections of this chapter, that utilize the same techniques of external and internal rigid fixation.

External fixation consisted of any method that immobilized the fractured maxilla by utilizing a stable extraoral form of fixation to a point on either the mandible or maxilla. One common method was *cranio-maxillary* rigid direct suspension that was similar to Karl Ferdinand von Graefe's headcap described earlier. This method utilized a maxillary tooth-borne cast that connected via rods to a plaster of Paris headwrap, immobilizing the fractured segment. Alternatively, a halo frame which was described in the 1950s for cervical traction was applied to maxillofacial injuries in the mid-1960s (Rowe and Kelly 1968). It was also commonplace to pass a "cheek-wire" which was a trans-buccal wire connecting the halo frame to the maxilla. The wire was passed through the soft tissues with a spinal needle. *Cranio-mandibular* fixation was a form of indirect support which stabilized the maxilla in occlusion by way of mandibular immobilization. The mandible could be immobilized in a similar fashion as just described.

Overall, early treatments all revolved around connecting the maxilla or mandible via a tooth-borne splint in place to *any* extraoral rigid point of fixation (plaster of Paris headframe, halo frame, or external skeletal pins) via metal rods or wires. There were creative ways to do so, many of which were quite bulky and cumbersome. Fortunately, these techniques quickly fell out of favor as more favorable treatment options developed.

Prior to "plates and screws." *internal fixation* consisted of either *trans-osseous wiring* (e.g., wiring across the zygomatico-frontal suture), *direct suspension* (e.g., wiring from the maxillary arch bar to a point superior to the fracture line), *indirect support* (e.g., wiring from the mandibular arch bar to a point superior to the fracture line), *direct support* (e.g., use of packing), or *trans-fixation* (e.g., Kirschner wires or Steinmann pins) (Dingman and Natvig 1964).

To accomplish internal wire fixation, the patient was placed into IMF. Second, the wire fixation was between either the maxillary arch bar (direct) or mandibular arch bar (indirect) and to a point superior to the fracture line, typically the infraorbital rim, lateral zygoma, or pyriform rims. An incision was made from the skin to the bone at the selected site, with drill holes completed via use of a hand-turned drill. A stainless steel wire was passed from the drill hole into the oral cavity, where it was secured to the selected arch such as the maxilla (Dingman and Natvig 1964). This allowed the maxilla to be positioned by occlusion with additional support by the fixation wire. Le Fort II and III fractures were treated with the same principles, with differing anchorage points depending where stable bone was. For Le Fort II fractures, wires were passed directly across the infraorbital area or from the zygomatic process of the frontal bone, referred to as "cranial suspension," to the mandibular arch bar, with the patient in IMF. Edentulous patients of note had dentures wired via suspension wires to the maxilla, superior to the fracture line, and then placed into IMF. Interestingly, it was commonplace for the anterior teeth to be removed from the denture for the patient to better accommodate eating and drinking during the healing phase.

3.1 Modern Treatment

In the last 40 years, rigid fixation has become the mainstay treatment for midface fractures. The concept of rigid fixation uses hardware in the form of bone plates and screws to absorb part or all of the functional load of the fracture site, thereby preventing any mobility of the fracture segments. The advent of rigid fixation started in the early nineteenth century. In 1866, German surgeon Carl Hansmann was the first to experiment with the plate and screw system on orthopedic fractures and was also the first advocate of rigid plate fixation in maxillofacial injury (Verbeek 1955). In the 1890s, Belgian surgeon Albin Lambotte was one of the first to publish on the technique of internal fixation of displaced orthopedic fractures. Lambotte coined the term "osteosynthesis" and outlined the tenets for the technique which includes limiting dissection and preserving the periosteal covering to maintain the bone's blood supply. The first plates Lambotte used were designed and milled by him in his private workshop. The initial design was a trapezoidal plate made of a copper alloy with nickel and zinc. However, due to the high rates of complications such as infection, osteosynthesis of orthopedic fractures was put on hold for many years until after the development of modern aseptic technique and the discovery of antibiotics in the early twentieth century (Lambotte 1987).

Rigid fixation found favor in orthopedic literature in the mid-twentieth century with a 1949 publication by Luhr who described compression of bony fragments as an important adjunct to fracture healing (Luhr 1982). Subsequently in 1958, Bagby and Janes published an article detailing the use of bone plates to achieve immobilization of the fracture and active compression which showed more favorable clinical outcome than closed reduction (Bagby and Janes 1958). Early literature on the application of rigid fixation for craniomaxillofacial fractures showed mixed results as most appliances available were designed for extremity fractures. In 1973, a landmark paper was published by Michelet et al. where they advocated for the use of small, malleable Vitallium (cobalt-chromium alloy) plates and detailed 300 clinical cases where miniaturized plates and screws were used in the reduction and immobilization of maxillofacial fractures (Michelet et al. 1973). Since then, many different systems and materials have been introduced and have evolved into the current systems we have today. The use of miniaturized plates ("miniplates") and screws in maxillofacial fractures is now considered the standard of care in the treatment of maxillofacial injuries.

Current techniques in the management of midface fractures involve the use of miniplate fixation, primarily along the facial buttresses for optimal stability and maintenance of the midface vertical height. This concept evolved from the description of facial buttresses by Gentry et al. in 1983 and multiple publications by Gruss et al. on the important role of facial buttresses in maxillofacial reconstruction (Gentry et al. 1983; Gruss and Mackinnon 1986). Rigid fixation with miniplates in the maxilla also allows for immediate function, forgoing of maxillomandibular fixation, and more predictable outcomes.

A split palatal fracture can occur in conjunction with other maxillary fractures resulting in issues with the transverse width of the midface. Treatment of such split palate fractures utilizes basic orthognathic surgery principles. Dental impressions of both arches are taken, and model surgery is carried out to re-establish the original occlusion. An occlusal splint is then made and wired to the maxillary dentition during open reduction and internal fixation of the fracture to correct the transverse width.

4 Zygoma and Zygomatic Arch Fractures

The first description of a fracture to the zygoma is from the *Edwin Smith Papyrus*, "If thou examines a man having a smash in his cheek…should it crepitate under thy fingers, while he discharges blood from his nostril…" (Breasted 1930). While for other injuries daily honey and lint applications are often recommended, for this injury the writer determines it is, "an ailment not to be treated."

As outlined previously, the historically established principal objectives of treating any fractures are to reduce the fragments in a way that restores form and function and to provide adequate support during the healing course. This was done via a wide variety of treatment options for zygomatic fractures over the past hundreds of years.

Dr. Guichard Du Verney, a French otologist, described what may have been the first formal treatment methods of zygomatic fractures in the modern era (Smith and Yanagisawa 1961). In his book published in 1751, he described three methods utilizing intraoral digital pressure, mechanical occlusal or masticatory forces, and external pressure. They are outlined as follows:

1. "I introduced my index finger of my left hand into the mouth of the patient and I placed it over the first molar tooth, the more forward that I could [push] with the finger within, outward and I realized that by the touch the zygomatic process was fractured and depressed" (Smith and Yanagisawa 1961).
2. "I told the patient to take a piece of wood slightly flattened thick as a finger, and put it over the last molar tooth and to close the mandible as much as he could. After having done this for a few hours he felt pulling; he kept on doing it, increasing the size of the size of wood and by this means the pieces came back into place by the action of the contraction of the temporal muscle, that pulls the process from inward outward" (Smith and Yanagisawa 1961).

3. "I applied the palm of the hand over the cheek, pressing a little and the process came into place" (Smith and Yanagisawa 1961).

Throughout the 1800s, with the advent of instruments, many novel methods were described. Utilizing a variety of direct incisions or wounds, a number of imaginative techniques were attempted. In 1878, Dr. David Agnew, an American surgeon from Philadelphia, published a three-volume series on surgery. He recognized the challenge of restoring facial harmony with digital pressure alone and utilized a screw elevator, functionally identical to the modern-day Carroll-Girard, to aid his reduction. He writes, "If there is displacement, it must be corrected by pressure applied inside of the mouth or outside of the cheek…If the body of the bone is depressed, which implies also a broken antrum, the screw elevator, bored into its substance, will be the most convenient method of restoring it to the proper position" (Agnew 1878). I think it is also important to appreciate that in 1878, surgical principles such as dependent drainage were already commonplace in practice—"When no wound is present, in incision must be made…it should be carried along the lower rather than along the upper margin of the zygomatic…although a few muscular fibers belonging to the masseter must be cut, we shall have a dependent wound for the escape of any collection of blood or pus" (Agnew 1878). He continues to advocate for wound care and pain control following the reduction with "lotion of lead-water and laudanum" (Agnew 1878).

One of the next major treatment approaches was written by Dr. Howard Lothrop, an American surgeon from Boston who was a Surgeon-in-Chief at Boston City Hospital. He advocated for an antral route via the canine fossa, utilizing direct elevator of the fragments from within the antrum by outward pressure (Dingman and Natvig 1964; Smith and Yanagisawa 1961; Keen 1909). He approached this by making, "a horizontal incision, about three quarters of an inch long…along the line of the junction of the mucous membrane of the alveolus and the cheek…the director should now be pushed through…into the antrum…then a 24 French sound is introduced… gradual increase in pressure should now be exerted…" (Smith and Yanagisawa 1961).

In 1909, Dr. William Williams Keen, an American surgeon, published three methods of operating, including an intraoral technique for reduction, which is an approach still commonly referred to today by his namesake. One method was a direct method, "an incision is made through the skin and the fragments pulled outward" (Keen 1909). However he commented that it was objectionable both due to scar formation and poor outcomes. His second method was "through the mouth by inserting blunt instruments beneath the bone from within and lifting the fragments up" (Dingman and Natvig 1964; Keen 1909). Of note, he does not describe an intraoral incision here; however to this day an intraoral approach for this fracture is still referred to by "Keen approach." For his third method, he refers to the method of Lothrop, which is described previously above.

In 1913, Dr. J.G. Manwaring, a surgeon from Flint, Michigan and a founder of the American College of Surgeons, published the use of dental cow-horn forceps for reduction of zygoma fractures in the *Journal of American Medical Association*

(Manwaring 1913). He writes "For elevating depressed fractures of the malar bone I have used an instrument always obtainable, the ordinary 'cow-horn' forceps of the dentist. One point of the forceps is placed over the orbital ridge and the other just under the margin of the body of the bone...no dressing is necessary…the holes in the skin are mere pricks" (Manwaring 1913). Understanding obvious skepticism he continues, "This is more readily appreciated when tried, than would be believed…[provides] sure control it leaves no scars, is quickly used, and does not enter through the mouth cavity" (Manwaring 1913).

In 1927, a novel temporal approach was described by Gillies, which is another technique that is still commonly practiced today and referred to by his namesake like the Keen intraoral approach (Figs. 1 and 2). Gillies writes, "Our technique…differs from those mentioned. A curved incision, 1.5 in. long, is made over the temporal muscle…an incision is made in the temporal fascia; and a long, thin

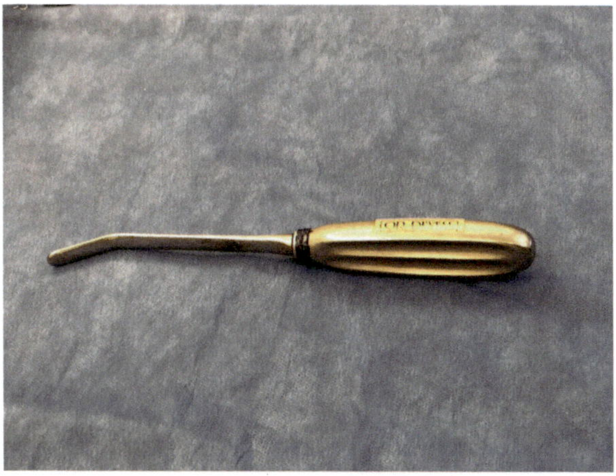

Fig. 1 Gillies zygoma elevator, designed for the temporal "Gillies" approach to zygomatic arch fractures

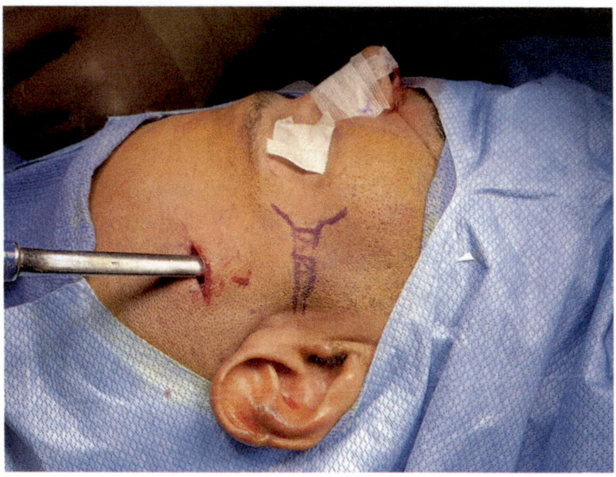

Fig. 2 Surgical photograph demonstrating the temporal "Gillies" approach and operative use of the Gillies zygoma elevator

elevator is passed downwards on the surface of the temporal muscle until it lies deep to the displaced bone" (Gilles et al. 1927). The advantages of this technique that are well known today were self-evident at that time as well: hidden scar location, safe dissection plane, and adequate leverage to reduce the fracture segments. In the same paper of note, the authors outline the importance of a "supero-inferior view of the skull" and technique for the radiograph to highlight and isolate the arch post repair (Gilles et al. 1927). This landmark publication has survived the standard of care for nearly a century.

In 1928, Dr. Sam Roberts described using a corkscrew instrument similar to Agnew's use of a screw elevator in 1878 for reduction (Roberts 1928). "A stab is made…about three-fourths of an inch directly below the external canthus… The screw is then inserted, with a half turned motion in a perpendicular plane with the flat surface of the bone. Considerable pressure may be necessary in older patients to penetrate the bone…as soon as one full turn of the screw has passed through the flat bone, it may be elevated to a normal position" (Roberts 1928).

Over the next few decades, multiple variations on the previously described methods were attempted. Various instruments, wires, and approaches were all used to reduce and stabilize the segments that only varied slightly. In 1931 a novel anatomical approach was introduced—A nasoantral route was proposed by making a window under the inferior turbinate and inserting a curved sound (Smith and Yanagisawa 1961). Kazanjian and others propose variations on plaster of Paris headcaps or a halo frame as described for Le Fort fractures, to which a screw or wire attached to the zygoma was fixed to, thus stabilizing the reduced segments (Dingman and Natvig 1964; Smith and Yanagisawa 1961; Kazanjian 1927; Flynn et al. 1958).

In the 1940s, internal rigid fixation via wires and pins began to be described. In 1946, a technique was introduced that was internal wire-pin rigid fixation for zygoma fractures (Brown 1946). After reduction, stainless steel pins were driven through the skin and zygoma in a transverse direction into solid parts of the maxilla or zygoma on the contralateral side (Brown 1946). They were removed at 4–6 weeks following an adequate or uncomplicated healing process.

However it was Dr. William Milton Adams from Tennessee in 1943 that made a major breakthrough and published one of the earliest reports on open reduction and internal wire fixation as a form of rigid fixation independent from external support (e.g., plaster headcaps) (Adams 1943). He acknowledged the limitations of all of the many treatments described above in this chapter and believed that his internal wire fixation "meets the requirements of facility of operation, complete immobilization, sound surgical principles, *and is applicable to practically every type of fracture of the facial bones*" (Adams 1943). With the benefit of time now, we can appreciate the genius and accuracy of his intuition. The benefits were obvious—since complete immobilization was achieved—repeated adjustments were unnecessary, and patients would not have to deal with bulky, complex extraoral appliances. The headwraps used as anchors for immobilization were imperfect, time-consuming, and required continual adjustments. Even in 1943, however, the importance of a large armamentarium was well understood by pioneers in facial surgery. Adams understood that with infected fractures, extraoral immobilization is critical, at least initially—"In the presence of infection…open reduction is definitely contraindicated…extraoral appliance may be required only for temporary immobilization; after the infection subsides, one may remove the appliance and wire the fragments together" (Adams 1943).

The advanced protocol in 1943 for a zygoma fracture started with incisions made over the frontal bone. A hole was bored to accommodate a 25- or 26-gauge wire. Next, "The wire is threaded through the opening, looped, and both ends are passed together along the anterior wall of the antrum into the upper sulcus over the second molar…" (Adams 1943). The fractures were reduced, and wires secured to the dentition as a stable point. The authors simplified the procedure to only requiring "minimum amount of time and equipment: a small drill, pair of pliers, spool of small stainless steel wire, and a dissecting set" (Adams 1943). Ultimately smaller fragments could be wired together via trans-osseous wires, and then larger segments such as malar fractures were immobilized to either the teeth in the maxilla or mandible via a suspension wire from the orbital rim, for instance. If the patent was edentulous, wires were attached to dentures, or in cases of no dentures, wax was molded around the ridges and wires were tied to each other over the palate in the midline (Adams and Adams 1956).

Finally, it was common practice to use packings, such as thin collagen tape or rubber dam packing to help support arch fractures, orbital floors, or anterior maxillary sinus wall fractures. This is not done routinely today. In the late 1930s through the war years, the text written by Norman Rowe and Wiley Kelly opened many avenues for the treatment of facial fractures from the 1960s to the early 1970s. One technique for the anterior maxillary fractures was the use of iodoform gauze coated with Whitehead's varnish to pack out the malar eminence. It was introduced through an inferior turbinate incision and packing the sinus and malar eminence. There were two types of external pin fixation—First is the Roger Anderson appliance, an erector set type external apparatus that was most useful in combat situations as being fast and easy to place and stabilize fractures until more definitive care could be undertaken. In the civilian world the Joe Hall Morris biphasic pin fixation tended to replace the Roger Anderson pin fixation. It used wider screws that were more stable. With the introduction of plates and screws made of noncorrosive metals and the top-down approach with rigid internal fixation, there were other methods introduced.

It is clear that zygomatic and midface fractures have seen multiple new techniques and instruments being introduced for their management. However, the basic principles largely remain the same. Each surgeon will always have their preferred approach, instrument, and technique, which will all hopefully be optimized for the finest patient care.

4.1 Modern Treatment

In the modern age, there now exist a number of new areas of technological development to help guide the surgeon in the management of midface fractures. Computer-assisted surgery in the form of presurgical analysis and planning and intraoperative navigation and assessment have revolutionized maxillofacial surgery for more predictable outcomes and shorter operating times. The age of three-dimensional imaging in medicine began in 1971 when Sir Godfrey Hounsfield developed the computed tomography scan, which allowed for unprecedented analysis of anatomy. Diagnostic imaging was advanced further in 1983 when Charles Hull developed 3D printing, allowing the first 3D milling of human anatomic structures in Germany and the USA in 1985 (Metzger et al. 2008). In the 1990s, intraoperative navigation system based on computed tomography technology was developed in Germany and quickly adopted in operative practice for numerous surgical specialties (Ewers et al. 2005). Coinciding with these technological advancements was the development and commercialization of software to analyze and manipulate 3D data which allowed for the application of this technology to virtual surgical treatment planning. Planning software can segmentalize the various facial subunits, provide better three-dimensional visualization of the injury, and guide the appropriate course of management. 3D printing offers the opportunity to manufacture accurate stereolithic models by steering a laser, guided by data from a conventional CT scan, onto selectively solidifying ultraviolet-sensitive liquid resin, creating an integrated solid counterpart of the CT slices (Schramm et al. 2006). From these stereolithic models, preformed customized hardware and cutting guides can be fashioned to assist the surgeon in complex reconstructions to produce more predictable and optimal results. 3D images and models also allow for a more interactive discussion with the patient and allow for better understanding of the extent of the injury and proposed treatment (Fig. 3). The same benefits can also be realized when training surgical residents in an educational environment.

Traumatic injuries cause significant alteration in both the soft and hard tissues of the face. These insults cause considerable distortion of the regional anatomy as well as destruction of surrounding structures, making the reconstruction a very challenging task. Over time, intraoperative navigation technology has become more readily accessible and user-friendly. The patient's anatomy is registered with a preoperative computed tomography scan with excellent accuracy. Virtual surgical planning software can be used to simulate the contralateral position of a fractured bone to give a planned position for reduction. This is especially useful in zygomatic fractures as the three-dimensional nature of a fractured zygomatic complex makes them challenging to orient during surgery to allow for optimal reduction. Real-time probe based on navigation systems can then be used to achieve and verify the desired position and is most useful in instances of positioning large orbital plates and comminuted zygoma pieces where surgical access may be restricted. Intraoperative computed tomography scans give surgeons the unprecedented ability to check fracture reduction and hardware positioning in the operative field, thereby improving

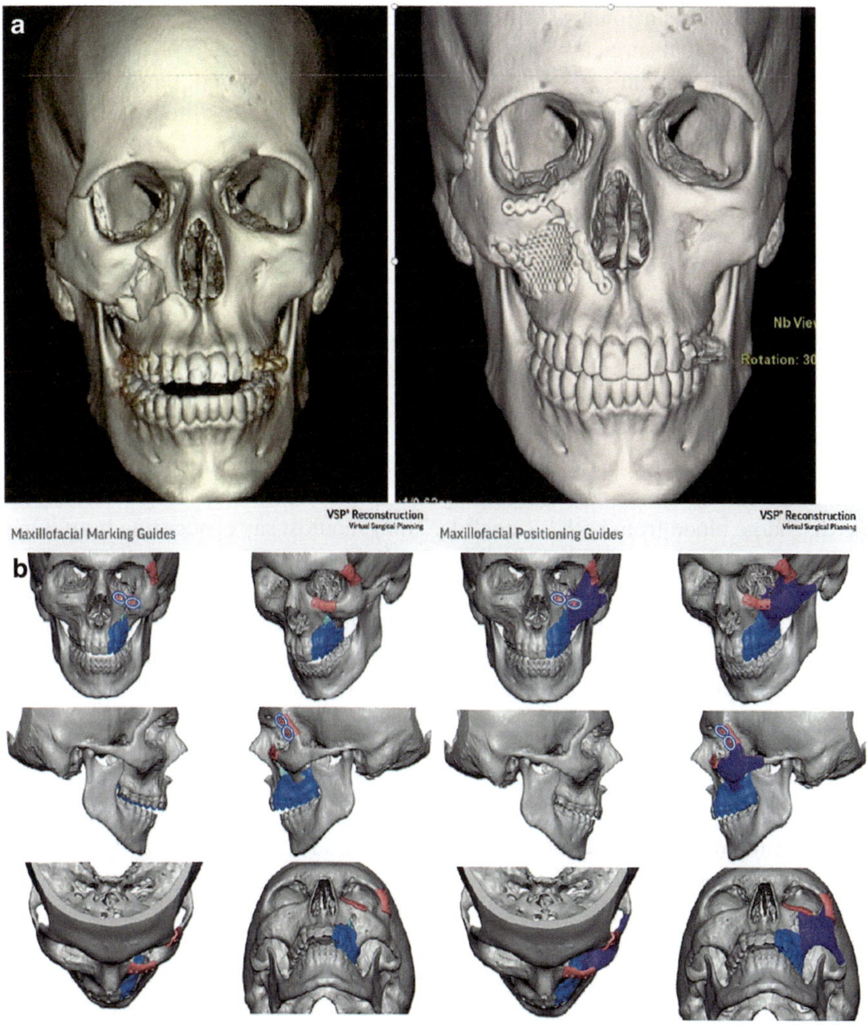

Fig. 3 (**a**) Three-dimensional reconstruction of pre- and postoperative CT maxillofacial imaging for a zygomaticomaxillary complex fracture. The postoperative image demonstrates the use of titanium miniplates across the fracture lines and a titanium mesh to maintain skeletal dimensions. (**b**) Virtual surgical plan with use of marking and positioning guides to reposition the left zygoma based on the uninjured, right zygoma

accuracy and reducing the need for take-back reoperations. In the setting of zygomatic fractures, this technology can be used to assess facial symmetry and orbital floor hardware positioning after the soft tissue retraction has been released (Klug et al. 2006).

With the development of miniplates and rigid fixation, increased points of fixation for zygomatic and associated mid to upper face fractures have allowed for improved three-dimensional stability and more accurate anatomical reduction. With the advent of virtual surgical planning, custom plates designed to provide accurate adaptation to the patient's post-reduction anatomy can be milled, thereby decreasing intraoperative time needed to contour the plates and providing more optimal outcomes.

5 Nasal Bone Fractures

Like the other facial fractures reviewed in this chapter, the treatment of nasal bone fractures was first described in the *Papyrus,* with techniques dating back to 1700 BCE (Breasted 1930). Among the near 50 cases, four (cases XI–XIV) are focused on isolated nasal injuries. In the first case, case XI, the book explains the diagnosis of a fractured nasal bone, "If thou examines a man having a break in the column of his nose, his nose being disfigured, and a depression being it…(and) he has discharge blood from both his nostrils. Thou shouldst say concerning him: 'One having a break in the column of his nose. An ailment which I will treat.'" The treatment involved in at least 1700 BCE, as translated in the *Papyrus*, was, "Thou should cleanse (it) for him [with] two plugs of linen. Thou shouldst place two plugs of linen saturated with grease in the inside of his two nostrils. Thou shouldst put [him] at his mooring stakes until the swelling is reduced. Thou shouldst apply for him stiff rolls of linen by which his nose is held fast. Thou shouldst treat him afterward [with] grease, honey (and) lint, every day until he recovers" (Breasted 1930). Of note, a few main treatment principles have carried through the last thousand years: utilizing a nasal packing, waiting for swelling to subside, and firm external, rigid support.

The principles of nasal bone fractures have not advanced significantly over the past few thousand years. Early texts advocated for reduction by inserting either fingers or firm instruments for manual manipulation and reshaping, followed by nasal packing and rigid support.

Other historical works with regard to the management of nasal bone fractures were discovered in 1844 when Francis Adams translated *The Seven Books of Paulus Aegineta* into English (Skoulakis et al. 2008). Paul of Aegina (CE 625–690) was a Greek physician and surgeon. His sixth book that was translated in 1844 focuses on surgery and medicine. Paul of Aegina understood that the nose had an "under part…being cartilaginous does not admit of fracture, but is liable to be crushed flattened, and distorted; but the upper part being of a bony substance is sometimes fractured" (Adams 1844). He advised against large bandaging of the nose which he observed contributed to distortion. He described his treatment as, "When, therefore, the nose is fractured in its under parts, having introduced the index or little finger into the nostril, he pushes the parts outwards to their proper position. When the fracture is of the inner parts, this is to be done with the head of a probe immediately, during the course of the first day, or not long afterwards, because the bones of the nose get consolidated about the tenth day. They are to be put into the proper position with the index finger and thumb externally. In order to prevent the bones from changing their position, two wedge-like tents, formed of a twisted, linen rag, are to be applied, one to each nostril" (Adams 1844). His solution for maintaining space for adequate respiration, he described, "sewing the quills of the feathers of a goose into the rags…they may preserve the parts in position without obstructing the respiration; but this is unnecessary, as respiration is carried on by the mouth" (Adams 1844). At the time they utilized natural anti-inflammatories such as diachylon, vinegar and oil, or a cataplasm of fine wheaten flour boiled with manna or gum (Skoulakis et al. 2008; Adams 1844). For comminuted fractures, he practiced opening the wound via incision and "…removed the small bones with a hair forceps, unite the divided parts with sutures…" (Adams 1844). Fascinatingly, all of the modern principles for closed reduction were practiced in ancient Greece. Further, a clear attention to detail for patient's postoperative comfort is eloquently written.

In 1898, a British surgeon, William Johnson Walsham, published in his textbook, "Nasal Obstruction: the diagnosis of the various conditions causing it, and their treatment," his modification of a previously introduced forceps that allows one to grasp and manipulate the nasal septum without crushing the columella (Walsham 1898). This convenient and useful forceps, referred to in present time as the "Walsham forceps," is still widely used for the same purpose.

In Keen's series of texts throughout the early 1900s, *Surgery, Its Principles and Practice,* similar treatments were advocated using manual reduction and splint placement. By this time, general anesthesia after being demonstrated in 1846 in the "Ether Dome," at the Massachusetts General Hospital, started to be well described in published texts. Further the author described that in the case of old fractures, "under general anesthetic, the nasal bones, together with the nasal process of the superior maxillae, broken away from their attachment by the use of a mallet and the handle of a chisel which is protected by, rubber jacket, and placed at the point where the fracture is desired. When the two sides have been treated, the nasal bones may be properly adjusted and held in place…" (Keen 1909).

Following reduction, a variety of methods were used to fixate the reduction. Previously described plaster of Paris was frequently utilized. Other nasal splints were designed with a heavy tin, lined by dental compound for molding the best fit. With certain depressed nasal bone fractures that require traction, two oval lead plates were contoured to a concave form and adapted to the sides of the nose. Subsequently, a horizontal mattress suture with soft stainless steel was thrown through the fractured fragment and septum and back to the original side (Rowe and Kelly 1968). All of these methods aided the development of modern techniques and treatments for the same injuries.

5.1 *Modern Treatment*

The bones and cartilage of the nose provide both aesthetic and structural support for the midface and airway; therefore, proper evaluation and management is necessary to prevent nasal deformity and nasal airway compromise. Modern approaches to nasal fracture repair emphasize accurate preoperative assessment of the extent of the nasal injury and compromised structures to allow for appropriate treatment planning. This is aided by advances in imaging technology such as the computed tomography scan and modern instruments such has the nasal endoscope. Advanced imaging techniques can be used to evaluate the extent of the comminution of the fracture and the involvement of the nasal septum and cartilage (Higuera et al. 2007). A nasal endoscope can be used to assess the involvement of the turbinates and ostiums of the sinuses. Based on the information obtained, the surgeon can determine if a closed reduction or open reduction is appropriate. Closed reduction is generally reserved for simple, noncomminuted nasal fractures where the key principle is to apply a force opposite to the vector of injury to achieve bone reduction (Verwoerd 1992). An important part of presurgical evaluation is to understand that certain nasal injuries cannot be sufficiently managed with a closed reduction. Comminuted fractures with severe loss of nasal support, severe septal injuries, and injuries with considerable soft tissue damage should be addressed with an open reduction. The greater exposure of anatomy allows for direct visualization and precise reduction of dislocated structures. In addition, any septal injury can be visualized via the traditional transfixion or hemitransfixion incision in the membranous septum. Development in rhinosurgery reconstructive techniques via various cartilage grafts has also improved the functional and esthetic outcomes in surgical repairs of nasal fractures (Rohrich and Adams Jr. 2000).

All reduced fractures, whether open or closed, should be splinted postoperatively. This may include internal as well as external splinting. Intranasal Doyle splints are recommended because they provide internal septal stabilization, aid in airway maintenance, and prevent synechiae after substantial manipulation. Extranasal splints such as a Denver splint made from aluminum and memory foam are now used as the modern counterpart of the lead plates used in the early twentieth century (Cox 3rd. 2000).

6 Conclusion

The diagnosis and treatment of midface trauma has been described for thousands of years. Many of the earliest principles still guide us today and have survived all of the technological advances we have seen. The evolution of the surgical treatment of midface trauma is also consistent with the evolution of oral and maxillofacial surgery as a specialty. Midface trauma is among the earliest surgeries oral and maxillofacial surgeons treated. Further, midface trauma treatment evolved in concert with the evolution of warfare, in particular ballistic warfare. In response to the need, World War I surgeons such as Gillies and Kazanjian developed techniques and principles of midface trauma management that are still in use today.

The surgical management of midface fractures has evolved throughout history to allow for more accurate reduction and fixation of fractured facial structures. With improved understanding of surgical technique and advances in anatomical imaging and rigid fixation, treatment of facial fractures has become increasingly predictable, customized, and refined. The use of computer-aided surgery continues to impact all areas of surgery, with maxillofacial surgery significantly benefiting from recent technological advancements. The ability to three-dimensionally visualize fractures and its influence on the surrounding anatomy allows the surgeon to accurately plan the reconstruction. With the development of software programs to manipulate image information and with the aid of the stereolithographic models made possible by advancements in 3D printing, a precise planning of the reconstruction can be transferred from the presurgical model surgery to the operating room. The optimization of the reconstructive component allows for not only decreased operating time and morbidity but also improved functional outcome and aesthetics.

References

Adams F. On Fracture and contusion of the nose (section XCI). The seven books of Paulus Aegineta (Book 6). London: Syndenham Society; 1844.

Adams WM. Internal wiring fixation of facial fractures. Am J Orthod Oral Surg. 1943;29(2):B111–B30.

Adams WM, Adams L. Internal wire fixation of facial fractures a fifteen-year follow-up report. Am J Surg. 1956;92(1):12–7.

Agnew DH. Principles and practice of surgery. Philadelphia: J.B. Lippincott Company; 1878. p. 838–40.

Bagby GW, Janes JM. The effect of compression on the rate of fracture healing using a special plate. Am J Surg. 1958;95(5):761–71.

Breasted J. The Edwin Smith surgical papyrus. Chicago: The University of Chicago Press; 1930.

Brown JB. Internal wire-pin fixation for fractures of upper jaw, orbit, zygoma, and severe facial crushes. Plast Reconstr Surg. 1946;9(3):276–83.

Claussen CD, Lohkamp FW, Krastel A. Computed tomography of trauma involving brain and facial skull (craniofacial injuries). J Comput Assist Tomogr. 1977;1(4):472–81.

Cox AJ 3rd. Nasal fractures--the details. Facial Plast Surg. 2000;16(2):87–94.

Dingman R, Natvig P. Surgery of facial fractures. W. B. Saunders; 1964.

Ewers R, Schicho K, Undt G, Wanschitz F, Truppe M, Seemann R, et al. Basic research and 12 years of clinical experience in computer-assisted navigation technology: a review. Int J Oral Maxillofac Surg. 2005;34(1):1–8.

Flynn E, Standerwick R, Trupp M. Skeletal head frame: a preliminary report. JAMA. 1958;167(4):442–3.

Gentry LR, Manor WF, Turski PA, Strother CM. High-resolution CT analysis of facial struts in trauma: 1. Normal anatomy. AJR Am J Roentgenol. 1983;140(3):523–32.

Gilles HD, Kilner TP, Stone D. Fractures of the malar-zygomatic compound: with a description of a new X-ray position. Br J Surg. 1927;14(56):651–6.

Gilmer T. Multiple fracture of the lower jaw complicated by double fracture of the upper jaw. JAMA. 1904;XLIII(1):8–9.

Gruss JS, Mackinnon SE. Complex maxillary fractures: role of buttress reconstruction and immediate bone grafts. Plast Reconstr Surg. 1986;78(1):9–22.

Higuera S, Lee EI, Cole P, Hollier LH Jr, Stal S. Nasal trauma and the deviated nose. Plast Reconstr Surg. 2007;120(7 Suppl 2):64S–75S.

Kazanjian VH. Treatment of injuries of the upper part of the face. J Am Dent Assoc. 1927;14(9):1607–18.

Keen WW. Surgery: its principles and practice. Philadelphia: W.B.Saunders; 1909.

Klug C, Schicho K, Ploder O, Yerit K, Watzinger F, Ewers R, et al. Point-to-point computer-assisted navigation for precise transfer of planned zygoma osteotomies from the stereolithographic model into reality. J Oral Maxillofac Surg. 2006;64(3):550–9.

Lambotte A. The Classic. Contribution to conservative surgery of the injured hand. By Dr. A. Lambotte. 1928. Clin Orthop Relat Res. 1987;(214):4–6.

Louis PJ, Morlandt AB. Advancements in maxillofacial trauma: a historical perspective. J Oral Maxillofac Surg. 2018;76(11):2256–70.

Luhr H. Oral and maxillofacial traumatology, compression plate osteosynthesis through the Luhr system. 1st ed. Chicago: Quintessence Publishing Company; 1982.

Manwaring JG. Replacing depressed fractures of the malar bone. JAMA. 1913;60:278–9.

McAuley JE. Charles Valadier: a forgotten pioneer in the treatment of jaw injuries. Proc R Soc Med. 1974;67(8):785–9.

Metzger MC, Hohlweg-Majert B, Schwarz U, Teschner M, Hammer B, Schmelzeisen R. Manufacturing splints for orthognathic surgery using a three-dimensional printer. Oral Surg Oral Med Oral Pathol Oral Radiol Endod. 2008;105(2):e1–7.

Michelet FX, Deymes J, Dessus B. Osteosynthesis with miniaturized screwed plates in maxillofacial surgery. J Maxillofac Surg. 1973;1(2):79–84.

Roberts S. Fracture of the malar Zygomatic arch-review of the literature-a simplified Operatice technic-case reports. Ann Otol Rhinol Larngol. 1928;37(3):826–38.

Rohrich RJ, Adams WP Jr. Nasal fracture management: minimizing secondary nasal deformities. Plast Reconstr Surg. 2000;106(2):266–73.

Rowe NL, Kelly HC. Fractures of the facial skeleton. 2nd ed. Great Britain: The Williams and Wilkins Compant; 1968.

Schramm A, Schon R, Rucker M. Computer-assisted oral and maxillofacial reconstruction. J Comput Inf Technol. 2006;14:71.

Seeram E. Computed tomography: an overview. Computed tomography—physical principles, clinical applications & quality control. Philadelphia: WB Saunders; 1994.

Simpson DA, David DJ. Herbert Moran Memorial Lecture. World War I: the genesis of craniomaxillofacial surgery? ANZ J Surg. 2004;74(1–2):71–7.

Skoulakis CE, Manios AG, Theos EA, Papadakis CE, Stavroulaki PS. Treatment of nasal fractures by Paul of Aegina. Otolaryngol Head Neck Surg. 2008;138(3):279–82.

Smith H, Yanagisawa E. Fracture-dislocations of Zygoma and Zygomatic Arch: historical development of surgical treatment. Arch Otolaryngol. 1961;73(2):172–85.

Tessier P. The classic reprint. Experimental study of fractures of the upper jaw. I and II. Rene Le Fort, M.D. Plast Reconstr Surg. 1972a;50(5):497–506 contd.

Tessier P. The classic reprint: experimental study of fractures of the upper jaw. 3. Rene Le Fort, M.D., Lille, France. Plast Reconstr Surg. 1972b;50(6):600–7.

Valadier AC, Whale HL. A report on oral and plastic surgery and on prosthetic appliances. Br J Surg. 1917;5(17):151–71.

van Middendorp JJ, Sanchez GM, Burridge AL. The Edwin Smith papyrus: a clinical reappraisal of the oldest known document on spinal injuries. Eur Spine J. 2010;19(11):1815–23.

Verbeek O. Osteosynthesis and the lane technic. Am J Surg. 1955;90(3):410–8.

Verwoerd CD. Present day treatment of nasal fractures: closed versus open reduction. Facial Plast Surg. 1992;8(4):220–3.

Walsham WJ. Nasal obstruction: the diagnosis of the various conditions causing it, and their treatment. Bailliere, Tindall and Cox: London; 1898.

Mandibular Trauma

Carlos R. Hernandez, Daniel E. Perez, and Edward Ellis III

1 Introduction

The earliest account of mandibular fractures is found in the *Edwin Smith Surgical Papyrus*, which was acquired by Smith at Luxor in 1862 and later translated by James H. Breasted in 1930 (Mukerji et al. 2006; Thoma 1944). The papyrus was written sometime in the Pyramid Age (3000–2500 BCE) (Thoma 1944). Breasted's translation of dealing with a mandibular fracture involves the following:

> If thou examines a man having a fracture in his mandible, thou shouldst place thy hand upon it. Shouldst thou find that fracture crepitating under thy fingers, thou shouldst say concerning him: One having a fracture in his mandible, over which a wound has been inflicted, thou will a fever gain from it. An ailment not to be treated. (Rowe 1971)

Therefore, the Egyptians at this time did not have much hope for patients with compound fractures of the mandible. This papyrus also illustrates how treatment of simple mandible fractures in these times consisted of the following:

> Applying bandages obtained from the embalmer, and soaked in honey and white of egg, while wounds were treated by the application of fresh meat on the first day, a method which may well have introduced tissue enzymes and thromboplastins without, one hopes, too many associated bacteria. (Rowe 1971)

C. R. Hernandez (✉) · D. E. Perez · E. Ellis III
Department of Oral and Maxillofacial Surgery, UT Health San Antonio,
San Antonio, TX, USA
e-mail: Hernandezc28@uthscsa.edu

E. M. Ferneini et al. (eds.), *The History of Maxillofacial Surgery*,
https://doi.org/10.1007/978-3-030-89563-1_12

2 The Hellenic Period

In 400 BCE, Hippocrates, also known as "the Father of Medicine," began devising his own methods to treat mandibular fractures. He advocated the use of gold or linen threads to tie teeth on either side of the fracture for fixation (Rowe 1971). He described the following regarding immobilizing and reapproximating fractures of the mandible:

> In fractures of the lower jaw, when the bone is not fairly broken across, and is still partially retained but displaced, it should be adjusted by introducing the fingers at the side of the tongue and making suitable counter-pressure on the outside; and if the teeth at the wound be distorted and loosened, when the bone is adjusted they should be connected together, not only two but more of them, with a gold thread if possible, but otherwise with a linen thread, until the bone is consolidated, and then the part is to be dressed with cerate, a few compresses, and a few bandages, which should not be very tight, but rather loose. (Thoma 1944)

Hippocrates not only taught ways of reducing and immobilizing a fractured mandible but is also credited with devising the technique of reducing a dislocated mandible (Thomaidis et al. 2018). This method, which is still used, is described as follows:

> The patient is put in a lying or sitting position, while an assistant must hold the head tightly in a steady position. The physician grabs the mandible with his two arms from inside and outside the oral cavity, from both sides, left and right, performing 3 manipulations simultaneously. He lifts up the mandible, pushes it backwards while closing the oral cavity, all at once. Painkillers should be given. The mandible should be fixed in its normal position with the aid of bandages. (Thomaidis et al. 2018)

3 The Early Medieval Period

In the period of the Roman Empire (23 BCE–CE 410), the Romans continued to rely on the principles of immobilization and repositioning established by Hippocrates (Rowe 1971). In 30 BCE, Aulus Cornelius Celsus recommended the following technique for fixation after setting the fractured segments of the mandible in place:

> Tie together the two teeth nearest the fracture with a silk thread, or else if these are loose, the next ones. After this a thick compress should be applied dipped in wine and oil and sprinkled with flour and powdered olibanum. This compress is to be fixed in place by means of a strip of soft leather with a longitudinal slit in the middle to embrace the chin, the two ends being tied together above the head. (Thoma 1944)

Furthermore, Celsus instructed his patients to not speak and to adhere exclusively to a liquid diet for several days (Mukerji et al. 2006; Thoma 1944). This is one of the earliest references of "closed treatment," a technique that we use today to manage non-displaced fractures.

Later, in about CE 500, Sushruta, an Indian physician, recorded a conservative method to treat mandibular fractures in his ancient Sanskrit text on medicine and surgery. He recommended using complicated bandaging, manual manipulation, and heat to treat fractures of the mandible (Mukerji et al. 2006; Qureshi et al. 2016).

4 Middle Ages–Early Eighteenth Century

During the Middle Ages, there was little advancement in the management of mandibular fractures. Around the year 1000 CE, Abu Al Qasim Al Zahrawi (Albucasis), one of the greatest surgeons of his time, illustrated principles for mandibular fixation using horizontal wiring adopted from Hippocrates (Thoma 1944).

From the Middle Ages to the early eighteenth century, "barber surgeons" had taken over the management of facial fractures when the Pope "ruled any operation involving the shedding of blood incompatible with the priestly office in 1163" (Mukerji et al. 2006). Therefore, these barbers became a one-stop shop by providing services such as cutting hair, extracting teeth, treating facial fractures, applying leeches, and performing minor surgeries (Mukerji et al. 2006). The barbers adhered to the Hippocratic principles of management of jaw fractures by manually reducing the fractured segments, wiring the teeth adjacent to the fracture site, and immobilizing the jaw with bandages (Mukerji et al. 2006) (see chapter Barber-Surgeons).

The importance of establishing proper occlusion when treating mandibular fractures was accentuated in a textbook written by Roger of Salerno in Italy in 1180 (El-Anwar 2017). Three centuries later, rigid MMF was introduced by Guglielmo Saliceto in 1492, when he described how the surgeon should "tie the teeth of the uninjured jaw to the teeth of the injured jaw" in patients with mandible fractures (Rowe 1971). Saliceto's groundbreaking concept of MMF, which is still used today, would later remain dormant for many centuries, with no accounts of its application until the late nineteenth century.

5 Eighteenth Century

Pierre Fauchard sparked the advent of scientific dentistry in 1728 when he wrote his book *Traité de Chirurgie dentaire* (Rowe 1971; Thoma 1944). Although he did not make direct contributions to management of mandible fractures, his comprehensive literature for the practice of dentistry, which included the development of dental prostheses, inspired others to develop prostheses or splints that would provide more stability in treating mandible fractures (Mukerji et al. 2006; Rowe 1971).

In 1743, Robert Bunon described a mandibular fracture case in which the mandibular bicuspids had been avulsed from the effects of trauma and there was subluxation of adjacent teeth (Thoma 1944). He replaced the empty space with a piece of ivory containing two holes and crossed threads from the second molar on one side of the fracture to the second bicuspid on the other side and tied it very tightly. By doing so he was able to create a single block and consolidate the loosened teeth, thereby curing the fracture in less than a month (Thoma 1944).

Later in 1779, Chopart and Desault stated in their book *Traite des Maladies Chirurgicale* that mandible fractures may occur at the chin, near the ramus, at the condyle, on one side, or on both (Thoma 1944). They recommended bandages made of "iron hooks previously covered with linen, cork, or lead leaf and placed over the lower occlusal table or the alveolar border and then clamped down with screws and nuts to a plate of sheet iron below the lower border of the mandible" (Thoma 1944). They also described the effects of elevator and depressor muscles on mandibular fragments in their book (Thoma 1944).

6 Nineteenth Century

During this century the importance of proper occlusion in fracture reduction and stabilization, inspired by Roger of Salerno, was elucidated. Its importance has been maintained since, and it is currently well known that there is an increase in postoperative complications if the occlusion is unstable when treating with rigid internal fixation (Ribeiro-Junior et al. 2020).

There was also wide use of splints and bandages in the nineteenth century. In 1805, Boyer recommended the use of cork splints to treat mandible fractures (Thoma 1944). Moreover, Barton recommended applying a bandage made of a roll that was five yards long as a form of fixation in 1819 (Fig. 1). The Barton bandage is still used at times today either pre- or postoperatively (Kademani et al. 2016). Gillespie, in 1836, used a piece of sole leather between the teeth on both sides and passed a bandage around the head and another one around the chin. Following the advent of ether anesthesia (1846), Gordon Buck became the first to apply metallic fixation to a mandible fracture by using intraosseous wiring in the United States in 1847 (Ellis 1993; Rowe 1971; Thoma 1944).

Hamilton introduced the gutta-percha splint in 1855, claiming improved stability over Boyer's cork splint (Thoma 1944). The gutta-percha was heated, molded into wedge-shaped blocks, and placed on each side between the teeth while the jaw was being reduced. Hamilton recommended its use together with a vertical bandage around the head for fractures occurring within the dental arch (Mukerji et al. 2006; Thoma 1944).

In 1858, Hayward designed a metal splint for severely dislocated fractures (Mukerji et al. 2006). The fabrication of this splint involved taking an impression of the lower jaw and making a cast. "The cast was sectioned at the fracture site and the occlusion was realigned. Then, the metal splint was made to the new occlusion and the fractured segments were forced into the splint" (Mukerji et al. 2006).

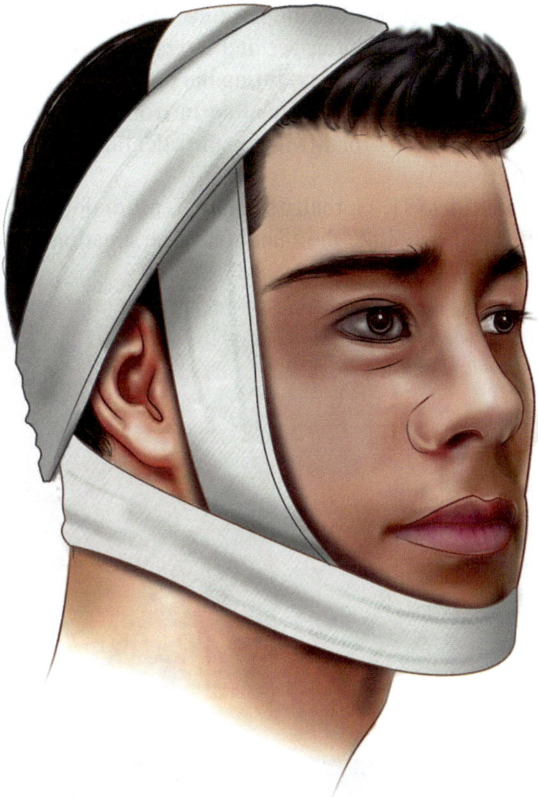

Fig. 1 Barton bandage

In the early nineteenth century, there was not much improvement in the treatment of mandibular fractures besides the use of splints fabricated from different materials and use of bandages. It was not until Kearney Rogers from New York applied bone sutures to fractures of long bones, which later prompted the use of bone sutures for mandible fractures as well (Fig. 2). The procedure involved a thread being passed inside the mouth through the gingiva and periosteum (Thoma 1944). In 1859, Kinloch describes a case, in the *American Journal of the Medical Sciences*, which involved a compound fracture just anterior to the masseter muscle (Thoma 1944). Treatment with wiring of the teeth and use of bandages was not effective for this case. Therefore, he administered chloroform and via a submandibular approach drilled a hole in each fragment. Then, he used a silver wire to bring the fractured segments together (Rowe 1971; Thoma 1944).

In 1865, Thomas Gunning designed the "Gunning splint" specifically for Mr. Seward, the Secretary of State to Abraham Lincoln who fell out of a carriage and fractured the body of his mandible bilaterally. The Gunning splint was a single piece of vulcanite with a space for eating that was attached to the hard palate and mandible using screws (Mukerji et al. 2006; Rowe 1971). The fabrication of this splint involved taking impressions of the upper and lower jaws and making casts. The model was sectioned at the fracture site and was realigned into proper occlusion. Then the casts of the upper and lower jaws were put in an articulator to make a model of the splint in wax, fitting the upper and lower jaws so they were partly open which allowed a hole for feeding in front (Rowe 1971). The Gunning splint also provides a means for MMF for the edentulous patient currently (Kademani et al. 2016) (Fig. 3).

Later in 1871, Gurnell Hammond, a London dentist, developed a wire ligature splint to immobilize the mandible. The creation of this splint involved taking an

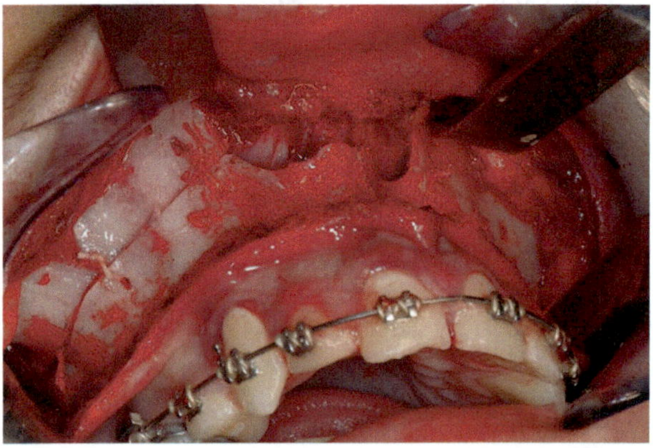

Fig. 2 Bone sutures in a Le Fort osteotomy. (*UT Health San Antonio*)

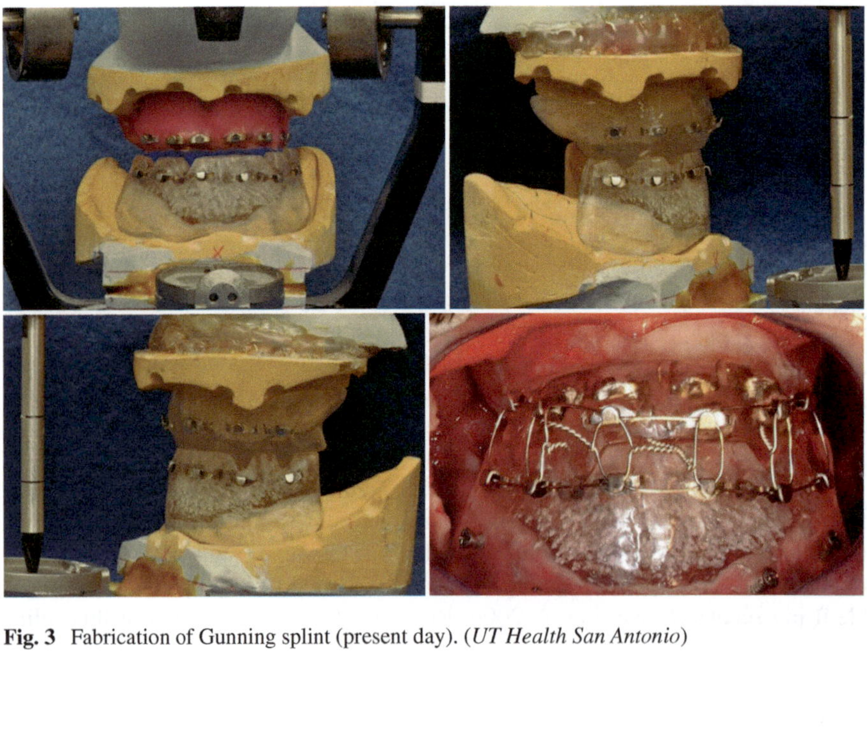

Fig. 3 Fabrication of Gunning splint (present day). (*UT Health San Antonio*)

impression of the lower jaw and casting it in stone. The fractured segments were realigned on the model and then an iron wire was secured to the teeth on the model. The bar was then wired to the patient's natural teeth. This technique is regarded as the predecessor of arch bars and model surgery used today (Mukerji et al. 2006).

Almost a decade later, in 1880, Kingsley of New York fabricated a horseshoe-shaped metal tray which fit the mandible. It had two wires that were soldered to it that extended out of the mouth so that a bandage could be adapted to the wires and pass beneath the mandible. The metal tray was filled with heated gutta-percha and applied over the mandibular teeth (Thoma 1944).

In 1887, intermaxillary ligation was reintroduced by Thomas L. Gilmer (Thoma 1944). He described applying this principle to a case in which his patient had a compound fracture of the right mandibular body and a comminuted fracture of the angle and a part of the lower half of the ramus on the left side. This is the first account in literature of fixation of a fractured mandible by holding the lower teeth in occlusion with the upper teeth by wire ligatures twisted together (Gilmer 1887; Mukerji et al. 2006). He pointed out the value of wiring the lower to the upper teeth in fixation of fractures of the mandible. Gilmer describes his procedure below:

> In each fragment a hole was drilled of suitable size to just admit a No. 16 (standard gauge) platinum wire, which was bent in the shape of a staple; the fragments having been put in place the two arms of the staple were inserted from the lingual surface. These arms were brought together on the buccal surface and tightly twisted, drawing the parts into close apposition. Next, a short steel wire, No. 27, was placed around the neck of each individual tooth of the lower jaw between the second bicuspid on the right and the second molar on the left and the corresponding teeth of the upper jaw. The ends of each wire were brought together and twisted, fastening it securely to the teeth. This being done, the teeth of the lower jaw were exactly articulated with those of the upper by bringing them together and twisting thus firmly lashing the lower to the upper jaw. To prevent lateral motion the wire of the upper left lateral was secured to the lower right lateral; this crossing being continued throughout, held the jaw immovable. (Gilmer 1887)

In 1890, Edward Angle, who is regarded as "the Father of American Orthodontics," contributed to the management of mandibular fractures by introducing special bands that could be placed around the teeth on either side of the fracture instead of using interosseous wiring (Rowe 1971; Thoma 1944). These bands had tiny knobs or tubes which accommodated wires and held the fractured segment in firm contact. For intermaxillary fixation, Angle placed bands on the upper and lower teeth on each side of the fracture and then fixed a wire along the short arms that held the upper and lower jaws together (Thoma 1944).

7 Early–Mid-Twentieth Century

During World War I and II, there were a myriad of soldiers who suffered extensive maxillofacial injuries from shrapnel, bullets, and shells. The fractures involved in these injuries were characterized by comminution and loss of bone in many cases (Fig. 4). Surgeons were put to the test to develop reduction and fixation methods that provided better results than ever before. Consequently, it has been noted that some of the greatest advancements in the development of treatment methods were made during periods of war. Hippocrates regards war as "the only proper school of the surgeon" (Mukerji et al. 2006).

The use of external fixation devices became popular in this era with many patients presenting with compound, comminuted infected fractures of the mandible (Fig. 5). "The Amex casque, popular with French and British military surgeons, had an adjustable steel band, fitting around the circumference of the head, with adjustable cranial bands and an adjustable perpendicular rod and horizontal face bow"

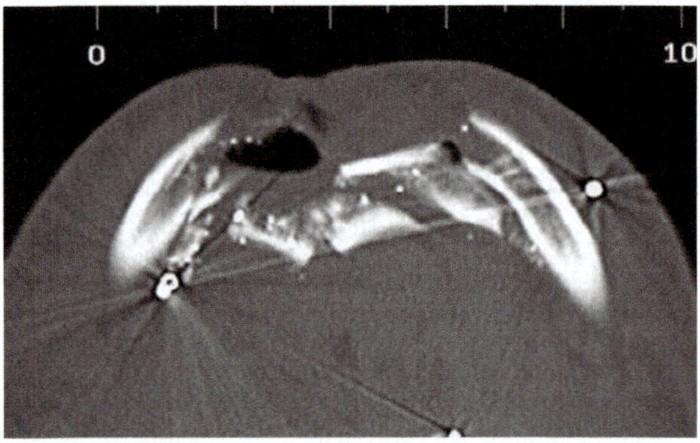

Fig. 4 Radiograph of comminuted fracture of the mandible. (*UT Health San Antonio*)

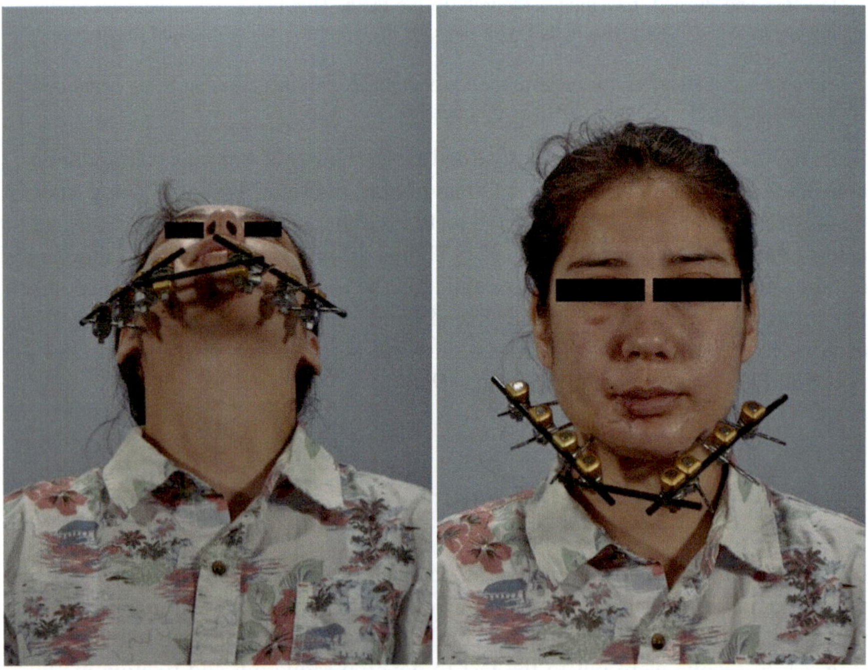

Fig. 5 External fixation devices. (*UT Health San Antonio*)

(Mukerji et al. 2006). Its use in facial and jaw reconstruction permitted absolute fixation for either soft tissue or osseous fragments (Mukerji et al. 2006).

During World War I, Varaztad H. Kazanjian used wire sutures through bone fragments and tied the wire to an arch bar for fixation. Kazanjian's method of suturing osseous fragments resulted in great success with managing severely comminuted fractures of the mandible. He also fabricated splints and "internal vulcanized rubber supports that prevented the face from contracting until surgeons were able to graft bone and skin onto the damaged areas" (Mukerji et al. 2006). The wire sutures were removed after about 3–4 weeks. Kazanjian is known for emphasizing the value of various types of prosthetic appliances, which he inserted immediately after injuries to support the tissues while they were still soft and flexible and to prevent unwanted adhesions (Thoma 1944).

Kazanjian is also known for classifying fractures of the mandible by the presence or absence of serviceable teeth in relation to the line of fracture. The classes include the following:

- Class I: teeth are present on both sides of the fracture line.
- Class II: teeth are present on only one side of the fracture line.
- Class III: patient is edentulous (Thoma 1944).

In 1922, Robert H. Ivy modified the intermaxillary fixation technique by creating a loop, or eyelet, in the wire ligature. Ivy loops are normally used for MMF of minimally displaced fractures when the patient has a full dentition, but can also be used when there are only a few stable teeth within the arch (Eusterman 2012; Ivy 1922; Kademani et al. 2016) (Fig. 6). Although percutaneous nailing of fractured longs bones was described by Parkhill in 1897, the use of Kirschner wires in the treatment of mandibular fractures was published in 1932 (Mukerji et al. 2006; Thoma 1944; Vero 1968). Once normal occlusion was achieved, the fractured segments were fixed with a pin inserted transcutaneously (Mukerji et al. 2006).

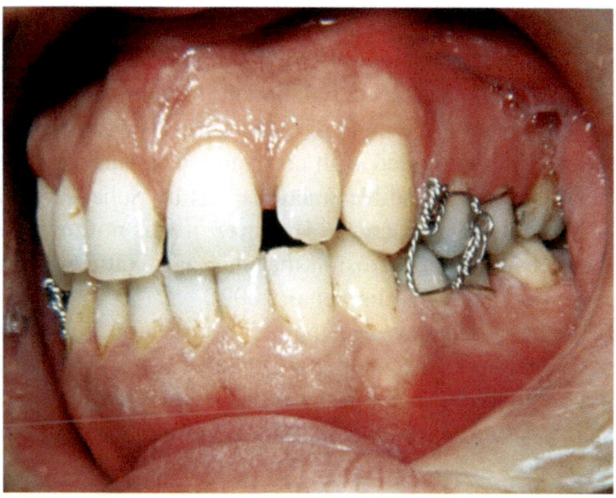

Fig. 6 Ivy loops. (*UT Health San Antonio*)

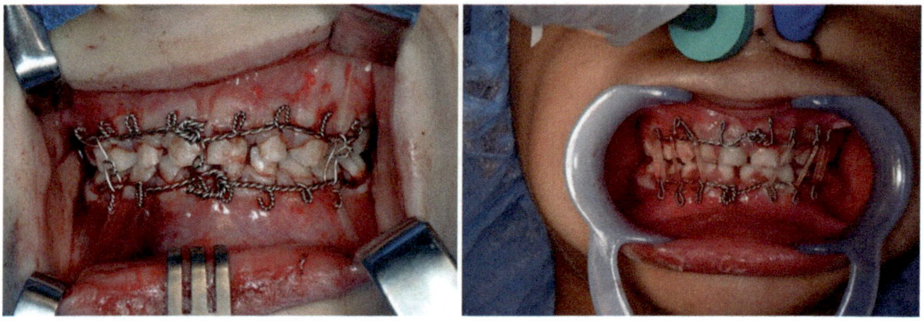

Fig. 7 Risdon wires. (*UT Health San Antonio*)

In 1936, E. Fulton Risdon described a twisted type of arch wiring for MMF (Fig. 7). He described using a wire that was twisted around the last molar tooth of the mandible. The ends were then twisted following the contour of the mandible at the cervical margin of the teeth to the midline. This was accomplished bilaterally. The two twisted ends were then twisted together in the symphyseal region to form a substitute arch bar. Ligature wires were then passed to secure the individual teeth to the bar. This was also done on the maxilla to allow MMF. Additionally, the Joe Hall Morris appliance, which consisted of biphasic external pin fixation, was extensively used during World War II for closed reduction of comminuted fractures of the mandible. This appliance was noninvasive and did not require concurrent MMF (Ellis 1993; Eusterman 2012). Prior to the development of antibiotics, open reduction techniques were not widely accepted due to the likelihood of osteomyelitis or other infections arising postoperatively, which consequently resulted in failure of treatment (Ellis 1993).

7.1 *Rigid Internal Fixation*

Despite the first application of rigid internal fixation with a plate and screws being credited to Hansmann in 1858, the most significant advances were brought on by Sir William Lane and Albin Lambotte (Gilardino et al. 2009). From 1893 to 1914, they experimented in the field of osteosynthesis with steel plates and screws for internal fixation but struggled with corrosion. The earliest account of the use of true bone plates to treat mandible fractures was by Schede, in 1888, who used a solid steel plate held by four screws. However, it was not until the development of materials more resistant to corrosion that internal fixation for mandibular fractures became more popular (Gilardino et al. 2009).

In 1943, Bigelow was the first to use Vitallium, an alloy of cobalt, chrome, and molybdenum, for mandibular fractures (Mukerji et al. 2006). In an effort to reproduce a material that had the inertness of Vitallium combined with the usability of stainless steel, Leventhal in 1951 proposed the use of titanium for fractures. Whereas many metals were tested and abandoned for use in treatment of mandibular fractures and facial fractures in general, stainless steel, titanium, and Vitallium became more widespread during the new era of internal rigid fixation for facial fractures (Gilardino et al. 2009).

Following this, in 1949, the Belgian general surgeon Robert Danis introduced the principle of axial compression of the fracture ends (Luhr 2000; Uhthoff et al. 2006). He recognized his goal of achieving compression between the fractured segments using a plate he called the *coapteur*, which "suppressed interfragmentary motion and increased the stability of the fixation." This principle influenced all subsequent plate designs (Uhthoff et al. 2006).

8 Late Twentieth Century

8.1 Compression Osteosynthesis

Luhr developed a compression plate in 1967 which adhered to Danis' principle of axial compression. He is known for performing the first compression plating of the maxillofacial area in the world. Furthermore, he set the foundation for osteosynthesis to be the generally accepted treatment for facial fractures (Luhr 2000). Luhr is also credited with developing self-threading screws, which no longer required pretapping before screw insertion (Ellis 1993; Luhr 2000).

In the 1970s, Spiessl recognized that "chewing tends to distract the dental border of a fracture line, whereas the basal border tends to be compressed." He learned that fixation at the basal border of the mandible does little to overcome the distracting forces occurring more superiorly (Kellman 1995). To address this problem, he advocated using a "tension band arch bar" so that forces applied during chewing could not pull this area apart. He then applied a compression plate along the basal border. In situations where there were no teeth to apply the tension band arch bar, or it was difficult to apply compression forces at the superior area without damaging the tooth roots, the use of an eccentric dynamic compression plate was advocated (Kellman 1995). This type of plate, introduced by Schmoker and Niederdellrnann in 1973, has compression holes directed both horizontally and superiorly (Ellis 1993; Kellman 1995). When applied properly this plate provides compression at the alveolar region through the superior directed screws, as well as the basal border via the horizontal compression screws (Kellman 1995).

An alternative to the use of plates and screws for compression fixation is the lag screw technique which was introduced in 1970 by Brons and Boering (Ellis 1993). This technique is used when fragments of the bone overlap, and it has been shown to work well in the symphyseal and parasymphyseal region of the mandible where there is cortical overlap due to the curvature of the mandible (Kellman 1995). In the case of oblique fractures, at least two screws are required to prevent rotational movements (Ellis and Ghali 1991). In 1991, Ellis and Ghali found that the lag screw technique results in a simple yet successful way to secure the fragments in a non-comminuted fracture of the anterior mandible (Ellis and Ghali 1991) (Fig. 8).

Finally, the mandibular reconstruction plate was designed to be strong enough to replace a missing segment of the mandible or for cases of comminution (Kellman 1995). These plates are usually placed along the inferior border of the mandible to avoid damaging teeth or neurovascular structures and are placed with bicortical screws to gain additional stability (Kademani et al. 2016) (Fig. 9).

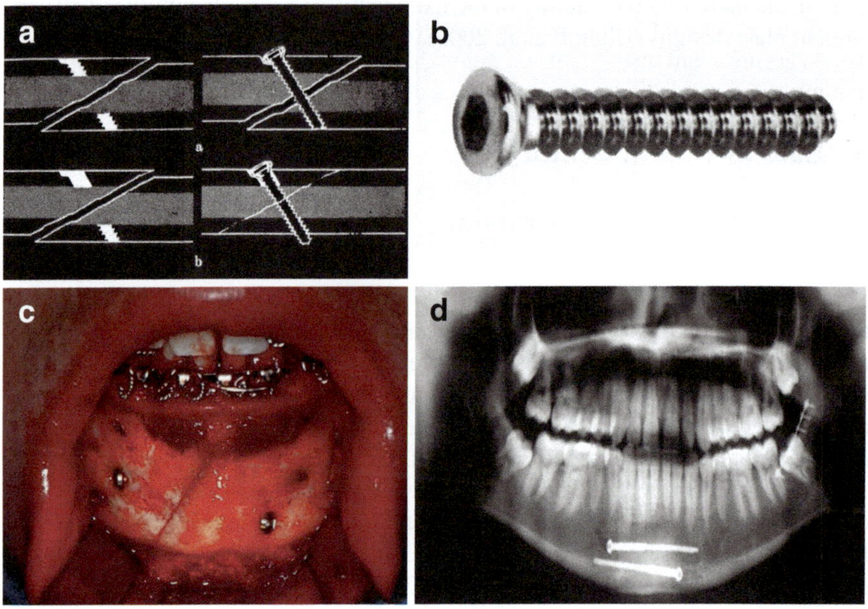

Fig. 8 Lag screws. (**a**) Technique, (**b**) lag screw, (**c**) intraoperative image of lag screw application, (**d**) postoperative radiograph. (*UT Health San Antonio*)

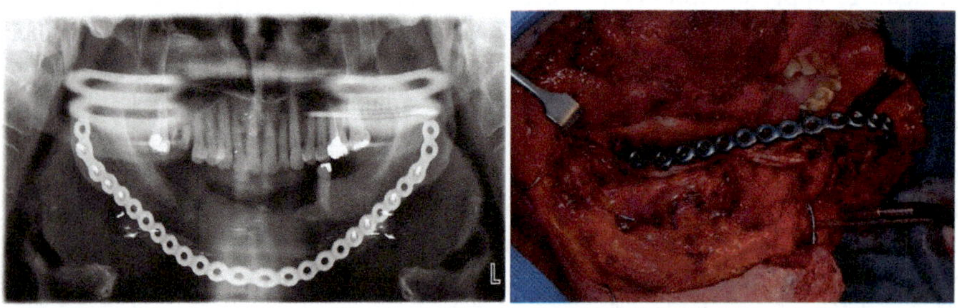

Fig. 9 Mandibular reconstruction plate. (*UT Health San Antonio*)

8.2 *Miniplate Osteosynthesis*

Michelet revolutionized the technique of internal fixation through his introduction of miniplate osteosynthesis in 1973. Before this, surgeons relied on an extraoral approach to treating mandibular fractures due to the large size of compression plates (Ellis 1993). Michelet's technique consisted of using small, non-compression bone plates placed juxta-alveolar and subapical via a transoral approach with monocortical screws.

In 1978, Champy et al., following along the technique of Michelet, advised against the use of compression plates due the following reasons:

1. There is a natural strain of compression existing along the lower border due to masticatory forces.
2. There is an inability to measure the amount of compression created between the two fragments which may lead to bone necrosis.
3. The use of a rigid lower border plate will result in the "shield effect."
4. There is difficulty in reestablishing normal occlusion with use of compression.
5. Compression osteosynthesis requires access through a transcutaneous approach.

Therefore, they advocated the use of very strong miniature and malleable screwed plates in the subapical position without compression. This miniplate is applied with monocortical screws in order to avoid damaging the tooth roots or the nerve (Champy et al. 1978; Ellis 1993).

Champy also described lines of tension along the mandible that correspond with biomechanically favorable regions for osteosynthesis (Champy et al. 1978; Koshy et al. 2010) (Fig. 10). He advised the use of one miniplate in all these areas of the mandible except for the symphyseal region where there are rotational or twisting forces during function (Kellman 1995). He recommended the use of two miniplates in this location. For mandibular angle fractures, he advocated the use of a miniplate along the vestibular osseous flat portion located in the third molar region (Champy et al. 1978) (Fig. 11).

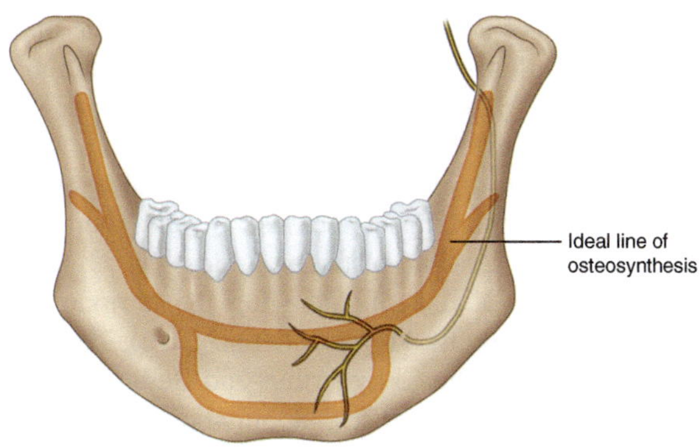

Fig. 10 Champy's ideal line of osteosynthesis

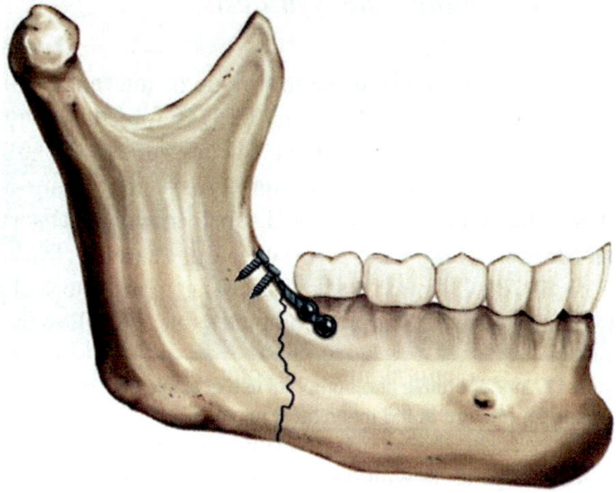

Fig. 11 Champy miniplate

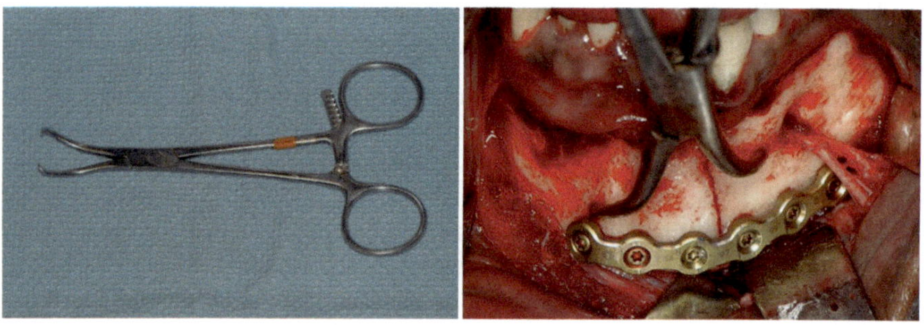

Fig. 12 Bone clamps. (*UT Health San Antonio*)

In 1973, Goode and Shinn described the use of a bone compression clamp, which would shorten or eliminate the need for intermaxillary wiring. It was found that this clamp held the fractured segments of the mandible in good position and promoted bone healing at 4 weeks (Fig. 12). These clamps were attached to the buccal and lingual cortices around the inferior border of the mandible. However, later studies showed how this device did not provide rigid fixation of the mandible and had some slippage (Ellis 1993; Goode and Shinn 1973).

The use of Erich arch bars provided an effective method for MMF prior to the development of open reduction and internal fixation (ORIF) (Fig. 13). However, there were shortcomings to their use as well. There is increased surgical time in both placement and removal of the arch bars, the surgeon bares the risk of penetrating injury, there is a risk of damaging the periodontium, and proper oral hygiene becomes compromised (Qureshi et al. 2016). Therefore, in 1989, self-drilling IMF screws were introduced by Arthur and Berardo to help overcome these shortcomings (Fig. 14). They used self-tapping bone screws that were 2 millimeters in diameter. The mandibular screws were placed between the root apices and the mental

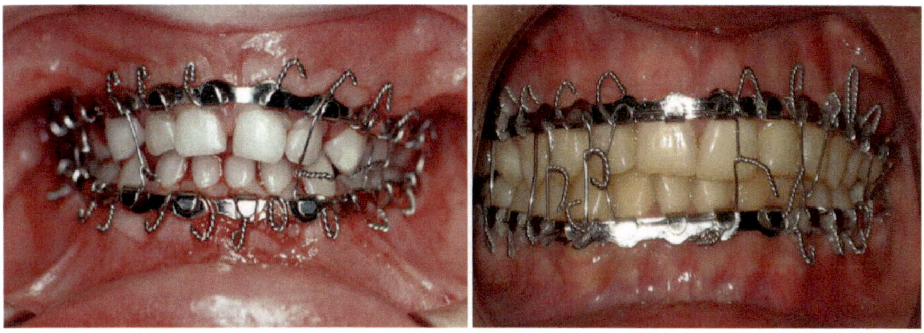

Fig. 13 Erich arch bars. (*UT Health San Antonio*)

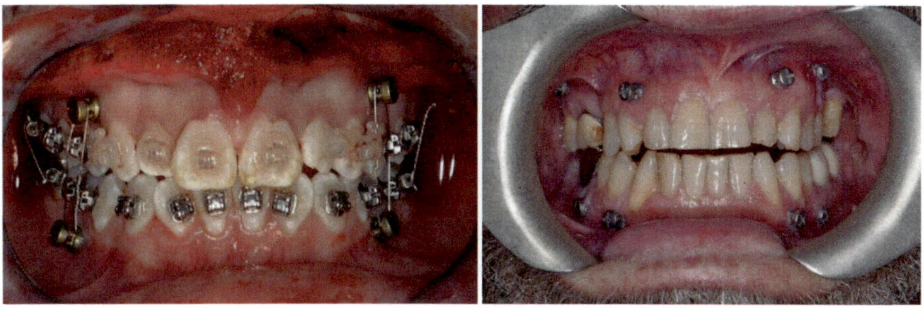

Fig. 14 IMF screws. (*UT Health San Antonio*)

foramen, whereas the maxillary screws were placed in the pyriform rim and zygomatic buttress areas (Qureshi et al. 2016). Some advantages of IMF screws were minimal use of hardware, decreased operation time, and no risk of needlestick injuries; however, there is still the risk of accidental root perforation (El-Anwar 2017; Qureshi et al. 2016). Ultimately, both Erich arch bars and IMF screws offer adequate temporary MMF intraoperatively to check occlusion (Qureshi et al. 2016).

9 Present Day

Currently, the most common treatment modality for mandible fractures is ORIF (Ellis and Miles 2007). In spite of this, closed reduction is still commonly used in some cases when surgery is not indicated. The location as well as the number and severity of fractures guides the anatomical approach and hardware that can be utilized. Research has also greatly expanded on the comparison of different techniques or armamentarium for treating mandible fractures. For instance, it is now known that the use of two miniplates results in more postoperative complications versus the use of one stronger plate for treatment of mandibular symphysis/body fractures (Ellis 2011).

Advances in plating osteosynthesis have also decreased the need for postoperative MMF (Ellis and Miles 2007). This is advantageous because it has been found that there are detrimental effects of mandibular immobilization on the masticatory apparatus (Ellis and Carlson 1989). Moreover, the ability to access fracture sites intraorally, or even endoscopically in some cases, has provided a significant improvement in aesthetic outcomes (Ellis and Miles 2007). Recently, resorbable polymer plates have been introduced as a management technique for mandibular fractures; however, they remain mostly used in non-load-bearing cranial and orbital regions (Hosein et al. 2013).

10 Conclusion

Despite the significant advances in management of mandible fractures, from the time of the ancient Egyptians to the present day, the goal of the surgeon of restoring form and function remains unchanged.

References

Champy M, Loddé JP, Schmitt R, Jaeger JH, Muster D. Mandibular osteosynthesis by miniature screwed plates via a buccal approach. J Maxillofac Surg. 1978;6:14–21.
El-Anwar M. Changing trends in the treatment of mandibular fracture. Int Arch Otorhinolaryngol. 2017;22(03):195–6.
Ellis E, Carlson DS. The effects of mandibular immobilization on the masticatory system. A review. Clin Plast Surg. 1989;16(1):133–46.
Ellis E, Ghali GE. Lag screw fixation of anterior mandibular fractures. J Oral Maxillofac Surg. 1991;49(1):13–21.
Ellis E, Miles BA. Fractures of the mandible: a technical perspective. Plast Reconstr Surg. 2007;120(Supplement 2):76S–89S.
Ellis E. A study of 2 bone plating methods for fractures of the mandibular symphysis/body. J Oral Maxillofac Surg. 2011;69(7):1978–87.
Ellis E. Rigid skeletal fixation of fractures. J Oral Maxillofac Surg. 1993;51(2):163–73.
Eusterman VD. Mandibular trauma. In: Resident manual of trauma to the face, head, and neck. Alexandria: American Academy of Otolaryngology—Head and Neck Surgery Foundation; 2012. p. 100–24.
Gilardino MS, Chen E, Bartlett SP. Choice of internal rigid fixation materials in the treatment of facial fractures. Craniomaxillofac Trauma Reconstr. 2009;2(1):49–60.
Gilmer TL. A case of fracture of the lower jaw with remarks on the treatment. Arch Dentistry. 1887;4:388–90.
Goode RL, Shinn J. A compression clamp for internal fixation of the mandible. Arch Otolaryngol Head Neck Surg. 1973;98(6):377–9.
Hosein KMM, Bhagol A, Singh V, Singhal R. Management of Mandibular Fractures. A textbook of advanced oral and maxillofacial surgery. London: InTech; 2013. p. 385–409.
Ivy RH. Observations on fractures of the mandible. J Am Med Assoc. 1922;79(4):295–7.
Kademani D, Tiwana PS, Yamashita D, Cho N. Techniques for maxillomandibular fixation. Atlas of oral & maxillofacial surgery. St. Louis: Elsevier; 2016. p. 638–45.

Kellman RM. Compression plating (compression osteosynthesis) of mandible fractures. Oper Tech Otolaryngol Head Neck Surg. 1995;6(2):80–5.

Koshy J, Feldman E, Chike-Obi C, Bullocks J. Pearls of mandibular trauma management. Semin Plast Surg. 2010;24(04):357–74.

Luhr HG. Evolution of rigid plate and screw fixation. Mund-Kiefer-Gesichtschirurgie. 2000;4(1):84–9. https://doi.org/10.1007/PL00022964.

Mukerji R, Mukerji G, Mcgurk M. Mandibular fractures: historical perspective. Br J Oral Maxillofac Surg. 2006;44(3):222–8.

Qureshi A, Reddy U, Warad N, Badal S, Jamadar A, Qurishi N. Intermaxillary fixation screws versus Erich arch bars in mandibular fractures: a comparative study and review of literature. Ann Maxillofac Surg. 2016;6(1):25. https://doi.org/10.4103/2231-0746.186129.

Ribeiro-Junior PD, Senko RA, Momesso NR, Izidoro JH, Padovan LEM, Viswanath A. Occlusal instability results in increased complication rates after treatment of mandibular fractures. J Oral Maxillofac Surg. 2020;78(7):1163.e1–7.

Rowe NL. The history of the treatment of maxillo-facial trauma. Ann R Coll Surg Engl. 1971;49(5):329–49.

Thoma KH. A historical review of methods advocated for the treatment of jaw fractures, with ten commandments for modern fracture treatment. Am J Orthod Oral Surg. 1944;30(8):C399–504.

Thomaidis V, Tsoucalas G, Fiska A. The Hippocratic method for the reduction of the mandibular dislocation, an ancient Greek procedure still in use in maxillofacial surgery. Acta Med Acad. 2018;47(1):139–43.

Uhthoff HK, Poitras P, Backman DS. Internal plate fixation of fractures: short history and recent developments. J Orthop Sci. 2006;11(2):118–26.

Vero D. Jaw injuries. The use of Kirschner wires to supplement fixation. Br J Oral Surg. 1968;6(1):18–30.

Part III
Advanced Procedures

Orthognathic Surgery

Christopher S. Midtling and Timothy A. Turvey

1 Introduction

The evolution of orthognathic surgery extends almost 200 years with contributions from generations of surgeons and clinicians across Europe and the United States. The culmination of creative minds, innovative research, and open dissemination of knowledge has led to the development of safe and efficient surgical treatment options. From the countryside of West Virginia to anatomy halls in Graz, Austria, all of the individuals who contributed to our understanding of the craniofacial skeleton, congenital or developmental deformities, diagnoses, treatment options and planning, and technical advances have exerted a profound influence on this amazing subspecialty.

Orthognathic surgery encompasses a broad range of procedures to correct minor and major skeletal and dental deformities. With the ability to correct misalignment of jaws and teeth; improve function in chewing, speaking, swallowing, and breathing; reduce muscle pain and improve TMJ mechanics; and enhance facial balance and cosmetics, it has evolved into one of the most powerful tools in the oral and maxillofacial surgeon's armamentarium.

A historical account of the evolution of orthognathic surgery must inevitably focus on the contributing surgeons and their introduction or impact on various procedures. A perfect chronological description of these events is complex. The multitude of operations to reposition the mandible, maxilla, and midface were often being developed simultaneously by surgeons on both sides of the Atlantic. This chapter journeys through more than 170 years to chronicle some of the milestones,

C. S. Midtling (✉) · T. A. Turvey
Department of Oral & Maxillofacial Surgery, University of North Carolina,
Chapel Hill, NC, USA

University of North Carolina, Chapel Hill, NC, USA
e-mail: Christopher.Midtling@unchealth.unc.edu; Tim_Turvey@unc.edu

E. M. Ferneini et al. (eds.), *The History of Maxillofacial Surgery*,
https://doi.org/10.1007/978-3-030-89563-1_13

pioneers, and breakthroughs in the evolution of orthognathic surgery, focusing on chronological history as best possible. The first section reviews its early history through pioneering surgeons who first addressed mandibular and maxillary deformities and established the specialty. The second section reviews the discovery, establishment, acceptance of orthognathic surgery, and refinement of techniques, with its rich history and future challenges.

2 The Pioneering Era (1850–1960s)

The origin of orthognathic surgery is traced to the mid-nineteenth century in the rustic mining community of Wheeling, West Virginia. In 1835, medically trained surgeon Simon P. Hullihen set out from Pittsburgh via steamboat to establish a new practice in Kentucky (Fig. 1). He fell ill while en route and was forced to disembark in Wheeling for medical attention. Following his recovery, he decided to settle in the community and devote his career to surgery of the oral cavity, head, and neck. For his exemplary work and leadership in maxillofacial surgery, he was awarded an Honorary Doctor of Dental Surgery by the Baltimore College of Dentistry in 1842 (Turvey 2017; Goldwyn 1973). The local medical community was at first skeptical of him, as dentists of this time were considered "barber-surgeons," but he soon established a reputation for surgical excellence (Aziz and Simon 2004).

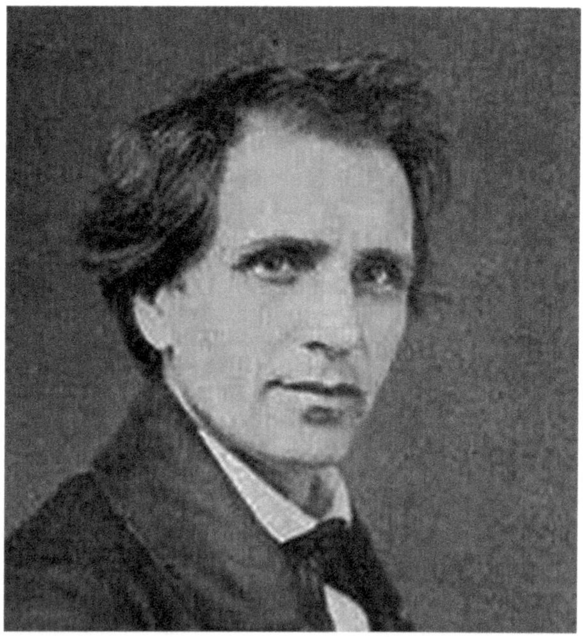

Fig. 1 Photograph of Simon P. Hullihen, "the father of orthognathic surgery" (Aziz and Simon 2004). (Reproduced with permission without alterations)

Hullihen was a meticulous recordkeeper, often publishing case reports in both medical and dental literature that described novel reconstructive techniques. Unbeknownst to him, his 1849 case report entitled *Case of Elongation of the Underjaw and Distortion of the Face and Neck, caused by a Burn, Successfully Treated*, would become his most influential publication (Aziz and Simon 2004). Hullihen described the case of the adolescent patient, Mary S., who suffered from prognathism and open bite as a result of scar contractures after severely burning her neck and chin at the age of five. His three-stage surgical plan included correction of the skeletal deformity via what is now known as an anterior subapical segmental osteotomy, followed by resection of scar tissue along the right face and neck, and concluding with correction of the lower lip defect. He emphasized the importance of correcting her malocclusion to provide restoration of function (Fig. 2).

The monumental milestones in this highly innovative series of operations should not be understated: Hullihen performed a novel procedure to reposition the dentoalveolus of the mandible; conducted the successful operation in a pre-antibiotic and pre-anesthetic era; and recognized that release of soft tissue scarring, which precipitated the skeletal deformity, was required to improve surgical outcome. As the first operation of its kind in medical literature, he demonstrated that malocclusion and jaw deformity could be treated with surgery, thus igniting the development of orthognathic surgery.

Widely acclaimed as "the father of oral and maxillofacial surgery" in the United States, Hullihen was the first surgeon known to limit his scope to the face and neck. Throughout his career in the Ohio River Valley, he conducted more than 1100 maxillofacial surgeries from oral cancer resections to cleft lip and palate repairs. His most lasting legacy in Wheeling, however, was the founding of Wheeling Hospital

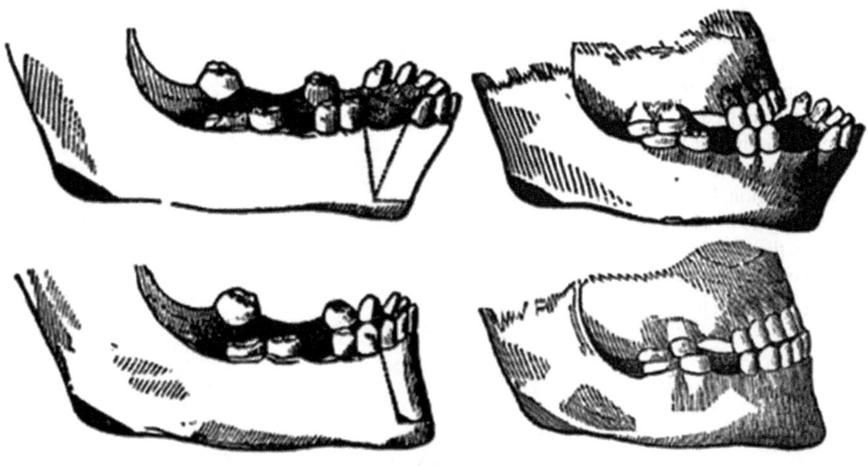

Fig. 2 Hullihen's illustration of the first anterior subapical segmental osteotomy for a 20-year-old patient, Mary S., who suffered severe malocclusion. Hullihen repositioned the anterior dentoalveolus to re-establish occlusion and restore function (Aziz and Simon 2004). (Reproduced with permission)

and the first dental unit in an inpatient facility. The revolutionary work of Simon P. Hullihen paved the way for future pioneers and the evolution of this subspecialty.

3 Early Mandibular Osteotomies

The ensuing decades saw little in the way of advances in mandibular reconstruction. It wasn't until 1897 when publications in Europe and the United States brought a new wave of innovative mandibular osteotomies. In Lyon, France, surgeons Jaboulay, Bérard, and Berger investigated the correction of prognathism via bilateral subcondylar osteotomies for mandibular setbacks using an extraoral approach (Jaboulay and Berard 1898; Berger 1897). The following year James Whipple and Edward Angle, two orthodontists in the United States, published case reports of prognathism corrected by surgeon Vilray Blair at Washington University (Whipple 1898; Angle 1898). In Blair's extraoral approach, later named the "St. Louis Operation," he opted to conduct mandibular body ostectomies in the premolar regions, removing the blocks of the bone to create space for a mandibular setback (Fig. 3). The two segments were then secured with copper wire ligation. Blair, a famed general surgeon, had soon developed a devotion for reconstructive surgery of the head and neck.

By 1907, Blair published various methods for the correction of maxillofacial deformities in the article *Operations on the Jaw-Bone and Face* (Blair 1907). He described a novel extraoral approach using bilateral osteotomies of the mandibular rami to protrude the mandible in a patient with retrognathia. Blair repositioned the

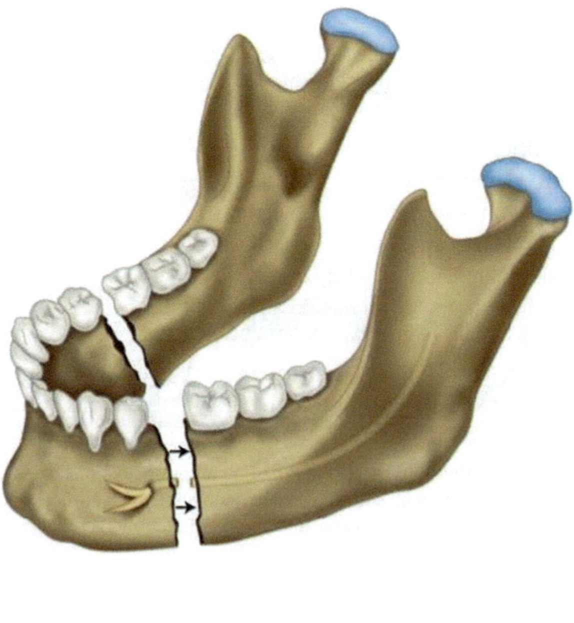

Fig. 3 A depiction of Vilray Blair's "St. Louis Operation" (1897). His approach consisted of bilateral mandibular body ostectomies in the premolar region. Following removal of the blocks of the bone, the anterior mandible was set back and secured with wire ligation

segments to achieve proper occlusion and secured the mandible by intermaxillary wiring and a plaster splint. While this approach resulted in visible scarring and damage to the inferior alveolar nerve (IAN), Blair's primary concerns consisted of relapse and nonunion. The three distinct problems he recognized in orthognathic surgery included cutting of the bone, positioning the jaw in proper orientation, and maintaining this placement postoperatively.

Ahead of his time in many respects, Blair's affinity for corrective jaw surgery awakened him to the importance of the role of orthodontists in obtaining successful outcomes. Though he never directly published with Edward Angle – the father of orthodontics – he often turned to him for his expertise, advice, and guidance in treatment planning. Blair's interest in operations of the jaw bones and face led to several editions of the text, *Surgery and Diseases of the Mouth and Jaws* (Blair 1912). Angle's own text on oral surgery, *Treatment of Malocclusion of the Teeth and Fractures of the Mandible*, also went into several editions and featured corrective surgery for malocclusion (Angle 1915). Each becoming pillars in their respective fields, Angle and Blair are recognized as the first surgeon-orthodontist duo to collaborate. They established a multidisciplinary approach in pre- and postoperative treatment planning, sequencing of procedures, and considerations for growth and development that would become the model for modern orthognathic surgery.

Detroit surgeon Max Ballin (1908) suggested preoperative extraction of teeth in the region of proposed mandibular body osteotomies several months prior to the reconstructive operation (Ballin 1908). This, he argued, would reduce contamination of the extraoral surgical sites from intraoral pathogens. Ballin published a report of a patient with class III malocclusion treated with this technique. The patient, who suffered from maxillary retrusion and mandibular prognathism, would have likely benefited from bimaxillary intervention; however, the ability to reposition maxilla in a stable manner had yet to be established. Consequently, many patients of this time underwent mandibular operations to correct even primary maxillary deformities. American orthodontist Rodrigues Ottolengui recognized this issue and warned that if the mandible is normal in size, an effort must be made to correct the abnormal part (i.e., maxilla), "thus making the abnormal fit the normal" (Ballin 1908). This principle was appreciated years later as surgeons continued to advance in the field of orthognathic surgery.

Matthew Cryer, a Professor of Oral Surgery at the University of Pennsylvania, is credited with the founding of the first hospital dental service in America (Cryer 1913). Cryer made several contributions to oral and maxillofacial surgery (OMFS) including "Cryer's elevators," which is still used in exodontia today (Naini 2017). In 1913, he suggested a semicircular osteotomy near the angle of the mandible to create a hinge effect (Fig. 4). This technique permitted vertical rotation of the mandible and did not require removal of any bone from the mandibular body, which Cryer felt would decrease infection rates. However, this method often resulted in posterior open bites and did not gain acceptance with other surgeons.

Attempts at mandibular reconstruction during the early 1900s brought universal challenges including high rates of postoperative scarring, open bites, relapse, and nonunions. This led to continued variations in mandibular osteotomies across

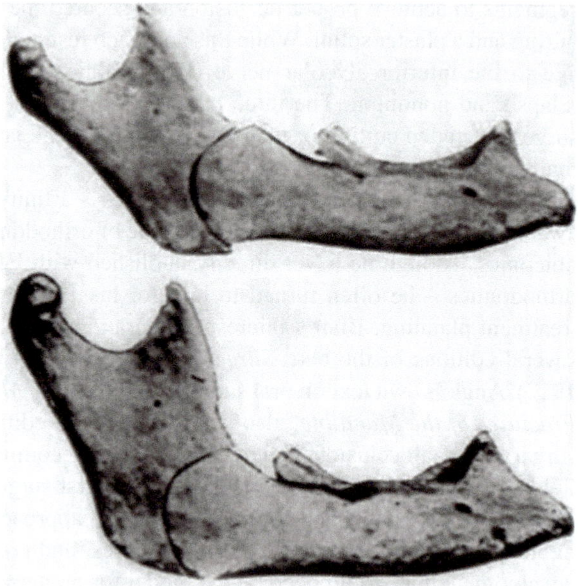

Fig. 4 A photograph of the semicircular mandibular osteotomy proposed by Cryer (1913) (Naini 2017). (Reproduced with permission)

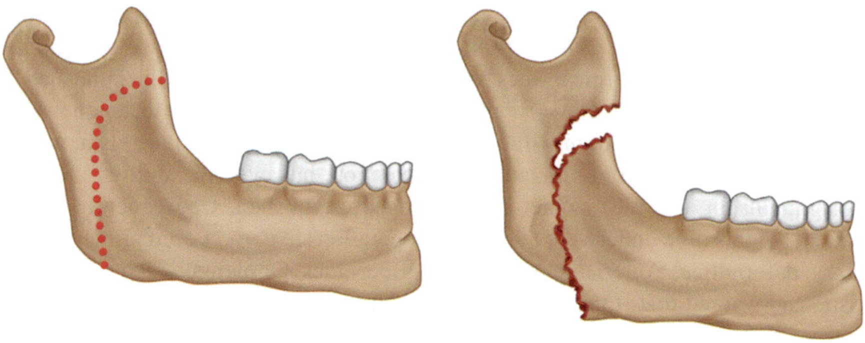

Fig. 5 Wassmund's inverted "L"-type osteotomy of the mandibular ramus (1927) (Naini 2017). (Reproduced with permission)

Europe and the United States between 1920 and 1940. Berlin surgeon Martin Wassmund (1927), who began the "German School" of maxillofacial surgery, published an inverted "L"-type ramus osteotomy using an extraoral approach (Wassmund 1927a). Wassmund's technique could be used for mandibular advancement or closing anterior open bites (Fig. 5). Frantisek Kostečka (1928), a Czech surgeon, described a closed osteotomy technique where he used a Gigli saw placed through limited stab incisions to avoid excessive scarring (Kostečka 1934). Referring to the technique as a "blind procedure," he placed the wire and completed the condylar neck osteotomy before setting back the mandible (Fig. 6). While the procedure was straightforward and avoided large facial scars, it had the same range of complications with relapse, open bite, nonunion, parotid fistulas, and nerve injuries.

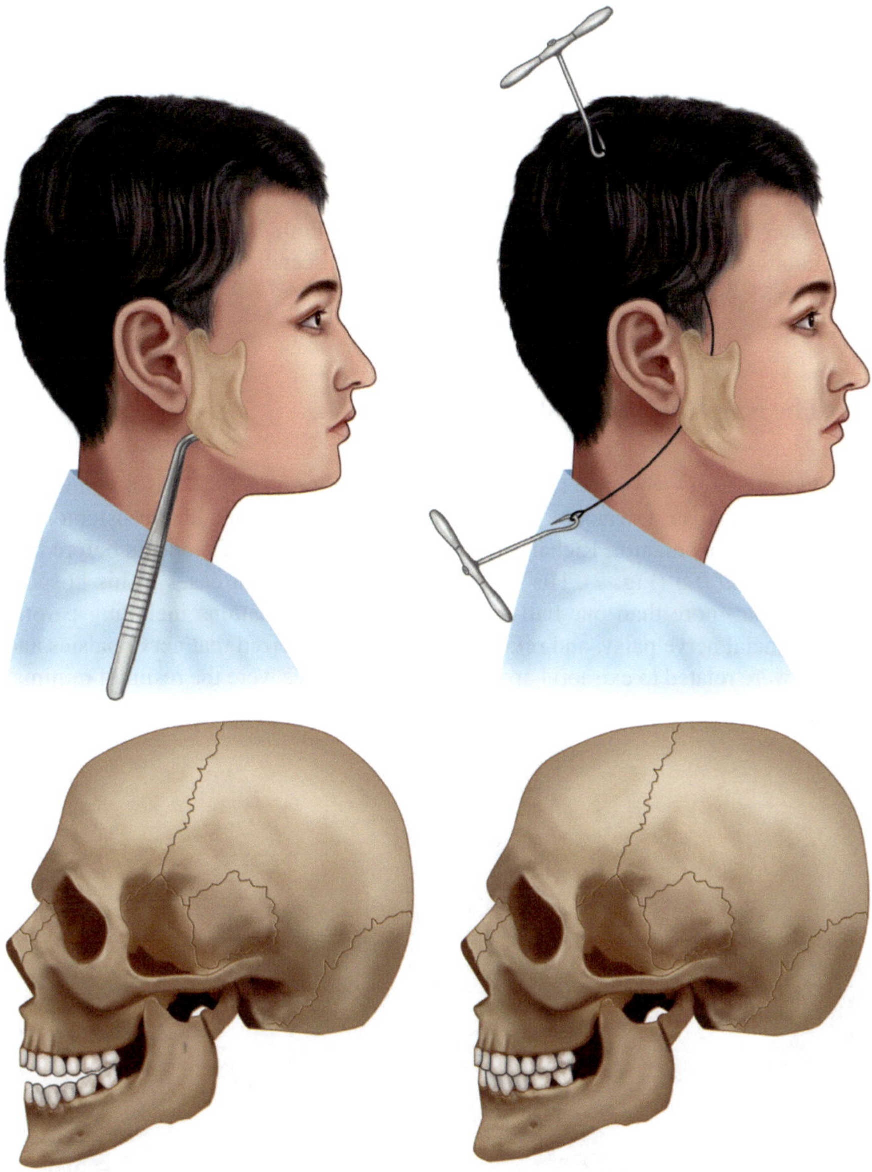

Fig. 6 Kostečka's 1934 modification to his Gigli saw technique. Kostečka utilized a curved needle to place a Gigli saw. The condylar neck osteotomy was completed allowing the mandible to be pushed up into occlusion. (Reproduced with permission without alterations)

In the United States, Armenian-born Varaztad Kazanjian (1932) was able to reduce the rate of infection and improve the overall outcome by performing the procedures in two stages through premolar extraction sites as opposed to the single-staged neck approaches of prior surgeons (Kazanjian 1932, 1939). In 1936, to address the problem of nonunion, he increased the contact area between the two segments of the mandible by using an oblique horizontal osteotomy of the ramus (Kazanjian 1936). Like those before him, Kazanjian preferred an extraoral approach.

By the 1940s, American surgeon Reed Dingman improved the method of mandibular body osteotomies. Importantly, he was one of the first to advocate for preserving the IAN (Dingman 1944). Dingman published more than 150 articles and textbook chapters in oral and maxillofacial surgery and plastic surgery. Several years later Sanford Moose and A.C. "Cuffy" Sloan, both Americans, devised other techniques to perform intraoral osteotomies of the ascending rami to correct prognathism (Moose 1945; Sloan 1951).

4 The Sagittal Split Osteotomy

Hugo Obwegeser – the father of modern orthognathic surgery – was a young surgeon in Graz, Austria, when he analyzed the techniques of mandibular osteotomies performed by his mentor, Richard Trauner, as well as those of pioneers before him (Obwegeser 2007) (Fig. 7). His 1952 review of 36 surgical cases in his hospital revealed that more than one-half suffered major complications including parotid fistulas, facial nerve palsy, and relapse. Obwegeser theorized that nerve palsies and fistulas were related to extraoral approaches and relapses were the result of minimal

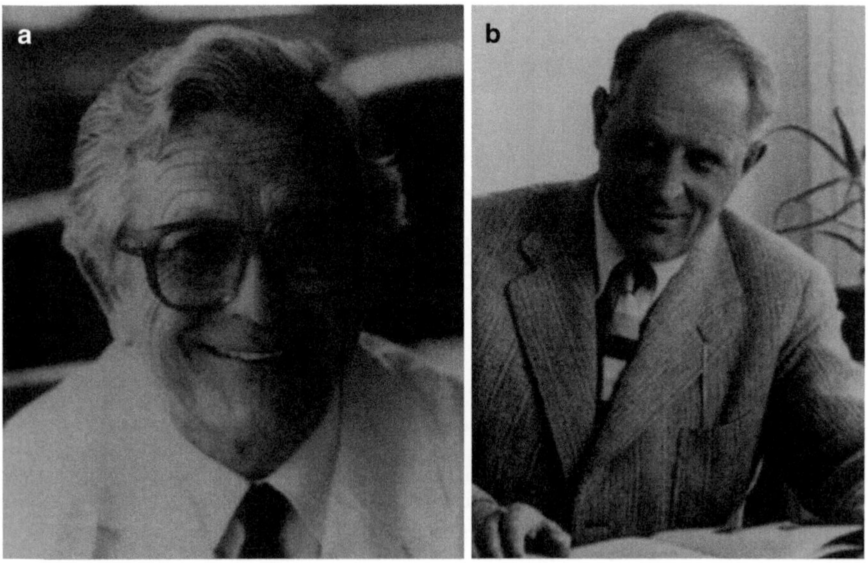

Fig. 7 (**a**) Photograph of Hugo Obwegeser, widely acclaimed as the father of modern orthognathic surgery. (**b**) Photograph of Richard Trauner, who helped train Obwegeser in Austria (Steinhauser 1996). Together, Obwegeser and Trauner eventually performed the first mandibular sagittal split osteotomy. (Photographs reproduced with permission)

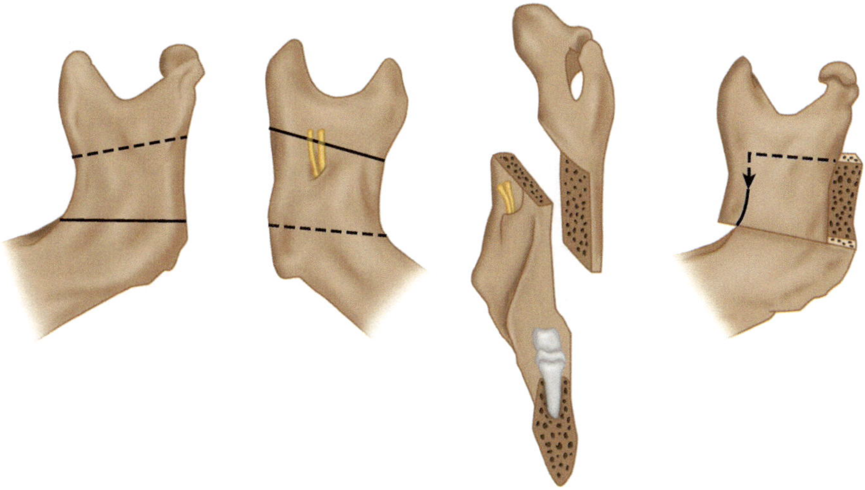

Fig. 8 Obwegeser's illustration of his first sagittal splitting osteotomy of the mandibular rami from his 1955 publication (Obwegeser 2007). (Reproduced with permission without alterations)

contact area between bony segments. From hours studying cadaveric mandibles and using experience from trauma patients who suffered sagittal plane fractures of the ramus, he developed and named the "sagittal splitting osteotomy," finding a solution to the many problems of mandibular surgery once and for all (Fig. 8).

With the assistance of Trauner, Obwegeser performed the first sagittal split osteotomy of the mandible on February 17, 1953 (Obwegeser 1957). He used an intraoral approach with local anesthesia for a 27-year-old woman with a protruding mandible. The procedure had been inspired by the work of Schlössmann, and descriptions of similar operations using an oblique horizontal osteotomy were described by Georg Perthes and Karl Schuchardt, but it was Obwegeser who performed and later described the complete operation in the medical literature (Schuchardt 1942a; Perthes 1922, 1924). Schuchardt was present to assist during Obwegeser's second sagittal split procedure.

Over the ensuing years, Obwegeser and others published modifications of the operation. Surgeons including Dal-Pont, Hunsuck, Epker, and Bell, among others in the United States and Europe, soon shared their experiences (Fig. 9) (Dal-Pont 1958; Hunsuck 1968; Epker 1977; Bell and Schendel 1977). To avoid stress on the neurovascular bundle, Hunsuck used an incomplete horizontal osteotomy along the medial ramus just posterior to the lingula and relied on vertical cleavage lines to complete the split. Epker advocated for a short split and developed figure-eight wire fixation of the two fragments, while Bell encouraged minimal soft tissue stripping to ensure wound healing, having investigated this with revascularization studies on rhesus monkeys. Primary advantages recognized by all surgeons included the intraoral approach which spared patients from facial scarring and bone-on-bone contact over a wide surface area that promoted healing without the need for grafting.

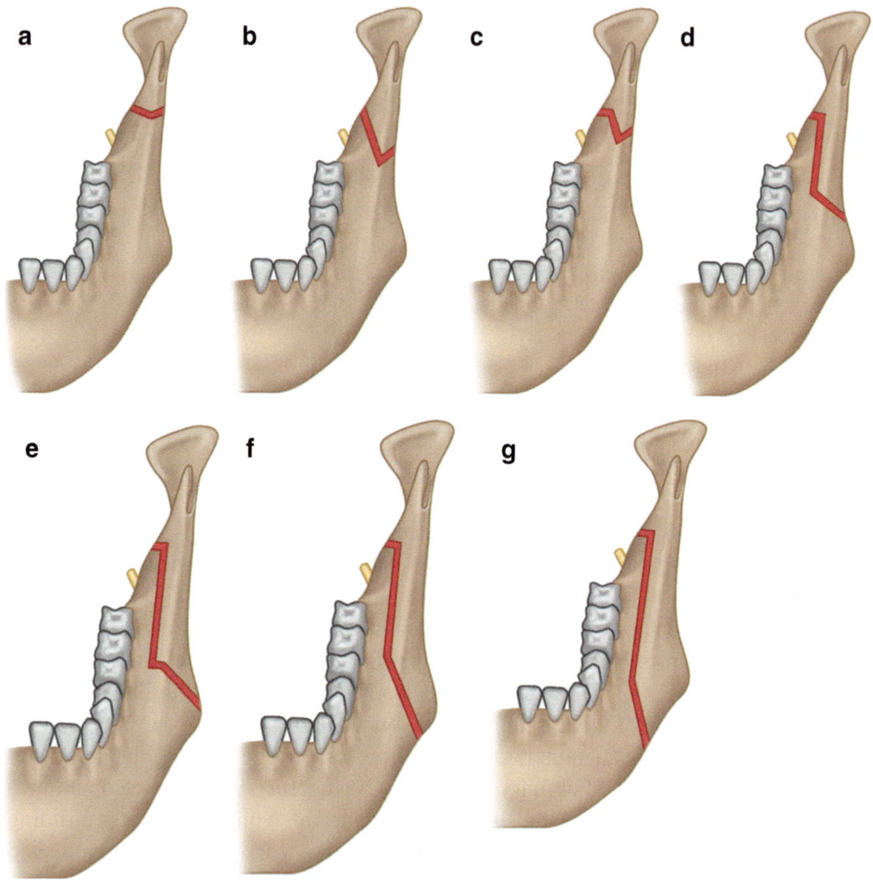

Fig. 9 Evolution of mandibular osteotomies through the 1960s, with date of publication. (**a**) Blair's initial proposal in 1907, (**b**) Schlossmann-Perthes-Kazanjian from 1922 to 1951, (**c**) Schuchardt 1954, (**d**) Obwegeser's first sagittal split osteotomy in 1955, (**e**) Obwegeser 1957, (**f**) Dal Pont 1958, (**g**) Obwegeser 1968 (Obwegeser 2007). (Reproduced with permission without alterations)

Throughout the 1950s, several surgeons continued to explore additional operations for mandibular setbacks. Inspired by Kostečka's condylar neck osteotomy, American military surgeons Caldwell and Letterman published a true vertical ramus osteotomy using an extraoral approach in 1954 (Caldwell and Letterman 1954). This vertical subsigmoid osteotomy (VSSO) was used for mandibular setbacks in severe prognathism cases. Other surgeons including Robinson (1956), Hinds (1958), and Thoma (1961) published very similar techniques using an extraoral approach (Robinson 1956; Hinds 1958; Thoma 1961).

5 Mandibular Subapical Osteotomies

While Simon Hullihen completed the first anterior subapical osteotomy in 1849, it wasn't until nearly a century later that the procedure was described further. German surgeon Otto Hofer reported his anterior subapical osteotomy to complete a mandibular dentoalveolar advancement in 1935 (Hofer 1936a). Unfortunately, he severed the bilateral mental nerves with his incision. The procedure was eventually popularized by Heinz Köle in 1959 after he published several new techniques for the operation (Köle 1959a, b, c). By positioning his incision within the anterior vestibule, he preserved the mental nerves and maintained mucosal coverage of the mobilized segment. Köle created his osteotomy 10 mm below the incisor apices to ensure preservation of the dental roots and to provide greater contact area for healing (Fig. 10). Köle demonstrated that variations of the procedure can correct open bites, protrusion, deep bites, or short face deformities. Common concerns by other surgeons remained including soft tissue healing, bone healing, survival of dentition, and maintaining adequate perfusion of the pedicle.

Segmental subapical osteotomies were documented extensively by notable surgeons including Wassmund, Axhausen, Immenkamp, Wunderer, Cupar, and others (Wassmund 1927b, 1935a; Axhausen 1934a; Immenkamp 1960; Wunderer 1962a; Cupar 1954). It was not until the 1970s that the operation was attempted to mobilize the *entire* mandibular dentoalveolus. Following his training at Henry Ford Hospital

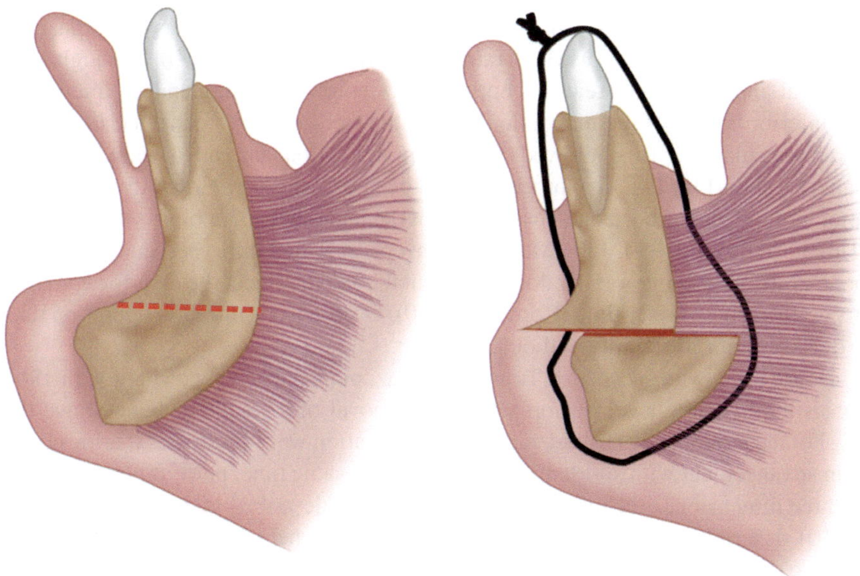

Fig. 10 Köle's anterior mandibular subapical osteotomy, allowing for advancement of the alveolar process. (Reproduced with permission)

in the 1960s, Robert B. MacIntosh spent several years training at Obwegeser's clinic in Zurich (MacIntosh 1973; MacIntosh and Carlotti 1975). Soon after, he published his successful experiences with total alveolar subapical osteotomies to correct apertognathic conditions. MacIntosh acknowledged that with these conditions, ramus height and masticatory muscle relationships preclude conventional osteotomies. His technique included vertical osteotomies posterior to the last molars and continued subapically around the mandibular arch, allowing for mobilization of the entire dentoalveolus.

Modifications continued to be explored by several surgeons including Booth, Buckley, and Turvey. Booth used the complete mandibular subapical osteotomy in combination with a sagittal osteotomy to correct class II malocclusions (Booth et al. 1976). Buckley and Turvey advocated for leaving the neurovascular bundle undisturbed and performing the subapical osteotomy between the nerve and the tooth roots, while the posterior vertical osteotomy was conducted through the third molar sockets (Buckley and Turvey 1987). These procedures continue to be used with considerable stability to correct dentoalveolar retrusion; however, it poses a threat to the inferior alveolar neurovascular bundle and blood supply to the osteotomized bone.

6 Genioplasty

In 1957, Hugo Obwegeser, with Trauner, performed the first osseous genioplasty in a living patient in Graz, Austria (Trauner and Obwegeser 1957a, b). Through their intraoral approach they created a horizontal osteotomy and descending fracture of the inferior border of the mandible, leaving the free segment connected to the lingual musculature. This allowed for the mobilization and advancement of the patient's chin (Fig. 11). This procedure had been described by Hofer 15 years prior, after he conducted a horizontal osteotomy of the mandibular symphysis on a cadaver (Hofer 1936b). In 1950, John Marquis Converse reported his experience using free bone grafts placed intraorally along the mental bone to project the chin forward, but his grafts resorbed over time (Converse 1950). Obwegeser's intraoral operation thus proved superior in stability and outcome.

Heinz Köle, who succeeded Trauner in Graz, published a new technique in 1968 consisting of a low-level genioplasty with removal of a wedge of bone above the level of the genioplasty (Köle 1968). Köle's operation was versatile as it allowed for chin advancement with shortening in height at the same time, permitting movement in three dimensions. Technical advances have been described including Schendel's (2010) description of a sagittal split genioplasty to help eliminate an hourglass esthetic deformity seen on frontal view (Precious and Delaire 1985). Other modifications to the genioplasty including publications by Precious (1985) and Triacca (2010) have been described, but the basic principles have remained for decades (Schendel 2010; Triacca et al. 2010).

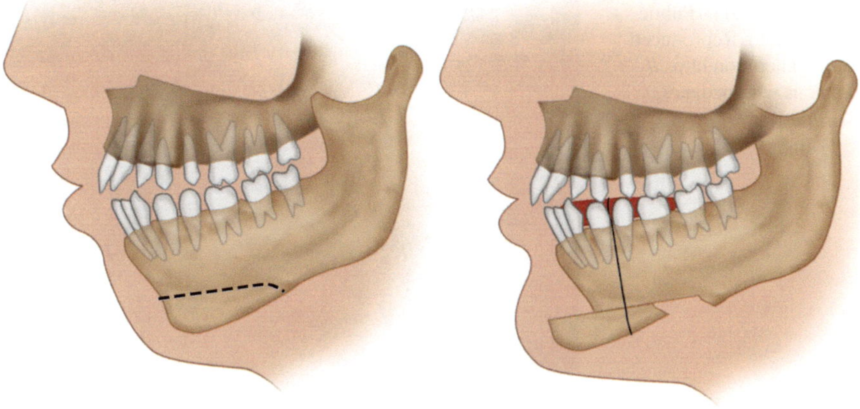

Fig. 11 Obwegeser's rendering of his sliding genioplasty to advance the chin. The horseshoe-shaped bone was slid forward and held in position by bilateral circumferential suturing tied over a bite-raising splint and broad contact with the mandible (Buckley and Turvey 1987). (Reproduced with permission without alterations)

7 The Introduction of Maxillary Osteotomies

Surgery to mobilize the maxilla lagged behind the development of mandibular operations. With more complex anatomy, the maxilla made surgical exposure more challenging and prone to blood loss. Nonetheless, the need for access to nasopharyngeal tumors and polyps inspired progress in the development of maxillary osteotomies. A decade after Hullihen shared his work on the mandible, the iconic German surgeon Bernhard von Langenbeck published the first description of a surgical osteotomy of the maxilla. Von Langenbeck (1859) completed the resection of nasopharyngeal tumors exposed through unilateral infracturing of the maxilla (Von Langenback 1859).

The surgical mobilization of the *entire* maxilla had its beginnings with David Cheever, a general surgeon in Boston, when he described the first maxillary downfracture in 1868 (Cheever 1870; Maloney and Worthington 1981; Halvorson and Mulliken 2008). Cheever's approach, known as the "double operation," was the first known procedure that could be described as a Le Fort I osteotomy. He completed the operation at Boston City Hospital to excise nasopharyngeal pathology and address complete nasal obstruction. Cheever later became chairman of the Department of Surgery at Harvard Medical School.

Reviewing the history of maxillary osteotomies is not possible without mention of the famed French surgeon and anatomist René Le Fort (Fig. 12). Le Fort's treatise *Étude expérimentale sur les fractures de la mâchoire supérieure* (1901) became a landmark of the medical literature (Le Fort 1901). Le Fort reproduced facial fractures in the heads of cadavers with the same implements used by street toughs in the streets of Paris: a wooden club, an iron rod, a kick, or a throw against a marble table.

Fig. 12 Photo of René Le Fort (1869–1951). (Public domain photo. Reproduced without alteration https://commons.wikimedia.org/wiki/File:Ren%C3%A9_Le_Fort.jpg)

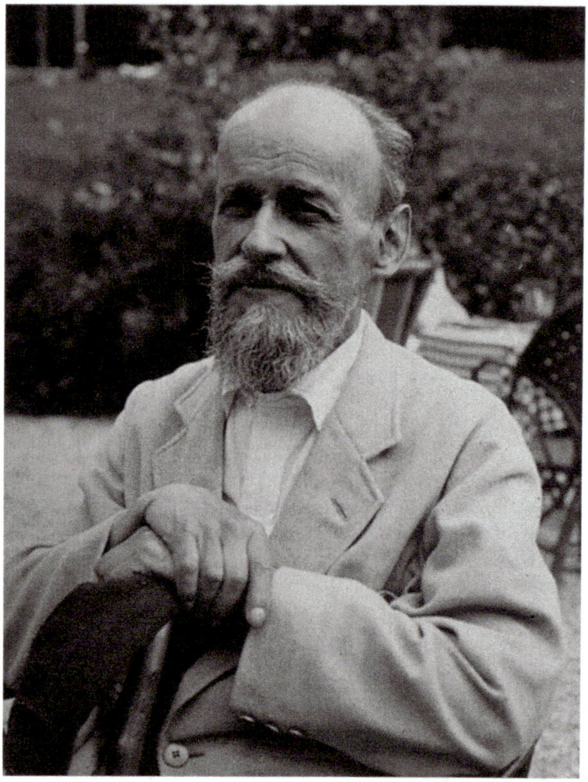

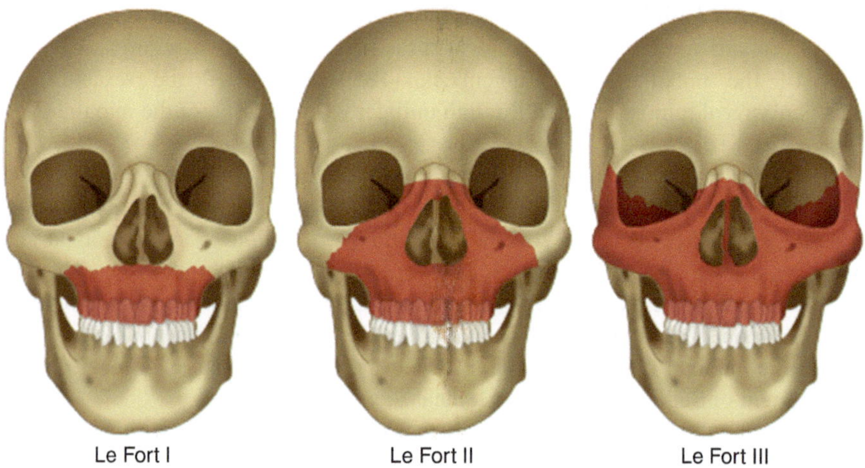

Fig. 13 René Le Fort's classification of the three predominant fracture patterns of the midface

By varying the degree of blunt forces, he discovered three predictable fracture patterns of the midface and classified them as Le Fort I (horizontal), Le Fort II (pyramidal), and Le Fort III (transverse) planes (Fig. 13) (Dyer 1999). Despite countless advances in medicine and maxillofacial surgery, his findings and classification system continue to be used and became important in orthognathic surgery.

One of the most common operations of the maxilla today, the Le Fort I maxillary osteotomy, was first performed a quarter century after Le Fort's publication by Martin Wassmund of Berlin. In 1927, he described the classic Le Fort I operation using the horizontal plane to correct post-traumatic malocclusion in a single-stage procedure (Wassmund 1927b, 1935b). Wassmund did not release the maxilla from the pterygoid plates to mobilize the osteotomy, preferring instead to use orthopedic traction to advance the maxilla postoperatively.

Another Berlin surgeon, Georg Axhausen, who was Wassmund's student and crosstown rival, was the first to describe a complete maxillary osteotomy with separation at the pterygoid plates in 1934 (Axhausen 1934b). This full release of the maxilla allowed for mobilization and advancement of a malunited maxillary fracture to correct an open bite deformity in a trauma patient. Most surgeons considered the operation too dangerous to attempt because of the difficulty with access and blood loss and the risks of relapse and postoperative necrosis. Axhausen and others found success through transfacial incisions, multiple vertical buccal incisions, or even palatal incisions in a staged approach to maintain adequate perfusion.

Trench warfare during World War I and the conflicts of World War II led to a dramatic increase in gunshot wounds and trauma to the head and face. Surgeons on both sides of the conflicts cared for soldiers with horribly disfiguring facial injuries, resulting in extensive experience and significant advancements in reconstructive surgery. Gillies, Schuchardt, Kazanjian, Ganzer, Rowe, Pichler, and others made substantial advancements from their wartime experiences, particularly in the development of facial osteotomies and reconstruction (Gillies and Rowe 1954; Bamji 2006; Schuchardt 1942b, 1955; Drommer 1986). The techniques developed for injured and disfigured soldiers were applied with success to patients with congenital dentofacial and craniofacial anomalies and malformations, which proved beneficial in the advancement of orthognathic surgery.

New Zealand-born British otolaryngologist Sir Harold Gillies, who helped open the Queen's Hospital in Sidcup, South-East London, developed many new techniques during World War I (Bamji 1993). He and his colleagues conducted over 11,000 procedures on more than 5000 patients, primarily soldiers with facial trauma. Gillies established an international reputation as a skilled surgeon; Kazanjian and Ivy, who were US Army surgeons in France, often collaborated with him on difficult cases. In 1942, Gillies built on his trauma experience treating a patient with Le Fort III fractures and became the first surgeon to publish an attempt at mobilizing the midface to treat a patient with craniofacial dysostosis (Gillies and Harrison 1950a). He published the case in 1950, and although Rowe was not included in the publication, Rowe was part of the surgical team. Gillies cautioned use of this approach because of the difficulties with surgery. Contributions were made by others including Moore, Ward (1949), and Converse (1952), though each documented their struggles with freeing the maxilla from the pterygoid plate region (Moore and Ward 1949; Converse and Shapiro 1952).

Schuchardt (1942) was among the first surgeons to report success releasing the maxilla at the pterygoid plates (Schuchardt 1942b). He conducted a staged Le Fort

I osteotomy, followed by pterygomaxillary separation, and used external traction with an overhead pulley and weights to advance the maxilla postoperatively. Converse and Shapiro documented their approach in 1952, raising extensive buccal and palatal flaps and resulting in incomplete soft tissue coverage over the maxilla at the conclusion of the operation (Converse and Shapiro 1952). This left many followers with doubts about the prognosis of the maxilla, with anticipated problems in healing and bony sequestrations, though he never reported loss of dentition or bone.

Despite the difficulty of mobilizing the maxilla from the pterygoid plates, Hugo Obwegeser thought it essential for success in maxillary surgery and made it a critical part of his operations in the 1950s (Obwegeser 1969a, 2007). By 1965, he described full mobilization as the key to success in this procedure and emphasized the importance of pterygomaxillary disjunction, advancement into preferred position, and the use of autogenous bone grafts to aid healing (Obwegeser 1965). By 1969, he described a circumvestibular incision and an intraoral approach to Le Fort I osteotomy that left no facial scars. He felt the approach improved skeletal stability with less risk of relapse. The bony facial structures were better positioned with improved aesthetic appearance (Fig. 14) (Obwegeser 1969b).

Le Fort I osteotomies were also described by surgeons Dingman and Harding (Dingman and Harding 1951) and Gillies and Rowe in the 1950s (Gillies and Rowe 1954). Gillies and Rowe (1954) discussed a segmental osteotomy in a cleft patient;

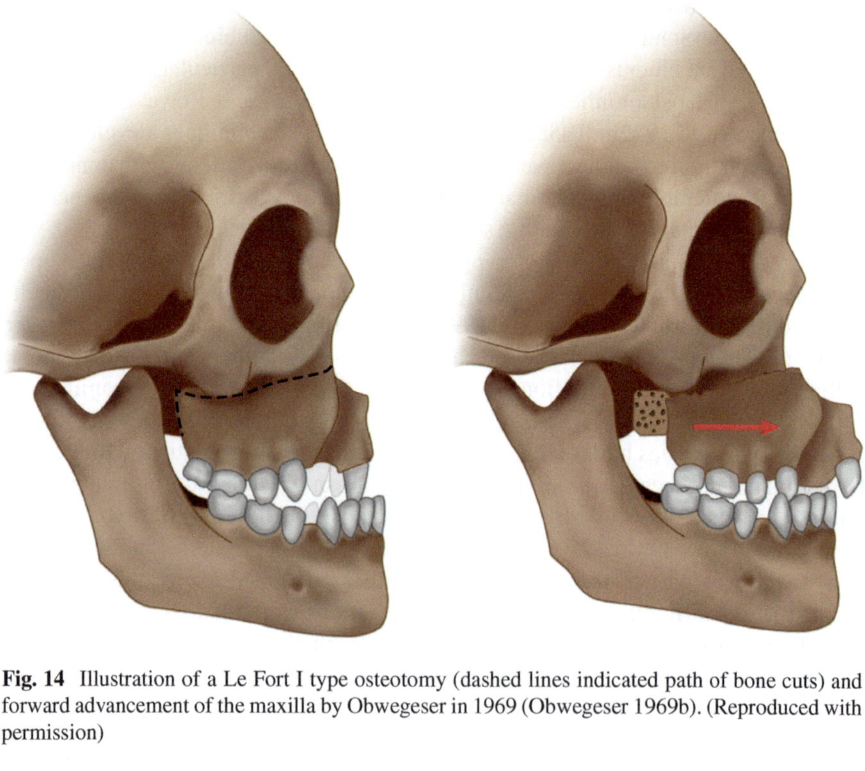

Fig. 14 Illustration of a Le Fort I type osteotomy (dashed lines indicated path of bone cuts) and forward advancement of the maxilla by Obwegeser in 1969 (Obwegeser 1969b). (Reproduced with permission)

however, they relied on postoperative elastic forces to guide repositioning of the maxilla. Swedish pioneer Karl-Erik Hogeman also applied Le Fort I osteotomies in patients with cleft lip and palate (Hogeman and Wilmar 1967). Hogeman and Willmar became so proficient with the procedure that they published a report on over 100 cases they operated in 1973 (Willmar 1974).

8 Isolated Anterior Maxillary Segmental Osteotomies

Osteotomies of a segment of the maxilla were traditionally more common in Europe in the early twentieth century. Berlin surgeon Günther Cohn-Stock (1921), considered by some to be the father of maxillary osteotomy techniques, sparked enthusiasm for anterior segmental osteotomies after publishing on retroclination of a proclined anterior maxillary dentoalveolus (Cohn-Stock 1921; Wolfe 1989). The technique began with extraction of premolars bilaterally, removal of a wedge of the bone from the anterior dentoalveolus with a palatal approach, and retroclination of the dentoalveolus (Fig. 15). Cohn-Stock, who was Jewish, safely left Germany for London in 1939 with the help of Prince Bernhard of Holland, who was fortunately one of his patients.

Martin Wassmund conducted his now famous segmental setback of the anterior maxilla in 1935 (Wassmund 1935b). His technique included two stages: first with a palatal approach to remove palatal bone and second with a buccal approach 4 weeks later to remove buccal bone and set back the anterior maxilla. By 1962, Siegfried Wunderer of Vienna developed modifications to this operation, describing a single-step procedure from the palatal approach to preserve the labial mucosa (Wunderer 1962b). Heinz Köle was responsible for several variations of segmental osteotomies and is credited with eventually popularizing the procedure (Köle 1959a, b, c, 1970).

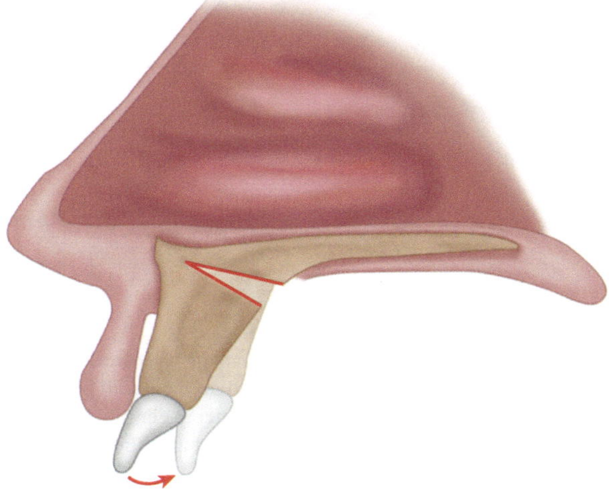

Fig. 15 Cohn-Stock's anterior maxillary segmental osteotomy for retroclination of the maxilla. Relapse occurred within 1 month (Cohn-Stock 1921; Wolfe 1989). (Reproduced with permission)

9 Isolated Posterior Maxillary Osteotomies

By the 1950s, Schuchardt, who gained experience from his training with Wassmund, recognized the complexity of closing open bites with only anterior maxillary osteotomies (Schuchardt 1955). Understanding the difficulty with aesthetics and lip support, he proposed maintaining the upper lip to incisor relationship by creating posterior maxillary osteotomies and moving the posterior maxilla superiorly in a two-stage technique (Fig. 16). Schuchardt began the first stage with a palatal flap to create bone cuts and closed the site for 3 weeks. Upon return for the second stage, buccal osteotomies and separation from the pterygoid plates were completed. He then used a wooden wedge and mallet to impact the posterior maxilla into the sinuses superiorly, asking the patient to forcefully bite to assist with mobilization. Remarkably these operations were conducted on awake patients using local anesthesia in a dental chair.

Five years following Schuchardt's report, a single-stage posterior maxillary osteotomy was introduced by Czech surgeon Josef Kufner to close an open bite (Kufner 1960, 1970). Kufner's contribution, which included a buccal approach with transantral palatal access, unfortunately went under the radar for nearly a decade as it was published in his native Czech language. After spending several years with Obwegeser in Zurich, he published his work in English and presented it at the International Congress on Oral Surgery in New York City in 1968. Kufner's transantral approach had proven advantageous for both access and stability of maxillary osteotomies, which was detailed by multiple other surgeons including Perko, West, Stoker, and Epker (Perko 1972; West and Epker 1972; Stoker and Epker 1974).

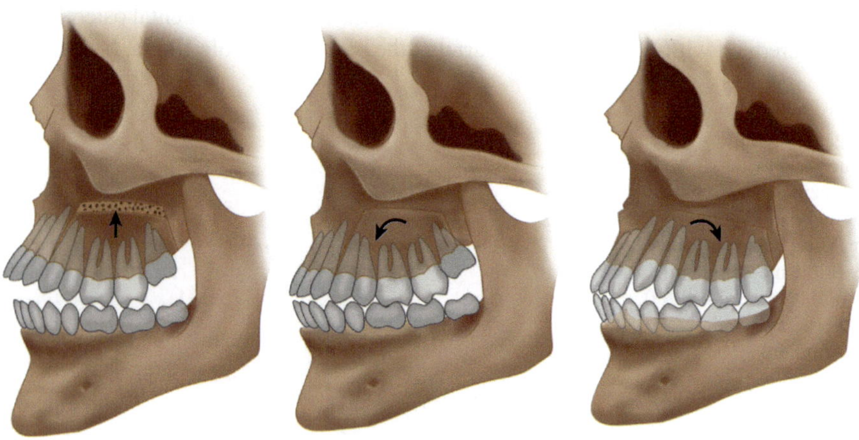

Fig. 16 Schematic drawing of Schuchardt's posterior segmental osteotomy in the 1950s. Schuchardt described a two-stage procedure, first with bilateral palatal alveolar osteotomies, followed by buccal osteotomies 3–6 weeks later to elevate the posterior dentoalveolar segments (Köle 1970). (Reproduced with permission without alterations)

10 Complete Simultaneous Mobilization of the Maxilla and Mandible

As advancements were made in both mandibular and maxillary osteotomies, the idea of simultaneous mobilization of both jaws developed. Heinz Köle was responsible for several innovations in orthognathic surgery and was first to describe bimaxillary alveolar osteotomies in the 1950s; however, he did not completely mobilize both jaws (Köle 1959a). American surgeon Alec Mohnac also shared his work with simultaneous osteotomies of both jaws, though like Köle his operations did not involve complete mobilization (Mohnac 1965). Eventually Hogeman and Obwegeser, two of the earliest pioneers of bimaxillary procedures, reported their experiences with full mobilization of the maxilla and mandible in a single operation (Hogeman and Wilmar 1967; Obwegeser 1970). Obwegeser was first to report the procedure in 1970 after completing both a Le Fort I osteotomy and bilateral sagittal split osteotomy (Fig. 17).

In the following decade, many surgeons in both Europe and the United States began publishing their experiences with simultaneous complete mobilization of the

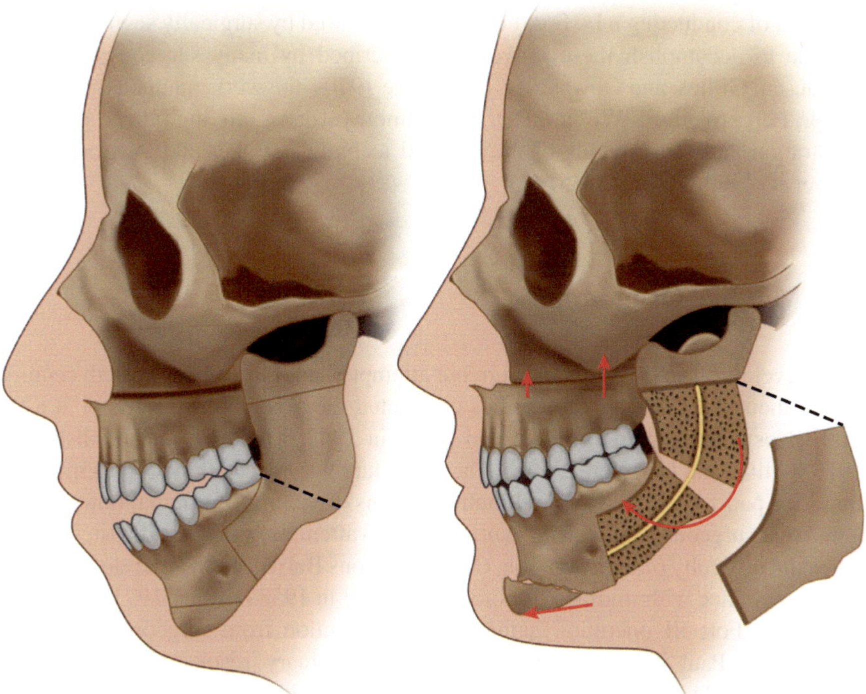

Fig. 17 Depiction of a simultaneous maxillary and mandibular surgical plan by Obwegeser, including superior maxillary impaction, mandibular angle osteotomy with clockwise rotation, and a sliding genioplasty (Obwegeser 2007). (Reproduced with permission)

maxilla and mandible. This included Americans Gross and James (1975), as well as Germans Helmut Lindorf and Emil Steinhauser (1978) (Gross and James 1978; Lindorf and Steinhauser 1978). This revolutionary procedure was recognized for its tremendous versatility and usefulness in correcting multiple dentofacial deformities, particularly open bites; sagittal, vertical, and transverse dysplasias; and cases of asymmetry. By the 1980s, simultaneous mobilization became well detailed and many Americans began adopting the procedures into their practice. Americans Turvey, Epker, and LaBanc documented their experiences with over 100 patients in 1982 (LaBanc et al. 1982). The use of study models and introduction of cephalometric tracings, face-bow transfers, interim splints, and semi-adjustable articulators aided surgeons as their understanding of timing and sequence of surgery expanded significantly.

11 Multipiece Segmental Maxillary Osteotomies

The early pioneers continued to recognize the essential need for widening, leveling, advancing, or closing spaces in the maxillary arch for both aesthetics and function. The earliest published case reports typically involved trauma or cleft palate patients. The idea of conducting a Le Fort I osteotomy followed by surgically segmenting the maxilla to accomplish these moves was described by many surgeons including Axhausen, Gillies, and Obwegeser. By the late 1970s, the work conducted by Bruce Epker, Larry Wolford, William Bell, and Timothy Turvey, among others, provided illustration and great details of the surgical technique (Epker and Wolford 1980; Bell et al. 1980; Turvey 1985).

12 Midface Osteotomies

High-level midface osteotomies were not attempted until the mid-twentieth century due to their sheer complexity. Gillies conducted the first recorded attempt at a Le Fort III osteotomy with Harrison and Rowe in 1942, which he later published in 1950 (Gillies and Harrison 1950b). The procedure was repeated by Gillies multiple times for patients with congenital malformations or victims of trauma; however, he noted that surgeons should heed caution prior to attempting Le Fort III osteotomies given the difficulty of the operation. Czech surgeons Burien and Kufner documented their experience with midface osteotomies as well in 1958 (Kufner 1971).

The Le Fort III operation gained notable attention from surgeons across the world after Paul Tessier showcased his extraordinary results in 1967 at the International Meeting of Plastic Surgery in Rome (Tessier et al. 1967; Tessier 1971a, b). Tessier further introduced the transcranial approach and demonstrated the use of Le Fort III operations in the treatment of midfacial trauma victims, correction of craniofacial deformities, and patients with Crouzon and Apert syndromes. Working alongside neurosurgeon Guiot, Tessier had spent years practicing on cadavers, planning every step, and anticipating each possible complication (Jones 2008). Together they worked to hone their skills and improve the functional and aesthetic outcomes in patients who previously had no surgical options available to treat their conditions. The enthusiastic response to Tessier's presentation was remarkable and inspired the foundation for the field of craniofacial surgery.

Encouraged by the work of Tessier and Obwegeser, many surgeons continued to develop and publish descriptions of high-level midface osteotomies. Joseph Murray, considered the father of craniofacial surgery in the United States, was chief of pediatric plastic surgery at Boston Children's Hospital in the 1970s when he emphasized the need to add dental training to medical education to bridge the knowledge gap in craniofacial surgery. Murray and Lennard Swanson, a prosthodontist and dentist-in-chief at Boston Children's, often published on the preoperative analysis, treatment planning, sequencing, and rehabilitation of children with craniofacial deformities (Fig. 18). As craniofacial surgery became more advanced, they underscored the importance of collaboration beyond surgeon and orthodontist, requiring the participation of neurosurgery, ophthalmology, radiology, anesthesiology, speech and language, and psychosocial disciplines (Murray et al. 1975).

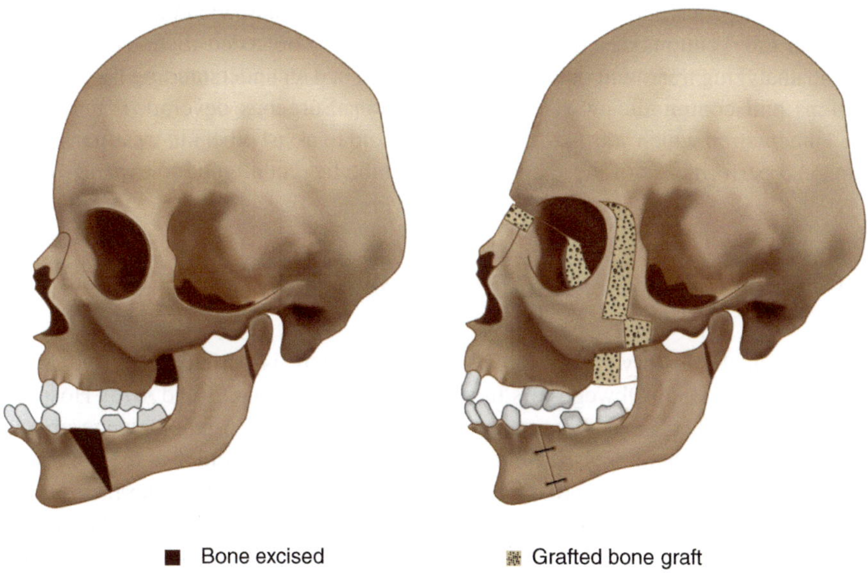

Fig. 18 Sketch of a treatment plan by Murray and Swanson, showing osteotomy sites (dotted lines in left drawing) along the maxillary, zygomatic, frontal, and nasal bones. A V-resection of the mandibular body was proposed to correct the mandibular prognathism. The shaded regions in the right drawing indicate areas for bone graft replacement using bone blocks from the root of the nose, lateral orbital walls, zygomatic arches, and posterior to the maxillary tuberosities, highlighting the complexity of these procedures (Murray et al. 1975). (Reproduced with permission without alterations)

Tessier also worked to break barriers between specialties and traveled across the world, inviting plastic surgeons, maxillofacial surgeons, pediatricians, neurosurgeons, and radiologists to his courses and symposiums. His philosophy that "no one man could master all techniques and be an island unto himself" inspired surgeons from all arenas to contribute in the development of craniofacial surgery (Ghali et al. 2014). Over the ensuing decades, the works of Murray, Epker, Wolford, Edgerton, and Psilakis, among others, contributed to a variety of new high-level osteotomies (Converse and Wood Smith 1971; Converse et al. 1970; Converse and Telsey 1971; Epker and Wolford 1979; Psillakis et al. 1963; Jabaley and Edgerton 1969). By the late 1990s, the simultaneous treatment of anterior open bite and midface advancement was described using a combination of Le Fort I and Le Fort III osteotomies by Sailer in Switzerland (Sailer 1997).

13 The Discovery Era (1960s–Present)

In the hundred years after Hullihen's first publication on surgical correction of skeletal deformities, pioneers from both sides of the Atlantic demonstrated the successful use of surgery to correct dentofacial deformities. From the mid-twentieth century to today, surgeons built on this foundation to discover new techniques and refine surgical interventions described by the pioneers who preceded them. As surgeons began analyzing treatment outcomes, they established an understanding for the indications and contraindications of each operation. Surgeons developed innovative instrumentation which was manufactured and sold to assist others in treatment planning and performance of these operations, and the field continued to expand.

14 Hugo Obwegeser and the Paradigm Shift

Throughout the history of orthognathic surgery, there is perhaps no event more influential than Hugo Obwegeser's June 1966 visit to the Walter Reed Army Hospital in Washington, D.C. Following an earlier lecture in Buenos Aires, Obwegeser was approached by General Robert Shira, who was serving as the chief of the US Army Dental Corps. Shira later invited Obwegeser to deliver a 3-day lecture series on the techniques of orthognathic and other maxillofacial procedures. With more than 500 awestruck surgeons in the audience, Obwegeser captivated the crowd, igniting an evolution in the field's scope of practice. His landmark presentations sparked a paradigm shift in focus among oral and maxillofacial surgeons and awakened the beginning of modern orthognathic surgery (Obwegeser 2017; Naini and Hugo 2017).

During his visit to Washington, D.C., Obwegeser illustrated the correction of craniofacial deformities using the new procedures and techniques he helped pioneer. These included the demonstration of mandibular setbacks and advancements using his revolutionary sagittal split osteotomy. His technique for Le Fort I maxillary osteotomies was presented, which further included lectures on segmenting the maxilla and mandible. In addition, he shared his work on patients with cleft lip and palate and explained applications for pre-prosthetic surgery (MacIntosh 2018).

Prior to his visit, US oral and maxillofacial surgery was considered a fledgling specialty and was often discredited by groups of disgruntled competitors. The work of maxillofacial surgeons was at times condemned, with desperate competitors denouncing practitioners and seeking to bar its practice throughout US hospitals. It was the exposition presented by Obwegeser that captured the energy of oral and maxillofacial surgeons and empowered the development of orthognathic surgery as a specialty within the healthcare system in the United States.

American surgeons, fascinated by the accomplishments shared by Obwegeser, quickly accumulated experience performing these operations. Notable practitioners including Bell, White, Walker, Costich, and dozens of others adopted his techniques, published their experiences, and incorporated more orthognathic surgery into their practices. By 1968, Raymond White shared his work following 17 patients he treated successfully with sagittal split osteotomies (White et al. 1969). The same year, Bell published his experiences with anterior maxillary osteotomies, which was soon followed by Kent and Hinds reporting their work with the same procedure (Bell 1968; Kent and Hinds 1971). In the words of Robert McIntosh, Obwegeser "initiated an indebtedness in [surgeons] for all generations that is so enormous as to be beyond reckoning" (MacIntosh 2018).

One of the most significant developments following Obwegeser's visit was recognition for the importance of interdisciplinary collaboration between surgeons and orthodontists. Pioneers Vilray Blair and Edward Angle realized the significance of this partnership decades prior, often seeking each other's advice. John Converse, a plastic surgeon, had published with orthodontists H.H. Shapiro in the 1950s and later with Sidney Horowitz (Converse and Shapiro 1952; Converse and Telsey 1971). It was after Obwegeser's visit, however, that this multidisciplinary approach became commonplace. Notable duos including Bell-Creekmore, White-Proffit, Epker-Fish, Ware-Poultan, Walker-Murphy, Wolford-Hilliard, and West-McNeil, among others, began publishing routinely and gained recognition in both specialties. By sharing a wealth of information and experiences, practitioners were able to modify new techniques, anticipate complications, develop innovative instruments, establish new treatment sequences, and ultimately improve outcomes.

15 The Specialty Is Named

The term "orthognathic surgery" (*Greek* "orthos" – straight; "gnathos" – jaws) is attributed to Harold Hargis who coined the term in the late 1960s (Turvey 2017). Hargis, an oral and maxillofacial surgeon in the US Army, was assigned to Obwegeser's clinic in Zurich in the mid-1960s to learn his innovative procedures. There he worked alongside Bruce MacIntosh, another American surgeon sent by Fred Henny of Detroit, US Naval officer Bill Terry, and Obwegeser's first trainee

Emile Steinhauser. Following his return from Europe, Hargis continued to refine orthognathic techniques, invent various surgical instruments, and would go on to become chairman of oral and maxillofacial surgery at the University of California-Los Angeles.

16 The Acceptance of Orthognathic Surgery

Skeptics of orthognathic surgery as an option for cranio- and dentofacial abnormalities pointed to concerns about the maxilla's vascular supply following complete mobilization. It was William Bell's investigations into blood supply and revascularization after surgery that proved critical to this understanding (Rhinelander et al. 1968; Bell 1969, 1973; Bell and Levy 1970; Bell et al. 1975). Bell investigated flap designs to aid maxillary osteotomies and studied bone healing using the microangiographic techniques described by Rhinlander. In 1970 he published his exploration on wound healing after completing maxillary osteotomies in adult rhesus monkeys. These successes paved the way for subsequent publications, including *Bone healing and revascularization after total maxillary osteotomy* authored by Bell and Fonseca in 1975. Bell's innovative contributions confirmed what had been clinically known: that vascular circulation to the osteotomized segment is maintained when a viable buccal or palatal pedicle remained intact (Fig. 19). These groundbreaking studies provided the biological basis of orthognathic procedures and led to its acceptance as a legitimate and safe treatment option for patients.

Another lingering concern in the 1970s was acceptance of orthognathic surgery by the orthodontic community and the long-term stability following surgery. The postoperative adaptations and stability of the maxilla and mandible were investigated extensively by world-renowned orthodontist William Proffit et al. (2003a). Proffit, among other orthodontists, published widely on the changes in bite forces, tongue and lip pressures, breathing patterns, speech and velopharyngeal function, and other neurosensory changes after orthognathic surgery. There is probably no one else more responsible for the explosive acceptance of orthognathic surgery by orthodontists than Proffit. In 1979, Proffit, Turvey, and biostatistician Ceib Phillips were awarded an NIH grant to analyze the long-term stability of orthognathic surgery (Turvey 2017). This grant extended for nearly four decades and produced hundreds of manuscripts and abstracts describing the topic. The efforts from this grant helped build a data bank at the University of North Carolina which includes records of more than 8000 patients treated with orthognathic surgery. Proffit, Turvey, and Phillips shared their extensive findings on the topic and produced a hierarchy of stability and predictability following orthognathic surgery (Proffit et al. 1996, 2007).

Throughout the early twentieth century, several publications of major textbooks dedicated to head and neck surgery were released. None, however, had been devoted to orthognathic surgery. Fundamental to the acceptance of orthognathic surgery as a surgical treatment was the release of several such textbooks. The 1964 text by Reichenbach, Köle, and Brückl titled *Surgical Orthodontics* is recognized as the

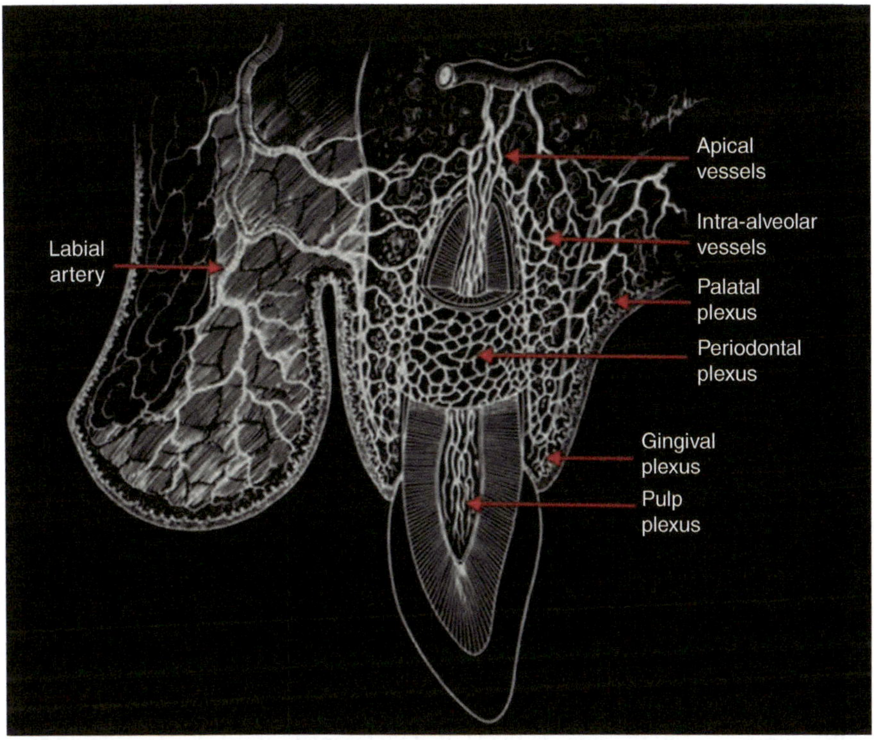

Fig. 19 Bell and Fonseca's schematic diagram of the vascular supply to the anterior maxillary dentoalveolus. Bell emphasized the various anastomosing vessels which permits maxillary osteotomies to be completed without compromising vascularity and allowing for adequate reperfusion postoperatively (Naini 2017). (Reproduced from Naini with permission)

first influential textbook for European maxillofacial surgeons and remains a standard work today (Reichenbach et al. 1964). Edward Hinds and Jack Kent, two surgeons from the University of Texas-Houston, co-authored *Surgical treatment of developmental jaw deformities* in 1972, the first orthognathic surgery textbook in the English language (Proffit and White 1991). Bell, Proffit, and White released a pivotal three-volume text in 1980, while Epker and Wolford published their distinguished textbook the same year (Epker and Wolford 1980; Turvey 1985). Four additional texts by Proffit and White as well as Epker, Fish, and Stella have documented the advances since that time (Proffit and White 1991; Proffit et al. 2003b; Epker and Fish 1986; Epker et al. 1999).

By 1986, Raymond White and orthodontist Robert Vanarsdale introduced *The International Journal of Adult Orthodontics and Orthognathic Surgery*, an interdisciplinary periodical dedicated to the subspecialty. The journal ran for nearly two decades, providing groundbreaking information, illustrating case history, explaining latest research results, and helping perfect clinical treatments. As of 2021, many texts have been dedicated to the review and practice of orthognathic surgery, including the notable *Essentials of Orthognathic Surgery* by Johan Reyneke of South Africa and the two-volume comprehensive review, *Orthognathic Surgery: Principles and Practice,* by Jeffrey Posnick (Reyneke 2010; Posnick 2014). These classic works, among others, have illustrated the various procedures and allowed other surgeons to follow the steps of orthognathic operations and avoid complications experienced by the early founders.

17 A Global Specialty

American surgeons grew hungry to experience and develop skills in orthognathic techniques following Obwegeser's visit. It was common for surgeons to travel to Europe to observe Obwegeser's work and to participate in surgeries with Paul Stoelinga and Henk Tiedeman in the Netherlands. Notable French surgeons such as Jacques Dautrey and Maxime Champy, who were strong advocates instrumental in the development of orthognathic surgery in France, were gracious hosts to visiting surgeons. The skilled cleft surgeon, Jean Delaire from Nantes, who developed methods for facial analysis and treatment algorithms, also commonly hosted visiting surgeons. The father of craniofacial surgery, Paul Tessier of Paris, was widely known to host fascinated visitors wishing to understand his techniques and learn orthognathic and craniofacial procedures.

In addition to those who traveled abroad to develop new skills and learn orthognathic surgery, many surgeons in the United States made efforts by developing continuing education courses (Fig. 20). William Bell, Bruce Epker, Raymond Fonseca, Raymond White, and Larry Wolford began conducting courses, lectures, and mini

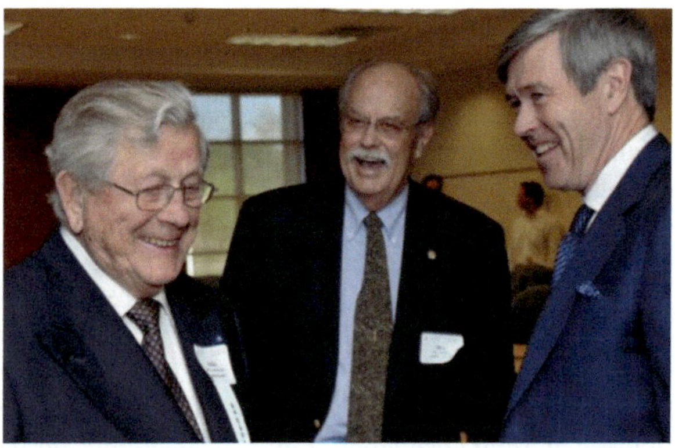

Fig. 20 Dr. Hugo Obwegeser with Drs. Bill Terry and Timothy Turvey at the 2011 annual meeting of the American College of OMFS in Las Vegas, NV. At the meeting, Dr. Terry presented a special tribute to Dr. Obwegeser commemorating his lifelong contributions to the field of oral and maxillofacial surgery. From *left to right*: Hugo Obwegeser, Bill Terry, Timothy Turvey. (Photo courtesy of Timothy Turvey)

residencies. These efforts were not exclusive to surgeons and included collaboration with orthodontists such as John Casko, Charles Fish, David Hall, Frank Hilliard, Harry Legin, William Proffit, and Robert Vanarsdale. The collaborative efforts made toward continuing education in orthognathic surgery have been unparalleled by any other area of interest in maxillofacial surgery.

18 Refinements of Orthognathic Surgery

Advancements in orthognathic surgery continued to develop throughout the late twentieth century. The work of Larry Wolford, a prolific surgeon, lecturer, inventor, and innovator in TMJ surgery, introduced the combination of orthognathic surgery in conjunction with TMJ procedures. Wolford eventually introduced total alloplastic joint replacements conducted at the same time as orthognathic surgical interventions. Talented surgeon Bruce Epker, a gifted writer and speaker, investigated surgical techniques, postoperative stability, and adaptations through statistical review and data analysis. He published over 200 peer reviews and manuscripts and contributed many chapters to various texts, including six of his own.

Robert V. Walker, a giant in the field of oral and maxillofacial surgery, founded the OMFS clinic at Parkland Memorial Hospital (University of Texas Southwestern Medical Center), which soon became the epicenter for orthognathic surgery in the United States. He recruited William Bell and Bruce Epker to faculty positions at UT-Southwestern in Dallas, Parkland Memorial Hospital, and John Peter Smith Hospital. This move proved instrumental in providing them the pathway, environment, and resources to blossom professionally and create a powerhouse for orthognathic surgery. Walker, Bell, and Epker's efforts sowed the seeds for the specialty, contributing to the training and development of an entire generation of leaders and specialists in orthognathic surgery. This includes the likes of Raymond Fonseca, Timothy Turvey, Douglas Sinn, Roger West, Stephen Schendell, Ghali Ghali, Richard Finn, Caesar Guerrero, and Scott Boyd, among others, who have collectively contributed to thousands of peer-reviewed articles, publications, and textbooks in craniomaxillofacial surgery and have left a profound impact on the surgeons they have trained.

Pivotal to provider success with orthognathic surgery was the development of useful and efficient instrumentation. Today, various companies produce and distribute instruments for surgeons worldwide. One of the first to do so in the United States was Walter Lorenz, who established his surgical instrument company in New York City in the 1960s (Turvey 2017). He initially traveled personally from practice to practice, marketing, selling, and servicing instruments for his clientele. Lorenz was a strong advocate for oral and maxillofacial surgeons, and his resilient support for the field developed into a mutual relationship. The *Walter Lorenz Instrument Company* soon became a leading maxillofacial instrument developer and distributor worldwide with high-quality, ergonomic instruments conducive to complex orthognathic procedures. Most equipment sold by Lorenz was manufactured in Tübingen,

Germany, and the Walter Lorenz Company was the exclusive distributor of Obwegeser's original instruments.

From the 1970s through 1990s, surgeons expanded the role of soft tissue procedures in conjunction with orthognathic surgery. John Hovell (1956) of London recognized the utility of simultaneous soft tissue procedures decades prior, noting the common problem of excessive submental fullness after mandibular setback procedures (Hovell 1956). Turvey and Epker (1974) acknowledged the improvement of facial balance through orthognathic surgery with adjunct soft tissue interventions, and Epker later published a textbook on such topics in 1994 (Turvey and Epker 1974; Epker and Wolford 1977; Epker 1994). Interest in cosmetic surgery among the OMFS community was further advanced when the American Academy of Facial Plastic Surgery and American Academy of Cosmetic Surgery began sponsoring educational training courses that allowed maxillofacial surgeons to learn new techniques. Procedures including rhinoplasty, rhytidectomy, blepharoplasty, submental liposuction, platysma plication, and forehead lifts were explored as interventions that could be done in conjunction with orthognathic surgery with minimal wound healing complications and quicker recovery. Adapting simultaneous soft tissue surgery became increasingly popular as surgeons like Epker, Sinn, Waite, Niamtu, Ghali, Griffin, and McBride began emphasizing the benefits (Waite and Matukas 1991; Niamtu 2011; Griffin and Kim 2010; Sinn and Ghali 1996).

Near the turn of the century, leaders in the field published works highlighting the approach to diagnosis and treatment planning for deformities encountered in clinical practice. This is illustrated beautifully through the works of Johan Reyneke of South Africa (Reyneke 2010). His most recent edition of *Essentials of Orthognathic Surgery* provides step-by-step protocols for facial analysis, interpretation of diagnostic data, and treatment planning and execution to obtain the most esthetically pleasing results. Reyneke stresses the relationship between soft and hard tissues and the benefits of rotating the maxillomandibular complex and explores the utility of distraction osteogenesis and vertical ramus osteotomies.

19 Bone Plates and Screws

Over the past 50 years, craniomaxillofacial surgery has been revolutionized by rigid or semirigid fixation of bony segments with plates and screws. With traditional orthognathic surgery, maxillomandibular fixation (MMF) for several weeks was often required for appropriate healing and postoperative stability. Advances in this technology have significantly influenced management of patient care by avoiding the need for MMF. This has allowed for orthognathic surgery to become a more attractive and feasible treatment option for patients.

The utilization of bone plates and screws has its origin in traumatology, with orthopedic surgeons using the system first. German surgeon Carl Hansmann shared his experiences using a self-developed plate and screw system for fixation of orthopedic fractures in 1886 (Sauerbier et al. 2008). His account included two mandible fractures, making him the first to report on the use of bone plating in the maxillofacial region. In 1917, German Johannes Soerensen shared his creativity after adapting a gold ring into a small bone plate for fixation of a comminuted mandible fracture (Soerensen and Warnekros 1917). Multiple surgeons developed primitive bone plates and screws for use in elective maxillofacial surgery, but the focus remained largely on trauma. Due to high complication rates, these methods fell out of favor in the facial skeleton for several decades.

Credit must be given to Bavarian plastic surgeon Bernd Spiessl, who applied rigid fixation to orthognathic surgery (Spiessl 1974). In 1974 he published his experience using compression screw fixation for sagittal split osteotomies with an intraoral approach (Fig. 21). Spiessl suggested that relapse, a known complication with all advancements or setbacks, was arguably impossible using this method. German surgeon Hans Luhr also worked extensively on the development of rigid osteosynthesis in both trauma and orthognathic surgery (Luhr 1967, 1968, 1990). Luhr first introduced chromium cobalt screws and plates for use in the mandible in 1967. By the early 1970s he improved upon miniplates developed by French surgeons Michelet, Festal, and Champy and by 1979 had introduced a compression screw miniplate set of his own, yielding excellent results in stabilization of the delicate midfacial bones (Fig. 22) (Michelet and Festal 1972; Luhr 1979). Similar to Spiessl, Luhr emphasized the principles of compression osteosynthesis for improvement in stabilization and healing.

Other surgeons including Champy, Lodde, and Steinhauser studied the biomechanics of the maxilla and mandible and developed stainless-steel bone plates and screws of their own (Champy and Lodde 1976, Luhr 1979; Steinhauser 1982). By 1986, Steinhauser had developed an all-titanium miniplate system for orthognathic surgery (Obwegeser 1957). Contrary to Spiessl and Luhr, they felt the application of compression screws and plates proved more difficult and hazardous for adjustments of occlusion. A long debate over compression osteosynthesis had continued, and by the twenty-first century it was widely accepted that compression is not imperative for bone healing in orthognathic surgery.

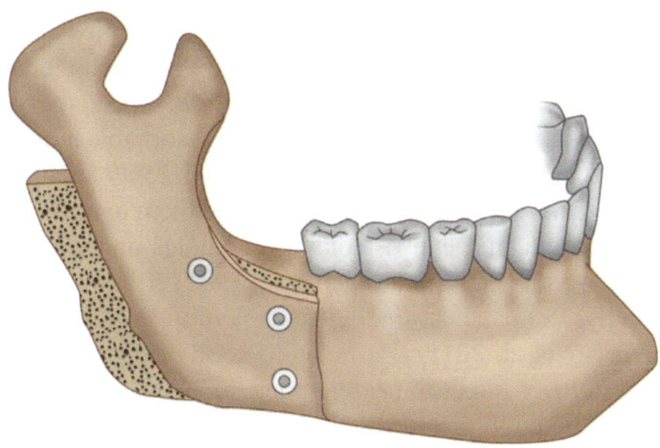

Fig. 21 Fixation of the mandible after a sagittal split osteotomy using three bone screws, according to Spiessl (Steinhauser 1982). (Reproduced with permission without alterations)

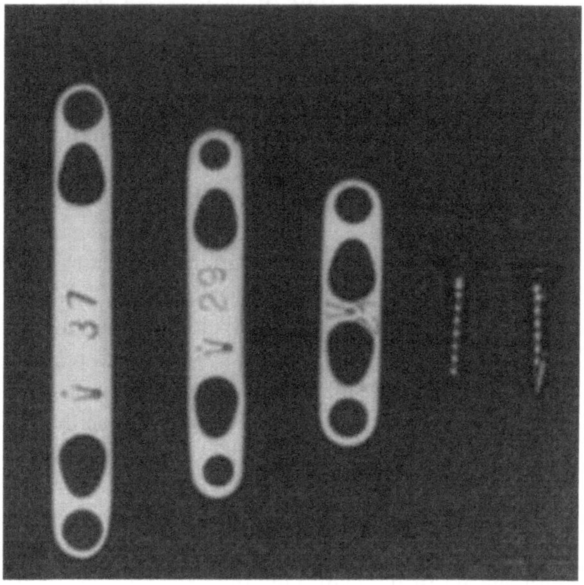

Fig. 22 Luhr's first set of miniplates that he designed for compression osteosynthesis in orthognathic surgical procedures, circa 1979 (Steinhauser 1982). (Reproduced with permission without alterations)

Many surgeons across the world, including Van Sickles, Jeters, Härle, Terry, and Tucker, among others, deserve recognition for contributions to the revolutionary breakthrough in the understanding of plates and screws, creating new instrumentation, and developing novel techniques for internal fixation (Jeters et al. 1984; Van Sickels et al. 1985a, b; 1999). The advantages of miniplates and screws are well established, and applying them has become rapid and relatively simple. Improvements in postoperative stabilization and reliability are recognized. Negating the need for MMF provides tremendous convenience for patients and their families. Internal fixation, most importantly, provides improved safety in the acute postoperative period as patients are able to open their mouth, allowing for assessment, suction, and control of the airway if required.

In the vast majority of cases, hardware will remain in place unless it becomes symptomatic or a source of infection. However, several countries have made it customary to perform a secondary operation to remove all metallic hardware following wound healing. These factors inspired the development of biodegradable plate and screw systems to negate the need for follow-up surgery. In the 1990s, Suuronen and Linquvist shared their development of resorbable polylactide bone plates and screws (Suuronen 1992; Suuronen et al. 1994). Further studies have focused on the efficacy and stability of such systems and found them to have similar success rates compared to titanium in facial osteotomies (Landes and Ballon 2006; Turvey et al. 2006; Blakey et al. 2014; Suuronen et al. 1999). Turvey (2011) reported his experience in nearly 750 patients, finding success in 94% of cases and bone healing at all sites (Turvey et al. 2011). He recognized advantages including gradual transference of physiologic forces to healing bone, reduced need for follow-up surgery, and potential to function as a medium to deliver bone-healing proteins to the osteotomy sites. However, improving this technology further has been limited by cost, complexity of handling and insertion, and instrumentation.

20 Technology Applied

The medical and surgical industries have been great beneficiaries of advancements in technology throughout the past half century. Since 1972 when Geoffrey Walker highlighted the use of digitized cephalometric radiographs in analysis of craniofacial growth and abnormalities, their use in preoperative analysis, treatment planning, and investigation of outcomes has seen tremendous progression (Walker 1972). Like all of radiology, plain film radiographs evolved into digital format, and ultimately three-dimensional analyses were capable through CT and MRI. Diagnostic and treatment planning capabilities have more recently benefited through the use of cone beam CT (CBCT) imaging. In recent years, tools such as 3D radiographs, MRI, and innovative 3D photography have developed into valuable instruments that will likely aid the future of orthognathic surgical planning.

Eisenfeld, Barker, and Mishelevich were some of the first to publish on the use of computers for facial analysis and studying the correction of dentofacial deformities in the 1970s (Eisenfeld et al. 1974; Eisenfeld and Mishelevich 1980). Since that time, software has been developed and commercialized by multiple companies to aid in treatment planning, case studies, and data analysis. Within the United States, companies such as Dolphin Imaging, Medical Modeling, Quintiles, and SAS Institute have established themselves as leaders in this arena. Similar companies have also been established in Europe.

In 2000, Jaime Gateno and James Xia from Houston published on computer-assisted 3D virtual surgical planning (VSP) for orthognathic surgery (Xia et al. 2000; Gatano et al. 2007). Using stereo eyewear, the surgeon held a virtual "scalpel" (computer mouse) to operate on a 3D visualized patient. This simulation was designed to help with presurgical osteotomy planning and prediction of bony segment movements. Belgian surgeon Gwen Swennen also pioneered 3D imaging to assist virtual planning (Swennen et al. 2007). This technology was soon expanded upon by entrepreneur Andy Christensen, who founded Medical Modeling Corporation in Golden, CO. Christensen's company worked diligently with surgeons including Bryan Bell to develop personalized anatomic modeling, virtual treatment planning, and custom surgical guides, making the technology widely available to surgeons. His company has allowed for the use of 3D reconstructions to create accurate and detailed stereolithic skull models, which aids in treatment planning from all dimensions (Fig. 23). This innovation permitted surgical planning without patient impressions, plaster study models, or hand-fabricated splints.

Orthognathic surgery with VSP took several years to make a significant breakthrough. Early obstacles with inadequate hardware for 3D image acquisition and meager software to diagnose, plan, and evaluate outcomes led to inefficiency in the clinical setting. This has been addressed through the introduction of more affordable CBCT scanners which permitted the technology to reach a wider base of surgeons. Many surgeons including Farrell (2014) have discussed methods to improve accuracy in virtual planning and execution of operations (Farrell et al. 2014). The recent development of intraoral optical scanners has allowed for detailed mapping of occlusal topography, permitting accurate final occlusion records and detailed surgical splint fabrication which can improve operative outcomes.

Inaccuracies with conventional model surgery are often not realized during preoperative lab work and are typically discovered intra- or postoperatively. VSP has allowed for early identification of such errors and opportunities to intercept discrepancies. Virtual manipulation of the maxilla and mandible can address midline or asymmetry deformities, anteroposterior or vertical movements, clockwise or counterclockwise occlusal rotations, yaw and cant corrections, and importantly any interferences requiring recontouring or anticipated needs for grafting.

Intraoperative efficiency is also improved with virtually planned custom-cutting guides, fabricated for accurate osteotomy location and orientation (Fig. 24). Prefabricated custom plates allow for patient-specific placement of screw holes, numbers, and positions while avoiding anatomic structures such as dental roots, nerves, and osteotomy margins. In lieu of traditional occlusal splints that reference the opposing arch, Polley introduced orthognathic positioning systems (OPS) to transfer virtual plans to the patient independent of occlusion (Polley and Figueroa 2013). The OPS allows for repositioning of the mobilized segment through reference from the stable maxilla or zygoma. Studies comparing accuracy and clinical outcomes of VSP to conventional orthognathic planning have been favorable and have led to a paradigm shift for many surgeons.

As orthognathic surgery progresses into the twenty-first century, surgeons continue to develop novel techniques to limit complications, facilitate safe procedures, and improve outcomes. This most recently includes intraoperative navigation, more commonly utilized in trauma and reconstruction, in hopes of improving accuracy of orthognathic surgery. Maria Troulis, among others, has published on the use of endoscopically assisted surgery for orthognathic procedures, which has benefits of reduced procedure time, minimal blood loss, decreased recovery times, and improvement in scarring (Troulis 2005).

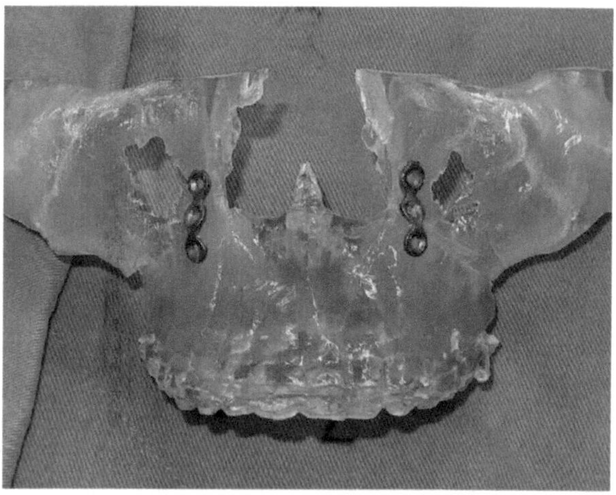

Fig. 23 3D printed stereolithic model of a patient's midface in the final position after a Le Fort I advancement. The model can be used intraoperatively to assist the surgeon with orienting the maxilla and for pre-bending plates (Lin et al. 2018). (Reproduced with permission without alterations)

21 Distraction Osteogenesis

Russian surgeon Gavriil Ilizarov developed a single-staged operation to lengthen long bones, repair skeletal limb deformities, and correct defects without the use of bone grafting through distraction osteogenesis (DO) in the 1940s and 1950s (Ilizarov 1989a, b, 1992). Applying his principles to craniomaxillofacial deformities was recognized as feasible decades later when Snyder (1973) utilized Ilizarov's methods and introduced DO for mandibular lengthening after creating an osteotomy (Snyder et al. 1973). Palatal expansion, which involves a naturally occurring symphysis, had been carried out for growing patients for many decades. By the 1990s many surgeons including McCarthy, Bell, and Guerrero endorsed DO as a viable treatment alternative to orthognathic surgery, highlighting the lack of need for bone grafting and minimal invasiveness (McCarthy 1999; Bell and Guerrero 2007). The biologic and physiologic principles of this technique are highlighted by McCarthy in his 1999 textbook, *Distraction of the Craniofacial Skeleton*. Guerrero, who has become a master of this technique, demonstrated the complexity in treatment planning, post-operative monitoring, and sophisticated analysis of esthetics and occlusion in his textbook co-authored with William Bell. Skilled surgeons from around the world including Walker, Chin, Polly, Rachmiel, Smith, Wangerin, Hoffmeister, MacCormick, and Cohen, among others, have contributed to the investigation of DO and are a testament to its success and popularity (Walker 2002; Chin and Toth

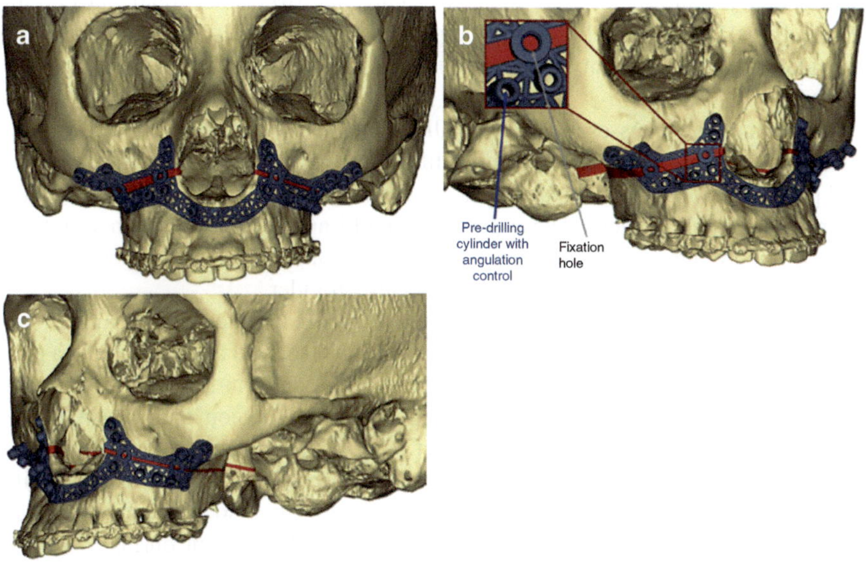

Fig. 24 (**a**) CT reconstruction with patient-specific cutting guide design. (**b**) Two fixation holes are located on each side of the cutting guide to secure it to the maxilla. (**c**) Le Fort I osteotomy markings are indicated in red. Bony wedge will be removed on the right maxilla to correct the occlusal cant (Greenberg et al. 2021). (Reproduced with permission without alterations)

1997; Polly and Figeroa 1997; Smith 2001; Rachmiel et al. 1995; Wangerin 2005; MacCormick et al. 1995; Hoffmeister et al. 1998).

Distraction osteogenesis continues to be investigated for its application to orthognathic surgery. Early on, its surgical devices were bulky, awkward, uncomfortable, and placed transfacially resulting in postoperative scarring. In the twenty-first century, most distraction devices can now be placed intraorally, hidden in hair-bearing regions of the scalp, and have a slimmer, more sleek appearance. In 1995, Molina projected that advancements in DO signaled a farewell to major facial osteotomies. While this has not been appreciated, it's application for cleft and syndromic patients and the benefits it provides for some must be realized (Molina and Ortez-Monasterio 1995).

22 Orthognathic Surgery, Health, and Well-Being

The versatility of orthognathic surgery has allowed for its application to treat multiple disease processes. Waite and Wooten (1989) reported their successes in treating patients with obstructive sleep apnea (OSA) through maxillomandibular advancements (Waite et al. 1989). Powell and Riley (2000), otolaryngologists by training, have continued to advocate for orthognathic surgery as a treatment option to improve symptoms and quality of life in patients with OSA (Riley et al. 2000). In the past decade, the work of Bundell (2012) and Boyd (2013) demonstrated that bimaxillary advancements have a superior cure rate over other treatment options (Bundell 2012; Boyd et al. 2013). The population of patients with OSA can find considerable improvement in symptoms and quality of life with orthognathic surgery.

Other disease processes are occasionally associated with dentofacial deformities such as sickle cell anemia, myopathies, fibro-osseous diseases, neurofibromatosis, and post-radiation growth disturbances, and these patients can benefit substantially from orthognathic surgery. These patients should not be denied treatment on the basis of their diagnosis. Many times, safe treatment algorithms can be developed in concert with their primary care or specialty care provider.

Orthognathic surgery has also provided a positive psychosocial impact for patients. There is no doubt that social conditions and societal attitudes create a profound impact on patients with noticeable dentofacial deformities, who often suffer from discrimination. Sir Archibald McIndoe, plastic surgeon and cousin of Sir Harold Gillies, demonstrated the impact of psychosocial issues in the treatment of patients with cranio- and dentofacial deformities in the 1940s (Pinney and Metcalfe 2014). Professor Frances Cooke Macgregor, a renowned social scientist, began researching and documenting patients with facial disfigurement during WWII in Columbia, Missouri (Naini 2011). She became the first scholar to describe the psychosocial impact of visible facial differences. Following WWII she met John Marquis Converse, and at her suggestion he conducted an exploratory research study of his patients with physical facial deformities (Thompson 1981). Macgregor's work eventually led to the recognition of facial disfigurement as a disability by the World Health Organization.

Since the 1980s, psychological and psychosocial changes in orthognathic patients have been investigated further by many physicians including Kiyak, Jacobson, Broder, Bennett, and Phillips (Kiyak et al. 1981, 1984, 1985; Jacobson 1984; Phillips and Bennett 2000; Phillips et al. 1997, 1998). Most studies have agreed that if the surgical outcome is perceived as positive, patients do experience a positive impact in self-concept, self-image, and confidence after surgery. Regardless of motive for pursuing orthognathic surgery, it seems to have a positive psychosocial impact on patients' quality of life.

23 Considerations for the Future of Orthognathic Surgery

Technology will drive the future of this exciting surgical subspecialty. Just as computers, bone plates and screws, and virtual planning and printing have brought us into the twenty-first century, the application of robotics, navigation, sensors, and many other developing technologies will mold our future. Surgeons must be open and receptive to these changes as we progress forward.

24 Conclusion

Orthognathic surgery has evolved into a vital component of not only oral, maxillofacial, and facial plastic surgery but also of the entire health care community worldwide. Generations of brilliant surgeons, anatomists, orthodontists, and researchers have led to the discovery of safe and effective treatment options. The accumulated knowledge and shared experiences of pioneers have helped us realize the functional, aesthetic, and psychosocial benefits of orthognathic surgery and will remain the foundation for future progress. The duration of time and expenses invested in treatment planning, preoperative care, and recovery is undoubtedly substantial. As the field continues to advance with new technology, surgeons must continue to improve accuracy, decrease treatment time, and limit cost to maintain orthognathic surgery as a viable and successful treatment option.

References

Angle EH. Double resection of the lower maxilla. Dent Cosmos. 1898;40:635.
Angle EH. Treatment of malocclusion of the teeth and fractures of the mandible, angles system. Philadelphia: White Dental Manufacturing; 1915.
Axhausen G. Zur Behandlung veralteter disloziert geheilter Oberkieferbruche. Dtsch Zahn-Mund-Kieferheilk. 1934a;6:582.

Axhausen G. Zur behandlung veralteter disloziert geheilter oberkieferbruche. Dtsch Zahn Mund Kieferheilk. 1934b;1:334–9.
Aziz SR, Simon P. Hullihen and the origin of orthognathic surgery. J Oral Maxillofac Surg. 2004;62(10):1303–7.
Ballin M. Double resection for treatment of mandibular protrusion. Dent Items. 1908;30:422–7. Discussion 427-31
Bamji AN. The Macalister archive: records from the Queen's Hospital, Sidcup, 1917-1921. J Audiov Media Med. 1993;16:76–84.
Bamji AN. Sir Harold Gillies: surgical pioneer. Trauma. 2006;8:143–56.
Bell WH. Surgical correction of anterior maxillary retrusion: report of a case. J Oral Surg. 1968;26:57.
Bell WH. Revascularization of bone healing after anterior maxillary osteotomy: a study using adult rhesus monkeys. J Oral Surg. 1969;27(4):249–55.
Bell WH. Biological basis for maxillary osteotomies. Am J Phys Anthropol. 1973;38:279–90.
Bell WH, Guerrero C. Distraction osteogenesis of the facial skeleton. Decker: Hamilton; 2007.
Bell WH, Levy BM. Revascularization and bone healing following total maxillary osteotomy. J Oral Surg. 1970;28:196.
Bell WH, Schendel S. Biological basis for the modification of sagittal split ramus osteotomy. J Oral Surg. 1977;35:362.
Bell WH, Fonseca RJ, et al. Bone healing and revascularization after total maxillary osteotomy. J Oral Surg. 1975;33:253.
Bell WH, Proffit WR, White RP. Surgical correction of dentofacial deformities. Philadelphia: Saunders; 1980.
Berger P. Du traitment chirurgical du prognathione. Med Trese. 1897.
Blair VP. Operations on the Jaw-Bone and Face. Surg Gynecol Obstet. 1907;4:67–8.
Blair VP. Surgery and diseases of the mouth and jaws. St. Louis: Mosby; 1912.
Blakey GH, Rossouw E, Turvey TA, et al. Are bioresorbable polylactate devices comparable to titanium devices for stabilizing Le Fort I advancement? Int J Oral Maxillofac Surg. 2014;43:437.
Booth DF, Dietz V, Gianeldy AA. Correction of class II malocclusions by combined sagittal ramus and subapical body oseteotmy. J Oral Surg. 1976;34:630.
Boyd SB, Walters AS, Song Y, et al. Comparative effectiveness of maxillomandibular advancement and uvulopalatopharyngoplasty for treatment of moderate to severe obstructive sleep apnea. J Oral Maxillofac Surg. 2013;71:743.
Buckley MJ, Turvey TA. Total mandibular subapical osteotomy; A report on long term stability and surgical techniques. Int J Adult Orthodont Orthog Surg. 1987;2(3):121–30.
Bundell JR. Primary and secondary telegnathic maxillomandibular advancement with or without adjunctive procedures for obstructive sleep apnea in adults. A literature review and treatment recommendations. J Oral Maxillofac Surg. 2012;70:1659–77.
Caldwell JB, Letterman GS. Vertical osteotomy in the mandibular rami for correction of prognathism. J Oral Surg. 1954;12:185–202.
Champy M, Lodde JP. Syntheses mandibulaires. Localisation des syntheses en function des contraintes mandibulaires. Rev Stomatol Chir Maxillofac Paris. 1976;77:971.
Cheever DW. Displacement of the upper jaw. Med Surg Rep Boston City Hosp. 1870;1:156.
Chin M, Toth BA. LeFort III advancement with gradual distraction using internal devices. Plast Reconstr Surg. 1997;100:819–30.
Cohn-Stock G. Die chirurgische immediatregulierung der kiefer, speciell die chirurgische behandlung der prognathie. Vierteljahrsschr Zahnheilk. 1921;3:320.
Converse JM. Restoration of facial contour by bone grafts introduced through the oral cavity. Plast Reconstr Surg. 1950;6:295–300.
Converse JM, Shapiro HH. Treatment of developmental malformations of the jaws. Plast Reconst Surg. 1952;10:473.
Converse JM, Telsey D. The tripartite osteotomy of the midface for orbital expansion and correction of the deformity in craniosynostosis. Br J Plast Surg. 1971;24:365–74.

Converse JM, Wood Smith D. An atlas and classification of midfacial and craniofacial osteotomies. In: Transactions of the 5th international congress of plastic surgery. Melbourne: Butterworth; 1971. p. 937.

Converse JM, Horowitz SL, Valouri AJ, Montandon D. The treatment of nasomaxillary hyperplasia. A new pyramidal naso-orbital maxillary osteotomy. Plast Reconstr Surg. 1970;45:527.

Cryer MH. Studies of the anterior and posterior occlusion of the teeth, with suggestions as to treatment. Dental Cosmos. 1913;55:673–91.

Cupar I. Die chirurgische Behandberg der Formund Stellungsverardeungen des oberkiefer. Osterr Z Stomat. 1954;51:565.

Dal-Pont G. L'osteotomia retromolare per la correzione della progenia. Minerva Chir. 1958;18:1138–41.

Dingman RO. Surgical correction of mandibular prognathism, an improved method. Am J Orthod. 1944;30:683.

Dingman RO, Harding RL. The treatment of malunited fractures of the facial bones. Plast Reconstr Surg (1946). 1951;7:505–19.

Drommer RB. This history of LeFort I osteotomy. J Maxillofac Surg. 1986;14:119.

Dyer PV. Experimental study of fractures of the upper jaw: a critique of the original papers published by Rene Le Fort. Trauma. 1999;1:81–4.

Eisenfeld J, Mishelevich DJ. Computer based research studies on the correction of dentofacial deformities. In: Bell WH, Proffit WR, White RP, editors. Surgical correction of dentofacial deformities. Philadelphia: Saunders; 1980.

Eisenfeld J, Barker DR, Mishelevich DJ. Iconic representation of the human face with computer graphics. Comp Graphics. 1974;8:9–11.

Epker BN. Modifications in the sagittal osteotomy of the mandible. J Oral Surg. 1977;35:157–9.

Epker BN. Esthetic Maxillofacial Surgery. Mahaven, PA: Lea & Febiger; 1994.

Epker BN, Fish LC. Dentofacial deformities/integrated orthodontic and surgical correction. St. Louis: Mosby; 1986.

Epker BN, Wolford LM. Reduction cheiloplasty: its place in the correction of dentofacial deformities. J Maxillofac Surg. 1977;5:134–41.

Epker BN, Wolford LM. Middle third facial advancement: treatment considerations in atypical cases. J Oral Surg. 1979;37:31–41.

Epker BN, Wolford LM. Dentofacial deformities surgical-orthodontic correction. St. Louis: Mosby; 1980.

Epker BN, Stella JP, Fish LC. Dentofacial deformities/integrated orthodontic and surgical correction, ed 2. St. Louis: Mosby; 1999.

Farrell BB, Franco PB, Tucker MR. Virtual surgical planning in orthognathic surgery. Oral Maxillofac Surg Clin N Am. 2014;26:459–73.

Gatano J, Xia JHH, Teichgraber JF. Clinical feasibility of computer aided surgical simulation (CASS) in the treatment of complex craniofacial deformities. J Oral Maxillofac Surg. 2007;65:728.

Ghali MGZ, et al. Craniosynostosis surgery: the legacy of Paul Tessier. J Neurosurg. 2014;36(4):E17.

Gillies HD, Harrison SH. Operative correction by osteotomy of recessed malar maxillary compound in a case of oxycephaly. Br J Plast Surg. 1950a;3:123–7.

Gillies H, Harrison SA. Operative correction by osteotomy of recessed malar maxillary compound in a case oxycephaly. Br J Plast Surg. 1950b;2:23–127.

Gillies H, Rowe NL. L'osteotomies des maxillaire superieur envisage essentiellement dans le cas de bec-de-lievre total. Reb Stomatol Chir Maxillofac. 1954;55:545.

Goldwyn RM. Simon P. Hullihen: Pioneer oral and plastic surgeon. Plast Reconstr Surg. 1973;52:250–7.

Greenberg S, et al. Three-dimensional repositioning of the maxilla in orthognathic surgery using patient-specific titanium plates: a case series. J Oral Maxillofac Surg. 2021;79(4):902–13.

Griffin JE, Kim K. Cosmetic surgery for the oral and maxillofacial surgeon. Chicago: Quintessence; 2010.

Gross BD, James RB. The surgical sequence of combined total maxillary and mandibular osteotomies. J Oral Surg. 1978;36:513–22.
Halvorson EG, Mulliken JB. Cheever's double operation: the first LeFort I osteotomy. Plast Reconstr Surg. 2008;121:1375–81.
Härle F, Champy M, Terry BC. Atlas of craniomaxillofacial osteosynthesis. Stuttgart: Thieme; 1999. p. 2009.
Hinds EC. Correction of prognathism by subcondylar osteotomy. J Oral Surg. 1958;16:209.
Hofer O. Die vertikale osteotomie zur verlangerung des einseitig verkurxten aufsteigenden unterkieferastes. Atschr Stomatol. 1936a;34:826.
Hofer O. Die vertikale Osteotomie des einseitig verkurzten aufsteigenden Unterkieferastes. Z Stomat. 1936b;34:826.
Hoffmeister B, Marcks CH, Wolff KP. The floating bone concept in intraoral mandibular distraction. J Craniomaxillofac Surg. 1998;26(1):76.
Hogeman KE, Wilmar K. Die Vorverlagerung des Oberkiefers zur Korrektur von GebiBanomalien. Fortschritte der Kiefer Gesichtschirurgie. Bd 12. Stuttgart: Thieme; 1967.
Hovell JH. The surgical construction of variations in the facial skeletal pattern. Proc R Soc Med. 1956;49:536–56.
Hunsuck EE. A modified intraoral sagittal splitting technique for correction of mandibular prognathism. Oral Surg. 1968;26:249.
Ilizarov G. The tension-stress effect on the genesis and growth of tissues. Part I. The influence of stability of fixation and soft-tissue preservation. Clin Orthop Relat Res. 1989a;238:249–81.
Ilizarov G. The tension-stress effect on the genesis and growth of tissues. Part II. The influence of stability of fixation and soft-tissue preservation. Clin Orthop Relat Res. 1989b;238:215–48.
Ilizarov G. Transosseous osteosynthesis. Theoretical and clinical aspects of the regeneration and growth of tissue. Berlin: Springer; 1992.
Immenkamp A. Beitraege zur maxilla-facielen chirugie unter besonderer beruecksuechtigung der korrehtur reon fihlbiddungen des mittelgieschtun. Dtsch Zahnaergtl Z. 1960;15:1073.
Jabaley ME, Edgerton MT. Surgical correction of congenital midface retrusion in the presence of mandibular prognathism. Plast Reconstr Surg. 1969;44:1.
Jaboulay M, Berard L. Traitement chirurgical du prognathisme inferieur. Presse Med. 1898;30:173–6.
Jacobson A. Psychological aspects of dentofacial esthetics and orthognathic surgery. Angle Orthod. 1984;54:18–35.
Jeters PS, Van Sickels JS, Dolwick FM. Modified techniques for internal fixation of sagittal ramus osteotomies. J Oral Maxillofac Surg. 1984;42:270–2.
Jones B. Paul Louis Tessier. BMJ. 2008;337(7661):118.
Kazanjian VH. Surgical correction of mandibular prognathism. Int J Orthod. 1932;18:1224.
Kazanjian VH. Surgical correction of deformities of the jaws and its relation to orthodontia. Int J Orthodont Oral Surg. 1936;22:259–82.
Kazanjian VH. Jaw Reconstruction. Am J Surg. 1939;3:249.
Kent JN, Hinds EC. Management of dental facial deformities by anterior alveolar surgery. J Oral Surg. 1971;29:13–21.
Kiyak HA, Hohl T, Sherrick RA, et al. Sex difference in motives for and outcomes of orthognathic surgery. J Oral Surg. 1981;39:757–64.
Kiyak HA, Hohl T, West RA, et al. Psychological changes in orthognathic surgery patients: a 24-month follow up. J Oral Maxillofac Surg. 1984;42:506–12.
Kiyak HA, McNeill RW, West RA. The emotional impact of orthognathic surgery and conventional orthodontics. Am J Orthod. 1985;88:224–34.
Köle H. Surgical operations on the alveolar ridge to correct occlusal abnormalities. Oral Surg Oral Med Oral Pathol. 1959a;12(3):277–88.
Köle H. Surgical operations on the alveolar ridge to correct occlusal abnormalities. Oral Surg Oral Med Oral Pathol. 1959b;12(4):413–20.

Köle H. Surgical operations on the alveolar ridge to correct occlusal abnormalities. Oral Surg Oral Med Oral Pathol. 1959c;12(5):515–29.

Köle H. Die chirurgische Behandlung von Formveranderungen des Kinss. Wien Med Wschr. 1968;118:331.

Köle H. Kinnostektomie nach Köle. In: Reichenbach E, Köle H, editors. Chirurgische Kieferorthopadie, 2. Leipzi: Aufl Joh Ambros Barth; 1970.

Kostečka F. A contribution to the surgical treatment of open-bite. Am J Orthodont Oral Surg. 1934;20:1082–92.

Kufner J. Nove otedy chirugickeho leceni otevrensho skusu. Cslk Stomat. 1960;60:5.

Kufner J. Experience with a modified procedure for correction of open bite. In: Walker RV, editor. Transactions of the third international conference of oral surgery. London: Livingston; 1970.

Kufner J. Four year experience with major maxillary osteotomy for retrusion. J Oral Surg. 1971;29:549–53.

LaBanc JP, Turvey T, Epker BN. Results following simultaneous mobilization of the maxilla and mandible for the correction of dentofacial deformities: analysis of 100 consecutive patients. Oral Surg Oral Med Oral Pathol. 1982;54(6):607–12.

Landes CA, Ballon A. Skeletal stability in bimaxillary orthognathic surgery. P(L/DL)LA-resorbable vs titanium osteofixation. Plast Reconst Surg. 2006;118:703.

Le Fort R. Étude expérimentale sur les fractures de la mâchoire supérieure. Revue chir de Paris. 1901;23:208–27, 360–79, 479–507.

Lin H-H, Lonic D, Lo LJ. 3D printing in orthognathic surgery – A literature review. J Formos Med Assoc. 2018;117:547–58.

Lindorf H, Steinhauser EW. Correction of jaw deformities involving simultaneous osteotomy of the mandible and maxilla. J Maxillofac Surg. 1978;6:239–44.

Luhr HG. The compression osteosynthesis of mandibular fracture in dogs. A histological contribution to "primary bone healing". Eur Sur Res. 1967;1:3.

Luhr HG. Zur stabilen osteosyntheses bei unterkiefer-frakturen. Dtsch Zahnarztl Z. 1968;23:754.

Luhr HG. Stabile Fixation von Oberkiefer-Mittelgesichtsfrakturen durch Mini-Kompressionsplatten. Dtsch Zahnarztl Z. 1979;34:851.

Luhr HG. Indications for use of a microsystem for internal fixation in craniofacial surgery. J Craniofac Surg. 1990;1:35–52.

MacCormick S, McCarthy J, Grayson B, et al. The effect of mandibular distraction on the temporomandibular joint, part I a canine study. J Craniofac Surg. 1995;6:358–63.

MacIntosh RB. Total mandibular alveolar osteotomy: encouraging experiences with an infrequently indicated procedure. J Maxilllofac Surg. 1973;2:210.

MacIntosh RB. Le Morte d'Arthur: a commentary on Hugo L. Obwegeser. J Maxillofacial Surg. 2018;76(1):6–7.

MacIntosh RB, Carlotti AE. Total mandibular alveolar osteotomy in the management of skeletal (infantile) apertognathia. J Oral Surg. 1975;33:921.

Maloney F, Worthington P. The origin of the LeFort I osteotomy: Cheevers operation. J Oral Surg. 1981;39:731.

McCarthy JG. Distraction of the craniofacial skeleton. New York: Springer; 1999.

Michelet FX, Festal F. Osteosynthese pur plaques visees dans les fractures de l'etage moyen. Sci Recherche Odonto-Stomat. 1972;2:4.

Mohnac AM. Surgical correction of maxillomandibular deformities. J Oral Surg. 1965;23:205–407.

Molina F, Ortez-Monasterio F. Mandibular elongation and remodeling by distraction: a farewell to major osteotomies. Plast Reconst Surg. 1995;96:825–40.

Moore FT, Ward TG. Complications and sequelae of untreated fractures of the facial bones and their treatment. Br J Plast Surg. 1949;1:257–67.

Moose SM. Correction of abnormal mandibular protrusion by intraoral operation. J Oral Surg. 1945;3:304.

Murray J, Swanson LT, Strand RD, Hricko GM. Evaluation of craniofacial surgery in the treatment of facial deformities. Ann Surg. 1975;182(3):240–65.

Naini FB. Psychological ramifications of facial deformities. In: Naini FB, editor. Facial aesthetics: concepts and clinical diagnosis. Oxford: Wiley-Blackwell; 2011.
Naini FB. Historical evolution of orthognathic surgery. In: Naini FB, Gill DS, editors. Orthognathic surgery: principles, planning and practice. Oxford: Wiley-Blackwell; 2017. p. 23–82.
Naini FB, Hugo L. Obwegeser (1920-2017) – The father of modern orthognathic surgery. J Orthod. 2017;44(4):317–9.
Niamtu J. Cosmetic facial surgery. St. Louis: Elsevier, Mosby; 2011. p. 1–11.
Obwegeser HL. Surgical procedures to correct mandibular prognathism and reshaping of the chin. In: Trauner R, Obwegeser HL, editors. The surgical correction of mandibular prognathism and retrognathia with consideration of genioplasty, Part I. Oral Surg Oral Med Oral Pathol, vol. 10; 1957. p. 677–89.
Obwegeser H. Surgery of the maxilla for correction of prognathism. SSO Schweiz Monatsschr Zahnheilkd. 1965;75:365–74.
Obwegeser H. Surgical correction of small or retrodisplaced maxillae. J Plast Reconstr Surg. 1969a;43:351.
Obwegeser HL. Surgical correction of small or retrodisplaced maxillae. The 'dish-face' deformity. Plast Reconstr Surg. 1969b;43:351–65.
Obwegeser H. Die einzeitige Vorbewegung des Oberkiefers und R flick bewegung des Unterkiefers zur Korrektur der extremen 'Progenie'. Schweiz Mschr Zahnheilk. 1970;80:305.
Obwegeser HL. Orthognathic Surgery and a tale of how three procedures came to be: a letter to the next generations of surgeons. Clin Plastic Surg. 2007;34:331–55.
Obwegeser HL. Orthognathic Surgery: A life's work. In: Naini FB, Gill DS, editors. Orthognathic surgery: principles, planning and practice. Oxford: Wiley-Blackwell; 2017. p. 1–20.
Perko M. Maxillary sinus and surgical movement of the maxilla. Int J Oral Surg. 1972;1:177.
Perthes G. Operative Korrektur der Progenie. Zentralbl Chir. 1922;49:1540.
Perthes G. Ueber fracturen und luxations-fracturen des kieferkopfchens und ihre operative behundlung. Berlin: Springer; 1924. p. 418–33.
Phillips C, Bennett ME. Psychological ramifications of orthognathic surgery. In: Fonseca RJ, editor. Oral and maxillofacial surgery. Philadelphia: Saunders; 2000.
Phillips C, Broder HL, Bennett ME. Dentofacial disharmony: motivations for seeking treatment. Int J Adult Orthod Orthognath Surg. 1997;12:7–15.
Phillips C, Bennett ME, Broder HL. Dentofacial disharmony: psychological status seeking treatment consultation. Angle Orthod. 1998;68:547–56.
Pinney J, Metcalfe AD. Sir Archibald McIndoe and the Guinea Pig Club. PMFA News. 2014;1:21–4.
Polley JW, Figueroa AA. Orthognathic positioning system: intraoperative system to transfer virtual surgical plan to operating field during orthognathic surgery. J Oral Maxillofac Surg. 2013;71:911–20.
Polly JW, Figeroa AA. Management of severe maxillary deficiency in childhood and adolescence through distraction osteogenesis with an external, adjustable rigid distraction device. J Craniofac Surg. 1997;8(3):181–5.
Posnick JC. Orthognathic surgery principles and practice. Philadelphia: Elsevier; 2014.
Precious DS, Delaire J. Correction of anterior mandibular vertical excess: the functional genioplasty. Oral Surg Oral Med Oral Pathol. 1985;59:229–35.
Proffit WR, White RP. Surgical-orthodontic treatment. St. Louis: Mosby; 1991.
Proffit WR, Turvey TA, Phillips C. Orthognathic surgery: a hierarchy of stability. Int J Orthod Orthognath Surg. 1996;11:191–204.
Proffit WR, White RP, Sarver DM. Contemporary treatment of dentofacial deformities. St. Louis: Mosby; 2003a.
Proffit WR, White RP, Sarver DM. Contemporary treatment of dentofacial deformities. Philadelphia: Elsevier; 2003b.
Proffit WR, Turvey TA, Phillips C. The hierarchy of stability and predictability in orthognathic surgery with rigid fixation; an update and extension. Head Face Med. 2007;3:21.

Psillakis JM, Lapa F, Spina V. Surgical correction of mid-facial retrusion (nasomaxillary hypoplasia) in the presence of normal dental occlusion. Plast Reconstr Surg. 1963;51:67.
Rachmiel A, Levy M, Laufer D. Lengthening of the mandible by distraction osteogenesis report of cases. J Oral Maxillofac Surg. 1995;53:838–46.
Reichenbach EH, Köle H, Schuchardt K. Brückl: Chirurgische Kieferorthopadie. Leipzig: JA Barth; 1964.
Reyneke JP. Essentials of orthognathic surgery. 2nd ed. Chicago: Quintessence; 2010.
Rhinelander FW, et al. Microangioplasty in bone healing. Displaced closed fracture. J Bone Joint Surg. 1968;50:643.
Riley RW, Powell NB, Li KK, et al. Surgery and obstructive sleep apnea. Long term clinical outcomes. Otolaryng Head Neck Surg. 2000;122:415–21.
Robinson M. Prognathsim corrected by open vertical condylotomy. J S C D Assoc. 1956;24:22.
Sailer HF. LeFort III osteotomy versus LeFort III and simultaneous LeFort I osteotomy in patients with clefts and craniofacial deformities. Transactions of the 8th International Congress on Cleft Palate and Related Craniofacial Anomalies. Singapore; 1997.
Sauerbier S, Schon R, et al. The development of plate osteosynthesis for the treatment of fractures of the mandibular body – A literature review. J Craniomaxillofac Surg. 2008;36(5):251–9.
Schendel SA. Sagittal split genioplasty: a new technique. J Oral Maxillofac Surg. 2010;68:931–43.
Schuchardt K. Ein beitraq zur chirurgischen kieferorthopadic unter beruchsichtigung ihrer bedentienq fur bihandlung angeloener und erworbener kieferdeform itaten ber soldaten. Dtsch Zahn Mund Kieferhlkd. 1942a;9:73.
Schuchardt K. Ein Betrag zur chirurgischen Kieferorthopadie unter Beruckssichtigung ihrer Bedeutung fur die Behandlung angeborener und erworbener Kieferdeformitaten bei Soldaten. Dtsch Zahn Mund Kieferheilkd Zentralbl. 1942b;9:73–89.
Schuchardt K. Formen des offenen Bisses und ihre operative Behandlungsmoglichkeiten. In: Fortschritte der Kiefer Gesichtschirurgie, Bd I. Stuttgart: Thieme; 1955.
Sinn DP, Ghali GE, editors. Combined orthognathic and esthetic surgery. Philadelphia: Saunders; 1996.
Sloan AC. Intraoral osteotomy of the ascending rami for correction or prognathism. Texas Dent J. 1951;69:375.
Smith KS. Internal distraction in neonates, treatment of obstructive apnea. In: Arnaud E, Dines P, editors. Third international congress on Cranio and facial bone distraction osteognesis. Paris, France; Bologna, Italy. Monduzzi Editore; 2001. p. 237–42.
Snyder CC, Levin GA, Swason HM, Browne EZJ. Mandibular lengthening by gradual distraction. Plast Reconstr Surg. 1973;51:506–8.
Soerensen J, Warnekros L. Befestigung von Goldschienen unter dem Periost. Chirurg u. Zahnarzt, Heft. Berlin: Springer; 1917.
Spiessl B. Osteosynthese bei sagittaler Osteotomie nach Obwegeser-Dal Pont. Fortschr Kiefer Gesichtschier. 1974;18:145–8.
Steinhauser EW. Bone screws and plates in orthognathic surgery. Int J Oral Surg. 1982;11:209.
Steinhauser EW. Historical development of orthognathic surgery. J Craniomaxillofac Surg. 1996;24:195–204.
Stoker N, Epker BN. The posterior maxillary osteotomy: a retrospective study of treatment results. Int J Oral Surg. 1974;3:153.
Suuronen R. Biodegradable self-reinforced polylactide plates and screws in fixation of osteotomies. PhD thesis, University of Helsinki. 1992.
Suuronen R, Laine P, Pohjonen T, et al. Sagittal ramus osteotomies fixed with biodegradable screws. A preliminary report. J Oral Maxillofac Surg. 1994;52:715.
Suuronen R, Haers PE, Lindquist C, Sailer HF. Update on bioresorbable plates in maxillofacial surgery. Facial Plast Surg. 1999;15:61–72.
Swennen GRJ, Barth EL, Eulger C, Schutyser F. The use of a new 3-D splint and double CT scan procedure to obtain an accurate anatomical virtual augmented model of the skull. Int J Oral Maxillofac Surg. 2007;36:146–52.

Tessier P. The definitive plastic surgical treatment of severe facial deformities of craniofacial synostosis: Crouzon and Apert disease. Plast Reconstr Surg. 1971a;48:419.
Tessier P. Total osteotomy of the middle third of the face for faceostenosis or for sequelae of LeFort III fracture. Plast Reconstr Surg. 1971b;48:533.
Tessier P, Guiot G, Rougerie J, et al. Cranio-naso-orbito-facial osteotomies (hypertelorism). Ann Chir Plast. 1967;12:103–18.
Thoma KH. Oblique osteotomy of the mandibular ramus. J Oral Surg. 1961;1:14.
Thompson N. John Marquis Converse 1909-1981. Chirurgia Plast. 1981;6:149–51.
Trauner R, Obwegeser H. The surgical correction of mandibular prognathism and retrognathia with consideration of genioplasty. Part I, Surgical procedures to correct mandibular prognathism and reshaping of the chin. Oral Surg Oral Med Oral Pathol. 1957a;10:677–89.
Trauner R, Obwegeser H. Surgical correction of mandibular prognathism and retrognathia with consideration of genioplasty. Part II, Operating methods for microgenia and distocclusion. Oral Surg Oral Med Oral Pathol. 1957b;10:899.
Triacca A, Minorelli R, Sculacic N. Mandibular wing osteotomy for correction of the mandibular plane: a case report. Br J Oral Maxillofac Surg. 2010;48:182–4.
Troulis M. Endoscopically assisted mandibular osteotomies. In: Fonseca RJ, Walker RB, Betts NJ, editors. Oral and maxillofacial surgery, ed 3, vol. 3. Philadelphia: Saunders; 2005.
Turvey TA. Surgical expansion of the maxilla. J Maxillofac Surg. 1985;13:51–9.
Turvey TA. The history of orthognathic surgery. In: Oral and maxillofacial surgery. Elsevier; 2017. p. 1–12.
Turvey TA, Epker BN. Soft tissue procedures adjunctive to orthognathic surgery for improvements of facial balance. J Oral Surg. 1974;32:572–7.
Turvey TA, Bell RB, Phillips C, et al. Self reinforced biodegradable screw fixation compared to titanium screw fixation in mandibular advancement. J Oral Maxillofac Surg. 2006;64:40.
Turvey TA, Proffit WP, Phillips C. Biodegradable fixation for craniomaxillofacial surgery: a 10-year experience involving 761 operations and 745 patients. Int J Oral Maxillofac Surg. 2011;40(3):244–9.
Van Sickels JS, Jeter TS, Aragon SB. Management of unfavorable fracture in sagittal split osteotomies. J Oral Maxillofac Surg. 1985a;43:808–9.
Van Sickels JS, Jeter TS, Thereot BA. Rigid fixation of maxillary osteotomies: a technique article. Oral Surg Oral Med Oral Pathol. 1985b;60:262–5.
Von Langenback BV. Bietriage zur osteoplastic die osteoplastische resection de oberkeafers. In: Goschen A, editor. Deutsche Klinck. Berlin: Reimer; 1859.
Waite PD, Matukas VJ. Indications for simultaneous orthognathic and septo-rhinoplastic surgery. J Oral Maxillofac Surg. 1991;49:133.
Waite P, Wooten V, Lachner J, et al. Maxillomandibular advancement surgery in 23 patients with obstructive sleep apnea syndrome. J Oral Maxillofac Surg. 1989;47:1256–61.
Walker GF. A new approach to the analysis of craniofacial morphology and growth. Am J Orthod. 1972;61:221–30.
Walker D. Vector planning and treatment visualization in distraction osteogenesis. J Craniomaxillofac Surg. 2002;20(1):61.
Wangerin K. Our concept of intraoral distraction. Stomatologie. 2005;102:59–66.
Wassmund M. Frakturen und Luxationen des Geishtschadels. Unter Berucksichtigung der Komplikationen des Hirnschadels. Ihre Klinik und Therapie. Praktisches Lehrbuch. Berlin: H. Meusser; 1927a.
Wassmund M. Frakturen und Luxationen des Gesichtsschadels. Leipzig: Muesser; 1927b.
Wassmund M. Lehrbuch der praktischen Chirurgie des Mundes und der Kiefer, Bd. I. Leipzig: Meusser; 1935a.
Wassmund M. Lehrbuch der prakitischen Chirurgie des Mundes und der Kiefer. Bd. I. Leipzig: Muesser; 1935b.
West RA, Epker BN. Posterior maxillary surgery: its place in the treatment of dentofacial deformities. J Oral Surg. 1972;30:562–3.

Whipple JW. Double resection of the inferior maxilla for protruding lower jaw. Dent Cosmos. 1898;40:552.

White RP, Peters PB, Costich ER, Page HL. Evaluation of sagittal split ramus osteotomy in 17 patients. J Oral Surg. 1969;27:851.

Willmar K. On LeFort I osteotomy. A follow up study of 106 operated patients with maxillofacial deformity. Scand J Plast Reconstr Surg. 1974;12:1–68.

Wolfe SA. G*ü*nther Cohn-Stock, M.S., D.D.S., father of maxillary orthognathic surgery. J Craniomaxillofac Surg. 1989;17:331–4.

Wunderer S. De prognathic operation mittels frontal gestieltem maxillofragment. Osterr Z Stomato. 1962a;59:98–102.

Wunderer S. Die prognathie-operation mittels frontal gestielten maxillafragment. Osterr Z Stomatol. 1962b;59:98–102.

Xia JHH, Samman N, Wang D, et al. Computer assisted three dimensional surgical planning and simulation: 3-D virtual osteotomy. Int J Oral Maxillofac Surg. 2000;29:11–7.

Radiation Oncology

Brett H. Diamond, Utkarsh C. Shukla, Mark H. Sueyoshi, and Kathryn E. Huber

1 Early History and Clinical Applications

The clinical application of radiation became possible with the characterization of X-rays by Wilhelm Roentgen in 1895 (Lederman 1981). Scientists across the globe began experimenting with this new technology and laid the foundation for the clinical use of X-rays both as a diagnostic and therapeutic tool. By January of 1896, Emil Grubbe reported the first treatment of an advanced breast cancer using X-rays, raising interest in the utility of X-rays as a treatment for cancer (Grubbe 1933). Likewise, early clinical experiments such as those in 1896 by brothers Gilman and Edwin Frost at Dartmouth College resulted in physicians being able to visualize the fractured wrist of a local schoolboy, Eddie McCarthy (Spiegel 1995). These early applications of X-rays for both diagnostic and therapeutic purposes inspired researchers around the globe to describe their findings characterizing this new and exciting discovery.

Similarly, the discovery of natural radioactivity by Henri Becquerel coupled with Marie and Pierre Curie's discovery of radium in 1898 established high energy photons or γ-rays ("gamma-rays") as another early tool for the clinical application of radiation (Blaufox 1996; Mould 1998). The major distinction between γ-rays and X-rays is their source: γ-rays are emitted by the atomic nucleus (or extra-nuclearly in electron-positron annihilation), while X-rays come from other sources, often from electrons transitioning between orbits of an atom or when electrons interact with the electric field of the nucleus. Of note, the distinction is not necessarily related to their energy and they are physically non-distinct. Soon, scientists were experimenting with radium as a source of γ-rays in both malignant and nonmalignant conditions. In 1901, Henri-Alexandre Danlos and Eugene Bloch used radium

B. H. Diamond · U. C. Shukla · M. H. Sueyoshi · K. E. Huber (✉)
Department of Radiation Oncology, Tufts University School of Medicine, Boston, MA, USA
e-mail: khuber@tuftsmedicalcenter.org

E. M. Ferneini et al. (eds.), *The History of Maxillofacial Surgery*,
https://doi.org/10.1007/978-3-030-89563-1_14

sent from the Curies to treat skin manifestations of lupus (Mould 2007). As early as 1903, physicians in St. Petersburg, Russia, described using radium to treat and cure basal cell carcinoma of the face (Kemıkler 2019).

During the early 1900s, scientists around the world continued experimenting with radium as a clinical tool. Shortly thereafter, the field of brachytherapy was born, as clinicians implanted radium directly into or near tumors, as opposed to external beam radiation where the therapeutic dose of radiation is delivered from outside of the body using a source that produces γ-rays or X-rays. Three general approaches to brachytherapy were developed: (a) an intracavitary approach that makes use of natural body cavities, (b) an interstitial approach where radioactive seeds are directly implanted into tissue or placed on the skin surface, and (c) an intraluminal approach where seeds are placed in a linear distribution within a luminal device that has been inserted into the body. The radioactive source placement of intracavitary and intraluminal brachytherapy is always temporary, while interstitial brachytherapy may be permanent or temporary. In 1903, Margaret Cleaves described the first case of cervical cancer cured by intrauterine radium (Aronowitz et al. 2007). Just a year later in 1904, Robert Abbe described early head and neck brachytherapy when he applied radium, first externally, and later internally, to treat a 17-year-old boy with a tumor of the lower jaw, likely representing the first interstitial use of brachytherapy (Aronowitz 2012). In the subsequent decades, both X-rays and radium-derived γ-rays were successfully applied in the treatment of a variety of malignant and benign conditions, solidifying the utility of radiation therapy as a practical clinical tool.

2 The Foundations of Radiobiology

Humans' understanding of radiation has grown immensely since its first clinical applications. Early discoveries of the clinical utility of radiation gave rise to an entirely new field of biology termed "radiobiology." Radiobiologists built upon early observations to establish principles which guide our understanding of the effect of radiation on both healthy and diseased tissues. In 1906, Jean Alban Bergonié and Louis Tribondeau theorized early principles of radiobiology by postulating that radiosensitivity was governed by the biologic properties of the tissue including cell division rate, dividing future, and an unspecialized phenotype (Table 1) (Bergonie and Tribondeau 1905). In other words, radiosensitivity of cells increased with increased mitotic activity and radiosensitivity decreased with greater cell differentiation. Similarly, scientists observing the biologic effect of radiation hypothesized that oxygenation may play an important role in radiosensitivity. This theory was studied by many including J.C. Mottram who in 1936 noted an increased sensitivity of tumor cells at the edge of masses, hypothesizing that an increased oxygen supply was correlated with increased radiosensitivity (Mottram 1936). Similarly, experiments by Louis Harold Gray throughout the 1950s provided further evidence of the presence of oxygen increasing tumor sensitivity to radiation (Gray et al. 1953).

Table 1 Overview of critical events in the early history of radiation and radiobiology

1895	Wilhelm Roentgen characterizes X-rays
1896	Emil Grubbe reports first treatment of breast cancer with X-rays
1896	Gilman and Edwin Frost utilize X-rays for diagnosis of fracture
1898	Marie and Pierre Curie discover radium and Henri Becquerel describes natural radioactivity
1901	Henri-Alexandre Danlos and Eugene Bloch utilize radium to treat skin manifestations of lupus
1903	Russian physicians utilize radium to cure basal cell carcinoma of the face
1903	Margaret Cleaves describe the first case of cervical cancer cure with intrauterine radium
1904	Robert Abbe describes the use of radium for early head and neck cancer used externally and then later internally
1906	Jean Alban Bergonie and Louis Tribondeau theorize early principles of radiobiology
1913	William Coolidge develops orthovoltage X-ray tube
1920s	Claudius Regaud demonstrates that radiation dose fractionation can kill rapidly dividing cells without death of non-rapidly dividing cells via ram sterility experiment
1925	G. Failla introduces an objective method for administration of X-rays
1934	Henri Coutard describes the use of radiation dose fractionation in head and neck cancer
1936	J.C. Mottram describes increased radiosensitivity of well-oxygenated tumor cells
1950s	Louis Harold Gray provides further evidence of the role of oxygen in radiosensitivity of tumors
1952	First megavoltage linear accelerator installed in Hammersmith Hospital in London, UK
1954	First US-based linear accelerator installed at Stanford Hospital in San Francisco, California
1956	Theodore Puck and Philip Marcus characterize radiation sensitivity by way of HeLa cells
1959	H.B. Hewitt and C.W. Wilson describe the radiation survival curve
1965	M.M. Elkind develops nascent rationale for fractionation which allows sublethal damage repair for normal tissue
1985	Ian Radford confirms that double-strand DNA breaks as the primary mechanism of cellular death by radiation
Late 1900s	Further elucidation of radiation-induced free radicals as predominant mechanism of DNA damage

Paramount to the understanding of modern radiobiology is the principle of fractionation, or dividing dose into multiple separate, smaller doses. In the early days of radiation, treatments were mostly given as large single doses by placing low-energy cathode ray tubes or radium-filled glass tubes in close proximity to tumors. These treatments were plagued by normal tissue toxicities and disappointing cure rates. Scientists such as Claudius Regaud began to experiment with delivery of smaller doses of radiation in his experiments on ram spermatogenesis in order to develop a technique to sterilize the animals with radiation. His experiments throughout the 1920s showed that dividing radiation doses into multiple smaller fractions targeting rapidly dividing cells could result in sterility of the ram without causing severe skin necrosis (Regaud 1977). Although the principle of dose fractionation was initially controversial, further clinical evidence as to its efficacy was demonstrated by Henri Coutard who described the use of fractionated radiotherapy in the treatment of head and neck cancers in 1934 (Coutard 1936). These basic observations enabled further study into developing optimal treatment regimens for a variety of cancers in subsequent decades. To this day, fractionation remains an important tool to optimize the therapeutic index of radiation.

With the development and refinement of cell culture techniques, it became possible for researchers to further analyze the effect of radiation on cells. Theodore Puck and Philip Marcus were among the early pioneers of this field with their experiments characterizing the radiation sensitivity of HeLa cells, the first immortal human cell line obtained from Henrietta Lacks's cervical cancer, and the development of early cell survival assays in their study published in 1956 (Puck and Marcus 1955). These assays allowed scientists to reproducibly study the effects of radiation on cell biology. In the subsequent years, advances including the first description of a radiation survival curve by H.B Hewitt and C.W. Wilson in 1959 allowed for further study into the biological effects of radiation (Hewitt and Wilson 1960). Cell culture allowed scientists to systematically study the effects of radiation to provide a biologic basis for the observations of their predecessors. For instance, in 1965 M.M. Elkind was able to provide an early explanation for the benefits of fractionation by describing how repair of sublethal damage in healthy tissue may account for the observed decreased toxicity profile of radiation when it is split into smaller doses rather than given as a larger single dose (Elkind et al. 1967).

As modern molecular biology techniques arose, contemporary studies confirmed the presence of DNA damage as a direct result of intracellular ionization events and subsequent free radical production to be the primary mediator of radiation therapy's lethality on tumor cells. In 1985, Ian Radford confirmed the role of double-strand DNA breaks as the primary mechanism for radiation-induced cellular death (Radford 1985). By the end of the twentieth century, radiobiologists were beginning to gain a deeper understanding of the highly complex signaling cascades that occurred as a result of this free radical-induced damage. These advancements led to further discoveries, including radiation sensitizers, targeted therapies, and strategic techniques in the delivery of radiation therapy which maximize its therapeutic benefit.

3 The Modernization of Radiation Delivery

In the years since the first therapeutic use of X-rays by Emil Grubbe to treat a patient with breast cancer in 1896, the field of radiation oncology has transformed dramatically. Early radiation therapy, referred to as external beam therapy or teletherapy, was limited by devices that could produce low-energy radiation energies of approximately 100 kiloelectron volts (keV). These energies were useful in the treatment of superficial tumors, but higher-energy beams were needed to reach deeper tumors inside the body. Although beyond the scope of this chapter, it is important to note that the maximum dose for a lower-energy X-ray beam deposits near the surface, while the maximum dose for higher-energy X-ray beam deposits deeper in tissue. Therefore, there is generally less superficial dose, and thus lower skin toxicity, from a higher-energy X-ray beam (Khan and Gibbons 2014). In 1913, an American physicist, William Coolidge, developed an X-ray tube which could produce X-rays on the order of 200 keV. For much of the 1920s, energies of 200 keV to 500 keV were utilized, later termed "orthovoltage." By 1952, the first "megavoltage" medical linear accelerator was installed at the Hammersmith Hospital in London, UK, which could generate energies up to 8 megavolts (MV) (Laurence and Livingston 1932; Bewley 1984). Shortly thereafter, in 1954, the first such linear accelerator in the United States was installed at Stanford Hospital in San Francisco, California (Weissbluth et al. 1959).

In order to transform radiation from an experimental therapeutic tool to a mainstay of head and neck cancer treatment, a deeper understanding of radiation physics proved to be essential. In the modern era, radiation physics allows for the careful application of reproducible doses of radiation. This arose from studies defining ways to model radiation dose such as early reports of primitive isodose diagrams in 1925 by G. Failla (Delaney 2005). Isodose diagrams help to visual the dose distribution within both the target of interest and nearby organs. More modern isodose diagrams take into account electron density based on CT imaging data to calculate dose distribution which will be discussed further in the next section.

This discussion has, thus far, covered foundational radiation therapies delivered via nuclear decay (brachytherapy), X-rays (external beam radiation therapy), and charged particles (electrons). There are numerous other modalities of radiotherapy that should be briefly mentioned for familiarization. For example, radiation therapy can be delivered by way of accelerated, and thereby energized, larger charged particle radiation (protons, carbon, etc.) and uncharged particles (neutrons). Additionally, within each modality there is further breakdown of technique. Consider the case of external beam radiation therapy that can vary by radiation dose per fraction, rate of radiation administration, as well as conformality of the radiation to the target of interest. The more pertinent aspects of radiation type and delivery in head and neck cancers will be discussed further in the following section.

4 Contemporary History of Head and Neck Radiation Oncology

In the modern era, radiotherapy remains a key modality in the treatment of cancer with approximately 50% of all cancer patients receiving radiation therapy during their treatment (Delaney 2005). Among head and neck cancer patients, it is estimated that radiotherapy is offered to nearly 75% of patients during the course of their management (Ratko et al. 2014). Patients may undergo radiation therapy alone in early-stage H&N cancers or in combination with chemotherapy in advanced cancers. In the field of head and neck oncology, radiotherapy has rapidly evolved to a highly technologically advanced, multidisciplinary field. Owing to advances in radiation treatment planning, image guidance, and treatment delivery technologies, radiation oncologists can deliver precise and reproducible doses of radiation while sparing normal tissues. This precision enables improved patient outcomes with better tumor control and lower toxicities for patients and is especially vital to the use of radiation in the head and neck region due to the intimate proximity of tumors and sensitive organs. A notable example of toxicity is xerostomia as a consequence of radiation to uninvolved salivary glands. The use of beam modulation often allows for lower doses and, in some cases, avoidance of these glands. Nonetheless, despite improved conformality of modern radiation delivery to the tumor and regions at risk, it remains vital that oral surgeons and/or dentists play a key role in the management of late effects of dry mouth on the health of the oral cavity even in the absence of surgical management of head and neck malignancies (Harrison et al. 2003).

Initially, target delineation for radiation therapy delivery was based on physical exam, plain radiographs, surgical findings, and any surgical clips placed during surgery, as well as an understanding of patterns of disease spread. Early forms of external beam radiation for head and neck cancers were of limited configurations. Typically, radiation beams were laterally opposed fields with or without a photon beam to cover the low anterior neck, or a "wedge pair" of 90 degree offset fields based on 2D fluoroscopic imaging. Given the large areas of exposure with these techniques, it was common for patients to experience severe mucositis, dermatitis, dysphagia, and odynophagia acutely, with xerostomia and fibrosis as late toxicities (Trotti et al. 2003).

In the late 1980s, there was a movement to reduce normal tissue irradiation with three-dimensional conformal radiation therapy (3DCRT) as imaging quality improved with the advent and increased availability of computed tomography (CT) scans, thus increasing confidence in target volume delineation and radiation planning. The integration of imaging for target localization at the time of treatment, referred to as image-guided radiation therapy (IGRT), improved the accuracy of treatment delivery. One such technique is through cone-beam computed tomography (CBCT), which reconstructs a 3D image from a series of 2D projection images of the patient while on the treatment table (Jaffray 2005).

Intensity-modulated radiation therapy (IMRT) was developed throughout the 1980s–1990s and revolutionized the way radiation oncologists could deliver conformal radiation. IMRT improved on the concept of conformality of radiation dose through the use of non-uniform radiation beam intensities that can be shaped by selectively and geometrically blocking components of the output beam as radiation is delivered from various angles. Such an approach improved the therapeutic ratio by increasing dose to the target tissue while simultaneously reducing dose to adjacent organs at risk (Hong et al. 2005). In 1994, the first commercially available

IMRT capable treatment machine, the NOMOS Peacock, was released which allowed for broader adaptation of IMRT throughout the radiation oncology community (Hong et al. 2005). The advances of 3D imaging, IGRT, and IMRT have allowed for the reduction of radiation planning target volume that is added to account for uncertainty in daily treatment alignment, thereby decreasing the amount of collateral radiation to adjacent normal tissues, which translates into significantly reduced toxicity.

Throughout the twentieth century, advances in particle physics gave rise to new radiation modalities that offer promise in the field of head and neck radiation oncology. Protons, which are positively charged particles in the nucleus, were initially described by Ernest Rutherford in 1919 (Peake 1989). Decades of research ensued before 1946 when Robert Wilson first proposed the use of protons as a potential new tool in radiation oncology (Wilson 1946). The first patient was treated with proton therapy at Berkeley Radiation Laboratory in 1954. After many years of clinical investigation and refinement of proton beam technology, protons were first approved by the FDA in 1988 (Smith 2009). The physical properties of protons result in a dose distribution in the tissue with minimal exit dose beyond the prescribed depth. This is particularly useful in the treatment of base of skull tumors, as its physical characteristics allow for the delivery of curative doses of radiation despite close proximity to structures with exquisite function such as the brainstem or optic chiasm. Today, proton therapy is under investigation for a variety of applications, and its use is likely to be expanded as this data matures and the cost of this technology declines.

As treatment delivery techniques have developed, the dose administered per fraction has also been investigated. Conventionally, treatment is delivered in 1.8–2 Gy per fraction (where 1 Gy refers to 1 joule per kilogram) with more fractions delivered to areas of higher risk for subclinical disease and the highest number of fractions to gross tumor. Patients are typically treated 5 days a week, one treatment per day in what is referred to as conventionally fractionated radiation. Hyperfractionation, or the use of a greater number of smaller treatment doses, has been proposed as a means of increasing total dose, and thus tumor control, without increasing permanent toxicities from the radiation. The hyperfractionated approach has shown promise in head and neck cancers with the seminal EORTC trial published in 1992 showing a tumor control benefit in the treatment of oropharynx cancer (Horiot et al. 1992). Another novel approach is hypofractionation, involving higher doses per fraction in fewer fractions. Hypofractionation has been used in a variety of cancer types and has recently shown promise in the treatment of head and neck cancers. Notably in 2006, there were noted improved outcomes using 2.25 Gy per fraction to treat early-stage laryngeal cancer (Yamazaki et al. 2006). However, hypofractionation in the head and neck region should be used with caution as this increases risk of severe toxicity such as necrosis of the bone, cartilage, and soft tissues. Ongoing clinical trials exist investigating the use of both hypofractionation and hyperfractionation to treat head and neck cancers.

5 Conclusion

Moving toward the future, the field of radiation oncology will continue to play an integral role in the management of cancer. The foundations of modern radiation oncology are a credit to the scientists and clinicians that have driven scientific progress allowing for radiotherapy to arise as a powerful clinical tool. Scientific progress will undoubtedly continue to drive the field of radiation oncology forward building upon its rich 130-year history.

References

Aronowitz JN. Robert Abbe: early American brachytherapist. Brachytherapy. 2012;11(6):421–8.

Aronowitz JN, Aronowitz S, Robison RF. Classics in brachytherapy: Margaret Cleaves introduces gynecologic brachytherapy. Brachytherapy. 2007;6(4):293–7.

Bergonie J, Tribondeau L. Aspermatogenèse experimentale apres une seule exposition aux rayons X. Compt Rend Soc de Biol. 1905;58:282–4.

Bewley DK. The 8 MeV linear accelerator at the MRC Cyclotron Unit Hammersmith Hospital, London. BJR. 1984;58(687):213.

Blaufox MD. Becquerel and the discovery of radioactivity: early concepts. Semin Nucl Med. 1996;26(3):145–54.

Coutard H. The conception of periodicity as a possible directing factor in the roentgentherapy of cancer. Am J Roentgenol. 1936;32:310–23.

Delaney G, Jacob S, Featherstone C, Barton M. The role of radiotherapy in cancer treatment: estimating optimal utilization from a review of evidence-based clinical guidelines. Cancer. 2005;104:1129–37.

Elkind MM, Sutton-Gilbert H, Moses WB, Kamper C. Sublethal and lethal radiation damage. Nature. 1967;214:1088–92.

Gray LH, et al. The concentration of oxygen dissolved in tissues at the time of irradiation as a factor in radiotherapy. Br J Radiol. 1953;26(312):638–648.2.

Grubbe EH. Priority in the therapeutic use of X-rays. Radiology. 1933;21:156–62.

Harrison JS, Dale RA, Haveman CW, Redding SW. Oral complications in radiation therapy. Gen Dent. 2003;51(6):552–60.

Hewitt HB, Wilson CW. Radiation survival curves. Br J Radiol. 1960;33(388):270.

Hong TS, Ritter MA, Tome WA, Harari PM. Intensity-modulated radiation therapy: emerging cancer treatment technology. Br J Cancer. 2005;92(10):1819–24.

Horiot JC, Le Fur R, N'Guyen T, et al. Hyperfractionation versus conventional fractionation in oropharyngeal carcinoma: final analysis of a randomized trial of the EORTC cooperative group of radiotherapy. Radiother Oncol. 1992;25(4):231–41.

Jaffray DA. Emergent technologies for 3-dimensional image-guided radiation delivery. Semin Radiat Oncol. 2005;15(3):208–16.

Kemıkler G. History of brachytherapy. Turk Onkol Derg. 2019;34(1):1–10.

Khan FM, Gibbons JP. Khan's the physics of radiation therapy. 5th ed. Lippincott Williams & Williams; 2014.

Laurence EO, Livingston MS. The production of high speed light ions without the use of high voltages. Phys Rev. 1932;40:19–35.

Lederman M. The early history of radiotherapy: 1895–1939. IJROBP. 1981:639–48.

Mottram JC. A factor of importance in the radio sensitivity of tumours. Br J Radiol. 1936;9(105):606–14.

Mould RF. The discovery of radium in 1898 by Maria Sklodowska-Curie (1867–1934) and Pierre Curie (1859–1906) with commentary on their life and times. Br J Radiol. 1998;71(852):1229–54.
Mould RF. Priority for radium therapy of benign conditions and cancer. Curr Oncol. 2007;14(3):118–22.
Peake BM. The discovery of the electron, proton, and neutron. J Chem Edu. 1989;66:738.
Puck TT, Marcus PI. A rapid method for viable cell titration and clone production with HeLa cells in tissue culture: the use of X-irradiated cells to supply conditioning factors. PNAS. 1955;41(7):432.
Radford IR. The level of induced DNA double-strand breakage correlates with cell killing after X-irradiation. Int J Radiat Biol Relat Stud Phys Chem Med. 1985;48(1):45–54.
Ratko TA, Douglas GW, de Souza JA et al. Radiotherapy treatments for head and neck cancer update. Agency for Healthcare Research and Quality (US). 2014.
Regaud C. The influence of the duration of irradiation on the changes produced in the testicle by radium (translated). IJROBP. 1977;2:565–7.
Smith AR. Vision 2020: proton therapy. Med Phys. 2009;36:556–68.
Spiegel P. The first clinical X-ray made in America—100 years. Am J Roentgenol. 1995;164:241–3.
Trotti A, Bellm LA, Epstein JB, Frame D, Fuchs HJ, Gwede CK, et al. Mucositis incidence, severity and associated outcomes in patients with head and neck cancer receiving radiotherapy with or without chemotherapy: a systematic literature review. Radiother Oncol. 2003;66(3):253–62.
Weissbluth M, Karzmark CJ, Steele RE, Selby AH. The stanford medical linear accelerator. Radiology. 1959;72(2):242–53.
Wilson RR. Radiological use of fast protons. Radiology. 1946;47(5):487–91.
Yamazaki H, Nishiyama K, Tanaka E, Koizumi M, Chatani M. Radiotherapy for early glottic carcinoma (T1N0M0): results of prospective randomized study of radiation fraction size and overall treatment time. Int J Radiat Oncol. 2006;64(1):77–82.

Head and Neck Tumor Surgery

Andrew Deek and Eric R. Carlson

1 Introduction

The practice of oral/head and neck tumor surgery represents an educational, technical, philosophical, and political transformation in the specialty of oral and maxillofacial surgery. Once practiced by a select few interested and passionate individuals, the subspecialty of oral/head and neck tumor surgery is now practiced by duly trained individuals in the twenty-first century who claim justifiable legitimacy and relevance with disruptive referral patterns and impressive clinical outcomes. The specialty of oral and maxillofacial surgery was once supported by its membership engaging in the routine diagnosis and occasional removal of benign and malignant pathologic processes of the oral cavity, oropharynx, facial skin, and neck. Over time, the development of bona fide and undisputed didactic and clinical blueprints has defined the unique ability of qualified members of our specialty to provide comprehensive ablative and functional/aesthetic reconstructive surgery of the oral/head and neck region while supporting patient safety (Carlson 2018).

The clinical repertoire of our specialty is perhaps best demonstrated in the international literature. It is true that we publish what we do, and our specialty's transformation is reflected in the literature that oral and maxillofacial surgeons have historically published. To that end, one can peruse the four issues comprising the first volume of the *Journal of Oral Surgery* in 1943 to appreciate the excitement of our specialty's membership for benign and malignant pathology of the oral/head and neck region. Forty-eight papers were published in this first volume, 19 of which focused on elements of pathology and tumor surgery of the oral and maxillofacial

A. Deek · E. R. Carlson (✉)
Department of Oral and Maxillofacial Surgery, University of Tennessee Medical Center, Knoxville, TN, USA
e-mail: adeek@utmck.edu; ecarlson@utmck.edu

E. M. Ferneini et al. (eds.), *The History of Maxillofacial Surgery*,
https://doi.org/10.1007/978-3-030-89563-1_15

region. By contrast, 15 papers focused on maxillofacial trauma diagnosis and management, part of our specialty's core practice in 1943. A case report of metastasizing ameloblastoma originating in the mandible and resulting in the death of a 27-year-old patient is representative of the benign pathology discussed in this first volume of the *Journal of Oral Surgery* (Schweitzer and Barnfield 1943). Other papers devoted to the treatment of benign neoplastic disease by oral and maxillofacial surgeons included those related to mixed tumors of the palate (Henny 1943; Wolfe and Hubinger 1943). Four of the 19 pathology papers published in this first volume of the *Journal of Oral Surgery* focused on malignant disease, including primary lymphosarcoma of the mandible (Penhale 1943), undiagnosed primary carcinoma of the gingiva with disseminated metastases (Burket 1943), adenocarcinoma originating from aberrant tissue in the gingiva (Loeb 1943), and carcinoma of the indifferent cell type of the maxilla (Gunter et al. 1943). The latter two papers contained specific comments regarding techniques of oncologic surgery, consistent with contemporary approaches observed and executed in the twenty-first century.

Decades following publication of these initial papers in our specialty's literature, our subspecialty realized its genesis with subspecialty fellowship education, accreditation, certification, and research in the arena of oral/head and neck oncologic and reconstructive surgery. Our subspecialty's involvement in benign tumor surgery has simultaneously evolved with recognition of evidence-based principles. The maturity of our subspecialty in benign and malignant oral/head and neck tumor surgery now represents a transformational and multidimensional process. This process has involved not only focused clinical and didactic training as its requisite framework but also precise and calculated national administrative oversight to effectively and legitimately create this subspecialty and introduce it to the forefront of our specialty. The waning enthusiasm of competing specialties in the arena of head and neck surgery, as well as the development of authentic training in this discipline within oral and maxillofacial surgery, has formidably positioned members of our specialty as the primary providers for patients with benign and malignant tumors of the oral/head and neck region. What began as a vision of greatness for the clinical care of patients with head and neck pathology in 1943 is now a well-recognized subspecialty supported by formal fellowship training, excellence in accreditation standards, board certification with a certificate of added qualifications, and an ongoing commitment to clinical and didactic continuing education. Our specialty's training and clinical appreciation for functional reconstruction of oral cancer patients, in addition to our commitment to ablative surgery, represents the road map to comprehensive care for these patients.

A review of the complete process of our subspecialty's development permits a deep understanding of the mechanics of such creation in oral and maxillofacial surgery. This chapter reviews this process in a dependent fashion of the development of didactic and clinical competencies through formal medical education, general surgery training, and fellowship training; accreditation of fellowship programs by the Commission on Dental Accreditation; the formal recognition of the subspecialty through the creation of dedicated committees within the American Association of

Oral and Maxillofacial Surgeons; the establishment of the Certificate of Added Qualification in oral/head and neck oncologic and reconstructive surgery by the American Board of Oral and Maxillofacial Surgery; and the publication of our research outcomes in the international oral and maxillofacial surgery literature.

2 Early Documents, Providers, Patients, and Essential Ancillary Services

The first medical documents with references to malignant disease are the *Ebers Papyrus* (Fig. 1), and the *Edwin Smith Papyrus* (Fig. 2). The *Ebers Papyrus* is a 110-page scroll written in hieratic Egyptian that measures approximately 20 meters in length and is among the oldest preserved medical documents. The papyrus discusses approximately 700 magical formulas and folk remedies, a treatise on the heart, a review of depression and dementia, contraception, dentistry, and the surgical treatment of abscesses and tumors. This voluminous record of ancient Egyptian medicine is currently stored at the library of the University of Leipzig in Germany.

The *Edwin Smith Papyrus* is an ancient Egyptian medical text and the oldest known treatise on trauma. The papyrus is a scroll written right to left in hieratic Egyptian and measures approximately 15 feet in length. The papyrus represents a surgical document discussing breast cancer, in part, and comprises 17 pages in length. Collectively, the *Ebers Papyrus* and *Edwin Smith Papyrus* are primarily

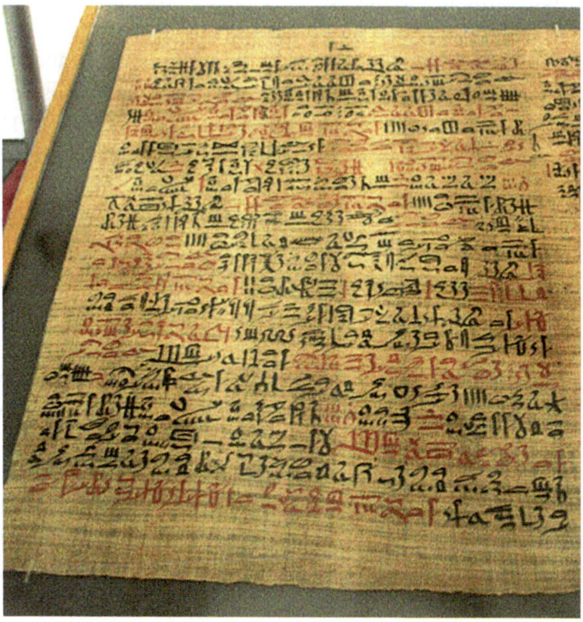

Fig. 1 The *Ebers Papyrus*. Accessed from www.wikipedia.org, 20 Sept 2020

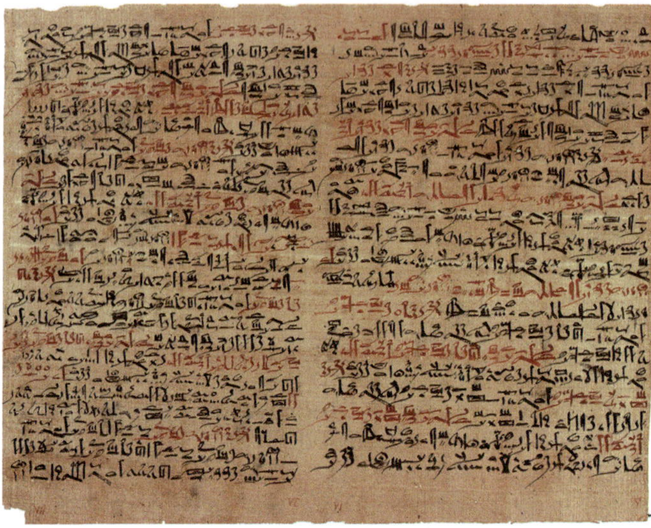

Fig. 2 The *Edwin Smith Papyrus*. Accessed from www.wikipedia.org, 20 Sept 2020

devoted to issues of trauma and dated between 1600 and 1550 BCE, although they contain descriptions of treatment from 3000 to 2500 BCE. According to the *Ebers Papyrus*, an example of gingival cancer, like other cancers of the oral mucosa discussed in this Papyrus, was noted to have been treated by the Egyptians with cinnamon, honey, and oil (Folz et al. 2008). Hippocrates (460–370 BCE) has been cited as the first to mention the terms "carcinos" and "carcinoma" to describe clinical conditions such as ulcerative and non-ulcerative tumors (Carlson 2018; Folz et al. 2008). He recommended the treatment of cancer with caustic pastes and cautery, and he recommended nonsurgical approaches to deeply invasive cancers, an approach that soon became known as the Doctrine of Hippocrates.

Aulus Cornelius Celsus (25 BCE–50 CE) has been cited as the first head and neck surgeon who described a surgical procedure for cancer of the lower lip in his medical text *De Medecina* (Goldstein and Sisson 1996). Although Celsus utilized the terms "carcinode" and "carcinoma," he recommended against the surgical treatment of cancer. Microscopic confirmation of the presence of cancer was first established in 1885 when Dr. George Elliott initiated interest in histopathology in his description of President Grant's cancer of the tonsil and tongue base (Carlson 2002; Goldstein and Sisson 1996). Surgery was never performed on Grant although the opinion of New York surgeon, Dr. George Shrady, was sought, and a radical surgical procedure was thought to be a reasonable approach for the former president. Moreover, radiation therapy was not considered a modality of treatment at that time. Grant resorted to sleeping upright after an initial episode of threatened suffocation. A severe hemorrhagic event and expectoration of part of the cancer relieved his partial airway obstruction although Grant died of his disease some 13.5 months following its original diagnosis.

3 Histopathology

The use of histopathology as part of diagnostic biopsies prior to cancer surgery was popularized in 1893 in the case of sitting US President Grover Cleveland, when incisional biopsies of his palatal lesion were procured by White House physician Major Robert Maitland O'Reilly. The diagnosis was thought to be consistent with squamous cell carcinoma, although some believe that the prognostically more favorable verrucous carcinoma was a more likely diagnosis. The microscopic diagnosis of President Cleveland's tumor was offered by Dr. William Welch from Johns Hopkins Hospital (Goldstein and Sisson 1996). This diagnosis occurred during a time of economic ruin in the United States such that President Cleveland's diagnosis and treatment were issues of national security. On June 30, 1893 President Cleveland boarded the Oneida, a yacht that was owned by Commodore Elias C. Benedict, along with Dr. Joseph Bryant, an eminent general surgeon of the day, who had previously published a history of 250 cases of maxillary resection, only two of which he personally performed. Providing assistance for the maxillary resection was neurosurgeon Dr. William Keen, and dentist Dr. Ferdinand Hasbrouck was assigned to the performance of necessary dental extractions and the administration of anesthesia. Dr. Edward Janeway, Dr. O'Reilly, and Dr. JF Eidmann, who assisted Dr. Bryant, were also present for the surgical procedure. The slightly longer than 1-h July 1, 1893 surgery was successful, and President Cleveland recovered from surgery and anesthesia aboard the Oneida that docked in Buzzards Bay. Shortly thereafter, Dr. Kason Gibson, a dentist, afforded the president with a vulcanized rubber obturator that permitted President Cleveland to address a session of Congress on August 7, 1893, only 5 weeks postoperatively. Cleveland passed away in June 1908, some 15 years following his cancer operation and at a time when he was undoubtedly cured of his disease.

4 Frozen Sections

The work of Christian Nezelof in frozen sections, later popularized by Dr. Thomas Cullen, further legitimized the value of microscopic tissue examination as part of tumor surgery and ushered in the routine evaluation of tissue as standard practice (Folz et al. 2008). In 1891, Dr. William Welch at Johns Hopkins Hospital used a carbon dioxide freezing microtome in the analysis of breast tissue removed by Dr. William Halstead (Gal 2005). As dictated by history, the frozen section analysis was excessively long for Dr. Halstead's preference such that the surgical procedure was completed before the results of the frozen sections were available. Dr. Cullen is credited with the first publication on the frozen section technique. The subsequent work of Dr. Louis B. Wilson of the Mayo Clinic ultimately ushered in a technique that is largely indispensable in contemporary cancer surgery, including that performed in the oral/head and neck region.

5 Antibiosis and Anesthesia

Advances in antibiosis and anesthesia represented new vistas for the practice of oral/head and neck surgery in the nineteenth century. The introduction of general anesthesia by Horace Wells and William Thomas Green Morton resulted in Dr. John Warren, a celebrated professor of surgery at Harvard Medical School and its dean, removing a tumor of the neck from Edward Gilbert Abbot. The patient was anesthetized with ether by Dr. Morton in a public demonstration at the yet to be named Ether Dome at Massachusetts General Hospital on October 16, 1846 (Fig. 3). When the patient emerged from anesthesia and indicated that he had felt no pain, Dr. Warren indicated that "this is no humbug." This successful surgical procedure exemplified the essential nature of anesthesia in the practice of oral/head and neck ablative surgery and surgery, in general (see Chapter "Anesthesia").

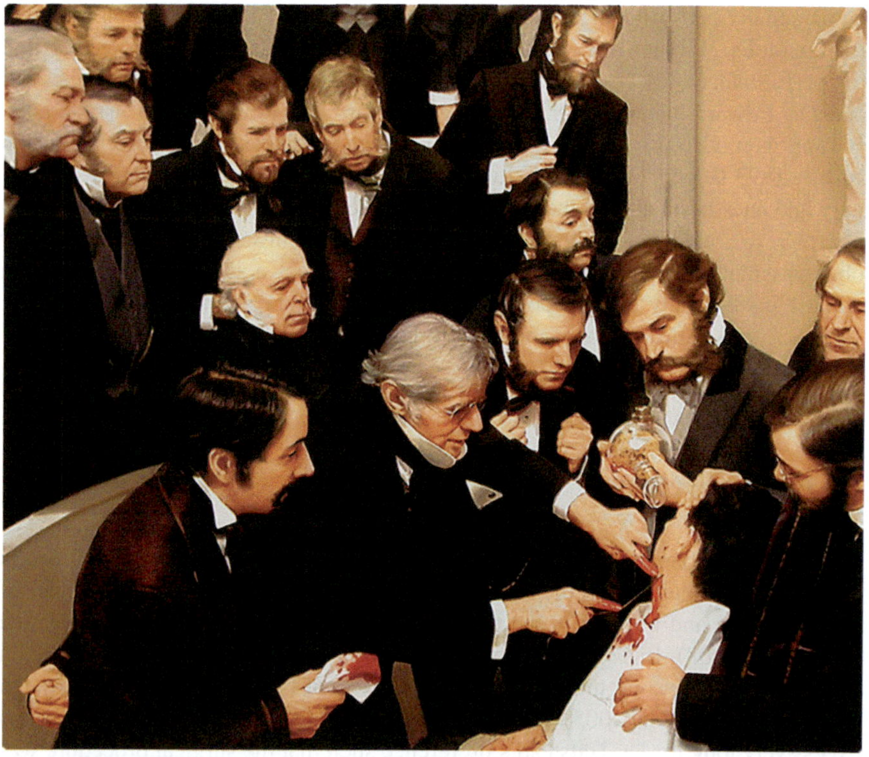

Fig. 3 Neck tumor surgery performed in 1846 at Massachusetts General Hospital by Dr. John Warren with administration of ether anesthesia by Dr. William Thomas Green Morton for patient Edward Gilbert Abbot. (Accessed from https://www.google.com/search?q=the+ether+dome+surgery&source=lnms&tbm=isch&sa=X&ved=0ahUKEwjknNqWnKzUAhUCPiYKHfPhCaEQ_AUIBigB&biw=1280&bih=899#imgrc=_&spf=1496855210893, 20 Sept 2020)

6 Paradigm Shift in Surgical Management of Oral/Head and Neck Cancer

The published works of George Crile (Fig. 4) in 1905 (Crile 1905) and 1906 (Crile 1906) represented a paradigm shift in the surgical management of oral/head and neck cancer, specifically related to isolated local surgery. As part of the acknowledgment of treatment failures in patients treated in the late nineteenth century, Crile advocated that surgical management of oral/head and neck cancer ought to consist of removal of the primary cancer as well as all associated cervical lymph nodes, including those that were visibly enlarged and/or palpably enlarged (Fig. 5). He emphasized that palpable cervical lymph nodes may be inflammatory and impalpable lymph nodes may contain cancer. He stressed that excision of a primary focus only of cancer in the head and neck region without addressing the regional lymphatic system represented an incomplete dissection and would provoke the dissemination of growth of the cancer. Crile indicated that incomplete operations do more harm than good. He therefore developed a technique for neck dissection that resulted in minimal hemorrhage and infection while removing all lymph nodes in the ipsilateral neck of patients with N+ necks and a more conservative approach to neck

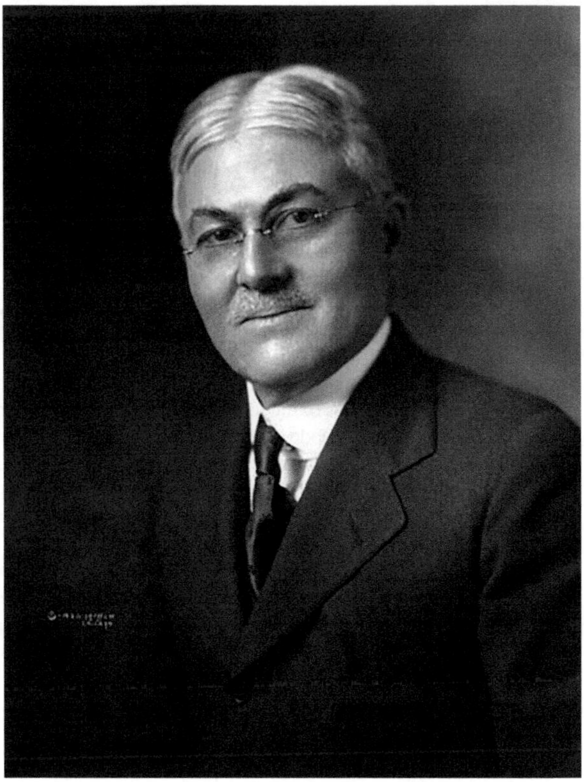

Fig. 4 Dr. George Crile (1864–1943). (Accessed from https://www.facs.org/about-acs/archives/pasthighlights/crilehighlight, 20 Sept 2020)

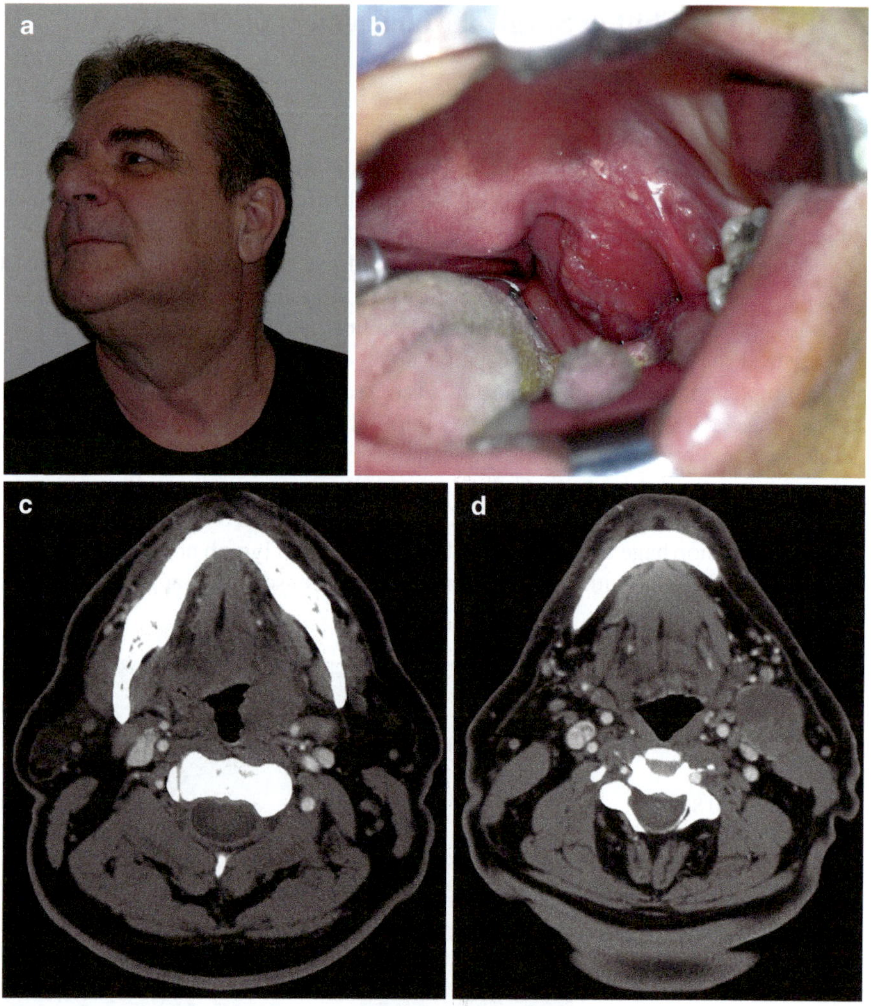

Fig. 5 A 60-year-old man presented with a 4-month history of a mass of the left neck (**a**). Physical examination revealed a mass of the left palatine tonsil (**b**). A diagnosis of squamous cell carcinoma of the left cervical lymph node was proposed based on fine needle aspiration biopsy. The CT images demonstrate the left tonsillar mass (**c**) and the enlarged and partially necrotic lymph node in level II of the left neck (**d**). The patient underwent left tonsillectomy (**e**) that identified squamous cell carcinoma on frozen sections. A left type I modified radical neck dissection was performed (**f**, **g**). Metastatic squamous cell carcinoma was identified in two of 62 lymph nodes in the left neck dissection specimen. The patient underwent postoperative radiation therapy and was without evidence of disease in the left neck (**h**) and tonsillar bed (**i**) at 6 years postoperatively. Patient consent obtained to publish his facial photographs without blocking out his eyes

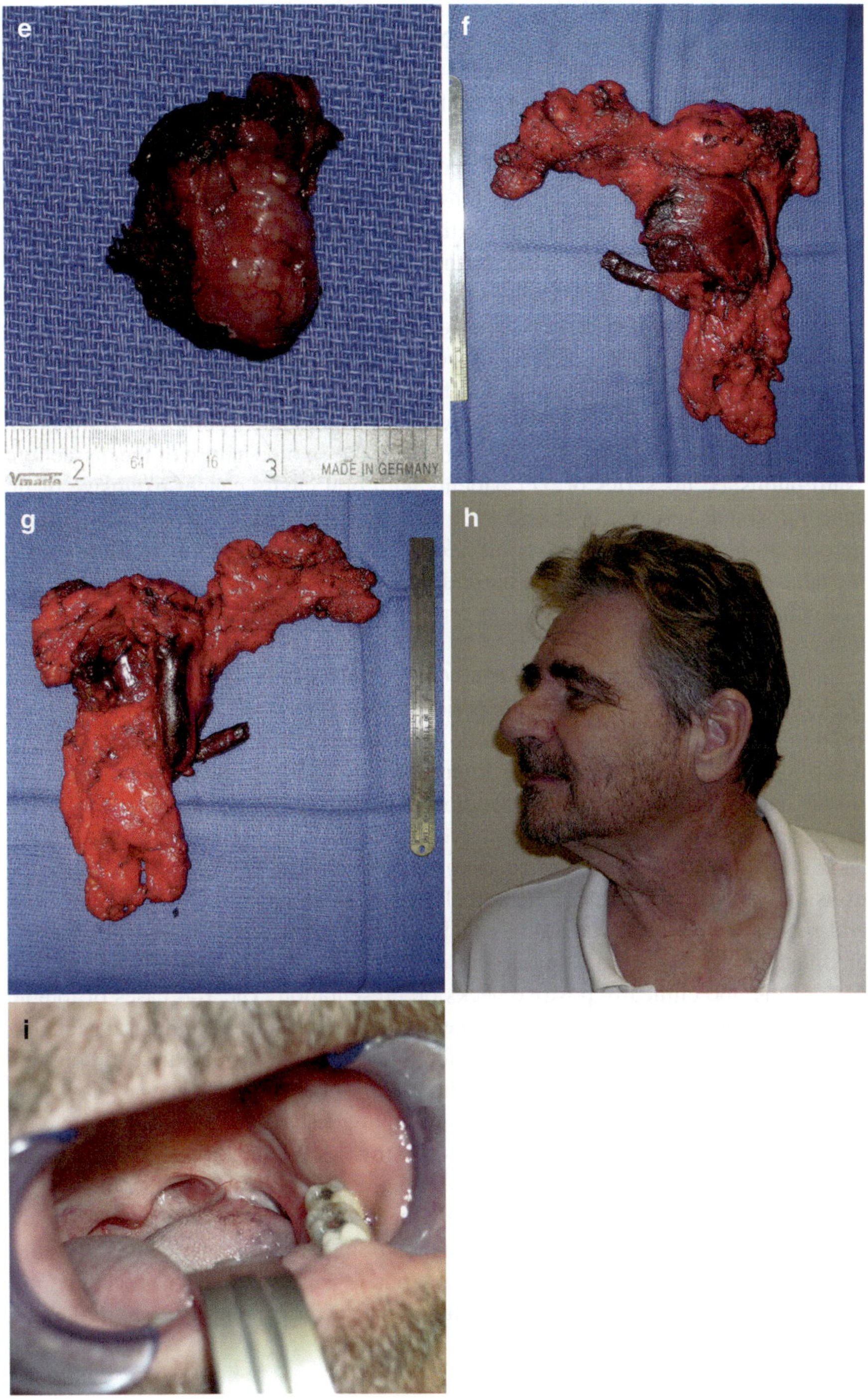

Fig. 5 (continued)

dissection in patients with N0 necks. Crile reported on 132 such operations, the last 63 of which were properly classified as N+ or N0. Thirty-one cases were identified as cancers of the lips, and 12 cases were reported in the tongue. With his technique, Dr. Crile decreed that since the regional lymphatics of the head and neck are accessible, applying the same comprehensive block dissection as utilized in breast cancer, the final outcomes in head and neck cancer should yield better results than cancer surgery of other anatomic regions of the body. Dr. Crile and his discussants emphasized the need to avoid handling the cancer during ablative surgery to reduce the dissemination of disease, a point further discussed in his 1923 paper (Crile 1923).

The terminology *composite operation* was first thoroughly discussed by Grant Ward in 1959 based on his first case performed in 1932 (Ward et al. 1959). Dr. Ward selected this term as it was felt to protect the humanity of the patient, rather than suggesting an assault on the patient or reflecting a dishonorable attitude by surgeons as might have been considered with the term, commando operation (Ward et al. 1959). In addition, this terminology exemplified the en bloc nature of the dissection. Ward published his series of 577 patients with oral cavity cancer exclusive of lip cancer operated between 1946 and 1958 including 453 patients treated by composite operation. He reported an overall 3.9% (18 cases) mortality in his series. This included one operative death with the enduring patients dying from any cause within 3 months of the operation. The 3-year survival rate was 51% and the 5-year survival rate was 35.5%.

In 1951, Hayes Martin (Fig. 6) et al. (1951) published a 59-page monograph on neck dissection that included his experience with 665 cases in 599 patients from 1928 to 1945. In this paper, radical neck dissection was defined as an en bloc resection of lymph nodes from inferior border of the mandible to clavicle along with the sternocleidomastoid muscle, submandibular gland, and internal jugular vein. No discussion of the spinal accessory nerve was offered by the authors. The radical neck dissection was distinguished from the partial neck dissection that involved excision of structures in the submandibular and supraomohyoid regions or the bilateral submental regions. The authors included outcomes from 144 tongue cancers, the most common anatomic site in the series, 127 cases of which corresponded to 25% of the 500 clinically positive necks on presentation. The 144 cases of tongue cancer were operated with 13 bilateral neck dissections and 131 unilateral neck dissections. It is noteworthy that Martin offered indications for neck dissection in this paper. Among them included definite clinical evidence that cancer was present in the cervical lymphatics, the primary lesion giving rise to the metastasis was controlled clinically either prior to or at the same time as the neck dissection, a reasonable chance existed of complete removal of the cervical metastases, the lack of clinical or radiographic evidence of distant metastases existed, and the neck dissection offered a greater chance of cure than radiation therapy. Remarkably, the author defined prophylactic neck dissection as a separate and independent procedure, not in conjunction with excision of the primary cancer, in patients for whom the primary cancer had already been surgically addressed.

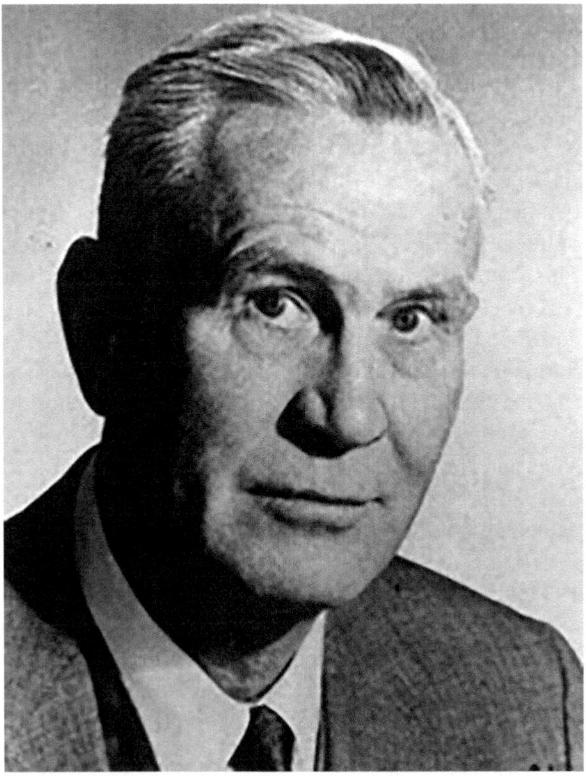

Fig. 6 Dr. Hayes Martin (1892–1977). (Accessed from https://www.ahns.info/about-ahns/past_presidents/martin/, 20 Sept 2020)

7 The Society of Head and Neck Surgeons

In 1954, Drs. Martin and Ward conceived the Society of Head and Neck Surgeons. Most of the society's membership was general surgeons or plastic surgeons, symbolic of the involvement of these surgeons in this subspecialty practice at that time. Many members had additional training in surgical oncology. In 1957, six otolaryngologists developed an organization composed primarily of otolaryngologists with an interest in head and neck surgery that became known as the American Society for Head and Neck Surgery in 1959. The first president was Dr. John Conley, and the society's mission was, in part, to encourage the training of otolaryngology residents in head and neck surgery. Specifically, it was this organization's goal to enable and advance knowledge relevant to surgical treatment of diseases of the head and neck, including reconstruction and rehabilitation; promote advancement of the highest professional and ethical standards as they pertain to the practice of major head and neck surgery; and to honor those who have made major contributions in the field of head and neck surgery or have aided in its advancement. In 1968, Dr. William

McComb, president of the Society of Head and Neck Surgeons, engaged a committee to investigate the educational training of head and neck surgeons. In December 1968, a similar committee appointed by the American Society for Head and Neck Surgery met in Pittsburgh. In October 1974, the Training Committee of the Society of Head and Neck Surgeons developed a course curriculum for fellowship training. In December 1975, a joint meeting of the Head and Neck Training Committee of the two head and neck societies was held in Chicago, and this combined training committee refined the course curriculum for training head and neck oncologic surgeons. This committee is contemporarily known as the Joint Council for Approval of Advanced Training in Head and Neck Oncologic Surgery. The course curriculum developed by this committee was approved by the Society of Head and Neck Surgeons in 1976 and by the American Society for Head and Neck Surgery in 1977 (Shah 1991). In 1998, the existence of two societies devoted to the same discipline was thought to be duplicative, such that the two societies merged into the American Head and Neck Society whose mission was to provide a unified voice to the advancement of research and education in head and neck oncology. This society remains dedicated to the common goals of its parent organizations. The International Federation of Head and Neck Oncologic Societies (IFHNOS) was established in 1987 with the purpose of creating channels of communication to enhance exchange of information, improve knowledge, and explore new directions in management of patients with head and neck cancer (Folz et al. 2008). Dr. Jatin Shah (Fig. 7) of Memorial Sloan Kettering Cancer Institute in New York conceived the idea of such

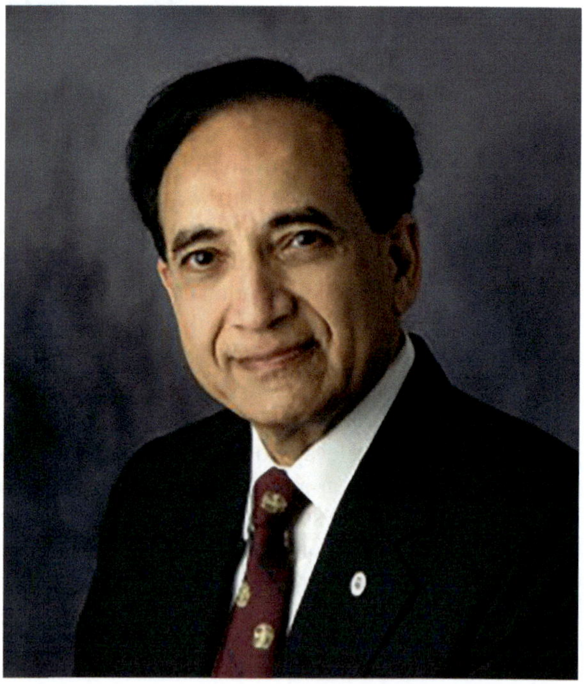

Fig. 7 Dr. Jatin Shah (1941). (Accessed from https://www.ahns.info/about-ahns/past_presidents/shah/, 6 Jun 2017)

an international body bringing together specialists involved in the care of patients with head and neck cancer worldwide. A steering committee was formed and met in London on May 1, 1987, with representation of 16 head and neck organizations from North America, South America, Europe, Africa, and Asia. The steering committee drafted the constitution and bylaws of the Federation that was subsequently ratified by the Governing Council, consisting of one member from each member organization in the Federation. The Federation has grown since its establishment, with a membership of 43 head and neck oncologic organizations, representing 65 countries. Quadrennial World congresses of the Federation have taken place since 1998. In recognition of his tremendous contributions to head and neck surgery, the IFHNOS has established the Jatin Shah lecture at its world congresses.

8 Disruptive Innovation: Enter Oral and Maxillofacial Surgery

The previous discussion serves to describe the organization of two societies in head and neck surgery and ultimately a single, unified society. While their specific educational objectives were unclear, including the existence of any accreditation standards, their voice was clearly heard. The Joint Council for Approval of Advanced Training in Head and Neck Oncologic Surgery was established in 1977 under the direction of Dr. John Lore, Jr. The Council was thereafter known as the Joint Training Council, and its objectives were to establish a program review process to create well-structured training programs with a specified didactic curriculum. The clinical influence of general surgeons and otolaryngologists in the management of patients with head and neck cancer was apparent. This notwithstanding, before and during this time, three oral and maxillofacial surgeons shared a career-long passion for oral cancer surgery, including Drs. Elmer Hume, Fred Henny, and Claude LaDow (Dierks 2002). These three individuals were passionately supportive of oral and maxillofacial surgery and trained future clinical and academic leaders of our specialty. Dr. Hume, who lived to the age of 98 years, was chairman of the Department of Oral Surgery at the Louisville College of Dentistry, later named the University of Louisville. He shared an office with his brother, a general surgeon, and later became chief of Maxillofacial Surgery at St. Joseph's Hospital in Louisville where he conducted an oral cancer clinic with his partner, Dr. James Skaggs. Dr. Hume frequently performed jaw resections, glossectomies, and orbital exenterations. Cases that involved a neck dissection were performed as a team effort with general surgery with Drs. Hume and Skaggs performing the ablative and reconstructive surgery of the primary cancer. Dr. Fred Henny became the chief of Oral Surgery at Henry Ford Hospital in 1952 and developed his institution as a referral center for the surgical management of oral cancer. During his 18-year administrative and clinical roles at Henry Ford Hospital, Dr. Henny became known for his educational and clinical prowess, training future leaders of our specialty, including Drs. Guy Catone,

Bruce Epker, William Grau, Bruce MacIntosh, and Ralph Merrill. Dr. LaDow served as chairman of the Department of Oral Surgery at the University of Pennsylvania from 1952 to 1974. He received formal training in head and neck surgery by Dr. John Gunter in Philadelphia and was involved in extensive head and neck surgical procedures under Dr. John Dorrance. Dr. LaDow served as chief of Oral Surgery at Episcopal Hospital in Philadelphia in the 1950s, and he also performed surgery at the American Oncologic Hospital of Philadelphia during that time. Dr. LaDow's comprehensive dedication to oncology was seen in his interest in placing radium needles and radon seeds into head and neck malignancies (LaDow 1984). He also placed carotid artery catheters through the superficial temporal artery for the intratumoral delivery of chemotherapy. The clinical presence of Drs. Hume, Henny, and LaDow established a reputable clinical base in oral/head and neck cancer surgery for the specialty of oral and maxillofacial surgery. Their strong leadership presence provided very favorable exposure of the specialty of oral and maxillofacial surgery in the management of patients with oral cancer. That notwithstanding, the 1960s ushered in changes in the practices of these surgeons due to the development and strategic vision of the two previously mentioned head and neck organizations that ultimately unified. In addition, the emphasis of oral and maxillofacial surgery changed during this time, in part due to the fascination that was developing in orthognathic surgery. Nonetheless, the establishment of oral/head and neck oncologic surgery fellowship programs by Dr. Robert Marx at the University of Miami in 1985 and by Dr. Eric Dierks at Legacy Emanuel Hospital in Portland, Oregon, in 1992 would lead to newfound enthusiasm for the development of subspecialty training in oral/head and neck oncologic and reconstructive surgery. Similar clinical and educational initiatives were established by Dr. Robert Ord at the University of Maryland in 1989 and Dr. Joseph Helman at the University of Michigan in 1994. Fellowships, once referred to as the third wave in oral and maxillofacial surgery, have been described as a contemporary mechanism that surgical specialties use to advance the art and science of their disciplines (Assael 2009a). They can be thought of as formal consolidation of clinical and educational tools to advance the art and science of a surgical discipline that became legitimized. The development of fellowships as the background of our subspecialty has been described as necessary to the future success of oral and maxillofacial surgery (Assael 2009a).

In 2001, Dr. Jesus Medina delivered his American Head and Neck Society Presidential address entitled "Tragic optimism vs learning on the verge of more change and great advances" (Medina 2001). As part of this address, Dr. Medina recognized the change that was inevitable in the practice of medicine, yet he emphasized the recent acceleration and greater change that was being observed at that time. Specifically, Medina mentioned the cost and reimbursement of head and neck surgical procedures, providing his forecast for medicine that the value for surgical services will be defined as the quality of surgical outcomes divided by their cost. In addition, Medina expressed concern for the decline in the number of applicants to head and neck fellowships, citing the number of general surgery residents considering head and neck surgery to be minimal. Shah (2005) further cited the insufficient job opportunities for head and neck surgeons and limited patient volumes accounting for the declining interest in these fellowship programs that would otherwise support a career in this discipline. In response to unfavorable pressures in the provision of head and neck surgical care to patients, Medina indicated that working harder to be successful in the subspecialty of head and neck surgery could lead to one or more preventable tragedies, including the bankruptcy of one's practice, the abandonment of head and neck oncologic surgery to practice more lucrative surgical procedures, or forfeiting one's role as a patient advocate. Lest the members of his specialty accept their call to action, tragic optimism might be the most applicable label of the ambivalence that might otherwise exist. The response of this published pessimism by the specialty of oral and maxillofacial surgery can only be called strategic opportunism (Carlson 2014) and what followed can only be referred to as a renaissance. Unambiguously, the clinical groundwork laid in oral/head and neck oncologic surgery by Drs. Hume, Henny, and LaDow, as well as the fellowship training programs of Drs. Marx and Dierks, was administratively supported by fellowship program accreditation and individual subspecialty certification that would follow. Collectively, every element of this surreptitiously calculated process is reminiscent of the business concept, disruptive innovation. Disruptive innovation describes a process where a previously considered inferior entity can challenge incumbent entities, specifically those controlling a market share of the industry under consideration. As stated by Christensen et al., as incumbent entities concentrate on improving their services for their most demanding customers, they exceed the requirements of some customers and ignore the needs of others (Christensen et al. 2009; Christensen et al. 2015). Entities that realize disruptive innovation initiate their process by addressing overlooked customers and their overlooked needs. The incumbents, chasing higher profitability in more demanding segments, tend to be slow or denying in their response, incorrectly believing that their momentum and stronghold on the market will forever be unencumbered. According to Christensen et al., disruptors then move upmarket, delivering the performance that the customers of incumbents require while also preserving the advantages that created their early success (Guralnick 1973).

9 Six-Year OMFS/MD Residency Programs and General Surgery Training

In 1973, Dr. Walter Guralnick (Fig. 8), then professor and chairman of the Department of Oral Surgery at the Harvard School of Dental Medicine and chief of Oral Surgery at Massachusetts General Hospital, published his philosophy and ethos regarding a transformation of the educational process in our specialty (Guralnick 1973). Dr. Guralnick pointed to the educational deficit that he recognized in our specialty's training programs, specifically that our residency programs consisted of insufficient medical and surgical training. In addition to high-quality oral surgical training, Dr. Guralnick believed that such deficits could be remedied

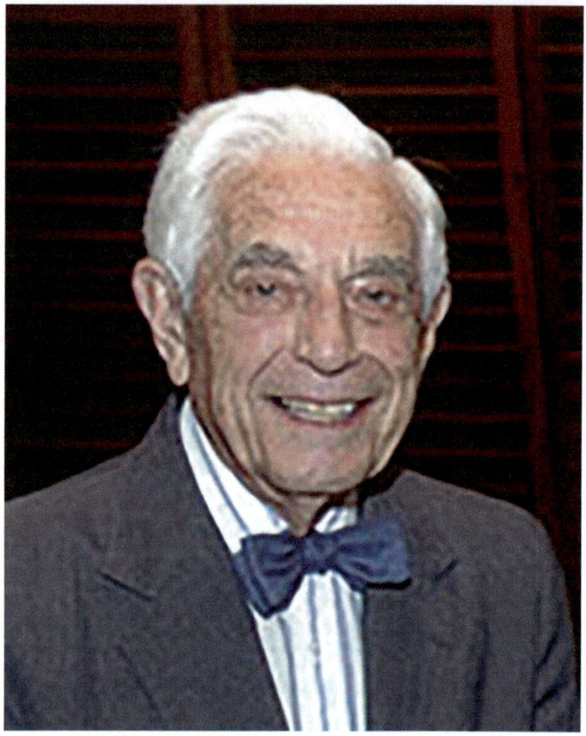

Fig. 8 Dr. Walter Guralnick (1917–2017). (Personal collection of ERC)

by residents obtaining a medical degree as well as general surgical training. He cited the sentiment of Dr. James Hayward at the time who indicated that two essential and complex requirements of oral surgery training in that era were to educate the educators of our specialty's needs while also gaining the respect of physician colleagues. Moreover, Guralnick considered the comments of General Robert Shira who indicated that while the medical degree would reduce administrative problems that were encountered by some members of our specialty in the 1970s, the added education would not improve the individual's surgical proficiency. Dr. Shira concluded that the addition of the MD, while imparting broad educational advantages, would not justify the added time and expense to obtain such education.

In his original paper, Dr. Guralnick disclosed the value-added nature of members of our specialty obtaining their medical degrees, specifically, their ability to also obtain general surgical training. He pointed to the renaissance in our specialty, as well as the leaders and innovators of this period who were oral surgeons who possessed general surgical training as well as oral surgery training. Guralnick elaborated that general surgery training would prepare the resident to care for the "whole patient." This educational process would permit the oral surgery resident to be able to perform equivalently to those in other surgical specialties, particularly regarding properly trained oral surgeons being able to manage the patient's care in the intensive care unit, perform a tracheotomy, remove a rib for reconstructive purposes, and ligate the external carotid artery. In the final analysis, three benefits would develop from such a dual degree training program. First, the expanded didactic and clinical curriculum would be beneficial to the overall education of the oral surgery resident. Second, oral surgery residents would be educationally qualified to serve as general surgery residents, thereby permitting the application of principles of medicine learned in medical school. Finally, graduates of the dual degree program would enter the mainstream of surgical specialists and narrow the political gap that fuels turf battles among competing surgical specialists. No mention was made of the benefits of the medical degree and general surgery training in permitting the resident to secure fellowship training in oral/head and neck oncologic and reconstructive surgery and to confidently care for compromised patients with neoplastic disease of this region.

With approval from the administrative board at the Harvard Medical School, the first student entered the program and graduated Harvard Medical School in 1972. In so doing, this first student's curriculum involved the first 3 years of the current dental curriculum of which the first 1.5 years were spent in the medical school completing the preclinical basic science curriculum with the medical students and the second 1.5 years involved the dental curriculum at the School of Dental Medicine. An oral surgery internship comprised the fourth year of the program followed by the principal clinical year at the medical school and its teaching hospitals. Thereafter, 6 months were spent as a resident in oral surgery and 6 months were spent as a general surgery intern. The seventh year of the program involved a general surgery year and the eighth year of the program involved an oral surgery year. In all, the 8-year program involved 2.5 years spent in medical school, 1.5 years were spent in dental school, 2.5 years were spent on the clinical oral surgery service, and 1.5 years were spent on the clinical general surgery service.

As should have been anticipated, the educational change implemented by the Harvard program was met with relative outcry, skepticism, and reported controversy within dentistry and oral surgery. In 1972, Dr. Morton Goldberg expressed his concerns with the new curriculum, indicating that our specialty was erroneously rushing onto an illusionary, exhausting, and self-destructive course in search of parity with other surgical specialties (Goldberg 1972). His letter to the editor generally represented a pessimistic discourse on the Harvard plan. This notwithstanding, Goldberg lamented that experimentation is necessary in science, even in the "science" of education. He concluded his letter to the editor by stating that the residency/MD programs represented a potential answer to our problems. Such programs, he stated, were short, inexpensive, educationally sound, and hopefully would be equally acceptable to organized oral surgery and the medical establishment. In retrospect, Dr. Goldberg indicated that his 1972 published statement was incorrect (personal communication, May 25, 2017). He now believes that double-degree education has not split our specialty. His experience and opinion with the general surgery year remains correct, per Dr. Goldberg. Greater than four decades later, he believes that the general surgery experience does not represent 1 year of retractor holding for carotid surgery, appendectomies, herniorrhaphies, etc., but a year of studying surgical metabolism, fluid-electrolyte balance, tissue healing, and general surgical principles. Thus, the general surgery experience provides caring for the whole patient, including their concerns, fears, and families, and that serious illness is a two-way street. Such general surgery experiences can properly prepare the resident for fellowship training in oral/head and neck oncologic and reconstructive surgery. As an example, lessons from the cancer ward include the essential nature of empathy and compassion in the management of sick patients, and these qualities ought to be reinforced during general surgical training and practiced during fellowship training (Assael 2008).

In 1972, Eisenbud presented an analysis of the potential impact of oral surgery-MD programs before the Section on Oral Surgery, Anesthesia, and Hospital Dental Service at the American Association of Dental Schools (Eisenbud 1973). From the perspective of turf battles, Eisenbud suggested that this new curriculum would create even greater conflict for the oral surgeon. He indicated that rather than expressing concern at the absence of the MD degree, the plastic surgeons would point to the absence of plastic surgery training and the head and neck surgeon to the absence of head and neck surgery training. He pointed out that such programs would produce a synthetic teratism: too good to extract teeth and not good enough to perform a radical neck dissection. Eisenbud was decades ahead of his time as future educational thought leaders in oral and maxillofacial surgery would create a solution to his perceived problem by creating fellowship programs in our subspecialty such that trainees *would* be good enough to perform a radical neck dissection.

In 2004, Dodson et al. (2004) provided a 30-year review of the Massachusetts General Hospital/Harvard Medical School Oral and Maxillofacial Surgery/MD Program. This retrospective cohort study assessed the outcomes of 56 graduates of the program from 1971 to 2000, specifically with regard to successful completion of the dual-degree program, performance on steps I and II of the US Medical Licensing Examination/National Board of Medical Examinations (USMLE/NBME), Harvard Medical School grades, and career trajectories such as full- or part-time academic practice or private practice. Of the 56 individuals who entered the combined program, all graduated from Harvard Medical School. Four individuals did not complete the OMFS portion of the combined program and chose non-OMFS career paths. Three graduates of the combined program completed additional specialty training, one in plastic surgery and two in otolaryngology. One of the 56 graduates of the program in this cohort entered fellowship training in oral/head and neck oncologic and reconstructive surgery, and two additional residents completed such fellowship training thereafter.

The introduction of formal medical school in oral and maxillofacial surgery training that leads to general surgery training is arguably one of the greatest controversies in the history of our exemplary specialty. No doubt, many of the pioneers of our specialty were singularly qualified, and their hard work and exceptional outcomes created an international level of respect and admiration for all members of our specialty. In addition, the technical expertise of members of our specialty was clearly derived from oral and maxillofacial surgery training rather than formal medical training. This notwithstanding, the Guralnick plan supports the training of those members of our specialty wishing to practice oral/head and neck tumor and reconstructive surgery at its highest level, the ability to do so resulting in part from their obtaining general surgery training. There are two obvious reasons that support this statement. First, as stated by Dr. Goldberg in 1972, he had never been questioned as to why his oral surgery colleagues did not possess an MD, but he was frequently asked why oral and maxillofacial surgery was the only surgical specialty where residents were not given a basic year of general surgery training. Fast forwarding to the twenty-first century, it is clear anecdotally and experientially proved that the general surgery year is invaluable in terms of being able to effectively and confidently assume daily care for sick patients for whom fellowship trained oral/head and neck oncologic and reconstructive surgeons are responsible. Second, medical school training followed by general surgery training overcomes a relatively deficient, abbreviated, and impractical medical curriculum in dental school. The dental graduate who enters a high-quality, accredited, and full-scope oral and maxillofacial surgery residency program will be afforded a valuable clinical education. Such a resident will undoubtedly benefit from the off-service experience on internal medicine, general surgery, and elective medical rotations. That said, there is no substitute for the full medical education that is afforded to residents in 6-year oral and maxillofacial surgery residency programs where full integration in comprehensive medical curricula occurs, leading to the MD degree, followed by a 1-year experience in general surgery. While this statement remains controversial after decades of recorded discussion and healthy debate, the value of the MD curriculum and general surgery training is undoubtedly meaningful and relevant to the individual wishing to practice our subspecialty at the highest level.

10 Accreditation by the Commission on Dental Accreditation

The Commission on Dental Accreditation (CODA) was established in 1975 and remains recognized by the US Department of Education. From 1938 to 1974 the Council on Dental Education of the American Dental Association was the accrediting organization for dental and dental-related education programs. In 1972, the Council recognized the need to provide the communities of interest with greater representation in accreditation policy issues and decisions such that CODA was ultimately established. Prior to formal accreditation of oral/head and neck oncologic and reconstructive surgery fellowship programs, the American Association of Oral and Maxillofacial Surgeons (AAOMS) conducted site visits of existing fellowship programs for recognition of the educational quality of these programs beginning in 1996. This fellowship recognition process occurred due to the realization of the lack of accrediting body status by the AAOMS. This led to the AAOMS approaching CODA, an approved accrediting body by the US Department of Education, concerning their willingness to assume responsibility for accrediting fellowship programs in oral and maxillofacial surgery. There was initial concurrence, in principle, that the Commission should assume such responsibility. The Commission first adopted proposed Accreditation Standards for Clinical Fellowship Training in Oral and Maxillofacial Surgery in January 1997 that included oral/head and neck oncologic and reconstructive surgery fellowships. At that time, the implementation date was planned for January 1999. After having circulated among the communities of interest for comment beginning in 1997, the Commission finally adopted and implemented the Accreditation Standards for Clinical Fellowship Training Programs in Oral and Maxillofacial Surgery on January 1, 2000.

Fellowship accreditation represents a voluntary process that ensures fellows, specialty boards, and the public that the training program follows published standards. Annual programmatic data from fellowship program directors and site visitor reports provides CODA the opportunity to establish accreditation actions. The Oral and Maxillofacial Surgery Review Committee, comprised of the Oral and Maxillofacial Surgery Commissioner as well as educators within our specialty appointed by the AAOMS and the ABOMS, provides administrative oversight of the accreditation process with the Commissioner reporting to the Commission the accreditation recommendations of the review committee. The Commission has the ultimate decision regarding a fellowship program's accreditation status. The Commission's primary objective in the accreditation of oral/head and neck oncologic and reconstructive surgery fellowship programs is to ensure that comprehensive clinical and didactic training is provided to fellows that will enable these individuals to serve as primary oral/head and neck oncologic and reconstructive surgeons in a cancer team following training.

In 2020, 14 institutions (Table 1) conduct fellowship programs in oral/head and neck oncologic and reconstructive surgery. Nine of these fellowships exist within academic oral and maxillofacial surgery departments that directly sponsor accredited residency programs. These fellowship programs are 12–24 months in length and offer fellows a comprehensive training in the management of oral and oropharyngeal tumors and microvascular surgery (Kademani et al. 2016). These programs originally participated in the maxillofacial oncology and reconstructive surgery match service (MORS match, https://www.MORSmatch.com) established in 2013. Effective in 2019, the fellowship match occurs in the American Academy of Craniomaxillofacial Surgeons (www.aacmfsmatch.org). The demand for oral/head and neck oncologic and reconstructive surgery fellowship programs remains robust as the number of applicants to these fellowship programs exceeds the number of available positions such that several candidates in the match process each year are not successful in securing a fellowship position (Table 2).

The recruitment of oral and maxillofacial surgeons into oral/head and neck oncologic and reconstructive surgery fellowships is intuitive. Such trainees are comfortable with bone plating; the management of soft tissues in the oral cavity, face, and neck; and the resection of the bone (Assael 2008). Moreover, these fellows possess proficiency in the principles of occlusion, arch form of the jaws, and orofacial function that lends to a unique understanding of orofacial reconstruction. Such fellows assume care for a patient with a benign or malignant tumor of the oral/head and neck region, provide effective resection with surgical management of cervical metastases, reconstruct the defect with a variety of flaps, and place implants in bone grafts, thereby providing comprehensive care for these patients whose ability to be functionally reconstructed is greatly enhanced (Hupp 2011).

Table 1 Oral/head and neck oncologic surgery fellowship programs in the United States in 2020

Program	Program director in 2020	Location	Date established	Date of most recent accreditation
John Peter Smith Hospital	Fayette Williams, DDS, MD	Ft. Worth, Texas	2014	
Louisiana State University	David Kim, DMD, MD	Shreveport, Louisiana	2006	2015
Minnesota Head and Neck Surgery	Deepak Kademani, DMD, MD	Minneapolis, Minnesota	2020	
North Memorial Hospital and Humbert Humphrey Cancer Center	Ketan Patel, DDS, PhD	Minneapolis, Minnesota	2012	2017
University of Alabama	Anthony Morlandt, DDS, MD	Birmingham, Alabama	2016	
University of Florida College of Medicine	Rui Fernandes, DMD, MD	Jacksonville, Florida	2008	2015
University of Maryland	Joshua Lubek, DDS, MD	Baltimore, Maryland	1989	2018
University of Miami	Ramzey Tursun, DDS	Miami, Florida	1985	
University of Michigan	Brent Ward, DDS, MD	Ann Arbor, Michigan	1994	2018
University of Tennessee	Eric Carlson, DMD, MD, EdM	Knoxville, Tennessee	2009	2017
University of California	Brian Woo, DDS, MD	Fresno, California	2018	
University of Texas Health Science Center	Jonathan Shum, DDS, MD	Houston, Texas	2016	
Boston University	Andrew Salama, DMD, MD	Boston, Massachusetts	2011	2025
Providence Portland Medical Center	R. Bryan Bell, DDS, MD	Portland, Oregon	2019	2020

11 The American Association of Oral and Maxillofacial Surgeons

In 2008, then American Association of Oral and Maxillofacial Surgeons president, Dr. W. Mark Tucker, established the Oral Cancer Task Force to assist in our specialty's management of patients with oral cancer. Under the leadership of Dr. Paul Lambert, the task force was charged with improving oral cancer care in the United States with three primary objectives: (1) to provide educational recommendations to

Table 2 The number of oncologic surgery fellowship programs and the number of applicants to these programs

Year	Number of institutions participating in the match (number of available positions)	Number of candidates submitting rank lists for the match
2013	7	8
2014	8	14
2015	7	13
2016	7	15
2017	7	17
2018	6	14
2019	10	18
2020	10	16

The competitive nature of these programs is noted with the number of applicants exceeding the number of available positions each year. Unmatched applicants have been realized due to the competitive nature of this process

the AAOMS Board of Trustees, (2) to realize the development of additional fellowship programs, and (3) to identify and support strategic areas of clinical and basic science research in oral cancer (Kademani et al. 2008). Such research findings were encouraged to be submitted to the *Journal of Oral and Maxillofacial Surgery*, *Oral Oncology*, and *Head and Neck* for consideration of publication. In June 2007 the Board of Trustees of AAOMS made the following recommendations and amendments to their strategic plan 2005–2008 by the third quarter of 2008, including the creation and dissemination of an oral cancer evaluation and treatment module for the National Curriculum Database; the development of educational material to enhance the skills of oral and maxillofacial surgeons in the detection and proper diagnosis of oral cancer; the development of educational materials for general dentists, dental hygienists, and primary medical providers to heighten the detection of oral cancer at an early stage; and the promotion of oral cancer screening, especially among high-risk populations. The Board also accepted the recommendation that the Oral Cancer Task Force be constituted as a special committee of the AAOMS to develop a plan with strategic implementation to improve the outcomes of patients with oral cancer. Further, the Board approved the recommendation to develop strategies on an oncology subsection for future AAOMS Research Summits in conjunction with the Advisory Committee on Research Planning and Technology Assessment. Finally, the Board approved the recommendation that the AAOMS provide support for the International Academy of Oral Oncology by encouraging AAOMS members and fellows to attend International Academy of Oral Oncology meetings, present educational programs, and submit manuscripts to their journal, *Oral Oncology*.

In 2012, Clark et al. (2012) conducted and distributed a survey to determine the prevalence and trends of the US oral and maxillofacial surgery residency programs in the arena of oral/head and neck oncologic surgery. Eighteen close-ended questions and one open-ended question comprised the survey that was distributed to 101 accredited oral and maxillofacial surgery residency programs. The questionnaire was grouped into the incidence of head and neck oncologic surgery-trained faculty and recruitment-related questions, caseload related questions, program-specific related questions, and academic productivity-related questions. Sixty-three of the 101 surveys (62.3%) were completed and returned. Ten program directors or chairs were noted to be fellowship trained in head and neck oncologic surgery. Programs with a fellowship-trained program director or chair were more likely to have another fellowship-trained faculty member and performed more malignant tumor resections, neck dissections, and microvascular free flap reconstructions than residency programs without program directors or chairs trained in head and neck oncologic surgery. Programs that regularly engaged in tumor board discussions performed more malignant tumor resections and neck dissections than programs that did not regularly attend their institution's tumor board meetings. Programs that presented oncologic surgery-related research at national meetings performed more malignant tumor resections and neck dissections than programs that did not present such research at national meetings. Programs that presented oncologic surgery research at national meetings were more likely to realize their residents entering fellowship training in this discipline than programs that did not present oncologic surgery research at these meetings. Finally, there was no difference in the prevalence of head and neck oncologic surgery-trained program directors and chairs between 6-year integrated and 4-year programs, and there was no difference in the number of malignant tumor resections or number of neck dissections performed between the 6-year integrated and 4-year programs studied in this report.

In 2016, the AAOMS Special Committee on Maxillofacial Oncology and Reconstructive Surgery published their survey results related to fellowship program graduates in our subspecialty (Kademani et al. 2016). The survey was sent to 64 oral and maxillofacial surgeons who completed their fellowship from 2000 to 2014. Thirty-four (53%) graduates responded, eight of whom completed the University of Maryland program; five trained each at Legacy Emanuel Hospital and the University of Tennessee; four trained at the University of Michigan; three trained each at the University of Florida, the University of California-San Francisco, Louisiana State University-Shreveport, and the University of Miami; and one trained at North Memorial Hospital. When asked how many patients they treated each year, nine respondents indicated greater than 100 and greater than 50% of the respondents indicated that they treated greater than 50 patients per year. Eighty-two percent of graduates were in academic positions, training fellows, and/or residents.

In 2019, the AAOMS established the standing Committee on Oral, Head and Neck Oncologic and Reconstructive Surgery (COHNORS), thereby replacing the MORS special committee. Of importance to the AAOMS was two issues including the conversion from a special committee to a standing committee in recognition of the importance of the committee's work to the specialty and subspecialty. In addition, the name change occurred to better align with its purpose and duties while also being consistent with the title of CODA-accredited fellowships and the American Board of Oral and Maxillofacial Surgery (ABOMS) Certificate of Added

Qualification (CAQ) examination, a discussion of which follows. The AAOMS Board approved the name change in March 2019 through a bylaw change in the AAOMS House of Delegates. In 2020, this committee is represented by board liaison, Dr. Mark Egbert; committee chair, Dr. Deepak Kademani; and committee members, Dr. Eric Carlson, Dr. Brent Ward, Dr. Mohammed Qaisi, Dr. Steve Schimmele, and Dr. Brian Woo. Dr. Paul Lambert serves as a consultant to the COHNORS, and AAOMS staff liaisons include Mary Allaire-Schnitzer and Jennifer Scofield.

12 Certification by the American Board of Oral and Maxillofacial Surgery

The American Board of Oral and Maxillofacial Surgery is approved and recognized by the Council on Dental Education of the American Dental Association and exists as the certifying board for the specialty of oral and maxillofacial surgery in the United States. In 1945, a committee congregated at the annual meeting of the American Society of Oral Surgeons to establish the American Board of Oral Surgery. In 1946, the American Board of Oral Surgery was incorporated under the laws of the State of Illinois. The Board was approved by the Council on Dental Education of the American Dental Association in 1947 with authorization to initiate the certification of specialists in our specialty. The Board was renamed the American Board of Oral and Maxillofacial Surgery in 1978 to reflect the scope of the specialty. The essence of the American Board of Oral and Maxillofacial Surgery is currently overseen by an eight-member Board of Directors including four directors, the secretary-treasurer, the vice-president, the president, and the past-president. Each member of the Board of Directors is board certified by the American Board of Oral and Maxillofacial Surgery and is a fellow of the American Association of Oral and Maxillofacial Surgeons. A new director is elected each year to an 8-year term by the House of Delegates of the American Association of Oral and Maxillofacial Surgeons. The Board of Directors appoint an examination committee that serves the purpose of administering the annual certification examination process.

Certifying boards in health-related professions exist to establish minimum standards of competency related to knowledge, experience, and training that result in the ability to effectively and safely provide care to patients (Hupp 2015). Board certification in medicine and dentistry was originally developed around recognized specialties that arose from clinical specialty training beyond medical and dental education. The certifying boards are designed to develop an examination process that reflects residency training within a specific discipline. In so doing, specialty education must be standardized for those future candidates of the board certification process. As this educational standardization is not always possible, board certification candidates will often participate in board review courses, and program directors will typically look for ways that their residents will receive clinical and didactic education in areas tested by the certifying board. In the final analysis, the awareness of a doctor's board certification status is beneficial to patients requiring healthcare services, hospitals, liability insurance companies, and third-party payers. The advent of subspecialty education in medicine and dentistry has been driven by the increasing complexity of patient diagnoses, as well as that of healthcare services, the burgeoning of biomedical technology, and the need to limit the length of residency education (Dodson et al. 2004).

13 Certificate of Added Qualification in Head and Neck Oncologic and Reconstructive Surgery

In 2014, the American Board of Oral and Maxillofacial Surgery initiated the process of establishing a certificate of added qualification (CAQ) in head and neck oncologic and reconstructive surgery. The CAQ is designed for oral and maxillofacial surgeons certified by the ABOMS who have established bona fide qualifications and experience in this subspecialty and who conduct a clinical practice committed to and focused on this subspecialty within oral and maxillofacial surgery. Possessing the CAQ does not endow special privileges related to the practice of head and neck oncologic and reconstructive surgery, does not bestow upon the certificate holder comprehensive qualification for surgical privileges, and does not imply the exclusion of other practitioners of either oral and maxillofacial surgery or other disciplines who do not hold this certification. Rather, the certificate of added qualification has been developed to inform the public and healthcare professionals that the oral and maxillofacial surgeon who possesses the certificate has completed subspecialty education, has completed a certification examination process, and is qualified to practice this subspecialty of oral and maxillofacial surgery. To be inclusive, the CAQ observes primary eligibility pathway criteria and alternate eligibility pathway criteria. Both pathways require that the candidate must hold full, active, unrestricted hospital staff privileges to provide head and neck oncologic and reconstructive surgery services, must submit a surgical case log, must be a diplomate in good standing of the American Board of Oral and Maxillofacial Surgery, and must successfully complete the CAQ 100-question examination. The results of the first three CAQ examinations is noted in Table 3. This examination will continue to be administered biennially going forward.

Table 3 Results of the certificate of added qualification examination in oral/head and neck oncologic and reconstructive surgery of the American Board of Oral and Maxillofacial Surgery

Year of CAQ	Number of candidates (primary pathway/alternate pathway)	Number of passing candidates
2016	17 (13 primary/4 alternate)	16
2018	5 (5 primary)	5
2020	9 (6 primary/3 alternate)	8

14 Section of Surgical Oncology and Reconstruction of the Journal of Oral and Maxillofacial Surgery

In 2011, newly appointed *Journal of Oral and Maxillofacial Surgery* editor-in-chief Dr. Jim Hupp reformatted the structure of the journal into multiple discipline-specific sections. One section is devoted to surgical oncology and reconstruction, exemplifying the prominence of our subspecialty of oral/head and neck oncologic and reconstructive surgery. In 2016, 1691 papers were submitted to the *Journal of Oral and Maxillofacial Surgery* including 247 papers being submitted to the surgical oncology and reconstruction section of the journal. A disposition for 198 of these papers was completed during 2017 including 120 papers devoted to surgical oncology and 78 papers devoted to reconstruction. The diversity of these publications is representative of the clinical scope of practice of our fellowship training programs and that of the individuals practicing our subspecialty in oral and maxillofacial surgery. The organization of the scholarly activity of our professional colleagues in surgical oncology and reconstruction in this section of the *Journal of Oral and Maxillofacial Surgery* provides formal consolidation of this scholarly effort.

15 The Provision of Microsurgical Reconstructive Surgery

Oral and maxillofacial surgery training has historically emphasized functional bone graft reconstructive surgery for patients with post-ablative and post-traumatic defects of the jaws. This commitment to this clinical service persists in the twenty-first century. In fact, oral and maxillofacial surgeons have emphatically recognized that reconstruction does not merely refer to an exercise where a hole is filled with tissue (Assael 2009b). Rather, our appreciation for orofacial form and function has translated to truly functional reconstructions of the head and neck region. With the introduction of predictable forms of soft and hard tissue free microvascular reconstruction of the head and neck, as well as an increased number of microvascular surgery trained members in our subspecialty, microvascular reconstructive surgery has become a common element of the armamentarium of oral/head and neck oncologic and reconstructive surgeons in oral and maxillofacial surgery. In addition to the well-accepted clinical advantages of immediate microvascular head and neck reconstruction, overall success rates exceeding 95% justify the application of these techniques to patients with oral/head and neck cancer (Fatahi and Fernandes 2013).

16 Future Opportunities and Directions

The development of the subspecialty of oral/head and neck oncologic and reconstructive surgery is now steeped in tradition with effective branding in oral and maxillofacial surgery. Our subspecialty is supported by excellence in clinical training, accreditation, certification, and overarching recognition by our parent surgical association. Our international prominence is well recognized and relevant. Our future, therefore, is unquestionably promising. While our primary challenge and opportunity for growth might seem to merely maintain what we have created and currently enjoy, improvement of the education of our trainees seems to be fertile ground. Engagement in the educational process by fellowship program directors, faculty, and fellows will enhance the ability for growth within our subspecialty. The millennial trainees, clearly gifted in terms of their ability to learn, nonetheless represent a challenge for seasoned faculty in our subspecialty to effectively engage in the educational process. It has been said that millennials will work to live, not live to work, as is the case with the baby boomer generation (Assael 2006). In addition, the existence of substantial educational debt might interfere with additional education following the completion of residency training. This notwithstanding, the millennials are particularly able to succeed (Assael 2005). They believe that integrity and honesty are the most important personality traits. As such, fellowship educators must seize the moment to properly and effectively educate this new generation of trainees.

Objective improvement in educational leadership (Carlson 2019; Carlson and McGowan 2019; Carlson and Tannyhill 2019a; Carlson and Tannyhill 2019b; Carlson and Tannyhill 2019c; Carlson and Tannyhill 2020) and outcomes by fellowship faculty and the introduction of innovation and emerging technologies by fellowship program directors and faculty will undoubtedly boost the fellowship educational process. Such enhancement will improve the graduates of our fellowship programs, likely rendering improved patient outcomes and safety. In addition, the diversity and increased availability of clinical trials and personalized medicine for thought-provoking and recurrent cancer cases will be value-added to patient care. Finally, the reassessment and broadening of the educational process with research opportunities in immuno-oncology and immunotherapy (Sim et al. 2019) is likely to pay great dividends in the realization of future growth and increased international prominence of our subspecialty of oral/head and neck oncologic and reconstructive surgery.

References

Assael LA. Distance traveled: the millennial generation enters oral and maxillofacial surgery. J Oral Maxillofac Surg. 2005;63:161–2.

Assael LA. A boomer specialty awaits a generational tsunami. J Oral Maxillofac Surg. 2006;64:1001–2.

Assael LA. Lessons from the cancer ward. J Oral Maxillofac Surg. 2008;66:1327–8.

Assael L. Fellowships: the third wave. J Oral Maxillofac Surg. 2009a;67:1159–60.

Assael LA. Mandibular reconstruction: expert opinion and outcome studies remain a fragile guide to treatment. J Oral Maxillofac Surg. 2009b;67:2557–8.

Burket LW. Undiagnosed primary carcinoma of the gingiva with widespread metastasis: report of case. J Oral Surg. 1943;1:309–16.

Carlson ER. Cancer in United States presidents. J Oral Maxillofac Surg. 2002;60:190–3.
Carlson ER. Strategic opportunism. J Oral Maxillofac Surg. 2014;72:1874–5.
Carlson ER. Oral/head and neck oncologic and reconstructive surgery: the creation of a subspecialty in oral and maxillofacial surgery. J Oral Maxillofac Surg. 2018;76:237–47.
Carlson ER. A foundational framework for andragogy in oral and maxillofacial surgery V: moving forward. J Oral Maxillofac Surg. 2019;77:1739–40.
Carlson ER, McGowan E. A foundational framework for andragogy in oral and maxillofacial surgery I: general considerations. J Oral Maxillofac Surg. 2019;77:891–3.
Carlson ER, Tannyhill RJ. A foundational framework for andragogy in oral and maxillofacial surgery II: interactive andragogies. J Oral Maxillofac Surg. 2019a;77:1101–2.
Carlson ER, Tannyhill RJ. A foundational framework for andragogy in oral and maxillofacial surgery III: emotional intelligence. J Oral Maxillofac Surg. 2019b;77:1324–6.
Carlson ER, Tannyhill RJ. A foundational framework for andragogy in oral and maxillofacial surgery IV: co-regulated learning. J Oral Maxillofac Surg. 2019c;77:1529–31.
Carlson ER, Tannyhill RJ. The growth mindset: a contextualization of faculty development. J Oral Maxillofac Surg. 2020;78:7–9.
Christensen CM, Grossman JH, Hwang J. The innovator's prescription. A disruptive solution for health care. New York: McGraw Hill; 2009. p. 1–36.
Christensen CM, Raynor M, McDonald R. What is disruptive innovation? Harv Bus Rev. 2015;
Clark PK, Markiewicz MR, Bell RB, Dierks EJ. Trends and attitudes regarding head and neck oncologic surgery: a survey of United States oral and maxillofacial surgery programs. J Oral Maxillofac Surg. 2012;70:717–29.
Crile GW. On the surgical treatment of cancer of the head and neck. With a summary of one hundred and twenty-one operations performed upon one hundred and five patients. Trans South Surg Gynecol Assoc. 1905;18:108–27.
Crile GW. Excision of cancer of the head and neck with special reference to the plan of dissection based on 132 operations. JAMA. 1906;47:1780–6.
Crile GW. Carcinoma of the jaws, tongue, cheek, and lips. General principles involved in operations and results obtained at Cleveland Clinic. Surg Gynecol Obstetr. 1923;36:159–62.
Dierks EJ. Surgeons of oral cancer and leaders of a young specialty: the role of 3 oral and maxillofacial surgeons. J Oral Maxillofac Surg. 2002;60:86–92.
Dodson TB, Guralnick WC, Donoff RB, Kaban LB. Massachusetts General Hospital/Harvard medical school MD oral and maxillofacial surgery program: a 30-year review. J Oral Maxillofac Surg. 2004;62:62–5.
Eisenbud L. An analysis of the potential impact of oral surgery-MD programs. J Oral Surg. 1973;31:277–82.
Fatahi T, Fernandes R. Value of microvascular surgery in academic oral and maxillofacial surgery. J Oral Maxillofac Surg. 2013;71:189–91.
Folz BJ, Silver CE, Rinaldo A, et al. An outline of the history of head and neck oncology. Oral Oncol. 2008;44:2–9.
Gal AA. The centennial anniversary of the frozen section technique at the Mayo Clinic. Arch Pathol Lab Med. 2005;129:1532–5.
Goldberg MH. J Oral Surg. 1972;30:157.
Goldstein JC, Sisson GA. The history of head and neck surgery. Otolaryngol Head Neck Surg. 1996;115:379–85.
Gunter JH, Novak AJ, Churchill HR. Carcinoma of the indifferent cell type involving the maxillae: report of case. J Oral Surg. 1943;1:360–5.
Guralnick WC. The combined oral surgery-MD program: the Harvard plan. J Oral Surg. 1973;31:271–6.
Henny FA. Mixed tumor of the palate presenting itself as a cyst: report of case. J Oral Surg. 1943;1:267–8.
Hupp JR. Maxillofacial surgical oncology and oral-maxillofacial surgery: a perfect fit. J Oral Maxillofac Surg. 2011;69:2941–3.

Hupp JR. Certification of head and neck oncologic surgeons – a new day. J Oral Maxillofac Surg. 2015;73:199–201.

Kademani D, Bell RB, Schmidt BL, et al. Oral and maxillofacial surgeons treating oral cancer: a preliminary report from the American Association of Oral and Maxillofacial Surgeons Task Force on Oral Cancer. J Oral Maxillofac Surg. 2008;66:2151–7.

Kademani D, Woo B, Ward B, et al. Oral/head and neck oncologic and reconstructive surgery fellowship training programs: transformation of the specialty from 2005 to 2015: report from the AAOMS Committee on Maxillofacial Oncology and Reconstructive Surgery. J Oral Maxillofac Surg. 2016;74:2123–7.

LaDow CS. Surgical aspects of oral tumors. In: Kruger GO, editor. Textbook of Oral and maxillofacial surgery. 6th ed. St. Louis: CV Mosby Co; 1984. p. 644–71.

Loeb MJ. Adenocarcinoma originating from aberrant tissue in the gingiva: report of case. J Oral Surg. 1943;1:347–51.

Martin H, Del Valle B, Ehrlich H, Cahan WG. Neck dissection. Cancer. 1951;4:441–99.

Medina JE. Tragic optimism vs. learning on the verge of more change and great advances. Presidential address, American Head and Neck Society. Arch Otolaryngol Head Neck Surg. 2001;127:749–55.

Penhale KW. Primary lymphosarcoma of the mandible. J Oral Surg. 1943;1:84–8.

Schweitzer FC, Barnfield WF. Ameloblastoma of the mandible with metastasis to the lungs: report of a case. J Oral Surg. 1943;1:287–95.

Shah JP. The making of a head and neck surgeon. Am J Surg. 1991;162:284–7.

Shah JP. Head and neck surgery in crisis. Preparing for the future. Arch Otolaryngol Head Neck Surg. 2005;131:556–60.

Sim F, Leidner R, Bell RB. Immunotherapy for head and neck cancer. Oral Maxillofacial Surg Clin N Am. 2019;31:85–100.

Ward GE, Edgerton MT, Chambers RG, McKee DM. Cancer of the oral cavity and pharynx and results of treatment by means of the composite operation (in continuity with radical neck dissection). Ann Surg. 1959;150:202–20.

Wolfe WC, Hubinger HL. Mixed tumor of the palate: report of case. J Oral Surg. 1943;1:256–8.

Surgical Flaps

Steven Halepas and Scott H. Troob

1 Introduction

Several factors have driven the evolution of tissue reconstruction, most significantly trauma from war, knowledge of anatomy, and technological advancements. Before discussing the history of tissue transfer, it is important to define terms to better understand how the field developed. Flaps are classified by blood supply, location, tissue content, and method of transfer. The flaps can be either random, axial, pedicled, or free. Random flaps are supplied by the dermal and subdermal plexus. Axial pattern flaps are supplied by a dominant vessel that is oriented along the axis of the flap. Pedicle flaps are tissues supplied by a named artery. Free tissues are harvested from a remote anatomic region, and the vascular connection is recreated at the defect site.

Tissue reconstruction can also be classified according to the relationship between the donor and recipient sites. Local flaps use adjacent tissues, regional flaps are located near the defect but not immediately adjacent, and distant flaps are harvested from different parts of the body. Flaps in the chapter will also be described based on the tissue contents. As examples, cutaneous contain skin, myocutaneous contain skin and muscle, fasciocutaneous contain skin and fascia, and osteocutaneous contain skin and bone. Finally, the method of tissue transfer is used in naming the type of flap. The methods of transfer include advancements, rotation, transposition, and interpolated. Advancement flaps are mobilized along a linear axis toward the defect.

S. Halepas
Division of Oral and Maxillofacial Surgery, NewYork-Presbyterian/Columbia University Irving Medical Center, New York, NY, USA

S. H. Troob (✉)
Department of Otolaryngology-Head & Neck Surgery, NewYork-Presbyterian/Columbia University Irving Medical Center, New York, NY, USA
e-mail: sht22@cumc.columbia.edu

E. M. Ferneini et al. (eds.), *The History of Maxillofacial Surgery*,
https://doi.org/10.1007/978-3-030-89563-1_16

Rotational flaps pivot around a point at the base. Transpositional flaps are when donor tissue is incised and lifted over an incomplete bridge of skin and placed into the defect, an example of which is a rhomboid flap. Interpolated flaps are mobilized either over or beneath a complete bridge of intact skin via a pedicle. The progression of this discipline has occurred from random local tissue advancements, followed by axial/pedicle regional rotational flaps, and ultimately to distant free flaps.

There are many instances that require reconstruction of defects in the head and neck region, with the most common being secondary to trauma and cancer resection. When deciding which option to use, one should progress from simple to complex options. Small defects can be closed primarily, moderately sized defects may require grafts or local flaps, and large or complex defects require regional or distant pedicled/microvascular free flaps. Reconstruction of the face is complex. The face is composed of esthetic subunits. Each of these subunits is composed of different tissue types that support vital functions such as mastication and vision. Different areas of reconstruction require different elements which is why no one flap technique is perfect for all scenarios and many techniques have evolved over time.

2 Random Tissue Advancements

Historically, punishment for adultery and theft was nose amputation in ancient Indian, Greek, and Roman societies. One of the first examples of reconstructive surgery dates to ancient India during the sixth–fourth century BCE when nose amputations were commonly practiced as a penalty for crimes. Nasal reconstruction was born to repair this damaging practice (Greco et al. 2010). Historians credit Sushruta of India with describing a regional pedicled flap for the nose in Samahita ca. 1000–800 BCE. In modern day, the paramedian flap is used for other nasal defects including those following cancer resections, burns, and trauma.

Many of the surgical techniques in the modern era have relied on the anatomical discoveries dating back to the ancient Greeks and Romans (for more on anatomical discoveries, see Chapter “Anatomists: The Basis of Surgery”). Celsus (25 CE) and Oribasius (325–403 CE) described pedicled flaps and local tissue rearrangement for the lips, nose, and ears (Fang and Chung 2014). As an example, Aulus Cornelius Celsus in 30 CE described paired quadrilateral advancement flaps for upper lip reconstruction. He stated “the method of treatment is as follows: the mutilation is enclosed in a square, from the inner angles of this, incisions are made across, so that the part on one side of the quadrilateral is completely separated from that on the opposite side. Then the two flaps, which we have freed, are brought together (Wallace 1978).” The fall of the Roman Empire resulted in the European Dark Age and few recorded advancements in reconstruction occurred.

Marie Antoinette, the Queen of France in 1774, once said “There is nothing new except what has been forgotten.” This concept will be a repeated theme throughout the discussion of many flap techniques. Specific flap designs have fallen out of favor over the years, only to regain popularity at later dates. Such an example comes from the fifteenth century, where European barber-surgeons "rediscovered" the flap techniques of ancient India. The barber-surgeons were the primary surgical providers from the eleventh to the seventeenth centuries in Europe. The guild of barbers had no formal medical education until beginning of the sixteenth century. The first secular European medical school was established in Italy at Salerno. Subsequent medical schools were then established at Montpelier, Bologna, Paris, Oxford, and Cambridge (Bagwell 2005) (for more on the barber surgeon era, see Chapter "The Barber-Surgeons"). The University of Bologna, in particular, always considered surgery an integral part of medicine, and the University of Bologna will play a key role in the evolution of tissue reconstruction.

It is not well known how the European surgeons of this era learned the techniques of ancient India. At this time, southern Italy was the center of Latin, Greek, and Arabic learning. Some believe that the Indian teaching of reconstructive surgery was found in the collections of the Roman Empire. Since Italy was the hub for this ancient collection, it is logical that Italian surgeons had the means to learn and utilize these techniques. Gustavo Branca was a surgeon in Sicily, born in the early 1400s. He is often considered the inventor of "the Italian method" of nasal reconstruction using skin from other parts of the body (see Fig. 1)[1]. There is no historical evidence telling us whether there were surgeons before Gustavo in the Branca family or why he was interested in nose reconstruction. It is also unclear how Gustavo learned the information of Sushruta. Regardless, Gustavo Branca began using the regional forehead flap technique of Sushruta for nose reconstruction. He later used a skin flap from the cheek for reconstruction. Antonio Branca, Gustavo's son, further developed his father's work using tissue from the arm for nasal reconstruction. This is believed to be the first documented use of the upper extremity as a donor site (Tomba et al. 2014). It is unclear whether the Branca family is the true inventor of "the Italian method." The Brancas had no successors and only worked in Sicily, never leaving the island. It is unclear if their work was ever picked up by others or "re-invented" independently. A historian in the 1400s, Bartholommeo Fazio, wrote: "Branca, the elder, was the inventor of an admirable and almost incredible thing. He conceived how he might repair and replace noses that had been mutilated and cut off, and developed his idea into a marvelous art. […] For he conceived how mutilated lips and ears might be restored, as well as noses. Moreover, whereas his father had taken the flesh for repair from the mutilated man's face, Antonius took it from the muscles of his arm, so that no distortion of the face should be caused (Wallace 1978)."

Another prominent Italian family was involved in nose reconstruction during this period. Vincenzo Vianeo was the first surgeon in his family, living in Calabria, Italy. He was born in the early 1400s and had a nephew, Bernardino Vianeo, who was

[1] Image from Wikimedia commons. Public domain image. Reproduced without alterations. https://commons.wikimedia.org/wiki/File:Indian_method_of_surgical_restoration_of_the_nose._Wellcome_L0017597.jpg Copyrighted work available under Creative Commons Attribution only license CC BY 4.0 http://creativecommons.org/licenses/by/4.0/ http://catalogue.wellcomelibrary.org/record=b1353614

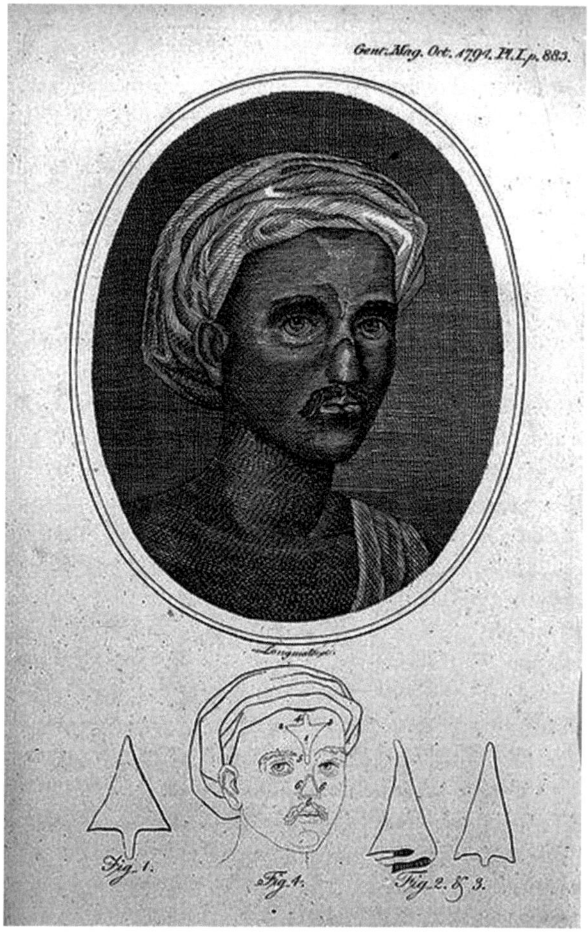

Fig. 1 The Indian method of rhinoplasty. Indian method of the restoration of the nose by plastic surgery, from article by BL to Mr. Urban concerning Cowasjee, a man who had his nose reconstructed with the aid of plastic surgery

born in 1464. Historians do not believe Vianeo had ever met the Branca family or heard of their work. There is also controversy as to which was born first. Although again it is unclear as to how Vincenzo learned his nasal reconstruction techniques, it is documented that he directly taught his nephew Bernardino (Greco et al. 2010). Some hypothesize that his techniques of arm-flap nasal reconstruction were influenced by religious documents from India kept in the archives of Basilian monasteries (Greco et al. 2010). The Vianeo family's nasal reconstruction was similar to the Branca family, using skin from the upper extremity. Bernardino would go on to educate his sons Pietro and Paolo of the surgical technique. Pietro and Paolo became well known throughout Italy for their surgical work. In 1561, a famous professor of philosophy at the University of Naples came to Tropea to have the surgical brothers restore his nose lost in an armed assault (Greco et al. 2010). It is said that the Viaeno family was secretive in its surgical technique. Leonardo Fioravanti, a surgeon in Bologna, wanted to learn Pietro and Paolo's surgeries. Legend says that he tricked

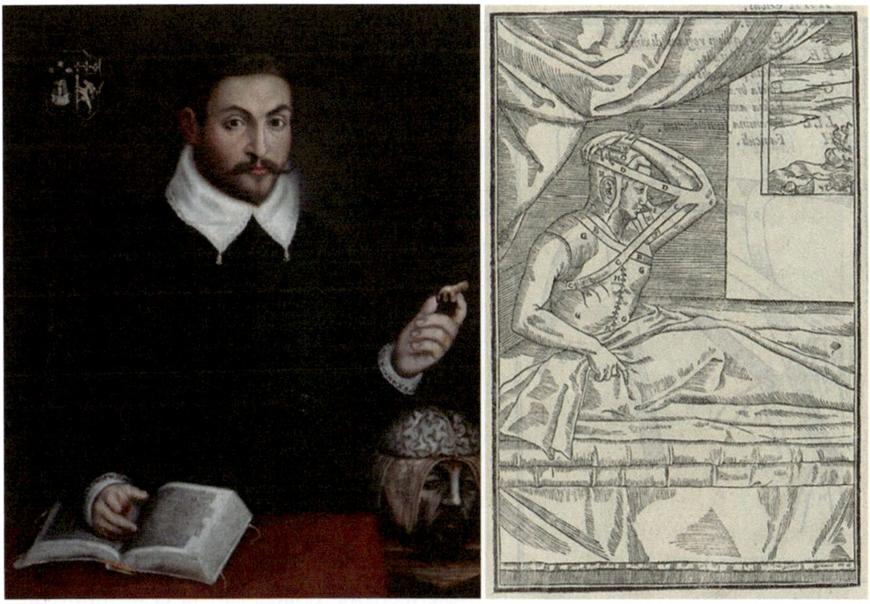

Fig. 2 Portrait of Tagliacozzi young. Circa 1580 (Ménard 2019) (left). Original illustration of the Italian method (right)

the Vianeo brothers into assisting in some operations. Years later he would describe the surgical technique in his work *Il Tesoro della Vita Humana* (Celani 2020; Greco et al. 2010; Santoni-Rugiu and Mazzola 1997).

Gaspare Tagliacozzi, was born in 1545 in Bologna, Italy. Tagliacozzi likely knew the methods of the Viaeno family from reading Leonardo Fioravanti's work as Tagliacozzi was a medical student while Fioravanti was a professor at College of Physicians at Bologna University. Tagliacozzi became a professor of surgery and anatomy at the Archiginnasio of Bologna. Among other contributions, he spent years improving and developing the "Italian method" for nasal reconstruction. He published a book entitled *De Curtorum Chirurgia per Insitionem in 1597* (On the Surgery of Mutilation by Grafting), where he described in great detail the technique and the original works of the Branca and Vianeo families, without mentioning their names (Santoni-Rugiu and Mazzola 1997). Tagliacozzi described nasal reconstruction using a flap of tissue from the upper arm (Ménard 2019). Soft tissue was taken from the skin and deep to the upper biceps fascia and rotated to the nasal defect. After healing of about 3 weeks the flap was divided (see Fig. 2).[2] The true founder

[2] This is a media file that Houghton Library believes to be in the public domain of the United States. This applies to a work published before January 1, 1923 or the unpublished work of an author who died more than 70 years ago. Houghton Library and Harvard University claim no rights in this photographic reproduction of the work, and the image is free to download and reproduce for any use, commercial or non-commercial, without any further permission required (Typ 525.97.820, Houghton Library, Harvard University).

of the "Italian method" is uncertain. The Vianeo and Branca family likely developed the technique independently, but it is more likely that the Vianeo family influenced Tagliacozzi work and publication.

One of the reasons that surgical technique in general took to develop and evolve prior to this period was due to the limitation in disseminating information. This is likely one of the reasons why two families in Italy were developing the same nasal reconstruction technique with no knowledge of each other. With the invention and proliferation of the printing press in the late fifteenth century, information began spreading rapidly across Europe. Fioravanti's work, *Il Tesoro della Vita Humana*, for example, was translated into French, German, and English and spread across Europe (Santoni-Rugiu and Mazzola 1997). With higher output printing, medical journals would arrive in the 1660s, increasing the efficiency of knowledge sharing (Fang and Chung 2014). In Europe, the mechanical movable printing press introduced the era of mass communication in the sixteenth and seventeenth centuries, and surgeons in Europe began to share information like never before. This allowed major strides in medicine, surgery, and anatomy. Most notably was an English physician named William Harvey, who made significant contributions in the understanding of anatomy and physiology. In addition to describing in detail the systemic circulation of the body, in 1682, he described the concept of arterial inflow and venous outflow in the extremities with his tourniquet experiment on the forearm and hand. This new understanding of vasculature would become instrumental in the development of flap reconstruction (Haddad and Khairallah 1936; Harvey 1928).

3 Local and Regional Flaps

European surgeons would continue to repair defects by taking skin from local areas until the fundamental understanding of the vascular system was developed. In 1743, in an attempt to reconstruct a lid defect in a 14-year-old boy, Henri Francois Le Dran described a sliding flap from the nose (Wallace 1978). In 1719, Renaulme de la Garanne placed an arm flap (from the Italian method) into a fresh surgical defect in the nose (Wallace 1978). Frank Hastings Hamilton, a surgeon in the 1840s, modified this and performed his cross-leg flap in treating a 15-year-old boy with chronic ulcers. In 1862, Wood reported on the first distant flap coverage for upper extremity defects with an axial groin flap in reconstructing a burn on the upper extremity of an 8-year-old girl (Wood 1863). Woods made direct reference to the Tagliacotian principal in his work. Francois Chopart of France (1743–1795) performed advancement flaps for lip reconstruction.

In 1855, a man named Iginio Tansini was born in Italy. He earned his medical degree from the University of Pavia in 1878. Following this, he stayed on staff at the Surgical Clinics and learned from Enrico Bottini before becoming professor of the Surgical Clinics at Modena in 1888 (Maxwell 1980). Tasini had many accomplishments as a surgeon. He was the first Italian surgeon to successfully perform a pylorogastric resection for cancer. He was also the first person to cauterize the stump of the trigeminal nerve following its transection in the treatment of trigeminal neuralgia (Maxwell 1980). Most notably for this work, he is credited with the first musculocutaneous flap. In 1896, he described a latissimus dorsi flap in the setting of breast cancer (Tansini. 1896) (see Fig. 3). When performing mastectomies, Tansini advocated for the excision of the skin to reduce the risk of recurrence of cancer after the mastectomy. In order to reconstruct this defect, he described the latissimus dorsi flap and highlighted the importance of vascularization for flap viability. Tansini consistently experienced necrosis of the distal one-third of his original flap. After further anatomical investigation with Professor Sala, an eminent anatomist from Pavia, he noted that the latissimus dorsi muscles needed to be included with the scapular circumflex. It is known now that he was mistaken only in his thinking that the scapular circumflex artery was more important than the subscapular and thoracodorsal arteries in this flap (Maxwell 1980). "We can only speculate why this popular and reliable procedure fell from favor, necessitating 'rediscovery' of musculocutaneous flaps and revival of the latissimus dorsi flap (Maxwell 1980)." Tansini's mastectomy was eventually replaced by that of Halsted's, and for reasons unknown his work

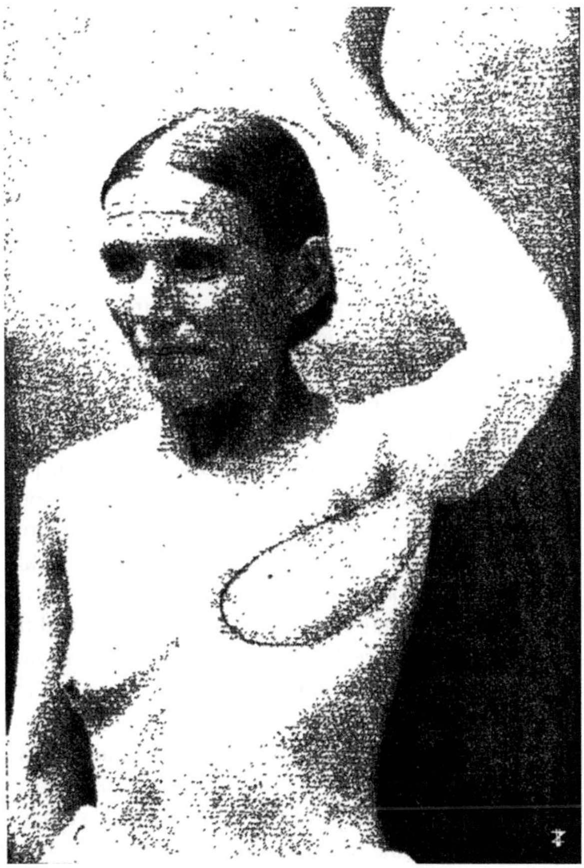

Fig. 3 Original photo of Tansini's latissimus dorsi flap reconstruction. Tansini method for the cure of cancer of the breast. Purpura, Francesco. The Lancet. 171(4409):634–637. (Figure 6 Reproduced with permission and without alteration)

with the latissimus dorsi flap failed to carry forward. "Halsted's mastectomy became accepted as the standard mode of management for this disease…Thus, widespread acceptance of Halsted's procedure put that of Tansini's to rest (Maxwell 1980)."

While substantial work took place in Italy, beginning in the nineteenth century, Italy began to be overshadowed by Germany in regard to medicine and surgery, especially because of their adoption of aseptic technique. Dr. Giuseppe Ruggi of Bologna said "Italy is the most indifferent of all nations, and seems as if she is neither interested herself nor wished to interest herself in this method of treatment [aseptic technique] which has been estimated so highly by the great surgical leaders of Germany (Maxwell 1980)." Much of the soft tissue work in the late 1800s was performed by German surgeons and ophthalmologists. In 1829, Fricke of Hamburg described many alternative facial flaps using the temple for upper eyelid repairs and tissue from the cheek for lower eyelid repairs (Wallace 1978). Jacques Lisfranc and Napoleon's surgeon Jean Dominique Larrey used the ancient technique of Celsus for upper lip reconstruction with wide undermining that has been recommended by Pierre Franco in 1561 (Wallace 1978). This would become known as the French method. Karl Heinrich August von Burow was a German surgeon and ophthalmologist born in 1830. He improved on the French method for lip repair when he developed a technique in which a triangle of skin and subcutaneous fat is excised so tissue can be advanced without buckling, referred as a "Burow's triangle." Burrow's triangle is utilized today, especially as an effective means for correcting "dog ears." Advancements in understanding of soft tissue handling are vital for the future use of surgical flaps.

The nineteenth century would lead to substantial breakthroughs in medicine by people like Louis Pasteur, the father of microbiology (1822–1895), and Joseph Lister (1827–1912), the father of modern surgery. Prior to the industrial revolution, most soft tissue injuries occurred due to warfare. Gunshot injuries became an increasing portion of battle wounds. During the American Civil War (1861–1865), 70% of traumatic injuries involved the limbs, just 3% underwent debridement with amputation as the preferred method of treatment (Fang and Chung 2014). With knowledge from Louis Pasteur and Joseph Lister, soldiers were less likely to die from infection after these injuries, thereby increasing the number of survivors with soft tissue defects. As an example of how gunshots provided the means for advancing flap reconstruction, in 1868, Carl Thiersch in Germany used a superiorly based nasolabial flap to close a palatal fistula resulting from a gunshot wound (Wallace 1978). The search for reconstruction options for facial defects would continue, with an emphasis on pedicles. Although he is best known for his discovery of paraffin and Vaseline, Robert Gersuny in Austria performed the first island flap reconstruction in 1887 (Wallace 1978). He used a random island of neck skin on a pedicle of subcutaneous tissue to provide lining for a defect in the mouth. More than a decade later, George Howard Monks in Boston would then use an axial island flap of forehead skin to reconstruct a lower eyelid (Wallace 1978).

Sir Harold Gillies was a New Zealand-born otolaryngologist, born in 1882, who is often considered the father of modern plastic surgery. He had many contributions, most notably in the field of craniofacial surgery and tissue repairs. During World

War I (1914–1918), he was working in the Royal Army Medical Corps as the medical director to a French-American dentist named Valadier. Auguste Charles Valadier attended the College of Physicians and Surgeons at Columbia University, graduating in 1895 followed by a dental degree from the Philadelphia Dental College (now the school of Dentistry at Temple University). When war broke out in August of 1914, he volunteered his services to the British Red Cross Society. The British Army would not have a separate commissioned dental corps until 1921. Gillies said "The credit for establishing the first plastic and jaw unit, which so facilitated the later progress of plastic surgery, must go to the remarkable linguistic talents of the smooth and genial Sir Charles Valadier (Cruse 1987)." Valadier worked on jaw repair and was using novel skin graft techniques. This interested Gillies who left his post with Valadier for Paris to work with Hippolyte Morestin.

Hippolyte Morestin was a French surgeon, known as the Father of Mouths. "Gillies described his meeting with Morestin thus: "In the space of a single moment he could reveal the gentleness of a kitten and the savagery of a tiger. He received me kindly, and I stood spellbound as he removed half of a face distorted with a horrible cancer and then deftly turned a neck flap to restore not only the cheek but the side of the nose and lip, in one shot. Although in the light of present-day knowledge it seems unlikely that this repair would have been wholly successful, at that time it was the most thrilling thing I had ever seen. I fell in love with the work on the spot (Lalardrie 1972)." Gillies was fascinated with this work, and when he returned to England, he started the facial injury ward at the Cambridge Military Hospital. As demand grew, this unit became inadequate and the Queen's Hospital, in Sidcup, opened in 1917. When faced with a horrific facial burn, Gillies invented the tube pedicle. He stated: "The process of thought on the problem led one to decide on a double pedicled chest flap, the pedicles to be tubed to prevent their being infected or exposed, to leave attached to these pedicles as large a chest flap as was deemed viable and then to place this large flap onto the face, excising the area covered by it [...] In regard to the raw area of the chest no attempt at closure was made and the main line of treatment carried out for this area was the use of paraffin No.7. At one stage hot fomentations were also applied to clean the surface. No grafting from the patient was attempted but three small grafts from another case were laid on the granulations, without success (Wallace 1978)." The waltzing tube pedicle, sometimes known as a walking-stalk skin flap, is a tubular pedicle connected from the donor site to the target, allowing blood flow through the pedicle. The connection is divided after the defected site heals (see Fig. 4).[3] Gillies treated over 8700 facial trauma patients at the Queens Hospital and the Park Prewett Hospital (Gebran and Nam 2020). Gillies was unaware that just 1 year prior, in 1916, Vladimir Petrovich Filatov, an ophthalmic surgeon in Odessa, would perform the first tube pedicle in a human after raising a tube pedicle on a rabbit and noting that the hair regrew after shaving, thereby assuming it had adequate blood supply (Wallace 1978). World War

[3] Marck KW, Palyvoda R, Bamji A et al. The tubed pedicle flap centennial: its concept, origin, rise, and fall. Eur J Plast Surg. 2017;40:473–78. https://doi.org/10.1007/s00238-017-1289-8 Image is of springer collection, need permission

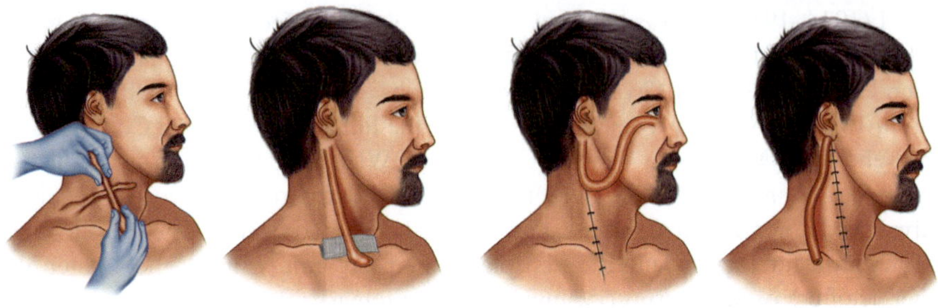

Fig. 4 Four drawings illustrating the first tubed pedicle flap of Filatov in 1916

I would provide a plethora of surgical patients in which the foundations of plastic reconstructive surgery would grow. (For more information on Gillies, see Chapters "The Legacy of Maxillofacial Surgery During The Great War" and "Midface Trauma").

4 Deltopectoral and Pectoral Flap

In 1945, Vahram Bakamjian, graduated from medical school at the American University of Beirut in Lebanon. He then came to the United States to attend an ear, nose, and throat residency at Columbia University in 1956 (Serletti et al. 2012). After residency, Dr. Bakamjian was recruited to Roswell Park Memorial Institute. In 1965, he performed one of the first modern deltopectoral flaps (Krishnamurthy 2015). While the deltopectoral flap sometimes is called the Bakamjian flap, the technique was first described by Aymard more than 40 years prior when he reported on raising a medially based fasciocutaneous flap from the shoulder skin for a nasal construction (Aymard 1917). Conley, another surgeon in New York, introduced the modified laterally based deltopectoral flap supplied by the lateral thoracic and thoracoacromial branches in 1953 (Hwang 2016). The deltopectoral flap did not gain much popularity until Bakamjian reported on his use with this technique. The deltopectoral flap which is a rotational flap that Bakamjian demonstrated was more dependable than a free skin graft. With this he developed the two-staged method for pharyngoesophageal reconstruction.

In 1969, Hueston in Melbourne, Australia, advanced the work of Aymard and Bakamjian, by including "the pectoralis major muscle in the chest skin flap and named it a compound pectoral flap. He was the first to combine a skin flap with the pectoralis major muscle, and used this technique to repair large defects of the chest wall (Hueston and McConchie 1968; Hwang 2016)." Ariyan's work in 1979 demonstrated the flap could be raised as an axial myocutaneous flap on the thoracoacromial artery. He described four cases, two were raised as a peninsular flap, one as an island flap, and one as a double paddle island (Ariyan 1979). In that same year, Baek described the anatomy, design, and blood supply of the pectoralis major myocutaneous island flap after dissecting 25 cadavers and performing the procedure on 26 patients (Baek et al. 1979). It is believed that these two surgeons developed the technique independently but simultaneously. This was a transition point in the world of head and neck reconstruction because it provided a large amount of well-vascularized tissue to cover defects from the neck up. The pectoral flap had major benefits over the deltopectoral flap with its rich vascularity, large skin area, increased bulk, and ease of harvest. This allowed coverage of almost anywhere in the oral cavity and became the workhorse of the 1980s and 1990s. Before the era of microsurgical free flaps, regional deltopectoral flaps and the pectoralis major myocutaneous flaps were most often utilized in the head and neck.

5 The Foundations of Vascular Surgery

The foundations of vascular surgery, the building block for microvascular surgery, begin with Alexis Carrel. Carrel was a French surgeon born in 1873. He attended the University of Lyon for medical school. His interest in vasculature is said to have initiated with the assassination of Sadi Carnot in 1894. Sadi Carnot was the president of the French Republic and was stabbed in the abdomen while visiting Lyon. At that time, it was believed that major vascular injuries were lethal, but Carrel felt that they could be repaired (Dente and Feliciano 2005). In 1903, he cared for a young woman dying of tuberculosis peritonitis. They took a trip to Lourdes where she was cured. The women proclaimed this miracle and named him as her primary witness. This was against Catholic teachings at this time and he was ridiculed by the French community. Due to this, and failing exams for faculty positions, he was unable to receive a hospital appointment in France requiring his immigration, first to Canada and ultimately to the United States. He accepted a position in Chicago in 1904. At Chicago University he met Charles Guthrie and together they perfected their vascular anastomotic technique. He pioneered new techniques like the triangulation of vessels and the use of sharp, round-bodied needles to minimize damage and irrigation with crystalloid solution. Carrel won the Nobel Prize in Physiology or Medicine in 1912 in recognition of his "work on vascular suture and the transplantation of blood vessels and organs" (Alexis Carrel – Biographical 2021; Dente and Feliciano 2005).

While Carrel and Guthrie's work was monumental, development of the surgical microscope was a truly pivotal moment in the history of microvascular surgery. Otologists were the first physicians to use such microsurgical techniques and Carl-Olof Siggesson Nylen is regarded as one of the founders of microsurgery. In 1921, he developed the first surgical microscope as a modification of the monocular Brinell-Leitz microscope (Schultheiss and Denil 2002). In 1922, Gunnar Holmgren created the binocular microscope. In the 1950s, Carl Zeiss further advanced Holmgren's binocular microscope seen in Fig. 5.[4]

[4]Reproduced without modification with permission from Zeiss

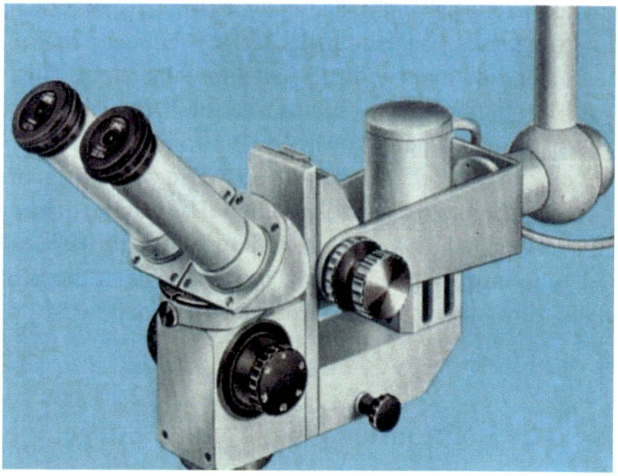

Fig. 5 OPMI1 was the first surgical microscope developed in cooperation with leading surgeons, Professor Hirst Wullstein and Professor Heinrich Harms. Source: Carl Zeiss archives

The foundation of microvascular surgery, the anastomosis of vessels using microscopic techniques, was first performed by Jules Jacobson in 1960 at the University of Vermont to couple small vessels of 1.4 mm diameter in dogs and rabbits (Jacobson et al. 1962; Rickard and Hudson 2014). Harry Buncke was an American plastic surgeon and often referred to as the "Father of Microsurgery" for his contributions to the field. Ronald Malt performed the first successful replantation of a forearm in 1962, as a chief resident at Mass General Hospital (Malt and McKhann 1964). In 1973, in the People's Republic of China, in Shanghai Sixth People's Hospital, the first successful distal forearm replantation was performed by Zhong-Wei Chen and coworkers. There is debate over who should receive credit for replantation first. "Ronald Malt performed the reattachment surgery on a boy who had an accident in 1962, but he published his case report two years later in 1964. Chen Zhongwei performed a similar surgery on a worker who cut off his forearm in 1963, but he published his case report the same year (Fan 2020)." Regardless, credit should be awarded to both surgical teams as it was truly a remarkable milestone. Yoshio Najayama et al. completed the first free flap transfer of the intestine to the head and neck region in 1964 (Fang and Chung 2014). Surgeons in China (Dong-Ye Yang and Yu-Dong Gu), unknown to the rest of the world at that time, would then perform the first extremity free flap of a human microvascular toe to thumb transfer in 1965 (Chang 1979; Fang and Chung 2014; Yang et al. 1977). In 1966, Buncke used microsurgery to transplant a primate's great toe to its hand (Buncke et al. 1966).

At the same time, Donagy and Tasargil organized the first microvascular surgery symposium, later published as Microvascular Surgery: Report of the First Conference, October 6–7, 1966 (Link et al. 2010). They outlined basic approaches to microvascular surgery: suture technique using silk, nylon, and metallic suture material; use of adhesive substances; the use of micro-staples; and electrocoagulation. As examples, they stated that a 1 mm vessel would require 10-micron flexible sutures which in 1960 were being manufactured by DuPont. They fabricated many different types of suture materials and experimented with different variations.

"Microfine manipulators of various shapes were fashioned by etching down stainless-steel wires mounted in 25 and 30 gauge hypodermic needles. These were used to handle the vessels atraumatically (Peardon Donaghy and Gazi Yaşargil 1966)." The Mark V instrument was developed to staple vessels between 1 and 2 mm in diameter. At this time, research was conducted to see if adhesive material could repair blood vessels or provide alternatives to conventional suture or staple repair. They used adhesives such as Eastman 910, a methyl 2-cyanoacrylate monomer, and M2C-2 a similar compound with methyl methacrylate.

John Cobbett was a plastic surgeon at Queen Victoria Hospital, East Grinstead, and Lewisham Hospital. As part of a research program at East Grinstead, he became interested in small vessel anastomosis. In 1968, Cobbett performed the first human microsurgical transplantation of the great toe to the thumb in the English-speaking world, 3 years after that of the Chinese (Cobbett 1969). He later went on to found the British Society for Surgery of the Hand.

Three events in the 1970s are believed to be the foundations that enabled the progression of flap surgery: the advancement of surgical equipment, the identification of flaps as a reliable option for reconstruction, and better understanding of anatomy. The development of microsurgical instruments by individuals like Acland in 1969 launched microsurgery into a more common practice (Acland 1969). These instruments included fine-tipped toothed forceps for minimal damage of delicate vessels, microsurgical scissors, and vessel dilators (Corlett et al. 2015).

In 1970, Milton, a plastic surgeon, debunked a long-believed myth by demonstrating that success of a flap was not dependent on the length to width ratio, but on the blood supply that is incorporated into the flap. This fact was coupled a year later with Strauch, Bloomberg, and Lewin at the Montefiore Hospital, who noted that mandibular replacement following mandibulectomy is challenging. There is often a limit of local tissue and rotational flaps often requiring multiple procedures based on the blood supply. They hypothesized that a better approach would be to insert a graft with its own blood supply. They reported on isolating a vascularized rib to the internal mammary vessels and successfully transplanted this to reconstruct the jaw in a dog (Strauch et al. 1971). Surgeons at this time realized the importance of the blood supply and the ability to use the microscopic anastomoses discovered by Jacobson and Buncke to use free flaps from distant donor sites, rather than just rotational flaps, in reconstruction.

G. Ian Taylor and Ronald Daniel, two plastic surgeons in Melbourne, Australia, identified a similar shortcoming to Strauch and his colleagues, specifically in reconstruction after trauma to the lower extremities. When the skin is lost, early flap coverage is often required, but local rotational flaps are often inadequate (see Fig. 6). They performed the first successful free flap transfer in a human in 1973 (Taylor and Daniel 1973). They used a large flap based on the superficial circumflex iliac vessel and superficial inferior epigastric vessels described by McGregor and Jackson, to repair the defect with microvascular anastomosis. They chose the 1.8 mm superficial inferior epigastric artery for anastomosis, and the superficial circumflex iliac artery was ligated (Taylor and Daniel 1973).

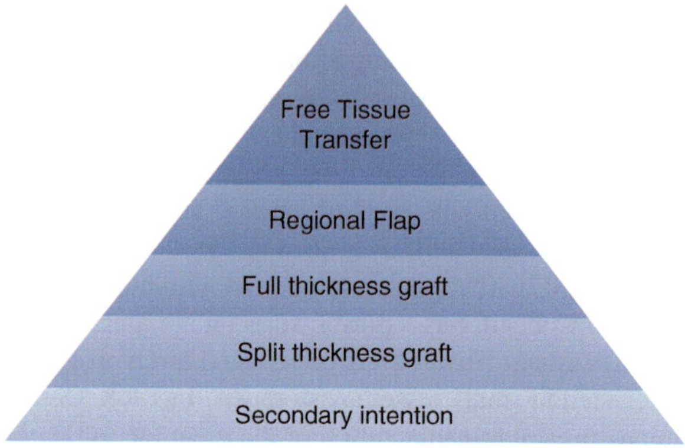

Fig. 6 The pyramid represents the escalation ladder for closing defects. More advanced closures are based on vasculature and the principles discovered by Buncke and others that a pedicled skin flap is more dependable than a free skin graft for large reconstructions

Free flap surgery could not have occurred without detailed understanding of the vascular system of the human body. Across the world, for over a century, numerous anatomists were involved in understanding this complex system (Taylor 2015). Unfortunately, many of these studies went unnoticed by the English-speaking world. The flap designs of the 1970s sent many surgeons back to anatomy labs to improve on their understanding of the architecture for better flap success. JB McCraw performed experimental studies in dogs using myocutaneous flaps based on the gracilis, sartorius, biceps femoris, trapezius, and rectus abdominis muscles in 1977 as well as in human cadavers (McCraw and Dibbell 1977). Taylor and colleagues performed many dissections and injected lead oxide into the arterial tree of more than 1000 fresh cadavers and over 3000 individual muscle studies. As their anatomical studies progressed, they moved from individual tissues such as skin to compound flaps supplied by a single vascular pedicle such as skin and muscle or skin muscle and bone (Taylor et al. 1979a; Taylor et al. 1983; Taylor and Ham 1976; Taylor and Townsend 1979). Their work reinforced the concept that a single vessel supplied multiple tissues types in a specific region, an understanding that we take for granted today. They further worked on investigating the venous system, and the lymphatics lead to the concept of the "angiosomes." "As a result of the total-body studies of the blood supply to the skin and underlying deep tissues, combined with reviews of previous works, especially those by Manchot and Salmon, it has been possible to divide the body into three-dimensional anatomical vascular territories. These three-dimensional composite blocks of tissue, supplied by a source artery and its accompanying vein that span between skin and bone, are defined as angiosomes (Taylor 2015)."

6 Radial Forearm Flap

The radial forearm flap was detailed by Yang et al. in 1981, for resurfacing the neck secondary to burn contractures (Yang et al. 1997). The blood supply of the forearm skin flap comes from the cutaneous branches of the radial, ulnar, posterior, and anterior interosseous vessels and was successful in 59 out of 60 flaps in his report.

The concept of this flap was first used in China in 1978, by Guo-fan, Baoqui, and Yuzhi for neck resurfacing after a burn (Yang et al. 1997). In 1982, Song et al. published in English their experience with this flap at the Beijing Plastic Surgery Hospital, in the *Clinics in Plastic Surgery*. The western surgeons at that time referred to it as "the Chinese flap (Song et al. 1982)."

Soutar provided the first English-language description of the use of the cutaneous and osteocutaneous forearm flap in the oral cavity reconstruction in 1983 (Soutar et al. 1983). This paper caused a paradigm shift. Prior to this, reconstruction in the oral cavity was done with the bulky pectoralis flap. Soutar et al. noted their radial forearm flap had several disadvantages as it is difficult to raise and produce a donor defect that restricts immediate postoperative mobilization. In 1985, Fenton and Roberts described a method to improve donor sites of the radial forearm (Fenton and Roberts 1985). The authors suggested placing the wrist in flexion to expose the tendon of the flexor carpi radialis. The skin edges of the defect can then be advanced and sutured to the forearm muscles. Once this is complete, the central muscle fibers of flexor pollicis longus can be sutured to the muscle belly of the flexor digitorum superficialis, thereby covering the tendon of flexor carpi radialis noting a better functional and cosmetic result. In 1986, Soutar et al. published on 60 flaps presenting uneventful primary healing with no fistula formation and return of oral function (Soutar and McGregor 1986). The average hospital course was 17.8 days. They had six microvascular failures. Most of the described patient morbidity was secondary to radiotherapy of the underlying malignancy. Flap reconstruction of the head and neck is often the result of malignancy, and the history of radiation oncology has been a major component in the evolution of head and neck reconstruction (for more on this, see Chapter "Radiation Oncology").

The harvest technique was further developed by Lutz et al. in 1999 where they described a suprafascial elevation of the radial forearm flap (Lutz et al. 1999). The 1990s saw a major change in the reconstruction of bony defects in the face. Large mandibular defects were repaired with a fibular, iliac crest, or scapular and large maxillary defects were mostly soft tissue via the rectus. In 2003, Villaret and Futran reported on 34 patients that were reconstructed with radial forearm osteofaciocutaneous free flaps in the maxilla or mandible (Villaret and Futran 2003). The donor site was rigidly fixated and a skin graft was placed at the site. The patients were followed for 10–54 months. Seven patients had anterior maxillectomy defects and 27 patients had lateral mandibulectomy defects. They reported no flap failures or donor site fractures. This was an important claim because at that point, 25% of published cases reported a radial bone fracture.

7 Deep Circumflex Iliac Artery Free Flap (DCIA)

The iliac crest was one of the first of three major donor sites for widespread use in reconstruction of the mandible. Early iliac crest harvesting was based on the use of the superficial iliac vessels. In 1979, Taylor, Townsend, and Corlett recommended the use of the deep circumflex system as a superior alternative for this technique (Taylor et al. 1979b). Their discovery was interestingly put:

During the dissection of the groin, the deep circumflex iliac vessels were encountered; because the bone graft was to be somewhat larger than usual, these vessels were dissected out as well and the graft was finally isolated on both vascular systems. Profuse bleeding was seen from all tissues. However, when the superficial system was temporarily occluded, there was copious arterial bleeding from the entire bone, but sluggish perfusion of the overlying skin. When the clip was removed and applied to the deep circumflex artery, the reverse situation occurred (Taylor et al. 1979b).

This observation in the operating room resulted in 40 dissections of the deep circumflex iliac vessel in cadavers and solidified the connection between the deep circumflex iliac artery (DCIA) and the superficial circumflex iliac artery (SCIA). Understanding the anatomical vascular supply allowed Taylor and colleagues to discover this new technique, which formed the foundation for the discoveries of the 1970s and 1980s. The benefit of the use of the deep circumflex iliac artery was confirmed by Sanders and Mayou in 1979 when they used an iliac crest artery free flap to reconstruct a compound fracture of the tibia and fibula in a 29-year-old man.

The following year, Franklin et al. reported the use of the DCIA free flap for mandibular bone and soft tissue reconstruction (Franklin et al. 1980). They acknowledged that no other flap to date so closely approximated both the mandibular thickness and curvature. Problematically, this flap is bulky and often requires many debulking procedures in the oral cavity. To remedy this, the internal oblique free muscle flap based on the ascending branch of the DCIA became the soft tissue component of the DCIA free flap. In 1989, Urken used the iliac crest bone flap with the internal oblique muscle in mandibular reconstruction (Urken et al. 1989). In 1996, Brown described the DCIA flap in which the internal oblique muscle was used for maxillary reconstruction (Brown 1996; Brown et al. 2002).

The DCIA flap is highly favorable as it provides excellent contour and can replace both the height and width of the native mandible. However, this flap is limited to about 16 cm which is not enough for complete mandibular reconstruction. The average pedicle size is 5–7 cm which can sometimes limit reconstruction. In addition, obesity is a relative contraindication as the bulky skin paddle becomes less reliable.

8 Fibula Free Flap

The fibula free flap has gained widespread use as a mainstay of reconstruction in the maxillofacial region. Building on the principals of microvascular design and free flaps, in 1975 Taylor described the first fibula free flap transfer in humans in the extremities (Taylor et al. 1975). It was not until 1989, however, when Hidalgo published the use of osteocutaneous fibula free flaps for use in mandibular reconstruction (Hidalgo 1989). He described 12 patients who underwent mandibular reconstruction with an average mandibular defect of 13.5 cm. He used a lateral approach to the dissection of the fibula in all patients, and most of the bone was harvested regardless of the amount needed for reconstruction. The bone was osteotomized first and then the peroneal artery and vein were divided and ligated distally. The anatomical basis and vasculature have been heavily studied to support the use of this technique. In 1986, Wei et al. described the reliability of the vasculature (Wei et al. 1986). There are four to eight perforators along the fibula making the vascularity of the bone highly dependable (Urken et al. 1998; Wei et al. 1994). A decade later, Hidalgo reported on 82 patients who underwent reconstruction with reliable outcomes (Hidalgo and Pusic 2002). The fibula became an attractive donor site as it has ample bone length available for reconstruction and has relatively uniform consistency and cross-sectional size, and osteotomies can be performed to shape to the intended position.

While numerous options exist for the reconstruction of the maxilla and mandible, the fibular free flap has become the workhorse because of its versatility and numerous other factors. One of the added benefits is its favorable bone quality for dental rehabilitation with dental implants (Patel et al. 2019). In 1993, Huryn et al. reported on the osseointegration of implants in microvascular free fibular reconstructed mandibles. In 2013, the first "Jaw in a day" surgery was performed by Levine, Hirsch, and colleagues using digital technology, placing dental implants into the fibular bone, allowing for immediate dental prosthetic rehabilitation (Levine et al. 2013).

9 Scapular Free Flap

The scapular free flap was first described by dos Santos in 1980 and is one of the most versatile flaps for the head and neck (Santos 1980). Bone, muscle, fat, fascia, and skin can be transferred via this flap design. Gilbert and Teot illustrated successful scapular free flaps in lower extremity reconstruction in 1982 (Gilbert and Teot 1982).

In the same year, Nassif et al. described an anatomical study of 20 fresh cadavers and found a constant artery descending along the lateral border of the scapula that was not previously described, which they referred to as the cutaneous parascapular artery (Nassif et al. 1982). The circumflex scapular artery is a branch of the subscapular artery which originates from the axillary artery. After the circumflex scapular artery travels through the triangular space, it branches into the transverse cutaneous scapular branch and a cutaneous parascapular branch. In 1987, Batchelor and Bardsley described the use of a bi-scapular free flap in a leg and noted that the whole flap was being adequately perfused by the single upper pedicle (Batchelor and Bardsley 1987). Deraemaecker et al. in 1988 reported on the angular branch of the thoracodorsal artery and vein as a potential additional blood supply for the caudal portion of the lateral scapular border (Deraemaecker et al. 1988).

In 1990, Sullivan et al. published their experience with five cutaneous scapular flaps and 31 osteocutaneous flaps for head and neck reconstruction (Sullivan et al. 1990). One hundred percent of the cutaneous and 90% of the osteocutaneous flaps were successful. One flap failed secondary to osteoradionecrosis and the second due to arterial insufficiency, also likely secondary to radiation. The third failed flap was caused by venous thrombosis. In 1991, Coleman and Sultan showed that the angular artery allowed the harvesting of two separate bone segments (Coleman and Sultan 1991). These can be independently harvested on separate branches of the subscapular artery and vein which was revolutionary at the time, most notably for the ability to harvest the scapular tip independently from the lateral border (Gibber et al. 2015). In 1994, Moscoso et al. preformed a comparative anatomic study of bone and noted that overall, 78% of harvested scapular bone segments were deemed for implant placement with a height of 10 mm and a width of at least 5 mm which supports the use of this flap design for dental rehabilitation after reconstruction (Moscoso et al. 1994).

Starting in the early 2010, the scapular tip free flap gained renewed interest as a modification of the scapular angle free flap. This flap design is often utilized in maxillary reconstruction. If the circumflex artery is scarified, the pedicle can be up to 20 cm long, much longer than alternative flaps (Ferrari et al. 2015).

10 Rectus Abdominis Free Flap (RAFF)

The rectus abdominis flap was described in 1977 by Mathes and Bostwick in the setting of abdominal reconstruction after trauma using a rotated pedicle (Mathes and Bostwick 1977). The rectus abdominis muscle flap was then described by Pairolero and Arnold in 1980 to reconstruct chest wall defects following sternotomy complications (Pairolero and Arnold 1984). In this case study, a total of 67 muscle transpositions were performed, 63 of which were pectoralis, three rectus, and one latissimus dorsi. The rectus abdominis was used as a rotational muscle flap. The anatomical premise of this flap was nicely described by Taylor and Boyd, who illustrated the cutaneous perfusion of the abdominal skin based on the deep inferior epigastric artery and vein through injections studies (Taylor et al. 1984). In 1985, Drever et al. used a rectus abdominis myocutaneous flap for breast reconstruction (Drever and Hodson-Walker 1985). When Drever first described this flap, he closed the donor site with mesh, but work of other surgeons resulted in a transition to closing the donor site directly. In 1986, Sakai et al. described the extended vertical rectus abdominis myocutaneous (VRAM) flap for breast reconstruction (Sakai et al. 1989). Prior to this the rectus abdominis myocutaneous flap was oriented as a lower abdominal transverse rectus flap. The authors noted that the defect is in the axillary region, and the lower abdominal transverse rectus abdominis myocutaneous flap was not reliable, hence the need for this modification. Over a decade later, Pennington and Pelly reported some of the first clinical applications of the free rectus abdominis musculocutaneous flap with a transfer for a facial defect in 1978, based on the inferior epigastric vessels (Pennington and Pelly 1980). This technique has proved advantageous as it has a reliable soft tissue donor and a long pedicle and can cover large defects.

Koshima and Soeda used the skin territory of the rectus abdominis muscle to reconstruct the floor of the mouth. This perforator vessel was followed toward the deep inferior epigastric vessel and dissected from the rectus abdominis muscle and resulted in a thin skin flap with an intact muscle left behind (Koshima and Soeda 1989). Allen, Treece, and Tucker worked to modify the rectus abdominis flap into the deep inferior epigastric perforator (DIEP) flap which is a technique where skin and tissue are taken from the abdomen to recreate a defect without the use of muscle (Allen and Treece 1994; Allen and Tucker 1995). In 2010, Masia et al. reported on 100 patients over a 10-year period using DIEP flaps in head and neck reconstruction (Masià et al. 2011). The overall flap survival rate was 97.1%. The DIEP flap is advantageous in that it can provide bulk if the rectus muscle is raised with the flap and it can allow easy molding if the cutaneous and muscular components are separated.

11 Anterolateral Thigh Flap (ALT)

This flap was first described by Song et al. in 1984 at the Beijing Plastic Surgery Hospital as a septocutaneous flap (Song et al. 1984). In 1979, Song found that although the cutaneous arteries were not suitable for vascular anastomosis, they could be traced to a more proximal vessel, and a free flap could be used off the intermuscular septal vessels. They described three thigh flaps, the anterolateral, the anteromedial, and the posterior. In 1990, Begue et al. described the vasculature of the descending branch of the lateral circumflex artery of the thigh and the principle behind this flap technique (Bégué et al. 1990). While the vasculature is not constant, Koshima et al. noted the technique is safe because there are usually accessory branches deriving from the lateral circumflex femoral vessels which can be included (Koshima et al. 1989). In most cases the flap relies only on musculocutaneous perforators. Malhotra et al. performed a cadaveric study that determined the musculocutaneous perforators to the ALT free flap entered the vastus lateralis muscle within 2 cm of the muscle border proving a good landmark when harvesting (Malhotra et al. 2008).

In the early 2000s the flap gained popularity in North America because of its use in extensive head and neck defects due to its bulk and low donor site morbidity. The ALT flap is a good replacement for oral cavity, pharyngeal, and cutaneous defects (Agostini and Agostini 2008). The ALT flap has also proved a good alternative to the radial forearm flap (Valentini et al. 2008).

The 1990s and early 2000s were a period of heavy utilization and focus on the recently developed vascular free flaps of the 1970s and 1980s, being used routinely in head and neck reconstruction. Since their inception, critics of free tissue transfer have detailed their downsides, namely, that they are long surgeries and resource intensive, can be associated with donor site morbidity. Partially as a response to these criticisms, there recently has been renewed interest in low-morbidity, highly versatile regional pedicled flaps. Examples of these were the supraclavicular, submental island, and facial artery musculomucosal flaps.

12 Supraclavicular Flap

In 1979, Lamberty et al. published an article describing 15 preserved cadaver and 22 fresh cadaver dissections in which they identify the thyro-cervical trunk and the associated vasculature of the transverse cervical artery and supraclavicular artery. The authors then used this information with two clinical patients in which they raised two axial flaps depending on the supraclavicular artery (Lamberty 1979). This flap was not heavily utilized until it was reintroduced in 1997, when Pallua et al. described the supraclavicular artery island (SAI) flap for reconstruction of cervicomental scars (Pallua et al. 1997).

During the following decade, supraclavicular flaps increased in popularity because of the good color and texture match of the recipient area and the simplicity of the technique. The literature was relatively quiet until in 2009 when Vinh et al. reported on 103 supraclavicular flaps over an 8-year period supporting the reliability (Vinh et al. 2009).

A 2012 review of 45 consecutive patients who underwent SAI flap reconstruction demonstrated success with the mean flap dimensions of 6.1 cm by 21.4 cm long. The review reported partial skin flap necrosis in eight patients with two having complete loss of the skin paddle. The authors noted that flap length greater than 22 cm was associated with flap necrosis (Kokot et al. 2013). The flap is relatively quick to harvest, with surgical times under an hour, reliable repair of defects without the need for performing microvascular anastomosis. However, one of the limitations of the SAI flap is the arc of rotation. A 2017 review demonstrated an overall success of 96.7% with only 10% of cases resulting in minor complications. The minor complications included distal flap necrosis, donor site dehiscence, recipient site dehiscence, fistula, and wound infection (Trautman et al. 2018).

13 Submental Island Flap (SIF)

Martin et al. first described a new axial-patterned island flap based on the submental artery in 1993 (Martin et al. 1993). The authors described a technique performed on 20 cadavers and eight patients who underwent radical neck dissection. The submental island flap consists of thin, pliable tissues with a good color match and wide arch of rotation, and the authors noted a reliable long pedicle of up to 8 cm that can be used as a cutaneous, musculofascial, or osteocutaneous flap.

The submental island flap is based on the submental artery which is a branch off the facial artery that has a typical diameter of 1–2 mm (9). In 1996, Sterne et al. described the retrograde variant and recommended that when a flap is raised in a reverse flow manner a separate venous anastomosis should be performed (Sterne et al. 1996). Sterne used this technique for oral squamous cell carcinoma. In 1997, Yilmaz et al. explained the de-epithelialized osteomuscular variant which is when the superficial epithelial layer of the flap was removed and only the bone and muscle were incorporated into the subcutaneous tunneled defect. The submental vessels run deep to the anterior belly of the digastric muscle in up to 70% of patients and should be included in the flap, but as stated in Yilmaz and Martins study, not including the anterior belly of the digastric muscle does not result in flap failure (Yilmaz et al. 1997). Kitazawa et al. in 1999 described the bipedicled flap, where the flap incorporated two vessels which is advantageous in that it provides a robust circulation of the flap and enabled them to reconstruct the upper lip as a unit safely. The drawback to this technique is the two pedicles result in a restricted range of rotation (Kitazawa et al. 1999). Patel et al. introduced the mylohyoid component to the flap harvest (Patel et al. 2007). The modification provides protection to the distal submental pedicle and cutaneous perforators adding reliability to the flap (Zenga et al. 2019).

Ramkumar et al. described the bi-paddled modification for increased bulk in 2012 (Ramkumar et al. 2012). There are two main uses for the submental artery flap. The first is de-epithelization of a portion of the flap and the second is a full-thickness flap that is split into two paddles. With the second method, the skin incision is made to ensure the perforators located on either side of the anterior belly of the digastric are included in the distal paddle. Ramkumar et al. find this advantageous to the de-epithelization of a portion of a flap, but there is waste of valuable skin area, less mobility, and de-epithelization and folding that can lead to inclusion cysts (Ramkumar et al. 2012). Today, this technique is used for many defects in the head and neck. Free flaps were mostly reserved for complex head and neck defects. SIF is quickly emerging as an important technique due to its shorter operation and patient recovery times (Jørgensen et al. 2019). This technique is comparable to the radial artery free flap with shorter length of hospital stay and has been recommended for defects in the oral cavity less then 40 cm (squared) (Conroy and Mahaffey 2009).

14 Facial Artery Musculomucosal Flap (FAMM)

Many intraoral techniques aided in the discovery and report of the facial artery musculomucosal flap. It began when Tipton first described the closure of large septal perforations with a labial buccal flap in 1965 (Tipton 1970). Years later, Jackson utilized buccal flaps for closure of a secondary palatal fistula in 1972 (Jackson 1972). Kaplan then used buccal transposition flaps to line the nasal surface of the soft palate in reconstruction in 1975 (Kaplan and Kaplan 1975). With the success of these surgeons, Rayner described the extended use of mucosal flaps in the midface with his patients (Rayner 1984). Finally, Bozola et al. provided the first description of an axial buccal musculomucosal flap based on the buccal artery for resurfacing oral mucosal defects in 1985 and again in 1989 (Bozola et al. 1989). In 1983, Sasaki et al. reported a case of a correction of cervical esophageal stricture using an axial island cheek flap (Sasaki et al. 1983). Sasaki's report led to Castens et al. to describe the anteriorly based buccinator myomucosal island flap for an oroantral fistula repair in 1991 (Carstens et al. 1991).

The term "facial artery musculomucosal flap" comes from Pribaz et al. who described it in 1992 based on this knowledge base (Pribaz et al. 1992). The FAMM flap consists of mucosa, submucosa, a small amount of buccinator muscle, the deeper plane of the orbicularis oris muscle, and the facial artery/venous plexus. The flap can be based superiorly (retrograde) or inferiorly (antegrade). When based superiorly, the FAMM flap can be used to close maxillary defects such as mucosal defects of the hard palate, alveolus, antrum, nasal floor, and septum as well as the orbit. Inferiorly, the flap can be used to close defects of the posterior hard palate, soft palate, tonsillar fossa, floor of the mouth, and even the lower lip. Pribaze et al. described this technique with success in 15 patients.

The FAMM has several advantages as it avoids an external scar, provides a great axis of rotation and range, is thin and pliable, provides a fully functional mucosal tissue, and is a suitable reconstructive option even in radiated patients (Berania et al. 2018). By 2013, a total of 441 FAMM flaps were reported in the literature with the most common site being the floor of the mouth. In a recent systematic review of 376 reported FAMM flaps, the rate of partial and complete flap necrosis was 12.2% and 2.9%, respectively, suggesting this flap is highly dependable (Ayad and Xie 2015). The FAMM flap has some disadvantages. Many recommend the utilization of a bite block after surgery to avoid biting of the pedicle by dentate patients. Two-stage procedure is required to section the pedicle in dentate patients although some modifications do exist to avoid a section procedure to section the pedicle. This is also a bulky flap that may hinder the use of dental prosthesis if used in vestibular reconstruction (Ayad and Xie 2015).

15 Tissue Engineering

While the concept of tissue engineering is outside the scope of this chapter, the authors felt it a necessary topic to discuss as the future of head and neck reconstruction. The history of tissue reconstruction began by borrowing or recruiting tissue from local, regional, and then distant sites to fill defects. With advances in molecular and cell biology, surgeons may 1 day be able to reconstruct these areas using tissues grown exclusively for this purpose, with exact matching form, function, and aesthetics of that area. Many methods are being studied, but current research uses skin tissue engineering with keratinocytes that are seeded onto bioactive scaffolds (Tarassoli et al. 2018). The scaffolds allow adequate perfusion and cellular proliferation/differentiation to produce tissue that mimics the defect site. With advancements in this technology, doctors will be able to regrow tissues that exactly mimic the tissue that was destroyed by resection or trauma.

16 Summary

Reconstruction of the head and neck is extremely challenging due to the limited access and complex anatomy. Fortunately, the robust vasculature has resulted in successful surgical flaps as excellent options to restore form and function. The surgical flap designs today rely on basic surgical technique and anatomical understanding that dates to almost 800 BCE.

Several factors have aided in the evolution of this discipline, most significantly trauma from war, knowledge exchange, and technological advancements in microsurgery. It is hard to believe that it was less than 50 years ago that G. Ian Taylor and Ronald Daniel did the first successful free flap transfer in a human in 1973. In 2021, with advanced computer-aided virtual surgical planning, microvascular reconstructive surgeons are benefiting from shorter operating room times, shorter hospital stays, and overall decreased morbidity and mortality. The next steps for tissue defect repair are with bioengineering.

References

Acland RD. Modified needleholder for microsurgery. Br Med J. 1969;1(5644):635.

Agostini T, Agostini V. Further experience with adipofascial ALT flap for oral cavity reconstruction. J Plast Reconstr Aesthet Surg. 2008;61(10):1164–9.

Alexis Carrel – Biographical 2021. Nobel Media AB. https://www.nobelprize.org/prizes/medicine/1912/carrel/biographical/. Accessed 10 Jan 2021.

Allen RJ, Treece P. Deep inferior epigastric perforator flap for breast reconstruction. Ann Plast Surg. 1994;32(1):32–8.

Allen RJ, Tucker C. Superior gluteal artery perforator free flap for breast reconstruction. Plast Reconstr Surg. 1995;95(7):1207–12.

Ariyan S. The pectoralis major myocutaneous flap. A versatile flap for reconstruction in the head and neck. Plast Reconstr Surg. 1979;63(1):73–81.

Ayad T, Xie L. Facial artery musculomucosal flap in head and neck reconstruction: a systematic review. Head Neck. 2015;37(9):1375–86.

Aymard JL. Nasal reconstruction: with a note on nature's plastic surgery. Lancet. 1917;190(4920):888–92.

Baek SM, Biller HF, Krespi YP, Lawson W. The pectoralis major myocutaneous island flap for reconstruction of the head and neck. Head Neck Surg. 1979;1(4):293–300.

Bagwell CE. "Respectful image": revenge of the barber surgeon. Ann Surg. 2005;241(6):872–8. discussion 878

Batchelor AG, Bardsley AF. The bi-scapular flap. Br J Plast Surg. 1987;40(5):510–2.

Bégué T, Masquelet AC, Nordin JY. Anatomical basis of the anterolateral thigh flap. Surg Radiol Anat. 1990;12(4):311–3.

Berania I, Lavigne F, Rahal A, Ayad T. Superiorly based facial artery musculomucosal flap: a versatile pedicled flap. Head Neck. 2018;40(2):402–5.

Bozola AR, Gasques JA, Carriquiry CE, Cardoso de Oliveira M. The buccinator musculomucosal flap: anatomic study and clinical application. Plast Reconstr Surg. 1989;84(2):250–7.

Brown JS. Deep circumflex iliac artery free flap with internal oblique muscle as a new method of immediate reconstruction of maxillectomy defect. Head Neck. 1996;18(5):412–21.

Brown JS, Jones DC, Summerwill A, et al. Vascularized iliac crest with internal oblique muscle for immediate reconstruction after maxillectomy. Br J Oral Maxillofac Surg. 2002;40(3):183–90.

Buncke HJ, Buncke CM, Schulz WP. Immediate Nicoladoni procedure in the Rhesus monkey, or hallux-to-hand transplantation, utilising microminiature vascular anastomoses. Br J Plast Surg. 1966;19(4):332–7.

Carstens MH, Stofman GM, Sotereanos GC, Hurwitz DJ. A new approach for repair of oro-antral-nasal fistulae. The anteriorly based buccinator myomucosal island flap. J Craniomaxillofac Surg. 1991;19(2):64–70.

Celani R. Fioravanti, Leonardo. In: Sgarbi M, editor. Encyclopedia of renaissance philosophy. Cham: Springer International Publishing; 2020. p. 1–8.

Chang TS. Experiences in microsurgery in the People's Republic of China. J Microsurg. 1979;1(2):154–7.

Cobbett JR. Free digital transfer. Report of a case of transfer of a great toe to replace an amputated thumb. J Bone Joint Surg Br. 1969;51(4):677–9.

Coleman JJ, Sultan MR. The bipedicled osteocutaneous scapula flap: a new subscapular system free flap. Plast Reconstr Surg. 1991;87(4):682–92.

Conroy FJ, Mahaffey PJ. Intraoral flap depilation using the long-pulsed alexandrite laser. J Plast Reconstr Aesthet Surg. 2009;62(11):e421–3.

Corlett R, Whitaker I, Ashton M. The microvascular anastomosis. In: Jones BA, editor. Operative microsurgery. McGraw Hill; 2015.

Cruse WP. Auguste charles valadier: a pioneer in maxillofacial surgery. Mil Med. 1987;152(7):337–41.

Dente CJ, Feliciano DV. Alexis carrel (1873–1944): nobel laureate, 1912. Arch Surg. 2005;140(6):609–10.

Deraemaecker R, Thienen C, Lejour M, Dor P. The serratus anteriorscapular free flap: a new osteo-muscular unit for reconstruction after radical head and neck surgery. In: Proceedings of the Second International Conference on Head and Neck Cancer, vol. 31; 1988. p. 133–7.

Drever JM, Hodson-Walker N. Closure of the donor defect for breast reconstruction with rectus abdominis myocutaneous flaps. Plast Reconstr Surg. 1985;76(4):558–65.

Fan KW. Ronald Malt or Chen Zhongwei: who performed the first surgical replantation? J Med Biogr. 2020;28(4):220–4.

Fang F, Chung KC. An evolutionary perspective on the history of flap reconstruction in the upper extremity. Hand Clin. 2014;30(2):109–22, v.

Fenton OM, Roberts JO. Improving the donor site of the radial forearm flap. Br J Plast Surg. 1985;38(4):504–5.

Ferrari S, Ferri A, Bianchi B. Scapular tip free flap in head and neck reconstruction. Curr Opin Otolaryngol Head Neck Surg. 2015;23(2):115–20.

Franklin JD, Shack RB, Stone JD, Madden JJ, Lynch JB. Single-stage reconstruction of mandibular and soft tissue defects using a free osteocutaneous groin flap. Am J Surg. 1980;140(4):492–8.

Gebran SG, Nam AJ. Sir Harold delf gillies-the surgeon artist. Ann Plast Surg. 2020;84(2):127–9.

Gibber MJ, Clain JB, Jacobson AS, et al. Subscapular system of flaps: an 8-year experience with 105 patients. Head Neck. 2015;37(8):1200–6.

Gilbert A, Teot L. The free scapular flap. Plast Reconstr Surg. 1982;69(4):601–4.

Greco M, Ciriaco AG, Vonella M, Vitagliano T. The primacy of the Vianeo family in the invention of nasal reconstruction technique. Ann Plast Surg. 2010;64(6):702–5.

Haddad SI, Khairallah AA. A forgotten chapter in the history of the circulation of the blood. Ann Surg. 1936;104(1):1–8.

Harvey W. Exercitatio Anatomica de Motu Cordis et Sanguinis in Animalibus (Translated): an anatomical study on the motion of the heart and blood in animals 1928.

Hidalgo DA. Fibula free flap: a new method of mandibule reconstruction. Plast Reconstr Surg. 1989;84(1):71–9.

Hidalgo DA, Pusic AL. Free-flap mandibular reconstruction: a 10-year follow-up study. Plast Reconstr Surg. 2002;110(2):438–49; discussion 450-431.

Hueston JT, McConchie IH. A compound pectoral flap. Aust N Z J Surg. 1968;38(1):61–3.

Hwang K. The origins of deltopectoral flaps and the pectoralis major myocutaneous flap. J Craniofac Surg. 2016;27(7):1845–8.

Jackson IT. Closure of secondary palatal fistulae with intra-oral tissue and bone grafting. Br J Plast Surg. 1972;25:93–105.

Jacobson JH, Wallman LJ, Schumacher GA, Flanagan M, Suarez EL, Donaghy RM. Microsurgery as an aid to middle cerebral artery endarterectomy. J Neurosurg. 1962;19:108–15.

Jørgensen MG, Tabatabaeifar S, Toyserkani NM, Sørensen JA. Submental Island flap versus free flap reconstruction for complex head and neck defects. Otolaryngol Head Neck Surg. 2019;161(6):946–53.

Kaplan EN, Kaplan EN. Soft palate repair by levator muscle reconstruction and a buccal mucosal flap. Plast Reconstr Surg. 1975;56(2):129–36.

Kitazawa T, Harashina T, Taira H, Takamatsu A. Bipedicled submental island flap for upper lip reconstruction. Ann Plast Surg. 1999;42(1):83–6.

Kokot N, Mazhar K, Reder LS, Peng GL, Sinha UK. The supraclavicular Artery Island flap in head and neck reconstruction: applications and limitations. JAMA Otolaryngol Head Neck Surg. 2013;139(11):1247–55.

Koshima I, Soeda S. Inferior epigastric artery skin flaps without rectus abdominis muscle. Br J Plast Surg. 1989;42(6):645–8.

Koshima I, Fukuda H, Utunomiya R, Soeda S. The anterolateral thigh flap; variations in its vascular pedicle. Br J Plast Surg. 1989;42(3):260–2.

Krishnamurthy A. A novel clinical application of the classical bakamjian flap in the reconstruction of a sternal chondrosarcoma defect. Indian J Surg. 2015;77(Suppl 3):1444–6.

Lalardrie JP. Hippolyte Morestin 1869–1918. Br J Plast Surg. 1972;25(1):39–41.

Lamberty BG. The supra-clavicular axial patterned flap. Br J Plast Surg. 1979;32(3):207–12.

Levine JP, Bae JS, Soares M, et al. Jaw in a day: total maxillofacial reconstruction using digital technology. Plast Reconstr Surg. 2013;131(6):1386–91.

Link TE, Bisson E, Horgan MA, Tranmer BI, Raymond MP. Donaghy: a pioneer in microneurosurgery. J Neurosurg. 2010;112(6):1176–81.

Lutz BS, Wei FC, Chang SC, Yang KH, Chen IH. Donor site morbidity after suprafascial elevation of the radial forearm flap: a prospective study in 95 consecutive cases. Plast Reconstr Surg. 1999;103(1):132–7.

Malhotra K, Lian TS, Chakradeo V. Vascular anatomy of anterolateral thigh flap. Laryngoscope. 2008;118(4):589–92.

Malt RA, McKhann C. Replantation of severed arms. JAMA. 1964;189:716–22.

Martin D, Pascal JF, Baudet J, et al. The submental island flap: a new donor site. Anatomy and clinical applications as a free or pedicled flap. Plast Reconstr Surg. 1993;92(5):867–73.

Masià J, Sommario M, Cervelli D, Vega C, León X, Pons G. Extended deep inferior epigastric artery perforator flap for head and neck reconstruction: a clinical experience with 100 patients. Head Neck. 2011;33(9):1328–34.

Mathes SJ, Bostwick J. A rectus abdominis myocutaneous flap to reconstruct abdominal wall defects. Br J Plast Surg. 1977;30(4):282–3.

Maxwell GP. Iginio tansini and the origin of the latissimus dorsi musculocutaneous flap. Plast Reconstr Surg. 1980;65(5):686–92.

McCraw JB, Dibbell DG. Experimental definition of independent myocutaneous vascular territories. Plast Reconstr Surg. 1977;60(2):212–20.

Ménard S. An unknown renaissance portrait of tagliacozzi (1545–1599), the founder of plastic surgery. Plast Reconstr Surg Glob Open. 2019;7(1):e2006.

Moscoso JF, Keller J, Genden E, et al. Vascularized bone flaps in oromandibular reconstruction: a comparative anatomic study of bone stock from various donor sites to assess suitability for enosseous dental implants. Arch Otolaryngol Head Neck Surg. 1994;120(1):36–43.

Nassif TM, Vidal L, Bovet JL, Baudet J. The parascapular flap: a new cutaneous microsurgical free flap. Plast Reconstr Surg. 1982;69(4):591–600.

Pairolero PC, Arnold PG. Management of recalcitrant median sternotomy wounds. J Thorac Cardiovasc Surg. 1984;88(3):357–64.
Pallua N, Machens HG, Rennekampff O, Becker M, Berger A. The fasciocutaneous supraclavicular artery island flap for releasing postburn mentosternal contractures. Plast Reconstr Surg. 1997;99(7):1878–84. discussion 1885-1876
Patel UA, Bayles SW, Hayden RE. The submental flap: a modified technique for resident training. Laryngoscope. 2007;117(1):186–9.
Patel A, Harrison P, Cheng A, Bray B, Bell RB. Fibular reconstruction of the maxilla and mandible with immediate implant-supported prosthetic rehabilitation: jaw in a day. Oral Maxillofac Surg Clin North Am. 2019;31(3):369–86.
Conference on Micro-vascular Surgery (1st: 1966: Burlington V. Micro-vascular surgery; report of first conference, October 6-7, 1966), Mary Fletcher Hospital, Burlington, Vermont/Edited by R.M. Peardon Donaghy and M. Gazi Yaşargil. 1966.
Pennington DG, Pelly AD. The rectus abdominis myocutaneous free flap. Br J Plast Surg. 1980;33(2):277–82.
Pribaz J, Stephens W, Crespo L, Gifford G. A new intraoral flap: facial artery musculomucosal (FAMM) flap. Plast Reconstr Surg. 1992;90(3):421–9.
Ramkumar A, Francis NJ, Senthil Kumar R, Dinesh Kumar S. Bipaddled submental artery flap. Int J Oral Maxillofac Surg. 2012;41(4):458–60.
Rayner CRW. Oral mucosal flaps in midfacial reconstruction. Br J Plast Surg. 1984;37(1):43–7.
Rickard RF, Hudson DA. A history of vascular and microvascular surgery. Ann Plast Surg. 2014;73(4):465–72.
Sakai S, Takahashi H, Tanabe H. The extended vertical rectus abdominis myocutaneous flap for breast reconstruction. Plast Reconstr Surg. 1989;83(6):1061–7. discussion 1068-1069
Santoni-Rugiu P, Mazzola R. Leonardo Fioravanti (1517–1588): a barber-surgeon who influenced the development of reconstructive surgery. Plast Reconstr Surg. 1997;99(2):570–5.
Santos D. Retalho escapular: um novo retalho livre microcirurgico. Rev Bras Cir. 1980;70:133–44.
Sasaki TM, Taylor L, Martin L, Baker HW, McConnell DB, Vetto RM. Correction of cervical esophageal stricture using an axial island cheek flap. Head Neck Surg. 1983;6(1):596–9.
Schultheiss D, Denil J. History of the microscope and development of microsurgery: a revolution for reproductive tract surgery. Andrologia. 2002;34(4):234–41.
Serletti JM, Cohen MN, Shedd DP, Vahram Y, Bakamjian MD. 1918 to 2010. Plast Reconstr Surg. 2012;129(5):1218–20.
Song R, Gao Y, Song Y, Yu Y, Song Y. The forearm flap. Clin Plast Surg. 1982;9(1):21–6.
Song YG, Chen GZ, Song YL. The free thigh flap: a new free flap concept based on the septocutaneous artery. Br J Plast Surg. 1984;37(2):149–59.
Soutar DS, McGregor IA. The radial forearm flap in intraoral reconstruction: the experience of 60 consecutive cases. Plast Reconstr Surg. 1986;78(1):1–8.
Soutar DS, Scheker L, Tanner N, McGregor IA. The radial forearm flap: a versatile method for intra-oral reconstruction. Br J Plast Surg. 1983;36:1–8.
Sterne GD, Januszkiewicz JS, Hall PN, Bardsley AF. The submental island flap. Br J Plast Surg. 1996;49(2):85–9.
Strauch B, Bloomberg A, Lewin M. An experimental approach to mandibular replacement island vascular composite rib grafts. Br J Plast Surg. 1971;24(4):334–41.
Sullivan MJ, Carroll WR, Baker SR, Crompton R, Smith-Wheelock M. The free scapular flap for head and neck reconstruction. Am J Otolaryngol. 1990;11(5):318–27.
Tansini. Nuovo processo per l'amputazione della maella per cancre. Refroma Medica. 1896;12(3)
Tarassoli SP, Jessop ZM, Al-Sabah A, et al. Skin tissue engineering using 3D bioprinting: an evolving research field. J Plast Reconstr Aesthet Surg. 2018;71(5):615–23.
Taylor G. Ives. The Angiosome concept. In: Jones BA, editor. Operative microsurgery. McGraw Hill; 2015.
Taylor GI, Daniel RK. The free flap: composite tissue transfer by vascular anastomosis1. Aust N Z J Surg. 1973;43(1):1–3.

Taylor GI, Ham FJ. The free vascularized nerve graft. A further experimental and clinical application of microvascular techniques. Plast Reconstr Surg. 1976;57(4):413–26.
Taylor GI, Townsend P. Composite free flap and tendon transfer: an anatomical study and a clinical technique. Br J Plast Surg. 1979;32(3):170–83.
Taylor G, Miller G, Ham F. The free vascularized bone graft. Plast Reconstr Surg. 1975;55(5):533–44.
Taylor GI, Townsend P, Corlett R. Superiority of the deep circumflex iliac vessels as the supply for free groin flaps. Clinical work. Plast Reconstr Surg. 1979a;64(6):745–59.
Taylor GI, Townsend P, Corlett R. Superiority of the deep circumflex iliac vessels as the supply for free groin flaps. Plast Reconstr Surg. 1979b;64(5):595–604.
Taylor GI, Corlett R, Boyd JB. The extended deep inferior epigastric flap: a clinical technique. Plast Reconstr Surg. 1983;72(6):751–65.
Taylor GI, Corlett RJ, Boyd JB. The versatile deep inferior epigastric (inferior rectus abdominis) flap. Br J Plast Surg. 1984;37(3):330–50.
Tipton JB. Closure of large septal perforations with a labial-buccal flap. Plast Reconstr Surg. 1970;46(5):514–5.
Tomba P, Viganò A, Ruggieri P, Gasbarrini A. Gaspare Tagliacozzi, pioneer of plastic surgery and the spread of his technique throughout Europe in "De Curtorum Chirurgia per Insitionem". Eur Rev Med Pharmacol Sci. 2014;18(4):445–50.
Trautman J, Gore S, Potter M, et al. Supraclavicular flap repair in the free flap era. ANZ J Surg. 2018;88(6):540–6.
Urken ML, Vickery C, Weinberg H, Buchbinder D, Biller HF. The internal oblique-iliac crest osseomyocutaneous microvascular free flap in head and neck reconstruction. J Reconstr Microsurg. 1989;5(3):203–14. discussion 215-206
Urken ML, Buchbinder D, Costantino PD, et al. Oromandibular reconstruction using microvascular composite flaps: report of 210 cases. Arch Otolaryngol Head Neck Surg. 1998;124(1):46–55.
Valentini V, Cassoni A, Marianetti TM, Battisti A, Terenzi V, Iannetti G. Anterolateral thigh flap for the reconstruction of head and neck defects: alternative or replacement of the radial forearm flap? J Craniofacial Surg. 2008;19(4):1148–53.
Villaret DB, Futran NA. The indications and outcomes in the use of osteocutaneous radial forearm free flap. Head Neck. 2003;25(6):475–81.
Vinh VQ, Van Anh T, Ogawa R, Hyakusoku H. Anatomical and clinical studies of the supraclavicular flap: analysis of 103 flaps used to reconstruct neck scar contractures. Plast Reconstr Surg. 2009;123(5):1471–80.
Wallace AF. The early development of pedicle flaps. J R Soc Med. 1978;71(11):834–8.
Wei FC, Chen HC, Chuang CC, Noordhoff MS. Fibular osteoseptocutaneous flap: anatomic study and clinical application. Plast Reconstr Surg. 1986;78(2):191–200.
Wei FC, Seah CS, Tsai YC, Liu SJ, Tsai MS. Fibula osteoseptocutaneous flap for reconstruction of composite mandibular defects. Plast Reconstr Surg. 1994;93(2):294–304; discussion 305-296.
Wood J. Case of extreme deformity of the neck and forearm, from the cicatrices of a burn, cured by extension, excision, and transplantation of skin, adjacent and remote. Med Chir Trans. 1863;46:149–59.
Yang D, Gu Y, Wu M. Thumb reconstruction by free second toe transplantation. Report of 40 cases. Zhonghua Wai Ke Za Zhi. 1977;15(1):13–8.
Yang GF, Chen PJ, Gao YZ, et al. Forearm free skin flap transplantation: a report of 56 cases. 1981. Br J Plast Surg. 1997;50(3):162–5.
Yilmaz M, Menderes A, Barutçu A. Submental artery island flap for reconstruction of the lower and mid face. Ann Plast Surg. 1997;39(1):30–5.
Zenga J, Emerick KS, Deschler DG. Submental Island flap: a technical update. Ann Otol Rhinol Laryngol. 2019;128(12):1177–81.

Microneurosurgery

Benjamin Palla, Preston Dekker, and Michael Miloro

"The patient is never to be abandoned to his sufferings."
– John Collins Warren (1829)

"Although the interests of clinicians in peripheral nerve injuries seems to wax in wartime and wane when peace comes, the peripheral nervous system has few rivals in the fascination it has exerted over the minds of workers in many fields of medical science."
– Sir Herbert Seddon (1943)

"The resolving power of the unaided eye does not permit an appreciation of the problem nor a true appraisal of nerve suture."
– James W. Smith (1964)

1 First Accounts of Peripheral Nerve Surgery

Prior to the twentieth century, most nerve injuries were left unrepaired. The surgical conditions were not ideal for such delicate and precise surgery required for suturing the epineurium, let alone in identifying the various neural layers. If a nerve injury received the attention of a surgeon, it was most likely for ablative purposes only. However, there have always been surgeons willing to endeavor on behalf of the treatment of patients with debilitating diseases, for which nerve damage is certainly one of these, with significant effects on quality of life.

Before nerves could be transected and repaired, they had to first be identified. **Herophilus of Chalcedon** (335–280 BCE) is credited for first identifying nerves, by differentiating nerves from tendons. The work was expanded further by the well-known physician, **Galen of Pergamon** (CE 121–200), who described nerve injuries in an interesting group of patients known as the gladiators (Galen of Pergamon 1576). Galen may also be the first physician to experiment on nerves as he transected the recurrent laryngeal nerve in pigs and described the weakening or loss of voice he observed after transecting unilateral or bilateral nerves.

B. Palla (✉) · P. Dekker · M. Miloro
Department of Oral & Maxillofacial Surgery, University of Illinois at Chicago, Chicago, IL, USA
e-mail: palla1@uic.edu

E. M. Ferneini et al. (eds.), *The History of Maxillofacial Surgery*,
https://doi.org/10.1007/978-3-030-89563-1_17

Courageous efforts were also made in a time when little was known of nerve physiology. **Ambroise Paré** (1510–1590) performed a nerve transection for King Charles IX after he developed a contracture from bloodletting. He took advice from surgeons such as **Guy de Chauliac** (1300–1368), physician to Pope Clement, and **Lanfranc of Milan** (1250–1306), the father of French surgery – first to suggest the primary repair of nerve injuries.

However, the first detailed description of peripheral nerve repair was provided by an Italian surgeon named **Gabriele Graf Von Ferrara** (1543–1627) in 1596 (Artico et al. 1996). During Ferrara's life, the Renaissance was blossoming across Europe, and the Italian Peninsula was the epicenter, with a significant study of anatomy and surgery. Just prior to Ferrara, **Leonardo da Vinci** (1452–1519) completed his anatomic works and dissections, and the year of Ferrara's birth, **Andreas Vesalius** (1514–1564) published his classic work, *De Humani Corporis Fabrica Libri Septem* (1543). Ferrara joined the Brothers Hospitallers of Saint John of God and worked at the Ospedale Fatebenefratelli in Milan in 1591, taking his vows and becoming known as "Fra Gabriello." Soon afterward, Ferrara published the first version of what would become his defining contribution to the study of peripheral nerve repair entitled, "Nova selva di cirugia di divisa in due parti," in 1596 (Ferrara 1596). This "due parti" soon became a "tre parti" with the release of his second edition, for which he provided details of the following: (1) surgery, (2) medicaments, and (3) figures of nerve treatment (Fig. 1).

Ferrara provided exquisite details of his surgical studies. Working 400 years ago, it is fascinating to read his descriptions now and imagine working in similar conditions (Fig. 2). In his work, Ferrara describes his stepwise process of identifying the nerve stumps, dissecting them away from surrounding soft tissues, and ensuring that the proper length of nerve was available so repair could occur without significant tension. Following the realignment of the nerve stumps, gentle suturing was done using a small needle and a suture made of turtle gut dipped in a concoction of red wine, roses, and rosemary. After, a hot oil mixture of herbaceous plants was applied. The surgery was followed by a period of rest and immobilization for the patient. In addition, like many nerve surgeons who would come after, Ferrara traveled to aid soldiers injured during war, which, for him, was at the Battle of White Mountain during the Thirty Years' War. He traveled extensively to aid patients, performing work in Rome, Krakow, Vienna, Prague, Trento, and Trieste. The skull of Ferrara can still be found at the Klosterkirche der Barmherzigen Brüder in Vienna, which he founded, in addition to the Hospital of the Barmherzigen Brüder, now the largest and oldest hospital in Vienna.

For centuries that followed, most surgeons avoided interventions related to maladies involving nerves. One of the first to advocate for surgical resection of neuromas was English surgeon **William Wood** (1783–1858), an audacious proposal at the time (Wood 1829). Yet, he was surpassed by fellow Englishman, **Joseph Swan** (1791–1874), and French surgeon, **Alfred L.M. Velpeau** (1795–1867), who would propose an even more radical idea for their time that divided nerves should be repaired (Swan 1834; Velpeau 1841).

John Collins Warren (1778–1856) provided an early publication on the treatment of peripheral nerves in the *Boston Medical and Surgical Journal* in **1829**

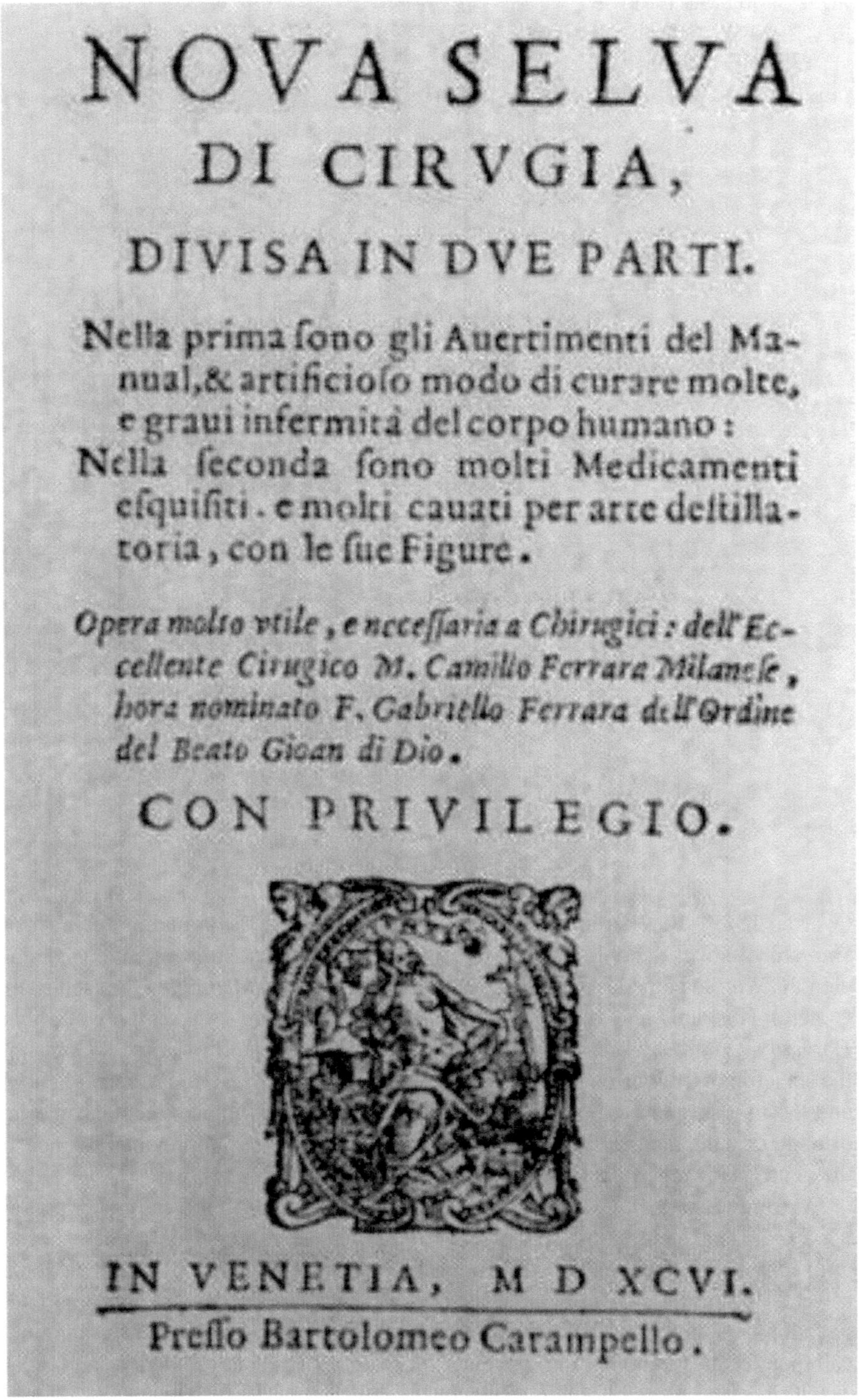

NOVA SELVA

DI CIRVGIA,

DIVISA IN DVE PARTI.

Nella prima ſono gli Auertimenti del Manual,& artificioſo modo di curare molte, e graui infermità del corpo humano:

Nella ſeconda ſono molti Medicamenti eſquiſiti. e molti cauati per arte deſtillatoria, con le ſue Figure.

Opera molto vtile, e neceſſaria a Chirugici: dell'Eccellente Cirugico M. Camillo Ferrara Milaneſe, hora nominato F. Gabriello Ferrara dell'Ordine del Beato Gioan di Dio.

CON PRIVILEGIO.

IN VENETIA, M D XCVI.

Preſſo Bartolomeo Carampello.

Fig. 1 The title page from Ferrara's 1596 "Nova selva di cirugia; divida in due parti"

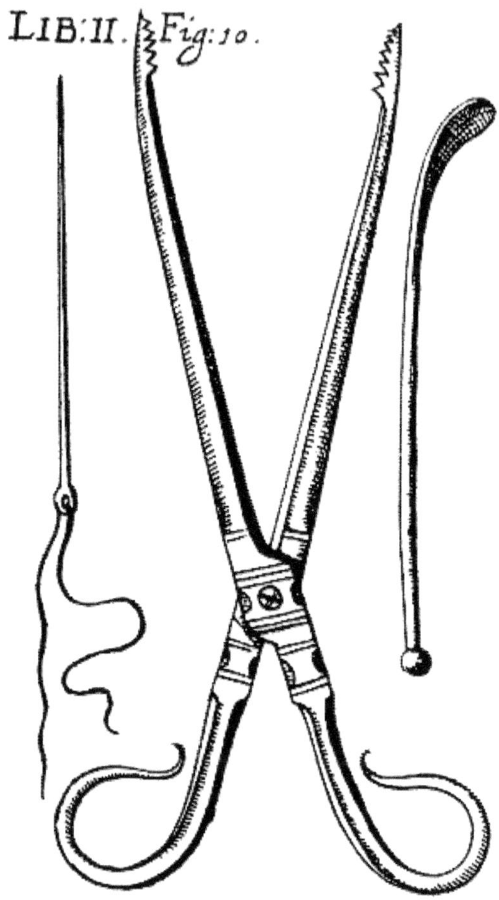

Fig. 2 Instruments used by Ferrara to perform his nerve repair

(Warren 1829). JC Warren, son of John Warren (1753–1815), founding member of Harvard Medical School, was himself a prolific physician, surgeon, and academician. JC Warren helped found *The New England Journal of Medicine*, Massachusetts General Hospital, and the Warren Anatomical Museum – currently housed in Harvard's Countway Library, which not only houses the skull of Phineas Gage but the skeleton of JC Warren as well. He was the first Dean of Harvard Medical School and the first surgeon to operate on a patient using general inhalational anesthesia, provided by the dentist **William T.G. Morton** (1819–1868), a previous partner to the dentist **Horace Wells** (1815–1848).

Warren was one of the first to describe a stepwise approach in treating peripheral nerve pain and neuralgias, specifically trigeminal neuralgia. This process began with identifying the specific nerve and then performing medical treatment for a 6-week duration – which included a combination of iron carbonate, iron sulfate, belladonna, conium, hyoscyamus, stramonium, opium, cinchona, sulfate of quinine, calomel, leeches, bloodletting, cupping, blistering, moxa, caustic potash, and other hot fomentations. In the cases of ongoing neuralgia, a surgeon should then intervene and excise a portion of the nerve, preferably a healthy portion, and the more proximal the better.

Similar to Ferrara, Warren noted observations that appeared almost prophetic despite the lack of knowledge related to nerve physiology during his era. Specifically, speaking on the temporal relation between injury and treatment, Warren said, "When the disease is of longstanding, neither excision nor amputation of the limb is to be relied upon: for the whole course of the nerve becomes diseased." He stated surgery would have better success if performed "within a few weeks of the origin of the disease." Yet, like others working before the availability of Nylén's surgical microscope, he was limited by magnification, stating that the "membrane lining the fibrils, -a part so minute, that we can scarcely expect to support the opinion by observation" (Warren 1829).

A breakthrough in the understanding of neurophysiology came with the observations of **Augustus Volney Waller** (1816–1870), an English neurophysiologist. It was his **1850** paper that described what is now known as "Wallerian degeneration." In the study, Waller transected the glossopharyngeal and hypoglossal nerves in frogs and studied the outcome histologically (Waller 1851). He observed that the distal nerve inevitably degenerated, while the proximal segment would remain healthy. Such a phenomena was noted in **1795** by surgeon **William C. Cruickshank** (1745–1800), but this observation was not fully appreciated by scientists of that era who believed that nerves are healed by "reunion" and not by this proposed cellular process of degeneration followed by "regeneration" (Cruikshank and Hunter 1795).

The credit for performing the first successful nerve resection for trigeminal neuralgia is given to **John Murray Carnochan** (1817–1887), an American surgeon practicing in New York (Carnochan 1859). He operated on three patients with unrelenting pain of the infraorbital region, all who had previously been treated with medical therapy similar to JC Warren's approach above. In **1856**, under chloroform anesthesia, Carnochan exposed the maxilla in these patients in an approach similar to the Weber Ferguson incision and resected the entirety of the maxillary branch of the trigeminal nerve up to the foramen rotundum. The first patient, a 69-year-old French physician, underwent surgery a day after meeting Carnochan. The surgery was successful, and seemingly immediate, as the French physician "ordered chicken broth, and wine and water" after resection. Remarkably, all three of these records of trigeminal nerve resection were successful, and no recurrence of trigeminal neuralgia was noted by Carnochan.

Significant advancement in the understanding of nerve repair is often attributed to the experiences working with injuries during the American Civil War (1861–1865), specifically to the work of **Silas Weir Mitchell** (1829–1914). Mitchell was a physician in Philadelphia and previous acquaintance to the Union's Surgeon General, **W.A. Hammond** (1828–1900). Hammond established a unit at the Turner's Lane Military Hospital in Philadelphia that would focus on nerve injuries and amputations. Hammond appointed Mitchell to what would colloquially be called "Stump Hospital." Mitchell is considered by many as the father of neurology and coined the term "causalgia," now known as complex regional pain syndrome (CRPS). Mitchell provided his experiences at "Stump Hospital" in two books, one in **1864** and the other in **1872**, that significantly impacted future physicians and surgeons (Mitchell et al. 1864; Mitchell 1872).

Across the Atlantic Ocean, **Jean Joseph Émile Létiévant** (1830–1884) was also publishing an immense 548-page treatise on nerves, published in **1873** (Létiévant 1873). In these pages, Létiévant cited articles in five different languages and described one of the first records of nerve repair. Prior to this, most surgeons dealt with nerves only as far as performing nerve resections for relief of neuralgia. Létiévant described the use of metallic sutures to repair nerve injuries, specifically one related to the ulnar nerve in **1869**. His book described nerve *sections*, *résections*, *suture*, *autoplasty*, and *greffe* as well as a "tingling sign" when percussing over some repaired nerves – but he neglected the significance of this as most during this time period did not believe nerves could regenerate. Shortly after, a German field surgeon **Bernhard von Langenbeck** (1810–1887) successfully repaired a median nerve in **1876** (Langenbeck 1876).

Although a growing number of surgeons were attempting nerve repair, the surgical technique was limited to re-aligning the proximal stump with the distal segment. In order to accomplish this, nerves were often stretched, liberated, and transposed, and the bony joints were flexed, sometimes allowing up to 8-cm gaps to be bridged (Davis and Cleveland 1934). These techniques showed little concern for the deleterious effects of tension on the nerve repair site. Performance of the first nerve graft is credited to **J.M. Philipeaux** and **Alfred Vulpian** (1826–1867), who performed their pioneering work in **1863** and **1870** (Philipeax and Vulpian 1863, 1870). In the initial study, the surgeons cut the hypoglossal and lingual nerves in a dog; then, using an optic nerve from a separate recently deceased puppy, they bridge the hypoglossal nerve to the lingual nerve. Although the connection was re-established and opened avenues of future practice, the dog unfortunately died. The second study by Philipeaux and Vulpian described seven attempts at nerve autografts, with two of these being reported as successes. In these dogs, a 2-cm segment of the hypoglossal and lingual nerves was excised. The lingual nerve segment was then utilized to reconnect the stumps of the hypoglossal nerve. In two puppies, movement was later reported in the distal tongue, both spontaneously and with the use of galvanized stimulation. Upon animal sacrifice and histologic examination, new nerve fibers were observed bridging the nerve repair sites.

In **1873**, a German surgeon named **Eduard Albert** (1841–1900) would attempt to advance the works of Philipeaux and Vulpian, attempting the first nerve graft in humans (Albert 1887). In his 1887 book, Albert describes two patients, one with a median nerve injury and the other with an ulnar nerve injury. Albert resected the nerve lesions back to a healthy proximal and distal stump and then used a recently amputated lower limb from separate patients to acquire a tibial nerve graft: a length of 3 cm in the first patient and 10 cm in the second patient. He sutured the nerve ends with catgut via a direct and indirect technique; however, as we may expect with our current knowledge of immunology, both grafts soon failed. Four years later,

Albert did perform a nerve graft experiment in dogs, exchanging the right and left sciatic nerves, in which case he reported success, with some recovery of motor function.

Building upon these creative techniques of nerve repair and nerve grafting, **Themistocles Gluck** (1853–1942) is credited with the first use of nerve entubulation, performed in **1881** (Gluck 1881). For this procedure, Gluck used an absorbable decalcified bone tube, developed by **Gustav Adolf Neuber** (1850–1932) initially for the use as a surgical drain in **1879** (Neuber 1879). Gluck described bridging a severed nerve with this Neuber tube, but unfortunately the attempt failed. A successful attempt was performed the same year however, but this was achieved by **Constant Vanlair** (1839–1914) (Vanlair 1882). On September 30, **1881**, Vanlair, who witnessed Gluck's procedure, resected a 3-cm segment of the sciatic nerve in a dog and bridged the defect with a 4-cm version of Neuber's decalcified bone tube. Vanlair reported the dog later regained mobility and a microscopic exam after the animal at time of sacrifice showed the presence of bridging nerve fibers.

Although some, such as the father of neurosurgery **Harvey Cushing** (1869–1939), would write about their experiences with peripheral nerve surgery, comments may be limited to a few case descriptions (Cushing 1983, 1903). A significant advancement body of work was when **Henry Head** (1861–1940) and **James Sherren (1872–1945)** began to focus on peripheral nerve injuries at the London Hospital in **1905** (Head and Sherren 1905). Focusing on peripheral nerve repair of the hand, they were among the first significant studies on a large population using objective criteria. Post-operative patients were evaluated utilizing instruments that remain extremely familiar to us in the twenty-first century: a cotton wool brush for detection of light touch, a compass to discriminate two points, a blunt pencil for pressure, a hot or cold glass tube for temperature, a tuning fork for vibration, and a sharp needle for pain.

Head and Sherren described in great detail the recovery pattern of injured nerves. After the initial anesthesia, pain and temperature sensation returned first, followed months later by "higher forms of sensibility" such as light touch. They took Weir-Mitchell's term "causalgia" and coined the term "hyperalgesia" to describe the "exaggeration of sensibility to pain" (Head and Sherren 1905).

Yet, Head was frustrated with what seemed to him to be unreliable patient descriptions of their pain and sensation. In his **1908** book with **William Halse Rivers Rivers** (1864–1922), Head relied on the only person he could definitely trust – himself. On April 25, 1903, Head allowed Mr. Sherren and an assistant Mr. Dean to make a 6.5-inch incision of his left forearm to remove a segment of the nerve from both his *N radialis and N cutaneous antebrachial lateralis*, placing two silk sutures in both nerves for realignment (Rivers and Head 1908). The book, which contained 450 pages and 19 photos of Head's hand, characterized the details of this experiment over the next 5 years (Fig. 3).

Through the work of Head and Sherren, surgeons began to differentiate various nerve insults and how they affected recovery – complete division, partial division, or blunt trauma. They were also adept in noting the sensation of "pins and needles" or "tingling" that some patients described after a nerve operation.

This later description is one which would be fully elucidated a decade later by two physicians during the WWI, although they were from opposite sides of the battlefield.

The German physiologist **Paul Hoffmann** (1884–1962) and the French neurologist **Jules Tinel** (1879–1952) described their observations only 6 months apart in **1915** during the WWI (Tinel 1915; Hoffmann 1915a). Their description became known as the "Tinel-Hoffmann Sign." Eager surgeons rounding on their patients only days after operation attempted various methods to determine the likelihood of successful repair and neurosensory recovery, a visual depiction of surgeons that remains true today. Both Hoffmann and Tinel noted that by tapping with light percussion just distal to the site of nerve injury and repair, some patients would experience a tingling sensation radiating in the distribution of the sensory nerve. If this occurred, it was considered a positive sign and a prognostic indicator that nerve regeneration was occurring across the site of repair or injury. In Hoffmann's paper, he even calculated a rate of regeneration based on the location of percussion and tingling, calculated as 2.25 mm/day in 1915 (Hoffmann 1915b). However, with the loss of Germany in WWI and WWII, much of Hoffmann's work was censored and unknown to the Western medical establishment for decades, finally translated to English in 1993 (Hoffmann et al. 1993).

Also performing nerve repair during WWI was **William Wayne Babcock** (1872–1963), an American surgeon (Babcock 1907). While operating on failed nerve repairs, Babcock noted a physical scar that seemed to mechanically obstruct the regenerating nerve fibers. This finding had been noted by prior surgeons, but Babcock was one of the first to give significant attention to preventing scar formation at the site of repair. He promulgated a belief of performing "nerve dissociation" in such cases, later termed "hersage," which involved incising the nerve sheath and separating out the individual nerve fibers or "skeletonizing" the nerve (Babcock 1907).

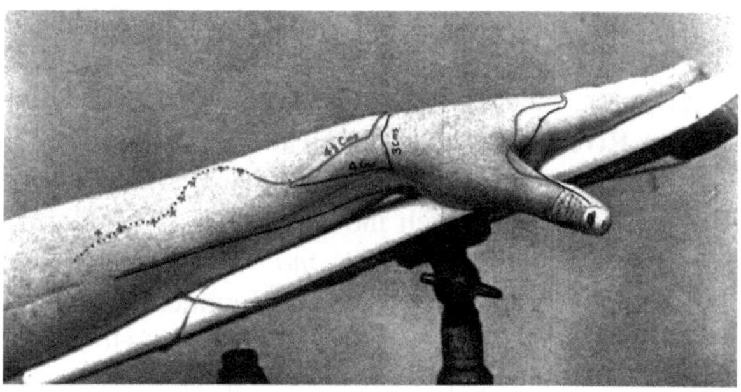

Fig. 3 Photograph from the 1908 book by Henry Head and William HR Rivers. This photo displays the left hand and forearm of Head, who allowed Rivers to perform a nerve resection so he could study the recovery pattern. Incision site and scar are visible on the proximal forearm

2 Development of Microneurosurgery

After WWI, advances in peripheral nerve surgery continued, in large part to the design and implementation of the first surgical microscope by **Carl-Olof Siggesson Nylén** (1892–1978). Nylén, in addition to being an Olympic tennis player, was an otolaryngologist and considered the father of microsurgery. Nylén described the development of what was first called an "otomicroscope" implemented in 1921 (Nylen and Person 1922).

Nylén first used a monocular microscope designed by Brinell to repair labyrinthine fistulas of the inner ear. The Brinell microscope had a magnification of 10–15X, but soon after Nylén designed a monocular microscope with an engineer **N. Person** (1922) that could achieve a magnification of 120X. The same year, **Zeiss** and **Gunnar Holmgren**, to whom Nylén was an assistant surgeon, designed the first binocular surgical microscope. The binocular microscope became widely popularized, and continual improvements to working distance, field of view, and illumination have occurred (Nylen 1954).

The implementation of the surgical microscope coincided with an immense increase in the knowledge of nerve physiology and regeneration. **Santiago Ramón y Cajal** (1852–1934), a 1906 Nobel laureate with Camillo Golgi, described the axonal cone, neurotropism, and the degeneration and regeneration model of nerves in his **1928** book (Ramon y Cajal 1928). In **1930**, **Sterling Bunnell**, the father of hand surgery, reported the first successful autogenous nerve graft of the facial nerve (Bunnell 1937). In 1934, **Loyal Davis** reviewed nerve repair techniques from nerve implants, nerve flaps, suture à distance, tubulization, nerve crossing, and nerve transplants or grafts (Davis and Cleveland 1934). Davis was keen to observe the difficulty in acquiring autogenous grafts of similar caliber that also had low donor site morbidity. He, like others, saw the potential in nerve allografts as an alternative, but it would be many years before an understanding of their immunogenicity progressed for this alternative to be realized.

In **1942**, **Herbert John Seddon** (1903–1977), an English orthopedic surgeon at Oxford, described a classification for nerve injuries that remains the foundation of modern practice today (Seddon 1942). Seddon initially described three types of lesions of nerves which were classified by morphologic and clinical behavior: first, "neurotmesis" (division of a nerve), a "cutting" or separation of the nerve with complete loss of sensation and motor function and low likelihood for spontaneous recovery; second, "axonotmesis" (lesion in continuity), a complete separation of nerve fibers with complete peripheral degeneration, but intact sheath and supporting structures, and high likelihood of spontaneous recovery; and third, "neuropraxia" (transient conduction block), a short-lived paralysis from disturbed nerve conduction without axonal degeneration. In his paper and speeches (Seddon 1943), Seddon also discussed treatments for each type of nerve injury and was an advocate for surgical exploration, even if only to incise the most fibrotic area in nerve lesions in order to evaluate for the presence of nerve fibers.

Seddon's classification of nerve injuries was soon updated by Australian **Sydney Sunderland** (1910–1993) in **1951** (Sunderland 1951). Sunderland, who was the Chair of Anatomy at the University of Melbourne, based the classification scheme on his detailed understanding of the peripheral nerve anatomy. Sunderland's main focus was to provide further clarification on the wide spectrum of Seddon's "axonotmesis" category. Sunderland provided "five degrees of nerve injury," from least to most severe, based upon the anatomy of the axon, axonal sheath (Schwann cell, neurilemma, endoneurium), funiculus (perineurium), and epineurium (Fig. 4).

"First-degree" injuries were associated with no anatomic disturbance, but simply a compromised conduction of the nerve, equivalent to Seddon's "neuropraxia." Seddon's "axonotmesis" was divided into second-, third-, and fourth-degree injuries. "Second-degree" injuries involved only the axons. "Third-degree" injuries disrupted the axon and the axonal sheath. "Fourth-degree" injuries disrupt the axons, axonal sheath, and funiculus, only leaving the epineurium intact. "Fifth-degree" injuries are a complete separation of all anatomical nerve structures, equivalent to Seddon's neurotmesis. Wallerian degeneration was described to be present in second-, third-, fourth-, and fifth-degree nerve injuries. Many years later, **Mackinnon** and **Dellon** would describe a "sixth-degree" injury that would account for the fact that some injuries may have mixed components of various degrees of injury (Mackinnon and Dellon 1988).

However, both Seddon and Sunderland should not simply be remembered for their classification systems. Both performed significant research related to nerve physiology and repair techniques that future generations would build upon. In 1943, Seddon already calculated the average nerve regeneration rate of 1.5 mm/day (Seddon 1943). Seddon established the Peripheral Nerve Injury Centre within the Department of Orthopedics at the University of Oxford, within which Peter Medawar started his career developing a plasma to connect nerves without the use of sutures; Medawar later received the 1960 Nobel Prize for his contributions to grafting and immune tolerance (Young and Medawar 1940). Sunderland also published

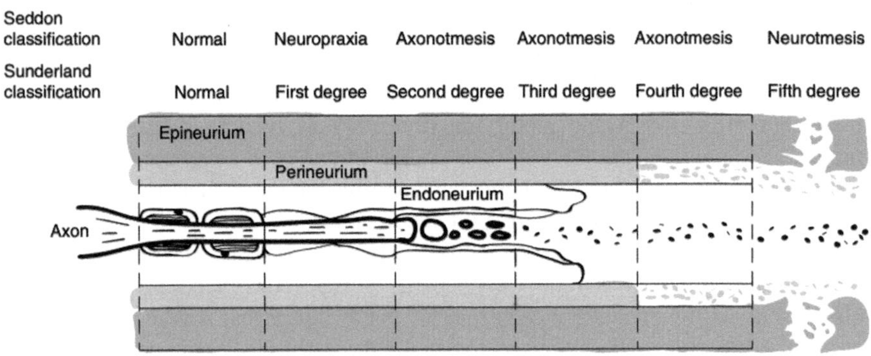

Fig. 4 Schematic representation of nerve anatomy and the various degrees of nerve injury. Above the figure are the classifications systems of Seddon and Sunderland with their associated degree of nerve damage

immensely and wrote a landmark text on nerve injuries and repair (Sunderland 1968). Both Seddon and Sunderland were knighted for their contributions.

Also working in Seddon's Peripheral Nerve Injury Centre was **W. Bremner Highet**, who contributed significantly to our understanding of how tension affected the outcomes of nerve repair (Highet and Holmes 1943; Highet and Sanders 1943). Prior to his studies in 1943, the standard technique of nerve repair was twofold: (1) preparation of healthy stumps and (2) tension-free, end-to-end alignment. This method is similar to that used today; however, prior to the 1940s, most large defects achieved tension-free closure via mobilization of the nerve and some degree of joint flexion. For instance, in the first article by Highet and Holmes, a patient required resection of an 11.5-cm segment of the lateral popliteal nerve. To close the nerve gap, Highet mobilized the nerve from the surrounding tissue (1.5-cm gain in nerve length), extended the hip (1-cm gain in nerve length), and then flexed the knee to 100° (9-cm gain in nerve length). The knee was held in this flexed position via a cast for 23 days, after which it was slowly straightened over 60 days. Highet noted that in five of their six cases treated by this methodology, no recovery occurred, and when histologic exam was performed, no nerve fibers crossed the repair site (Fig. 5).

Highet and Sanders confirmed this study in dogs, removing a portion of the external popliteal nerve and then flexing the knee to achieve an end-to-end

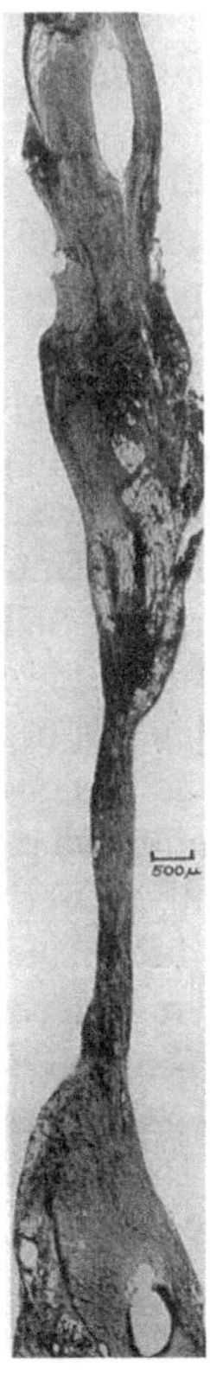

Fig. 5 Working in Seddon's Peripheral Nerve Injury Center, W Bremner Highet displayed the poor results from joint flexion and the subsequent extension of nerves that lead to significant tension, failure, and scarring

re-approximation. The dogs were placed in casts for 14 days, after which a rapid or passive extension of the knee was performed. In both groups, the postoperative stretching of nerves led to separation of the stumps, edema, fibrosis, and degeneration. Nerves did not lengthen, and the fibrosis around the repair site became adherent to the surrounding tissues in all animals. The authors discussed two future possibilities. First, implement the use of amnioplastin, which in **1941 Robert Lambert** had used to prevent scarring of peripheral nerves to the surrounding tissue (Rogers 1941). Secondly, improve and implement novel nerve grafting techniques.

Yet, despite this progress, results from surgical interventions did not occur initially, and nerve repair outcomes at this time remained poor. **Mackenzie** and **Woods** showed in **1961** that only 50% of patients recovered from repair of the median nerve (Mackenzie and Woods 1961), which were similar to findings of the **Medical Research Council** in **1954** under Seddon (1954).

In the 1960s, a varied group of peripheral nerve surgeons, most working in the upper extremities and hands, began to inquire about ways to improve nerve repair techniques. Surgeons saw the improvement their peers in microvascular surgery were experiencing with the use of the surgical microscope. Microscopes had not been used in peripheral nerve surgery up to this time. **James W. Smith** was an early advocate for the implementation combined with new instruments used by those in the jewelry and diamond cutting field (Smith 1964). At this time 7-0 silk and 8-0 nylon sutures were being used, cutting needles, and methylene blue for contrast. Smith seemingly proved the benefit of the surgical microscopes by performing the repair of the sciatic nerve in rabbits, one side by the unaided eye and the other by microscope.

Hanno Millesi (1927–2017) was an Austrian plastic surgeon who spent his career focusing on repair of peripheral nerves of the arm (Millesi 1973). Like Smith, he was also an early proponent of using the surgical microscope for nerve repair. Millesi is often credited with first describing the interfascicular suture technique in 1968 (Millesi 1968). At this time, Millesi proposed using only perineurial nerve sutures, and the epineurium at the stumps was removed to prevent scarring.

Nerve repair of the head and neck specifically benefited from the work of a German group led by **Jarg-Erich Hausamen**, a German oral and maxillofacial surgeon. Along with Berger, Meissl, Samii, and Schmidseder, this group focused on the repair and reconstruction of the facial nerve, inferior alveolar nerve (IAN), accessory nerve, and lingual nerve. In one study, Hausamen took five groups of rabbits to compare IAN repair and reconstruction techniques (Hausamen et al. 1974). The results were overwhelming and clearly showed that the autologous nerve graft group performed significantly better compared to the other four (nerves cut or resected with and without direct suture re-approximation). This study supported previous findings showing a high success of the use of the sural nerve as a graft for IAN reconstruction (Hausamen et al. 1973).

Bruce Donoff and **Walter Guralnick** from Harvard School of Dental Medicine and Massachusetts General Hospital discussed repair of the IAN and lingual nerve in 1982 (Donoff and Guralnick 1982). Using previous studies with dogs, they discussed the benefit of delayed primary repair (1–3 weeks after injury) and secondary repair (several weeks to months after injury) based upon the degeneration and regeneration nerve models.

3 Contemporary Practice of Microneurosurgery

The practice of peripheral nerve surgery as it is performed today consists of the cumulative work and endeavors of the pioneers mentioned above. Many advancements continue to occur in contemporary practice, with new innovative techniques specific to peripheral nerve repair in the hand and extremities that are beyond the scope of this chapter. However, with regard to peripheral nerve repair of the head and neck region, and specifically of the trigeminal nerve and its terminal branches, other surgical specialties have balked at addressing these injuries. The field of oral and maxillofacial surgery has stepped into this void and accepted responsibility for this complex anatomic field and difficult surgical environment. Perhaps one reason oral and maxillofacial surgeons may have become interested in these injuries is due to the significant number which occur iatrogenically within the field of dentistry, most commonly from the third molar removal in the mandible (Pogrel and Thamby 1999). Due to the unexpected nature of many of these injuries, a large aspect of recent research endeavors has been aimed to better evaluate the risks associated with nerve injury. It has been estimated that nearly 40% of patients with trigeminal nerve injuries are involved with medico-legal litigation (Pogrel and Thamby 1999).

First, a comment on the current terminology in practice today. "Nerve repair" refers to the procedure when two native nerve ends are sutured directly to each other head to head, such as in a direct repair after neurolysis. The term "nerve reconstruction" is a nerve surgery that uses a nerve graft, either autogenous nerve graft or allograft nerve, that is placed between two native nerve ends to bridge and reconstruct a defect. Finally, the term anastomosis is more specific to the repair of arterial or venous vessels and not appropriate for use with nerves.

In current dentoalveolar surgery practice, the vast majority of nerve injuries occur following third molar surgery. The risk of injury is estimated at 0.5–5.0% for the IAN and 0.6–2.0% for the lingual nerve during third molar extraction (Pogrel and Thamby 1999). Patients undergoing orthognathic surgery, maxillofacial trauma, or oncologic reconstruction may have a higher incidence, but oftentimes these patients are more accepting and understanding of sensory deficits. In recent decades, the development of dental implants has been associated with another iatrogenic cause of neurosensory injury pertaining specifically to the IAN.

In order to evaluate the proximity between the inferior alveolar nerve and the mandibular third molar, a landmark study was published in 1990. **Rood** and **Shehab** presented seven radiographic signs visible on panoramic radiographs that are associated with a close proximity between the roots of the mandibular third molar and IAN (Rood and Shehab 1990). Three of the seven radiographic signs were significantly associated with nerve injury, which included diversion of the canal, interruption of the corticated white line of the mandibular canal, and darkening of the root – the latter being the most significant.

Efforts were also made to determine the location of the lingual nerve. In 1984, **John Kiesselbach** and **Jack Chamberlain** performed dissection on cadavers, finding the lingual nerve located at 2.28 mm inferior and 0.58 mm medial from the lingual crest and plate in the third molar region (Kiesselbach and Chamberlain 1984). The authors also reported direct contact with the lingual plate in 62% of cadavers, with the nerve located above the level of the crest in 17.6% of cadavers. This article was followed in 1997 by **Michael Miloro**, whose group used MRI in ten living subjects that displayed the average lingual nerve that was located 2.75 mm inferior and 2.5 mmmedial to the lingual crest and plate, with 10% above the crest and 25% in contact with the lingual plate (Miloro et al. 1997).

In recent years, an additional cause of nerve injury that has become more prominent is the occurrence of nerve injury after routine nerve blocks. A significant amount of research initially went to distinguishing the relevance of two potential causes, namely, the trauma that occurs from needle penetration of a nerve and that of the toxicity from the local anesthesia drug. Using rat sciatic nerve however, **Hillerup** and colleagues displayed significant evidence indicating that the primary factor of injury was related to the high concentration of local anesthesia (4%), rather than from needle trauma alone (Hillerup et al. 2011).

In 1989, **G.E. Ghali** and **Bruce Epker** provided a high-impact article on clinical neurosensory testing (NST) as it relates to the trigeminal nerve (Ghali and Epker 1989). Later studies by **John Zuniga** have evaluated the accuracy of these various methods for NST: two-point discrimination and brush stroke direction (Level A), static light touch (Level B), and nociception via temperature or pinprick (Level C) (Zuniga et al. 1998). **Roger Meyer**, who speculated on the poor outcomes of nerve repair when delayed over 1-year at the American Association of Oral and Maxillofacial Surgery Meeting in 1991, later provided the evidence base in 2010 with Zuniga (Bagheri et al. 2010). Interestingly however, **M. Anthony Pogrel** showed only 10% of these patients undergo surgical intervention (Pogrel 2002).

The work of both **Susan Mackinnon** and **A. Lee Dellon** has brought significant advancement to nerve repair starting in the 1980s. Although innovating new techniques for nerve repair particularly for limbs, Mackinnon and Dellon modified the British Medical Research Council Scale for assessing nerve repair, originally published in 1954 by Sir Seddon (1954). They specifically developed the guidelines for assessing sensory function in the extremities (Mackinnon and Dellon 1988). This guideline was later adapted and applied to assessing the recovery of the trigeminal nerve by **Thomas Dodson** and **Leonard Kaban** (1997). The assessment will provide a grading scale ranging from S0 (no recovery) to S4 (complete recovery).

Mackinnon and Dellon are also credited with advancing the entubulation method developed in 1881 by **Themistocles Gluck**, implementing polyglycolic acid bioabsorbable tubes and comparing the results of the repair with autogenous sural nerve grafts (Pogrel 2002; Mackinnon and Dellon 1990). Prior to this, autogenous nerve grafts were the most common means of nerve repair and are still considered by many to be the gold standard. Given the diameter of the trigeminal nerve, the graft most often used for reconstruction was the sural nerve. Recent research from these authors have shown great benefit in the use of processed human nerve allograft and connected-assisted repair. The nerve allografts can now be ordered in a variety of lengths and diameter.

Today, nerve reconstruction of the head and neck with the use of allograft is slowly replacing autogenous grafts. Allografts have a few noted benefits, most notably avoiding a second surgical site and the associated morbidity. In addition, improvement in grafting materials and techniques has led to nearly equivalent or improved results between allografts and autografts (Safa et al. 2020; Miloro et al. 2015).

The work of **Ralph Merrill** and **Phillip Worthington**, who attended a course by Dr. Hausamen and Dr. Reuter at the University of Washington in Seattle in 1979, could be seen as a new era for the study of trigeminal nerve injuries and repair (Merrill 1979). These surgeons educated a lineage that has been proficient in the literature over the last 40 years and is still active today. In January 2018, the first oral and maxillofacial surgeons joined the American Society of Peripheral Nerve Surgery, those being **Shahrokh Bagheri**, **Michael Miloro**, and **John Zuniga**.

In recent decades, the field of microneurosurgery for the trigeminal nerve has experienced a significant expansion in evidence base. However, the field still remains in its infancy in many ways. The future of peripheral nerve repair will likely involve regeneration of the peripheral nerves through neurotropic factor manipulation in the microenvironment and other still unseen avenues of treatment. The knowledge in this field is now enough to comprise the first edition of the textbook in itself in 2013, "Trigeminal Nerve Injuries," with future editions to follow the progress of this field (Miloro 2013).

References

Albert E. Lehrbuchder Chirurgie und Operationslehre Vorlesungenftir praktische Arzte und Studierende, vol. 1. Leipzig: Urban & Schwarzenberg; 1887. 527 p.

Artico M, Cervoni L, Nucci F, Giuffré R. Birthday of peripheral nervous system surgery: the contribution of Gabriele Ferrara (1543-1627). Neurosurgery. 1996;39(2):380–2.

Babcock W. Nerve dissociation: a new method for the surgical relief of certain painful or paralytic affections of nerve trunks. Ann Surg. 1907;46(5):686–93.

Bagheri SC, Meyer RA, Khan HA, Kuhmichel A, Steed MB. Retrospective review of microsurgical repair of 222 lingual nerve injuries. J Oral Maxillofac Surg. 2010;68(4):715–23.

Bunnell S. Surgical repair of the facial nerve. Arch Otolaryngol. 1937;25(3):235–59.

Carnochan JM. Exsection of the trunk of the second branch of the fifth pair of nerves, beyond the ganglion of Meckel, for severe neuralgia of the face, with three cases. Am J Dent Sci. 1859;9(2):253–69.

Cruikshank W, Hunter J. Experiments on the nerves, particularly on their reproduction; and on the spinal marrow of living animals. Philos Trans R Soc Lond. 1795;85:177–89.

Cushing HI. The surgical treatment of facial paralysis by nerve anastomosis. Ann Surg. 1903;37(5):641–59.

Cushing H. Landmark article April 28, 1900: a method of total extirpation of the Gasserian ganglion for trigeminal neuralgia. By a route through the temporal fossa and beneath the middle meningeal artery. By Harvey Cushing. JAMA. 1983;250(4):519–28.
Davis L, Cleveland DA. Experimental studies in nerve transplants. Ann Surg. 1934;99(2):271–83.
Dodson TB, Kaban LB. Recommendations for management of trigeminal nerve defects based on a critical appraisal of the literature. J Oral Maxillofac Surg. 1997;55(12):1380–6.
Donoff RB, Guralnick W. The application of microneurosurgery to oral-neurologic problems. J Oral Maxillofac Surg. 1982;40(3):156–9.
Ferrara G. Nova selva di cirugia divisa in due parti. Venice: Bartolomeo Carampello; 1596.
Galen of Pergamon. Omnia quae extant opera in Latinum sermonem conversa. Venice: Apud Juntas; 1576.
Ghali GE, Epker BN. Clinical neurosensory testing: practical applications. J Oral Maxillofac Surg. 1989;47(10):1074–8.
Gluck T. Ueber transplantation, regeneration und entzündliche neubildung. Berl Klin Wochenschr. 1881;18:554–7.
Hausamen JE, Samii M, Schmidseder R. Repair of the mandibular nerve by means of autologous nerve grafting after resection of the lower jaw. J Maxillofac Surg. 1973;1(2):74–8.
Hausamen JE, Samii M, Schmidseder R. Restoring sensation to the cut inferior alveolar nerve by direct anastomosis or by free autologous nerve grafting. Experimental study in rabbits. Plast Reconstr Surg. 1974;54(1):83–7.
Head H, Sherren J. The consequences of injury to the peripheral nerves in man. Brain. 1905;28(2):116–338.
Highet WB, Holmes W. Traction injuries to the lateral popliteal nerve and traction injuries to peripheral nerves after suture. Br J Surg. 1943;30(119):212–33.
Highet WB, Sanders FK. The effects of stretching nerves after suture. Br J Surg. 1943;30(120):355–69.
Hillerup S, Bakke M, Larsen JO, Thomsen CE, Gerds TA. Concentration-dependent neurotoxicity of articaine: an electrophysiological and stereological study of the rat sciatic nerve. Anesth Analg. 2011;112(6):1330–8.
Hoffmann P. Uber eine Methode, den Erfolg einer Nervennaht zu beurteilen. Med Klin. 1915a;11:359–60.
Hoffmann P. Weiteres uber das Verhalten frisch regenerierter Nerven und uber die Methode, den Erfolg einer Nervennaht fruhzeitig zu beurteilen. Med Klin. 1915b;11:856–8.
Hoffmann P, Buck-Gramcko D, Lubahn JD. The Hoffmann-Tinel sign. 1915. J Hand Surg. 1993;18(6):800–5.
Kiesselbach JE, Chamberlain JG. Clinical and anatomic observations on the relationship of the lingual nerve to the mandibular third molar region. J Oral Maxillofac Surg. 1984;42(9):565–7.
Langenbeck B. Archiv für klinische chirurgie, vol. 19. Berlin; 1876.
Létiévant E. Traité des sections nerveuses: physiologie pathologique, indications – procédés opératoires. 1st ed. Paris: JB Baillére; 1873.
Mackenzie I, Woods C. Causes of failure after repair of the median nerve. J Bone Joint Surg. 1961;43(3):465–73.
Mackinnon SE, Dellon AL. Surgery of the peripheral nerve. New York: Thieme Medical Publishers; 1988. 638 p.
Mackinnon SE, Dellon AL. Clinical nerve reconstruction with a bioabsorbable polyglycolic acid tube. Plast Reconstr Surg. 1990;85(3):419–24.
Merrill RG. Prevention, treatment, and prognosis for nerve injury related to the difficult impaction. Dent Clin N Am. 1979;23(3):471–88.
Millesi H. On the problem of overbridging defects of the peripheral nerves. Wien Med Wochenschr 1946. 1968;118(9):182–7.
Millesi H. Microsurgery of peripheral nerves. Hand. 1973;5(2):157–60.
Miloro M. Trigeminal nerve injuries. 1st ed. Berlin Heidelberg: Springer-Verlag; 2013. 366 p.

Miloro M, Halkias LE, Slone HW, Chakeres DW. Assessment of the lingual nerve in the third molar region using magnetic resonance imaging. J Oral Maxillofac Surg. 1997;55(2):134–7.
Miloro M, Ruckman P, Kolokythas A. Lingual nerve repair: to graft or not to graft? J Oral Maxillofac Surg. 2015;73(9):1844–50.
Mitchell SW. Injuries of nerves and their consequences. Philadelphia: J.B. Lippincott & Co; 1872. 377 p.
Mitchell SW, Morehouse GR, Keen WW. Gunshot wounds and other injuries of nerves. Philadelphia: J.B. Lippincott & Co; 1864.
Neuber G. Ein antiseptischer Dauerverband nach gründlicher Blutstillung. Arch Für Klin Chir. 1879;24:314–30.
Nylen CO. The microscope in aural surgery, its first use and later development. Acta Otolaryngol Suppl. 1954;116:226–40.
Nylen CO, Person N. An otomicroscope. A review of the possibilities of making a microscope for examining the labyrinth and its surrounding and also for ear operations. Swed Manuscr. 1922.
Philipeax J, Vulpian A. Recherches experimentales sur la reunion bout a bout de nerfs de fonctions differentes. J Physio Homme Anim. 1863;6:421–55, 474–516.
Philipeux J, Vulpian A. Note sur des essais de greffe d'un troncon du nerf lingual entra les duex bouts du nerf hypoglosse, apres excision d'un segment de ce dernier neft. Arch Physiol Norm Pathol. 1870;3:618–20.
Pogrel MA. The results of microneurosurgery of the inferior alveolar and lingual nerve. J Oral Maxillofac Surg. 2002;60(5):485–9.
Pogrel MA, Thamby S. The etiology of altered sensation in the inferior alveolar, lingual, and mental nerves as a result of dental treatment. J Calif Dent Assoc. 1999;27(7):531, 534–8.
Ramon y Cajal S. Degeneration and regeneration of the nervous system. New York: Oxford University Press; 1928. 769 p.
Rivers WHR, Head H. A human experiment in nerve division. Brain. 1908;31(3):323–450.
Rogers L. Experiences in treatment of peripheral nerve injuries with amnioplastin. Br Med J. 1941;1(4189):587–9.
Rood JP, Shehab BA. The radiological prediction of inferior alveolar nerve injury during third molar surgery. Br J Oral Maxillofac Surg. 1990;28(1):20–5.
Safa B, Jain S, Desai MJ, Greenberg JA, Niacaris TR, Nydick JA, et al. Peripheral nerve repair throughout the body with processed nerve allografts: results from a large multicenter study. Microsurgery. 2020;40(5):527–37.
Seddon HJ. A classification of nerve injuries. Br Med J. 1942;2(4260):237–9.
Seddon HJ. Peripheral nerve injuries. Glasgow Med J. 1943;139(3):61–75.
Seddon H. Peripheral nerve injuries. Medical Research Council special report. London: Her Majesty's Stationery Office; 1954. 452 p.
Smith JW. Microsurgery of peripheral nerves. Plast Reconstr Surg. 1964;33:317–29.
Sunderland S. A classification of peripheral nerve injuries producing loss of function. Brain J Neurol. 1951;74(4):491–516.
Sunderland S. Nerves and nerve injuries. Baltimore: Williams and Wilkins Co; 1968. 1116 p.
Swan J. Treatise on diseases and injuries of the nerves. A new edition considerably enlarged. London: Longman; 1834. 356 p.
Tinel J. Le signe du fourmillement dans les lésions des nerfs périphériques. Presse Med. 1915;47:388–9.
Vanlair C. De la régénération des nerfs périphériques par le procédé de la suture tubulaire. Arch Biol (Liege). 1882;3:379–496.
Velpeau A. Nervomes. In: Lecons orales de clinique chirurgiicale. Paris: G. Bailliére; 1841. p. 408–24.
Waller A. Experiments on the section of the glosso-pharyngeal and hypoglossal nerves of the frog, and observations of the alterations produced thereby in the structure of their primitive fibres. Edinb Med Surg J. 1851;76(189):369–76.

Warren JC. Cases of neuralgia, or painful affections of nerves. Boston Med Surg J. 1829;2(12):178–85.

Wood W. Observations on neuromas. With cases and histories of the disease. Trans Med Chir Soc Edinb. 1829;3(Pt 2):367–434.

Young JZ, Medawar PB. Fibrin suture of peripheral nerves: measurement of the rate of regeneration. Lancet. 1940;236(6101):126–8.

Zuniga JR, Meyer RA, Gregg JM, Miloro M, Davis LF. The accuracy of clinical neurosensory testing for nerve injury diagnosis. J Oral Maxillofac Surg. 1998;56(1):2–8.

Temporomandibular Joint Surgery

Kenneth Kufta, Peter D. Quinn, and Eric J. Granquist

1 Introduction

The history of temporomandibular joint (TMJ) surgery encompasses a list of many successful and unsuccessful attempts at re-establishing form and function and decreasing pain in the orofacial region. The first TMJ surgeries were thought to be performed in BC, primarily for treatment of pathologies such TMJ ankylosis and dislocation (Indresano and Mobati 2006). The first documentation of an intra-articular TMJ procedure is by Annandale in 1887, during which he performed a disc repositioning procedure for treatment of closed lock (Annandale 1887). Over the next several hundreds of years, the pendulum of surgical tenets, approaches, and options offered to patients with TMJ disease swung widely. This included a strong movement that promoted nonsurgical treatments after many catastrophic outcomes, followed by the use of alloplastic implants which had previously been shown to have poor biocompatibility. More recently, oral and maxillofacial surgeons (OMS) have played a major role in innovating devices and techniques in TMJ surgery through appropriately designed clinical trials, demonstrating highly effective surgical options for patients. Some of these procedures include TMJ disc excision with or without autogenous replacement, TMJ disc repositioning, autogenous costochondral TMJ reconstruction, stock and custom prosthetic TMJ replacement, as well as minimally invasive procedures such as arthrocentesis and arthroscopy. In this chapter, we will explore the history of different TMJ surgical techniques, as well as highlight landmark articles that resulted in the field of contemporary TMJ surgery that continues to evolve today with the advent of advanced technology. While we

K. Kufta · P. D. Quinn · E. J. Granquist (✉)
Department of Oral and Maxillofacial Surgery, Hospital of the University of Pennsylvania, Philadelphia, PA, USA
e-mail: Kenneth.Kufta@pennmedicine.upenn.edu; Peter.Quinn@pennmedicine.upenn.edu; Eric.Granquist@pennmedicine.upenn.edu

E. M. Ferneini et al. (eds.), *The History of Maxillofacial Surgery*,
https://doi.org/10.1007/978-3-030-89563-1_18

attempt to arrange this chapter in chronological order in regard to when the techniques were developed, the history of TMJ surgery is convoluted, and thus organization is quite challenging.

2 Gap Arthroplasty/Discectomy/Disc Repositioning

While ancient cultures were familiar with certain TMJ pathologies such as ankylosis of joints and jaw dislocation, there was no documentation of surgical treatment of these disease processes until the late 1800s. TMJ ankylosis was first treated via simple gap arthroplasty, but this procedure was often complicated by re-ankylosis (Topazian 1966). John Murray Carnochan, a prominent New York surgeon, is praised for his ideology of inter-posing a material (a block of wood) between the bony surfaces of the mandible and temporal bone after gap arthroplasty for treatment of TMJ ankylosis (Carnochan 1860). Soon thereafter, many different surgeons used this same principle of gap arthroplasty with inter-positional grafting for treatment of TMJ ankylosis.

While Gluck first made use of an Ivory prosthetic stabilized with cement to bridge the gap in 1891 (Gluck 1891), Murphy was the first to use temporalis fascia as an inter-positional graft for gap arthroplasty (Murphy 1913). In 1914, he published a case series in which he described his use of an axial rotational inter-positional flap of temporal fat and fascia to line the TMJ with the goal of restoring joint function and preventing re-ankylosis (Murphy 1914). Since then, surgeons have attempted to use many different types of inter-positional materials to restore function and range of motion, including temporalis muscle (Risdon 1933), gold foil (Risdon 1933), tantalum foil (Eggers 1946), stainless steel (Smith and Robinson 1952), dermis (Georgiade et al. 1957), full thickness skin (Popescu and Vasiliu 1977), and in the modern era, silastic and polytetrafluoroethylene (PTFE) a.k.a. Teflon materials.

Perhaps one of the darkest ages of TMJ surgery lies in the years during which silastic and Teflon implants began to be placed within the joint in the 1960s. At the time, silastic materials were known for their high thermal stability as well as their relative inertness within the human body (Mercuri 2016). Silicone was first used as an inter-positional material in 1968 during reconstructive hand surgery (Swanson 1997). Subsequently, Brown et al. reported on the use of silicone material to serve as a barrier in preventing TMJ ankylosis after gap arthroplasty (Brown et al. 1963), and others reported similar techniques (Robinson 1968). Short-term studies revealed that the silicone implants would incite formation of a reactive fibrous capsule that could possibly serve as a new disc while helping to prevent re-ankylosis (Brown et al. 1963; Spagnoli and Kent 1992).

Unfortunately, by the 1980s, studies began to describe significant complications related to silastic materials placed within the TMJ. Severe inflammatory foreign body reactions with associated regional lymphadenopathy as well as erosion of condylar heads were described in multiple reports (Dolwick and Aufdemorte 1985;

Eriksson and Westesson 1986; Hartman et al. 1988). Further studies even revealed that fragmented silicone particles had migrated within the regional lymphatics (Hartman et al. 1988). Additional follow-up studies were published conveying poor results associated with silastic implants within the TMJ (Eriksson and Westesson 1992). After review of a multitude of studies demonstrating the negative consequences of the implantation of silicone materials into the joint space, the American Association of Oral and Maxillofacial Surgeons (AAOMS) published a consensus paper recommending that the use of permanent silastic implants be discontinued (American Association of Oral and Maxillofacial Surgeons 1993a). The publication of these results was preceded by a workshop in 1992, during which AAOMS organized a meeting consisting of OMS experts, nonsurgical clinician experts in managing TMJ disorders, and biomaterial experts tasked with developing a consensus on the use of alloplastic inter-positional materials within the TMJ. The experts developed a consensus stating that silastic implants should no longer be *permanently* placed in the TMJ as an inter-positional material (American Association of Oral and Maxillofacial Surgeons 1993a). However, silastic implants have continued to be used as temporary spacers after arthroplasty and disc excision. The workshop also made detailed recommendations regarding the need for removal of implants and follow-up intervals (American Association of Oral and Maxillofacial Surgeons 1993a).

Around the same time that silastic materials began to be used for reconstruction of the TMJ, surgeons such as Small also began to report on their use of PTFE as a material for joint reconstruction after large mandibular resections (Small et al. 1964). PTFE was found to have a high density as well as a self-lubricating property, which was believed to be suitable for a ginglymoarthrodial joint such as the TMJ. Despite prior studies demonstrating Teflon fragmentation under loading that resulted in significant foreign body reactions (Charnley 1963), Cook proceeded to use Teflon as an alloplastic inter-positional material in the TMJ in 1972 (Cook 1972).

Later in that decade, Vitek Inc. (Houston, TX) began to fabricate implants in which Teflon was combined with other materials. In the 1960s, a chemical engineer by the name of Charles Homsy designed a material named Proplast, which was originally intended for use in orthopedic surgery. Given its porous nature and thus potential for tissue ingrowth and implant stabilization, it was thought to be suitable for use as an inter-positional material in TMJ surgery (Homsy 1970; Homsy et al. 1972). Proplast I (PTFE + carbon/graphite) was first developed, followed by Proplast II (PTFE + aluminum oxide) to allow for more neutral coloration of implants placed superficially (Westfall et al. 1982). Again, despite several studies demonstrating the presence of giant cells and macrophages around these intra-joint materials (Homsy et al. 1973), others continued to use Proplast implants within the TMJ and reported short-term successful outcomes (Kirsch 1984; Wade et al. 1986; Bee and Zeitler 1986). However, it was not long until there were widespread studies reporting on the deleterious effects of Teflon-based materials placed within the TMJ.

The most notable complications included severe condylar degeneration (Florine et al. 1986; Bronstein 1987), remodeling/erosion of condylar and glenoid fossa bony structures (Heffez et al. 1987), implant fragmentation (Heffez et al. 1987), and foreign body giant cell reactions in regional lymph nodes (Lagrotteria et al. 1986). Additional longer-term studies demonstrated similar negative clinical and radiographic outcomes in patients with prior implantation of Teflon materials within the TMJ (Morgan 1988; Kaplan et al. 1988; Schellhas et al. 1988). As clinical symptoms were delayed compared to radiographic signs, patients soon began reporting symptoms including preauricular pain and swelling, limited mouth opening, occlusal changes, lymphadenopathy (Wagner and Mosby 1990), and even perforation into the middle cranial fossa (Fig. 1) (Berarducci et al. 1990).

Eventually, studies published by El-Deeb et al. and Valentine et al. demonstrated evidence of fragmentation of the Proplast implants with associated significant

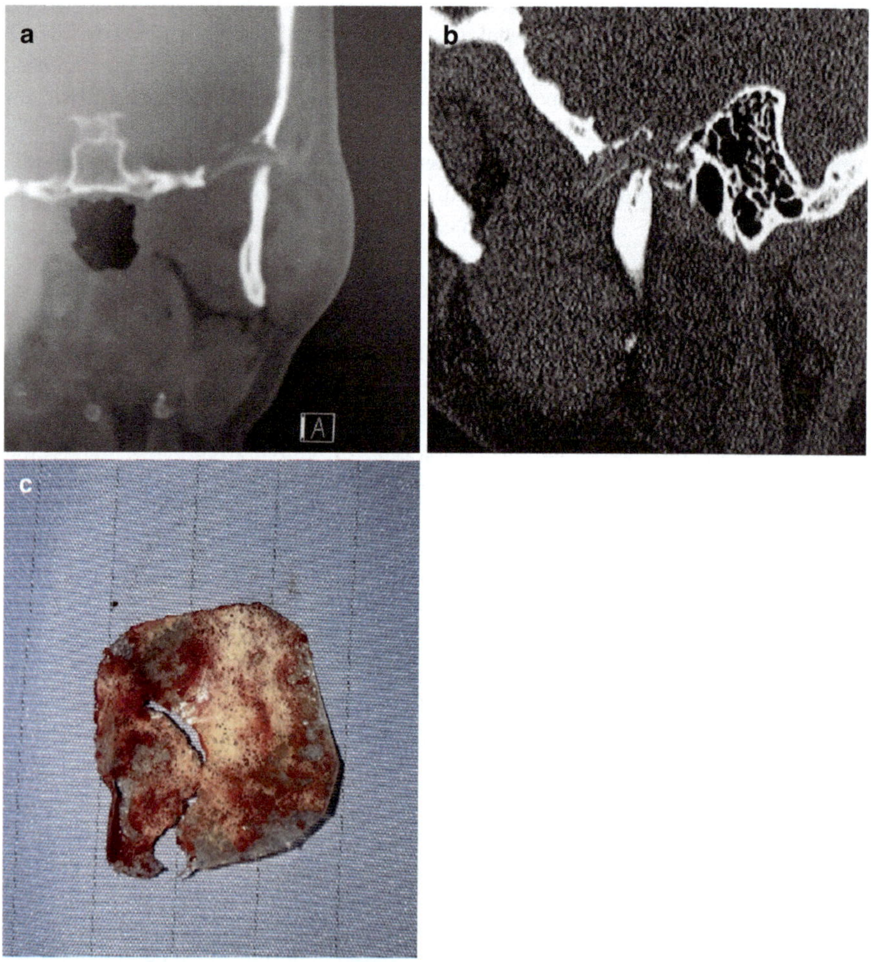

Fig. 1 (**a**) Coronal and (**b**) sagittal view of a CT scan demonstrating a Proplast implant within the TMJ resulting in erosion into the middle cranial fossa. (**c**) Explanted Proplast with evidence of significant wear leading to material perforation and implant fragmentation

foreign body reactions composed of active giant cells/osteoclasts that resulted in severe degeneration of adjacent bony structures (El Deeb and Holmes 1989; Valentine Jr. et al. 1989). Wagner and Mosby also published a long-term study revealing 95% of patients with Proplast implants reporting severe pain, along with 100% of cases with condylar degeneration (Wagner and Mosby 1990). In light of the plethora of studies revealing potential negative consequences associated with implantation of Teflon substances in the TMJ, the FDA and Center for Devices and Radiological Health issued a Public Health Advisory in September 1991 regarding the recall and close monitoring of patients with previously placed Teflon implants within the joint (Johnson 1991). In 1992, this was followed by the release of a TMJ Implant Advisory sent to all OMS regarding the published data revealing the negative outcomes seen in patients implanted with Proplast-Teflon materials (American Association of Oral and Maxillofacial Surgeons 1992). Further evaluation of published studies on the topic resulted in an AAOMS-sponsored workshop that published recommendations for discontinuation of Proplast-Teflon as an inter-positional implant for the TMJ, as well as either removal of the implant with reconstruction using autogenous tissue or close monitoring with yearly CT and/or MRI evaluation (American Association of Oral and Maxillofacial Surgeons 1993b). As a result of these devastating results associated with Teflon-Proplast implants, very strict measures have appropriately been put in place to rigorously investigate the use of any further materials to treat pathologies of the TMJ. Furthermore, these failed materials were shown to having lasting consequences, as it has been shown that TMJR outcomes are less likely to be successful after Proplast-Teflon implant failure (Henry and Wolford 1993).

In addition to treatment of ankylosis, surgical methods and approaches began to focus on treatment to improve symptoms of internal derangement of the TMJ. As such, discectomy became one surgical treatment modality, originally described by Lanz in 1909 (Lanz 1909) and further popularized by Pringle (1918) and Ashhurst (1921). Although the discectomy procedure was found to have favorable results in follow-up studies (Boman 1947; Dingman and Moorman 1951), there was a significant amount of controversy over its use given the uncertainty regarding the pathophysiology of disease within the TMJ. It wasn't until Bowman published his dissertation (Bowman 1947), and other long-term follow-up studies were published (Eriksson and Westesson 1985; Holmlund et al. 1993; Silver 1984) that discectomy became a broadly accepted, effective treatment modality for TMJ pathologies.

Although the discectomy became standard of care by the 1970s (Dingman and Moorman 1951; Kiehn and Desprez 1962), there was still controversy regarding the necessity of replacing the disc with autogenous versus alloplastic materials to prevent recurrent disease/ankylosis. Several long-term follow-up studies have shown success with discectomy without replacement of the disc (Holmlund et al. 1993; McKenna 2001). However, surgeons continued to search for a disc replacement material due to concerns regarding persistent joint noise, crepitus, and condylar resorption seen in patients who had underwent discectomy without replacement (Dimitroulis 2011a). In 1958, Gordon had described his technique of replacing the intra-articular disc with polyethylene caps to prevent re-ankylosis and collapse of vertical dimension (Gordon 1958). In addition to their use as inter-positional materials for gap arthroplasty, alloplastic materials such as silastic and Teflon were also used to replace discs. In light of the disastrous complications resulting from inserting these materials within the TMJ, surgeons began to search for autogenous grafts to serve as an articular disc replacement (Dimitroulis 2011a). Expanding upon Murphy's use of the temporalis fat-fascia axial flap for management of TMJ ankylosis (Murphy 1913, 1914), Dimitroulis introduced the use of abdominal dermis-fat as an inter-positional graft for use in ankylotic patients (Dimitroulis 2004). Given its relative success, Dimitroulis also introduced the concept of using abdominal dermis-fat grafting after TMJ discectomy and demonstrated its ability to survive and withstand the intra-articular forces (Dimitroulis et al. 2008). Fat grafting alone after discectomy was not shown to prevent additional bony morphological changes in the mandibular condyle (Dimitroulis 2011b), and it has been found to significantly decrease in size over time in orthopedic studies (Kanamori et al. 2001). While dermis-fat grafting has been shown to resist the reduction in size of the grafting as seen with fat alone (Dimitroulis et al. 2008), prevent ankylosis (Dimitroulis et al. 2008), and result in overall improvement in quality of life (Dimitroulis et al. 2010), severe condylar changes after its placement in the joint have prevented its regular use (Dimitroulis 2011b).

Additional autogenous materials used as a disc replacement include temporalis muscle flaps (Feinberg and Larsen 1989; Pogrel and Kaban 1990), auricular cartilage (Matukas and Lachner 1990), and dermis grafts (Meyer 1988; Dimitroulis 2005). Given studies that have shown fragmentation of the grafts, low survivability, and inability to prevent condylar changes, there has not been a graft that has shown adequate strength or biologic compatibility in serving as a replacement for the TMJ articular disc (Dimitroulis 2005; Yih et al. 1992; Sandler et al. 1997). Animal studies comparing meniscectomy alone versus different disc replacement grafts have largely demonstrated similar clinical outcomes in regard to pain relief, improvement in mouth opening, and osteoarthritic changes of the condyle with or without replacement. Histologic studies revealed that discectomy alone does not result in regeneration of the disc, but rather arthritic condylar changes along with replacement of the articular surfaces by infiltration of adjacent fibrovascular tissue (a pseudo-disc) (Tong and Tideman 2000). Discectomy with replacement using autogenous grafting demonstrated an extensive fibrotic response without survival of the graft. Given these results and similar clinical outcomes in human studies comparing discectomy alone versus discectomy plus replacement with graft, the decision whether or not to replace the disc remains controversial (Dimitroulis 2011a).

In addition to complete removal of the disc, other approaches including repositioning of the disc were attempted. While Annandale performed the first disc repositioning procedure in 1887, the concept of this surgical method for the treatment of internal derangement was not well-supported until Wilkes described the form and function of the TMJ in his arthrographic studies (Mehra and Wolford 2001; Wilkes 1978a, b). McCarty described the classic disc repositioning method of performing a high condylar shave with disc release and repositioning by suturing to the posterior attachments (McCarty and Farrar 1979). Leopard described posterior repositioning of the disc via suturing of the disc to the inferior aspect of the temporalis fascia (Leopard 1984). Walker and Kalamchi recommended condyloplasty with freeing of the articular disc, which allowed for suturing of the disc to the lateral capsule in a new position atop the condylar head (Walker and Kalamchi 1987). Eventually, Weinberg demonstrated successful outcomes in meniscocondylar plication for disc repositioning, which provided the foundation for the idea of the Mitek mini anchor (Weinberg and Cousens 1987). In 1993, Wolford et al. developed a technique in which a bone anchor, named a Mitek mini anchor (DePuy Synthes Mitek Anchor, Raynham, MA, USA), is implanted into the posterior condylar head and subsequently sutured to reposition and stabilize the articular disc (Fig. 2) (Cottrell and Wolford 1993). Since this time, the FDA has approved its use in patients for the treatment of internal derangement of the TMJ. Additional bone anchors, including the JuggerKnot Mini Soft anchor (Zimmer BioMet, Warsaw, IN, USA) (Hanley et al. 2015) and the Arthrex Corkscrew anchor (Arthrex Inc., Naples, USA) (Ryba et al. 2015), have also been developed for use in TMJ disc repositioning surgery.

TMJ ankylosis, along with internal derangement, served as the primary pathologies that led to the development of partial and total reconstruction of the joint. Although gap arthroplasty with inter-positional grafting for TMJ ankylosis has been shown to promote improved joint range of motion compared to gap arthroplasty alone (Ma et al. 2015), many studies have shown variable results in regard to re-ankylosis and restoration of function (Topazian 1966) (Ramezanian and Yavary 2006; Zhi et al. 2009). This, along with incomplete resolution of symptoms after

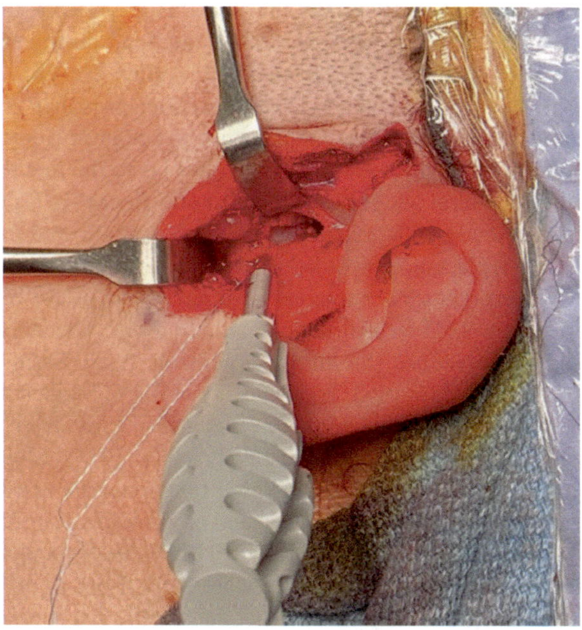

Fig. 2 Insertion of JuggerKnot Mini Soft anchor into the condylar head for the purpose of TMJ disc repositioning

discectomy/disc repositioning in the case of internal derangement, inspired surgeons to develop techniques for excision with TMJ reconstruction of joint articulation with both autogenous and alloplastic materials.

3 TMJ Reconstruction: Autologous and Alloplastic

The history of TMJ reconstruction includes unfortunate catastrophic failures and recent success. The goal of TMJ reconstruction is to restore form and function. In addition, the primary goal should focus on improving quality of life for the patient. Loss of TMJ functionality most often results from ankylosis, internally deranged joints/osteoarthritis, high inflammatory arthritides, as well as less common etiologies such as congenital abnormalities and neoplastic processes. The constant daily use of the TMJ, as well as the complex physiology of a joint that is capable of both rotational and translational movements, creates a significant hardship in effectively restoring form and function via reconstruction. A plethora of both autologous and alloplastic materials have been used to partially and totally reconstruct the TMJ.

3.1 Autogenous

Several different autologous grafts have been used to attempt to reconstruct the TMJ (Lindqvist et al. 1986; MacIntosh and Henny 1977). In 1909, Lexer was the first to describe the use of "joint allotransplantation," during which he used a costochondral graft to reconstruct a proximal tibia after excision of a sarcoma (Lexer 1909; Nikolaou and Giannoudis 2017). Bardenheur is then credited as the first surgeon to replace the mandibular condyle with an autograft (fourth metatarsal) in 1909 (Lexer 1925), while Gillies is well-known for being the first to reconstruct the TMJ with a costochondral allograft (MacIntosh and Henny 1977; Gillies 1920). The use of an osteochondral allograft was promising, as it allowed for the use of an avascular tissue to replace both hyaline cartilage and a significant bony deficiency.

Since this time, surgeons have attempted to use many different types of autografts for TMJ reconstruction, including iliac, metatarsal, tibial, fibula, and sternoclavicular tissues (Smith and Robinson 1952; Entin 1958; Dingman and Grabb 1964; Plotnikov 1965; Ware and Taylor 1966; Snyder et al. 1971). The uses of these autografts have had variable results, specifically given their inconsistent adaptability and lack of growth potential (Poswillo 1974). Most surgeons have collectively agreed that the costochondral graft functions best as a replacement of the mandibular condyle given its biological and physiological similarities, along with low donor site morbidity (Lindqvist et al. 1986; Freihofer and Perko 1976; Kennett 1973). Furthermore, biologic studies were carried out to prove superiority of the costochondral graft compared to other autografts, given its proliferative nature as well as its remodeling and growth properties (Poswillo 1974; Blackwood 1966; Durkin et al. 1973). Long-term follow-up studies have also confirmed the efficacy of costochondral grafts for TMJ reconstruction (Lindqvist et al. 1988; Perrott et al. 1994; Figueroa et al. 1984). Resnick et al. also recently developed a consensus regarding the use of costochondral grafts and other surgical modalities in the specific treatment of patients with juvenile idiopathic arthritis (JIA) (Resnick et al. 2019).

3.2 *Alloplastic*

The safety and efficacy of alloplastic joints in the orthopedic literature encouraged the OMS community to seek alloplastic implant options for their patients with severe TMJ disease (Charnley 1961). While alloplastic TMJ replacement is now a widely accepted procedure within the scope of OMS today, the history of placing alloplastic implants within the TMJ is fraught with publications describing drastic failures of materials such as the Kent-Vitek prosthesis (Vitek, Houston, TX, USA) as well as the Christensen, Osteomed, and Delrin-Timesh prostheses (Mercuri 2016; Driemel et al. 2009). One of the major advantages of alloplastic joint reconstruction is that it afforded the surgeon the ability to efficiently and predictably restore form and function to the TMJ without any donor site morbidity or need for maxillomandibular fixation (Donlon 2000).

Eggers was the first to describe placement of an alloplastic material between the mandible and cranium when he placed tantalum foil in the intra-joint space for the treatment of ankylosis (Eggers 1946). Subsequently, Smith and Robinson published on the use of a stainless steel fossa (Robinson 1960; Smith and Robinson 1957), while Henry published on the use of stainless steel as a means of replacing the mandibular condyle (Henry 1960). Ward, who also popularized the modified condylotomy approach for the treatment of TMJ internal derangement, published on the use of cobalt-chrome alloy to reconstruct the TMJ (Ward 1961). Notably in 1963, based on Robinson's method of creating a fossa prosthesis, Christensen designed a 0.5-mm Vitallium-based glenoid fossa eminence prosthesis to reconstruct the TMJ as well as provide a mechanical barrier for prevention of re-ankylosis (Christensen 1963, 1964). With this method, Christensen fabricated castings of 20 different-sized glenoid fossae prostheses made of rigid, polishable Vitallium that can be sized intraoperatively and anchored to the zygoma. Eventually, he expanded the stock of casted prostheses to 33 per side and then 44 to broaden the surgeons' reconstructive options for anatomic variations (Fig. 3) (Christensen 1964). Eventually, Christensen went on to describe the first total joint replacement device for the TMJ. The device consisted of his previously described Vitallium fossa prosthesis along with a condylar component made of cobalt-chrome (Co-Cr) alloy and a molded polymethylmethacrylate (PMMA) condylar head (Driemel et al. 2009; Christensen 1971). In 1996, he eventually discontinued the use of the PMMA head given reports of material resorption under function (Mercuri 1996). Almost 5000 Christensen prostheses had been implanted between 1993 and 2003, and their use continued until the FDA ordered a cease and desist order in 2015 due to non-compliance with 522

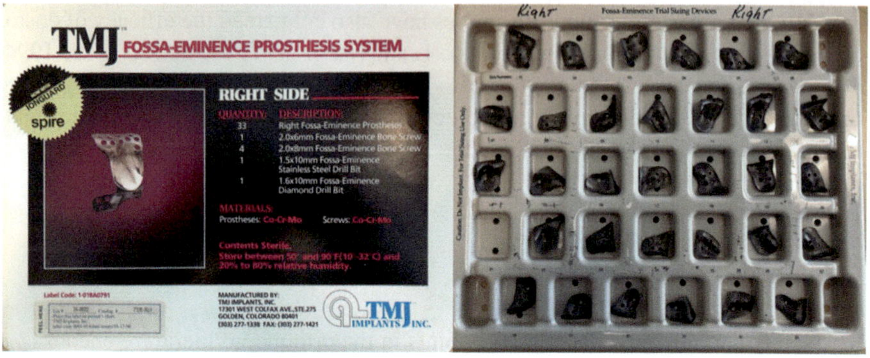

Fig. 3 Original set of Christensen set containing 33 variations of stock prostheses for reconstruction of the TMJ

post-market surveillance studies (Christensen 1971; TMJ 2021). Christensen also eventually developed an all-cast-Vitallium custom total joint prosthesis using CAD/CAM technology to treat more surgically and anatomically complex patients (Garrett et al. 1997).

In 1971, Morgan described alternative fossa eminence prostheses that consisted of a Vitallium eminence and eventually added a silastic articulating component given the degenerative changes seen within the condylar head (Morgan 1971; Morgan and Hall 1985). Eventually, the use of permanent silastic implants for TMJ surgery was discontinued given the significant foreign body reaction observed in patients (Eriksson and Westesson 1986; American Association of Oral and Maxillofacial Surgeons 1993a). Soon thereafter, Morgan went on to develop his own ramus-condyle replacement that consisted of an acrylic condylar head (House et al. 1984; Morgan 1992). Kiehn is also credited for the development of a Vitallium condylar-fossa prosthesis reinforced with PMMA (Kiehn et al. 1974).

Others had also reported on the idea of hemiarthroplasty, in which an alloplastic condylar component functions against a natural disc/fossa without an alloplastic fossa component. Authors have reported on the use of custom cast gold ramus-condyle units (Tauras et al. 1972), methyl methacrylate (Kameros and Himmelfarb 1975), Delrin (polyoxymethylene)-titanium (Boyne et al. 1987), Vitallium (Kiehn et al. 1974; Silver et al. 1977; Hahn 1964), Vitallium with PMMA cement (Silver et al. 1977), as well as the controversial Proplast-coated Ticonium condylar prosthesis (Hinds et al. 1974). Despite studies on TMJ hemiarthroplasty demonstrating successful outcomes with low complication rates (Marx et al. 2008), other studies have discredited its use given the potential dreadful complication of severe bony erosion into the cranial base (Lindqvist et al. 1992; Westermark et al. 2006).

In 1976, Spiessl attempted to decrease the risk of glenoid fossa resorption by altering the condylar head design in his AO/ASIF system (Spiessl 1976). He designed both short and long models of a condylar reconstruction plate (Prein 2002), although reports were still made describing erosions into the glenoid fossa (Lindqvist et al. 2002). Attempts were made to make use of the AO/ASIF system while preserving the articular disc or in conjunction with lining the glenoid fossa with a pedicled flap (Prein 2002; Klotch et al. 1998).

In 1972, Kent et al. published a pilot study describing the use of a condylar prosthesis with its head coated with Teflon-Proplast (Kent et al. 1972). Accordingly, Kent added a Teflon-Proplast fossa prosthesis consisting of a Proplast superior layer with a Teflon inferior layer (Kent et al. 1983), which collectively with the condylar unit became known as the Vitek-Kent I (VK-I) total joint prosthesis. The Vitek-Kent II (VK-II) was then subsequently described, which also included PTFE within the fossa component (Kent et al. 1986).

Throughout the 1980s the Vitek-Kent prosthesis was commonly used as a means for alloplastic joint reconstruction. During this time, Rooney et al. published a study with concerning findings of significant foreign body reaction to PTFE resulting in condylar degeneration (Rooney et al. 1988). Given the concerns for fracturing of the Teflon-Proplast fossae resulting in significant foreign body reactions, the Teflon portion of the Vitek-Kent prosthesis was eventually replaced with polyethylene. Kent subsequently reported an update on the follow-up of the VK-I and VK-II prostheses, which had 80% success rate at 6 years and 20% success rate at 10 years (Kent et al. 1993). Given the material failure of the Proplast-Teflon with associated foreign body giant cell reaction, patients who had undergone reconstruction with these devices underwent frequent imaging and follow-up to evaluate for the need for device removal (Spagnoli and Kent 1992; Feinerman and Piecuch 1993). These complications resulted in millions of dollars in claims and the official revoking of prior FDA approval (Speculand et al. 2000). As such, TMJ devices were reclassified as class III devices, suggesting the high risk posed to the patient and thus necessitating stringent pre- and post-market approval processes (FDA 2021).

After the devastating material failure of the Teflon-Proplast system, several other surgeons set out to develop other materials for alloplastic reconstruction, including ceramic implants (Szabo et al. 1990), titanium-based implants (Raveh et al. 1984; MacAfee and Quinn 1992; Butow et al. 2001), and titanium-polyethylene combinations (Sonnenburg et al. 1984; Sonnenburg and Sonnenburg 1990). Van Loon reported biomechanical studies demonstrating the acceptable wear resistance of metal-on-UHMWPE total TMJ prostheses (Van Loon et al. 1999, 2000). Others attempted to expand upon the AO/ASIF with adjustable/add-on condylar prostheses, but placement and positioning of the device proved to be quite technically difficult (Driemel et al. 2007; Raveh et al. 1980; Vuillemin et al. 1989).

In the early 1990s, Mercuri made use of the emerging advanced technology by developing the TMJ Concepts Prosthesis (Techmedica model) (Mercuri et al. 1995). This model made use of pre-operative CT scanning and CAD/CAM technology to fabricate custom condylar and fossa prostheses designed to fit the specific anatomy of each patient. Its condylar component consisted of a titanium alloy mandibular shaft with a cobalt-chromium-molybdenum (Co-Cr-Mo) condylar head, while its fossa component consisted of a titanium mesh with an articulating surface composed of ultra-high-molecular-weight polyethylene (UHMWPE) that is designed to maximize contact with the condylar head (Fig. 4) (Mercuri 2000). Given the extensive pre-operative surgical planning resulting in precise device fitting, the TMJ Concepts facilitated the reconstruction of TMJs that have been undergone multiple operations resulting in distorted anatomy (Mercuri et al. 2002; Wolford et al. 1994). After long-term follow-up studies demonstrating successful results, the TMJ Concepts prosthesis obtained FDA approval in 1999 (Driemel et al. 2009; Mercuri et al. 2002). Others such as Butow (Butow et al. 2001) and Hoffman and Pappas (Fig. 5) (Hoffman and Pappas 2000) had prostheses in development at the same time, but ultimately did not receive FDA clearance. These devices had titanium nitride at the condylar and fossa contacting surfaces to produce more wear-resistant components.

Also in the 1990s, Quinn and Van Loon built upon the ideology of a stock metal-on-polyethylene prosthesis to produce a more cost-effective, wear-resistant stock prosthesis (van Loon et al. 2000, 2002; Quinn 2000). In 1995, Quinn introduced the Biomet-Lorenz total joint stock prosthesis, which consisted of Co-Cr condylar heads with titanium plasma spray coating of different lengths and widths and a UHMWPE fossa of multiple flange sizes (Figs. 6 and 7) (Quinn 2000). This led to

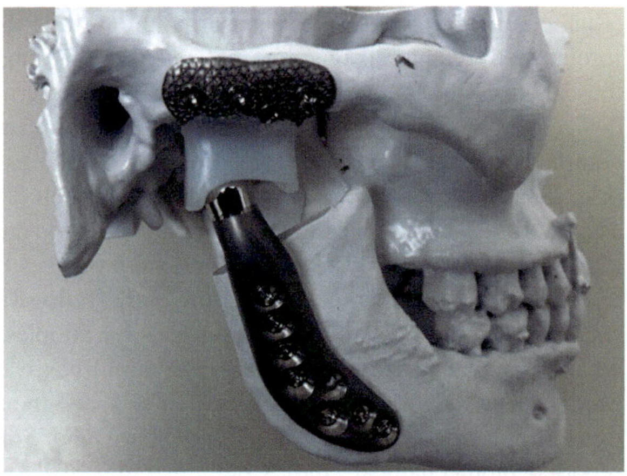

Fig. 4 Custom TMJ Concepts prosthesis with Co-Cr-Mo condylar head and titanium mesh + UHMWPE fossa component

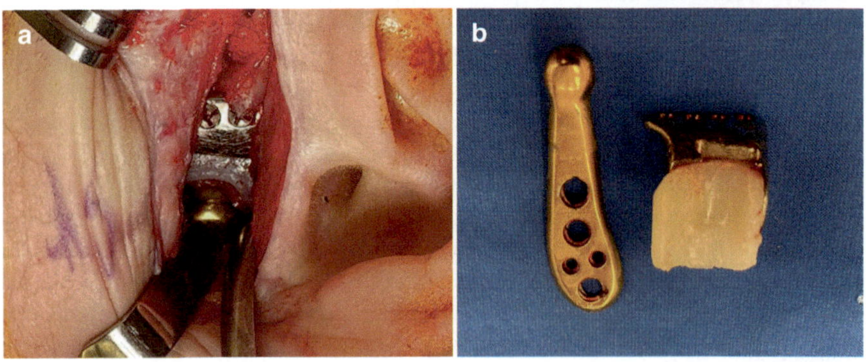

Fig. 5 Hoffman-Pappas device (**a**) implanted within the patient and (**b**) explanted

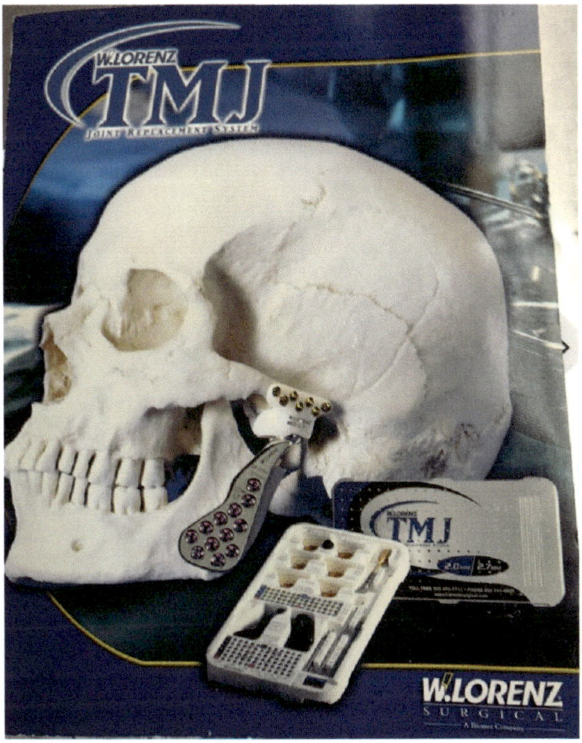

Fig. 6 Original Biomet-Lorenz TMJ replacement set

an investigational device exemption study published in 2012 demonstrating the safety and efficacy of the Biomet-Lorenz stock prosthesis (Giannakopoulos et al. 2012), and the device was approved by the FDA in 2010. A recent FDA post-market study by Granquist et al. revealed a similar survivorship rate and subsequent surgical intervention rate to that of other orthopedic joint replacements (Granquist et al. 2020).

4 Arthroscopy

As TMJ surgery continued to evolve throughout the 1900s with many successes and failures, OMS began to take notice of the orthopedic surgery literature and their minimally invasive techniques of treating diseased joints. A long history of endoscopic procedures exists in the orthopedic literature, dating back to the first use of an endoscope 1853. A French surgeon named Antoine Jean Desormeaux, now known as the “Father of Endoscopy,” first demonstrated the use of an endoscope (named the Lichtleiter) in a patient for a urology procedure (Indresano and Mobati 2006; Figdor 2004). The endoscope primarily functioned as a cystoscope until 1918, when Japanese surgeon Kenji Takagi described the use of a 3.5-mm

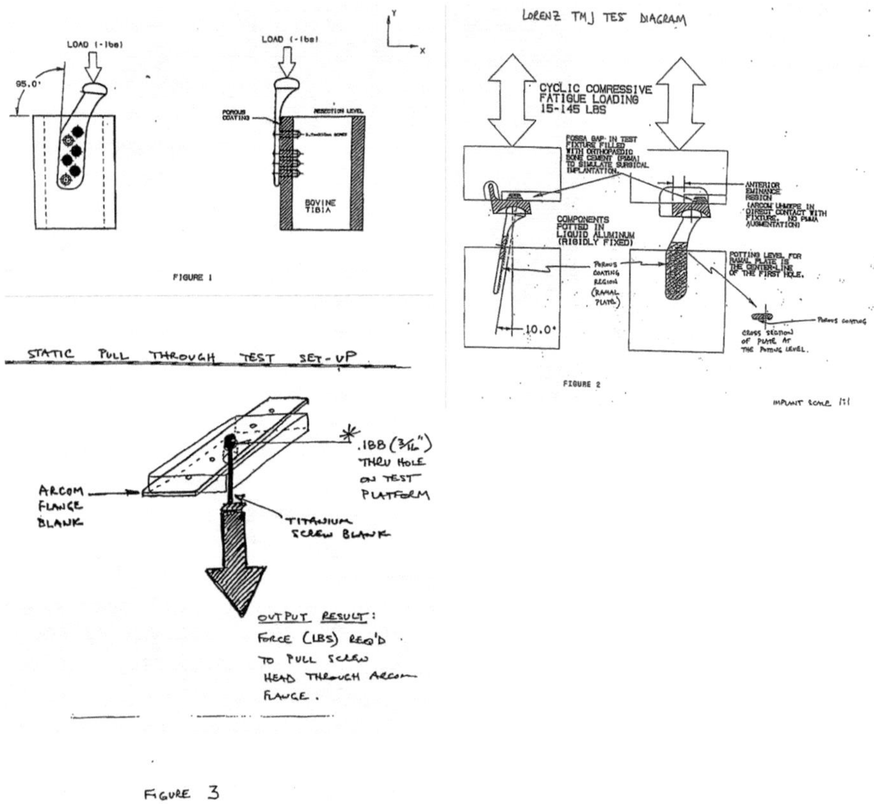

Fig. 7 Original design sketches by Dr. Peter Quinn demonstrating the biomechanical testing of the load and cyclic compressive fatigue for the Biomet-Lorenz TMJ prosthesis

cystoscope to perform diagnostic arthroscopies of cadaver knee joints (de Mello Granata Jr 2012). He subsequently helped design an arthroscope in 1920 and then published a case series including photos of his knee arthroscopies (Indresano and Mobati 2006; de Mello Granata Jr 2012). As additional studies were published describing diagnostic techniques using the arthroscope (Kreuscher 1925) and technologic advances allowed for the development of smaller arthroscopes with improved optics, TMJ surgeons took notice of this minimally invasive technique.

After the development of the small joint arthroscope by Watanabe in 1958 (Watanabe 1986; Watanabe and Takeda 1960) (Fig. 8), a Japanese surgeon by the name of Ohnishi was the first to describe its use for performing a TMJ arthroscopy in 1975 (Onishi 1975). As additional studies out of Japan by Murakami had described arthroscopy as a minimally invasive, useful adjunct in the treatment of patients with TMJ disorders (Murakami and Ono 1986; Murakami et al. 1986;

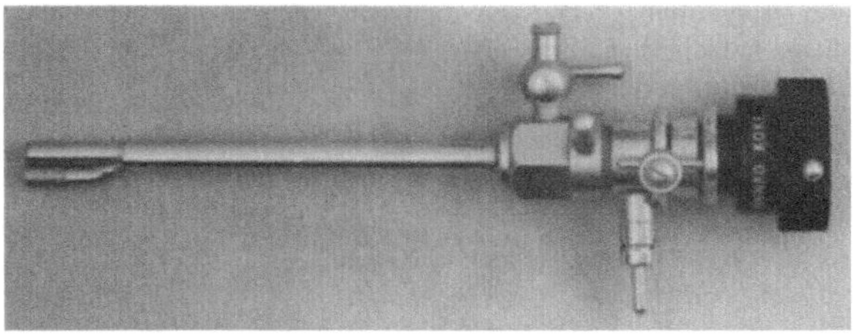

Fig. 8 The original no. 21 arthroscope developed by Watanabe in 1958 (Watanabe and Takeda 1960)

Murakami and Ito 1981, 1984), Sanders introduced the technique of TMJ arthroscopy in the United States (Sanders 1986).

Subsequent clinical studies carried out by Sanders, Murakami, and McCain evaluated the efficacy of arthroscopy of the TMJ and solidified its diagnostic and therapeutic use in the United States (Murakami et al. 1986; Sanders and Buoncristiani 1987; McCain 1988; McCain et al. 1989). In particular, Murakami published on the use of arthroscopy to evaluate joint adhesions (Murakami and Segami 1993), and Bronstein demonstrated its use in determining disc position (Bronstein 1989). McCain also published on advanced operative techniques in which the disc could be manipulated and repositioned using arthroscopy (McCain et al. 1992a). McCain and Sanders subsequently published a study describing high success rate of arthroscopies of over 4800 TMJs in 1992 (McCain et al. 1992b), with additional studies demonstrating high efficacy (Sanders and Buoncristiani 1993). Additional advanced techniques including the use of sclerotherapy (Merrill 1993) and laser treatments (Indresano and Bradrick 1993) were also developed and described. Further significant technological advances have also been made to develop state-of-the-art arthroscopes specifically designed to improve upon visualization of the temporomandibular joint space (Fig. 9). In a controversial surgical field troubled by the recent failure of alloplastic materials in TMJ replacements, TMJ arthroscopy served as an initial, safe, inexpensive, effective means of treating TMJ disease via lysis and lavage and offered an option to patient to potentially spare an open procedure.

5 Arthrocentesis

Evidence of the first "arthrocentesis" as a treatment for intra-joint fluid accumulation dates to the sixteenth century, during which it was described in the Aztec literature. During this time, the technique of simple paracentesis was often performed to treat joint effusions (Emmart 1940; Rodnan et al. 1966). In 1792, a French surgeon by the name of Jean Gay described the successful outcomes associated with his technique of paracentesis along with injection of "medication" into a knee joint. With the intention of decreasing inflammation, Gay injected a mixture of wine, brandy, and rum into the knee joint of two separate patients, noting a significant post-operative improvement in symptoms (Rodnan et al. 1966).

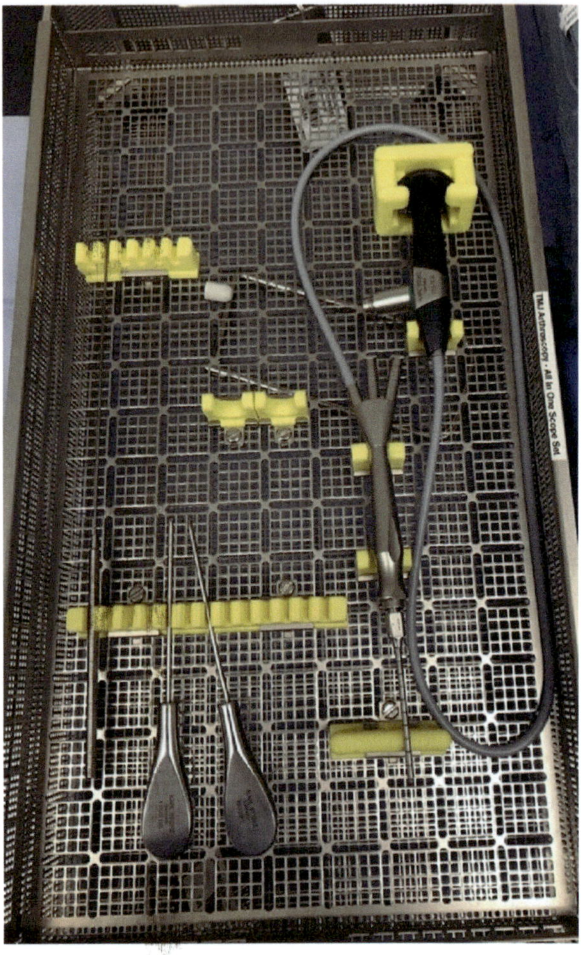

Fig. 9 Contemporary Karl Storz model all-in-one TMJ arthroscope system

In 1947, Schultz was the first to describe injection into the TMJ. He injected sodium psylliate into the periarticular region with the intent of stimulating a fibrotic response to limit condylar mobility in order to treat joint hypermobility (Schultz 1947). In 1950, McKelvey demonstrated successful patient outcomes of his own by injecting sclerosing solutions into the periarticular region of the TMJ to treat subluxation (McKelvey 1950). Later in 1987, Murakami et al. published on their use of arthrocentesis in the treatment of closed lock. Their team described a technique of readjusting the mandible while inducing hydraulic pressure with lidocaine in the upper joint space with a 21-gauage needle (Murakami et al. 1987). Nitzan, Dolwick, and colleagues then built upon Murakami's technique by describing the lavage of the TMJ with lactated ringers by placing two separate needles (one used for inflow, the other for outflow) into the superior joint space. They described successful results in patients with trismus, with lavage resulting in improvement in pain scores, improvement in maximal incisal opening, and lasting symptom relief (Nitzan et al.

1991). Although initially only used for acute closed lock, TMJ arthrocentesis is now used for a variety of conditions associated with the joint including disc displacement, synovitis, rheumatoid arthritis, disc adhesions, and hemarthrosis, with other medications such as steroids, anti-inflammatories, and lubricating agents commonly being injected.

References

American Association of Oral and Maxillofacial Surgeons. TMJ implant advisory. August 1992.

American Association of Oral and Maxillofacial Surgeons. Recommendations for management of patients with temporomandibular joint implants. Temporomandibular Joint Implant Surgery Workshop. J Oral Maxillofac Surg. 1993a;51(10):1164–72.

American Association of Oral and Maxillofacial Surgeons. Recommendations for management of patients with temporomandibular joint implants. Temporomandibular Joint Implant Surgery Workshop. J Oral Maxillofac Surg. 1993b;340:510–3.

Annandale T. Displacement of the interarticular cartilage of the lower jaw and its treatment by operation. Lancet. 1887;8:411.

Ashhurst AP. Recurrent unilateral subluxation of the mandible excision of the interarticular cartilage in cases of snapping jaw. Ann Surg. 1921;73(6):712–5.

Bee D, Zeitler D. The Proplast-Teflon implant in TMJ reconstruction following meniscectomy. 68th annual meeting of the American Association of Oral and Maxillofacial Surgeons New Orleans, LA. 1986.

Berarducci JP, Thompson DA, Scheffer RB. Perforation into middle cranial fossa as a sequel to use of a Proplast-Teflon implant for temporomandibular joint reconstruction. J Oral Maxillofac Surg. 1990;48(5):496–8.

Blackwood HJ. Growth of the mandibular condyle of the rat studied with tritiated thymidine. Arch Oral Biol. 1966;11(5):493–500.

Boman K. Temporomandibular joint arthrosis and its treatment by extirpation of the disc. Acta Chir Scand. 1947;95:1.

Bowman K. Temporomandibular joint arthrosis and its treatment by extirpation of the disk: a clinical study. Acta Chir Scand Suppl. 1947;118:225 p.

Boyne PJ, Mathews FR, Stringer DE. TMJ bone remodeling after polyoxymethylene condylar replacement. Int J Oral Maxillofac Implants. 1987;2(1):29–33.

Bronstein SL. Retained alloplastic temporomandibular joint disk implants: a retrospective study. Oral Surg Oral Med Oral Pathol. 1987;64(2):135–45.

Bronstein SL. Diagnostic and operative arthroscopy: historical perspectives and indications. Oral Maxillofac Surg Clin North Am. 1989;1:59–68.

Brown JB, Fryer MP, Kollias P, Ohlwiler DA, Templeton JB. Silicone and Teflon prostheses, including full jaw substitution: laboratory and clinical studies of Etheron. Ann Surg. 1963;157:932–43.

Butow KW, Blackbeard GA, van der Merwe AE. Titanium/titanium nitride temporomandibular joint prosthesis: historical background and a six-year clinical review. SADJ. 2001;56(8): 370–6.

Carnochan J. Mobilizing a patient's ankylosed jaw by placing a block of wood between the raw bony surfaces after resection. Arch Med. 1860:284.

Charnley J. Arthroplasty of the hip. A new operation. Lancet. 1961;1(7187):1129–32.

Charnley J. Tissue reaction to the polytetrafluoroethylene. Lancet. 1963;2:1379.

Christensen RW. The correction of mandibular ankylosis by arthroplasty and the insertion of a cast Vitallium glenoid fossa. South Calif Dent Assoc. 1963;31:117–8.

Christensen RW. Mandibular joint arthrosis corrected by the insertion of a cast-Vitallium glenoid fossa prosthesis: a new technique. Report of a case. Oral Surg Oral Med Oral Pathol. 1964;17:712–22.

Christensen RW. The temporomandibular joint prosthesis eleven years later. Oral Implantol. 1971;2(2):125–33.

Cook HP. Teflon implantation in temporomandibular arthroplasty. Oral Surg Oral Med Oral Pathol. 1972;33(5):706–16.

Cottrell DA, Wolford LM. The Mitek mini anchor in maxillofacial surgery. J Oral Maxillofac Surg. 1993;57(3):150.

de Mello Granata GS Jr. A hundred years of knee arthroscopy. Rev Bras Ortop. 2012;47(6):684.

Dimitroulis G. The interpositional dermis-fat graft in the management of temporomandibular joint ankylosis. Int J Oral Maxillofac Surg. 2004;33(8):755–60.

Dimitroulis G. The use of dermis grafts after discectomy for internal derangement of the temporomandibular joint. J Oral Maxillofac Surg. 2005;63(2):173–8.

Dimitroulis G. A critical review of interpositional grafts following temporomandibular joint discectomy with an overview of the dermis-fat graft. Int J Oral Maxillofac Surg. 2011a;40(6):561–8.

Dimitroulis G. Condylar morphology after temporomandibular joint discectomy with interpositional abdominal dermis-fat graft. J Oral Maxillofac Surg. 2011b;69(2):439–46.

Dimitroulis G, Trost N, Morrison W. The radiological fate of dermis-fat grafts in the human temporomandibular joint using magnetic resonance imaging. Int J Oral Maxillofac Surg. 2008;37(3):249–54.

Dimitroulis G, McCullough M, Morrison W. Quality-of-life survey comparing patients before and after discectomy of the temporomandibular joint. J Oral Maxillofac Surg. 2010;68(1):101–6.

Dingman RO, Grabb WC. Reconstruction of both mandibular condyles with metatarsal bone grafts. Plast Reconstr Surg. 1964;34:441–51.

Dingman RO, Moorman WC. Meniscectomy in the treatment of lesions of the temporomandibular joint. J Oral Surg (Chic). 1951;9(3):214–24.

Dolwick MF, Aufdemorte TB. Silicone-induced foreign body reaction and lymphadenopathy after temporomandibular joint arthroplasty. Oral Surg Oral Med Oral Pathol. 1985;59(5):449–52.

Donlon WC. Total temporomandibular joint reconstruction. Philadelphia: W.B. Saunders Company; 2000.

Driemel O, Carlson ER, Muller-Richter U, Moralis A, Lienhard S, Wagener S, et al. New condylar head system for temporary condylar reconstruction in ablative tumour surgery. Mund Kiefer Gesichtschir. 2007;11(4):193–9.

Driemel O, Braun S, Muller-Richter UD, Behr M, Reichert TE, Kunkel M, et al. Historical development of alloplastic temporomandibular joint replacement after 1945 and state of the art. Int J Oral Maxillofac Surg. 2009;38(9):909–20.

Durkin JF, Heeley JD, Irving JT. The cartilage of the mandibular condyle. Oral Sci Rev. 1973;2:29–99.

Eggers GW. Arthroplasty of the temporomandibular joint in children with interposition of tantalum foil. J Bone Joint Surg Am. 1946;28:603–6.

El Deeb M, Holmes RE. Zygomatic and mandibular augmentation with Proplast and porous hydroxyapatite in Rhesus monkeys. J Oral Maxillofac Surg. 1989;47(5):480–8.

Emmart EW. The Badianus manuscript (Codex Barberini Latin 241). Baltimore: The Johns Hopkins Press; 1940.

Entin MA. Reconstruction in congenital deformity of the temporo-mandibular component. Plast Reconstr Surg Transplant Bull. 1958;21(6):461–9.

Eriksson L, Westesson PL. Long-term evaluation of meniscectomy of the temporomandibular joint. J Oral Maxillofac Surg. 1985;43(4):263–9.

Eriksson L, Westesson PL. Deterioration of temporary silicone implant in the temporomandibular joint: a clinical and arthroscopic follow-up study. Oral Surg Oral Med Oral Pathol. 1986;62(1):2–6.

Eriksson L, Westesson PL. Temporomandibular joint diskectomy. No positive effect of temporary silicone implant in a 5-year follow-up. Oral Surg Oral Med Oral Pathol. 1992;74(3):259–72.
FDA. Temporomandibular joint implants. Silver Spring: US Food and Drug Administration; 2021. Available from: https://www.fda.gov/medical-devices/temporomandibular-disorders-tmd-devices/temporomandibular-joint-tmj-implants#implants.
Feinberg SE, Larsen PE. The use of a pedicled temporalis muscle-pericranial flap for replacement of the TMJ disc: preliminary report. J Oral Maxillofac Surg. 1989;47(2):142–6.
Feinerman DM, Piecuch JF. Long-term retrospective analysis of twenty-three Proplast-Teflon temporomandibular joint interpositional implants. Int J Oral Maxillofac Surg. 1993;22(1):11–6.
Figdor PP. The development of endoscopy in the 19th century. Tuttlingen: Endo Press; 2004.
Figueroa AA, Gans BJ, Pruzansky S. Long-term follow-up of a mandibular costochondral graft. Oral Surg Oral Med Oral Pathol. 1984;58(3):257–68.
Florine B, Gatto D, Wade M. Pre- and post-surgical tomographic analysis of TMJ arthroplasties. J Oral Maxillofac Surg. 1986;44(11):M3.
Freihofer HP, Perko MA. Simultaneous reconstruction of the area of the temporo-mandibular joint including the ramus of the mandible in a posttraumatic case. A case report. J Maxillofac Surg. 1976;4(2):124–8.
Garrett WR, Abbey PA, Christensen R. Temporomandibular joint reconstruction with a custom total temporomandibular joint prosthesis: use in the multiply operated patient. Surg Technol Int. 1997;6:347–54.
Georgiade N, Altany F, Pickrell K. An experimental and clinical evaluation of autogenous dermal grafts used in the treatment of temporomandibular joint ankylosis. Plast Reconstr Surg (1946). 1957;19(4):321–36.
Giannakopoulos HE, Sinn DP, Quinn PD. Biomet Microfixation Temporomandibular Joint Replacement System: a 3-year follow-up study of patients treated during 1995 to 2005. J Oral Maxillofac Surg. 2012;70(4):787–94; discussion 95–6.
Gillies HD. Plastic surgery of the face. London: Oxford University Press; 1920.
Gluck T. Referat Uber die Durch das Moderne Chirurgische Expierment Gewonnenen Positven Resultate, Betreffenddie Naht und den Ersatz von Defecten Hoerer Gewebe, Sowie Uber die Verwerthung Resorbirbarer und Bebendiger Tampons in der Chirgurie. Arch Klin Chir. 1891;4:186.
Gordon SD. Surgery of the temporomandibular joint. Am J Surg. 1958;95(2):263–6.
Granquist EJ, Bouloux G, Dattilo D, Gonzalez O, Louis PJ, McCain J, et al. Outcomes and survivorship of Biomet microfixation total joint replacement system: results from an FDA postmarket study. J Oral Maxillofac Surg. 2020;78(9):1499–508.
Hahn G. Vitallium mesh mandibular prosthesis. J Prosthet Dent. 1964;14:777–84.
Hanley C, Martin SR, Sullivan S. Utilization of the all-suture Biomet Juggerknot Soft Anchor for disc repositioning in the surgical management of internal derangements of the temporomandibular joint. Oral Surg Oral Med Oral Pathol Oral Radiol. 2015;119(5):e254.
Hartman LC, Bessette RW, Baier RE, Meyer AE, Wirth J. Silicone rubber temporomandibular joint (TMJ) meniscal replacements: postimplant histopathologic and material evaluation. J Biomed Mater Res. 1988;22(6):475–84.
Heffez L, Mafee MF, Rosenberg H, Langer B. CT evaluation of TMJ disc replacement with a Proplast-Teflon laminate. J Oral Maxillofac Surg. 1987;45(8):657–65.
Henry T. Prosthetic restoration of the left temporomandibular joint in a case of partial ankylosis. In: Transactions of the 2nd congress international society of plastic surgeons. London: Livingstone; 1960. 159 p.
Henry CH, Wolford LM. Treatment outcomes for temporomandibular joint reconstruction after Proplast-Teflon implant failure. J Oral Maxillofac Surg. 1993;51(4):352–8; discussion 9–60.
Hinds EC, Homsy CA, Kent JN. Use of a biocompatible interface for binding tissues and prostheses in temporomandibular joint surgery. Follow-up report. Oral Surg Oral Med Oral Pathol. 1974;38(4):512–9.

Hoffman D, Pappas M. Hoffman-Pappas prosthesis. Oral Maxillofac Surg Clin North Am. 2000;12(1):105–24.

Holmlund AB, Gynther G, Axelsson S. Diskectomy in treatment of internal derangement of the temporomandibular joint. Follow-up at 1, 3, and 5 years. Oral Surg Oral Med Oral Pathol. 1993;76(3):266–71.

Homsy CA. Bio-compatibility in selection of materials for implantation. J Biomed Mater Res. 1970;4(3):341–56.

Homsy CA, Cain TE, Kessler FB, Anderson MS, King JW. Porous implant systems for prosthesis stabilization. Clin Orthop Relat Res. 1972;89:220–35.

Homsy CA, Kent JN, Hinds EC. Materials for oral implantation--biological and functional criteria. J Am Dent Assoc. 1973;86(4):817–32.

House L, Morgan DH, Hall WP, Vamvas SJ. Temporomandibular joint surgery. Report of a 14 year joint implant study. Laryngoscope. 1984;94:537–8.

Indresano AT, Bradrick J. Arthroscopic laser procedures. Philadelphia: WB Saunders; 1993.

Indresano AT, Mobati DA. History of temporomandibular joint surgery. Oral Maxillofac Surg Clin North Am. 2006;18(3):283–9, v.

Johnson RM. Public health advisory on Vitek Proplast TMJ implants. 1991.

Kameros J, Himmelfarb R. Treatment of TMJ ankylosis with methyl methacrylate interpositional arthroplasty. J Oral Surg. 1975;33:282–91.

Kanamori M, Kawaguchi Y, Ohmori K, Kimura T, Md HT, Matsui H. The fate of autogenous free-fat grafts after posterior lumbar surgery: part 1. A postoperative serial magnetic resonance imaging study. Spine (Phila Pa 1976). 2001;26(20):2258–63.

Kaplan PA, Ruskin JD, Tu HK, Knibbe MA. Erosive arthritis of the temporomandibular joint caused by Teflon-Proplast implants: plain film features. AJR Am J Roentgenol. 1988;151(2):337–9.

Kennett S. Temporomandibular joint ankylosis: the rationale for grafting in the young patient. J Oral Surg. 1973;31(10):744–8.

Kent JN, Homsy CA, Gross BD, Hinds EC. Pilot studies of a porous implant in dentistry and oral surgery. J Oral Surg. 1972;30(8):608–15.

Kent JN, Misiek DJ, Akin RK, Hinds EC, Homsy CA. Temporomandibular joint condylar prosthesis: a ten-year report. J Oral Maxillofac Surg. 1983;41(4):245–54.

Kent JN, Block MS, Homsy CA, Prewitt JM 3rd, Reid R. Experience with a polymer glenoid fossa prosthesis for partial or total temporomandibular joint reconstruction. J Oral Maxillofac Surg. 1986;44(7):520–33.

Kent JN, Block MS, Halpern J, Fontenot MG. Update on the vitek partial and total temporomandibular joint systems. J Oral Maxillofac Surg. 1993;51(4):408–15; discussion 15–6.

Kiehn CL, Desprez JD. Meniscectomy for internal derangement of temporomandibular joint. Br J Plast Surg. 1962;15:199–204.

Kiehn CL, DesPrez JD, Converse CF. A new procedure for total temporomandibular joint replacement. Plast Reconstr Surg. 1974;53(2):221–6.

Kirsch T. The use of Protoplast-Teflon implants for meniscectomy and disc repair in the temporomandibular joint. Annual meeting of the American Association of Oral and Maxillofacial Surgeons. 1984.

Klotch DW, Lindqvist C, Schusterman MA, Prein J. Reconstructive tumor surgery in the mandible. Berlin: Springer; 1998.

Kreuscher P. Semilunar cartilage disease. A plea for early recognition by means of the arthroscope and early treatment of this condition. Ill Med J. 1925;47:290.

Lagrotteria L, Scapino R, Granston AS, Felgenhauer D. Patient with lymphadenopathy following temporomandibular joint arthroplasty with Proplast. Cranio. 1986;4(2):172–8.

Lanz A. Discitis mandibularis. Zentralbl Chir. 1909;36:289–91.

Leopard PJ. Anterior dislocation of the temporomandibular disc. Br J Oral Maxillofac Surg. 1984;22(1):9–17.

Lexer E. Uber Gelenktransplantation. Arch Klin Chir. 1909;90:263.

Lexer E. Joint transplantations and arthroplasty. Surg Gynecol Obstet. 1925;40:782.

Lindqvist C, Pihakari A, Tasanen A, Hampf G. Autogenous costochondral grafts in temporomandibular joint arthroplasty. A survey of 66 arthroplasties in 60 patients. J Maxillofac Surg. 1986;14(3):143–9.
Lindqvist C, Jokinen J, Paukku P, Tasanen A. Adaptation of autogenous costochondral grafts used for temporomandibular joint reconstruction: a long-term clinical and radiologic follow-up. J Oral Maxillofac Surg. 1988;46(6):465–70.
Lindqvist C, Soderholm AL, Hallikainen D, Sjovall L. Erosion and heterotopic bone formation after alloplastic temporomandibular joint reconstruction. J Oral Maxillofac Surg. 1992;50(9):942–9; discussion 50.
Lindqvist C, Söderholm A-L, Hallikainen D. Problems related to mandibular condylar prosthesis. Berlin: Springer; 2002.
Ma J, Liang L, Jiang H, Gu B. Gap arthroplasty versus interpositional arthroplasty for temporomandibular joint ankylosis: a meta-analysis. PLoS One. 2015;10(5):e0127652.
MacAfee KA, Quinn PD. Total temporomandibular joint reconstruction with a Delrin titanium implant. J Craniofac Surg. 1992;3(3):160–9.
MacIntosh RB, Henny FA. A spectrum of application of autogenous costochondral grafts. J Maxillofac Surg. 1977;5(4):257–67.
Marx RE, Cillo JE Jr, Broumand V, Ulloa JJ. Outcome analysis of mandibular condylar replacements in tumor and trauma reconstruction: a prospective analysis of 131 cases with long-term follow-up. J Oral Maxillofac Surg. 2008;66(12):2515–23.
Matukas VJ, Lachner J. The use of autologous auricular cartilage for temporomandibular joint disc replacement: a preliminary report. J Oral Maxillofac Surg. 1990;48(4):348–53.
McCain JP. Arthroscopy of the human temporomandibular joint. J Oral Maxillofac Surg. 1988;46(8):648–55.
McCain JP, de la Rua H, Le Blanc WG. Correlation of clinical, radiographic, and arthroscopic findings in internal derangements of the TMJ. J Oral Maxillofac Surg. 1989;47(9):913–21.
McCain JP, Podrasky AE, Zabiegalski NA. Arthroscopic disc repositioning and suturing: a preliminary report. J Oral Maxillofac Surg. 1992a;50(6):568–79; discussion 79–80.
McCain JP, Sanders B, Koslin MG, Quinn JH, Peters PB, Indresano AT. Temporomandibular joint arthroscopy: a 6-year multicenter retrospective study of 4,831 joints. J Oral Maxillofac Surg. 1992b;50(9):926–30.
McCarty WL, Farrar WB. Surgery for internal derangements of the temporomandibular joint. J Prosthet Dent. 1979;42(2):191–6.
McKelvey L. Sclerosing solution in the treatment of chronic subluxation of the temporomandibular joint. J Oral Surg (Chic). 1950;8(3):225–36.
McKenna SJ. Discectomy for the treatment of internal derangements of the temporomandibular joint. J Oral Maxillofac Surg. 2001;59(9):1051–6.
Mehra P, Wolford LM. The Mitek mini anchor for TMJ disc repositioning: surgical technique and results. Int J Oral Maxillofac Surg. 2001;30(6):497–503.
Mercuri LG. The Christensen prosthesis. Oral Surg Oral Med Oral Pathol Oral Radiol Endod. 1996;81(2):134–5.
Mercuri LG. The TMJ concepts patient fitted total temporomandibular joint reconstruction prosthesis. Philadelphia: Saunders; 2000.
Mercuri LG. Temporomandibular joint total joint replacement – TMJ TJR. Cham: Springer; 2016.
Mercuri LG, Wolford LM, Sanders B, White RD, Hurder A, Henderson W. Custom CAD/CAM total temporomandibular joint reconstruction system: preliminary multicenter report. J Oral Maxillofac Surg. 1995;53(2):106–15; discussion 15–6.
Mercuri LG, Wolford LM, Sanders B, White RD, Giobbie-Hurder A. Long-term follow-up of the CAD/CAM patient fitted total temporomandibular joint reconstruction system. J Oral Maxillofac Surg. 2002;60(12):1440–8.
Merrill R. Arthroscopic temporomandibular joint lysis, lavage, and manipulation and chemical sclerotherapy for painful hypermobility and recurrent mandibular dislocation. Philadelphia: WB Saunders; 1993.

Meyer RA. The autogenous dermal graft in temporomandibular joint disc surgery. J Oral Maxillofac Surg. 1988;46(11):948–54.
Morgan D. Dysfunction, pain, tinnitus, vertigo corrected by mandibular joint surgery. J South Calif Dent Assoc. 1971;39:505–7.
Morgan DH. Evaluation of alloplastic TMJ implants. Cranio. 1988;6(3):224–38.
Morgan DH. Development of alloplastic materials for temporomandibular joint prosthesis: a historical perspective with clinical illustrations. Cranio. 1992;10(3):192–204.
Morgan DH, Hall WP. Addition of a Silastic and metal implant to a metallic condyle. Cranio. 1985;3:179–83.
Murakami K, Ito K. Arthroscopy of the temporomandibular joint: arthroscopic anatomy and arthroscopic approaches in the human cadaver. Arthoscopy. 1981;6:1–13.
Murakami K, Ito K. Arthroscopy of the temporomandibular joint third report; clinical experiences. Arthoscopy. 1984;9:49–59.
Murakami K, Ono T. Temporomandibular joint arthroscopy by inferolateral approach. Int J Oral Maxillofac Surg. 1986;15(4):410–7.
Murakami K, Segami N. Intra-articular adhesions of the temporomandibular joint: arthroscopic views and clinical perspectives. Philadelphia: WB Saunders; 1993.
Murakami KI, Lizuka T, Matsuki M, Ono T. Diagnostic arthroscopy of the TMJ: differential diagnoses in patients with limited jaw opening. Cranio. 1986;4(2):117–26.
Murakami KI, Iizuka T, Matsuki M, Ono T. Recapturing the persistent anteriorly displaced disk by mandibular manipulation after pumping and hydraulic pressure to the upper joint cavity of the temporomandibular joint. Cranio. 1987;5(1):17–24.
Murphy J. Bony ankylosis of jaw with interposition of flaps from temporal fascia. Surg Clin. 1913;2:659.
Murphy J. Arthroplasty for intra-articular bony and fibrous ankylosis of temporomandibular articulartion. J Am Med Assoc. 1914;62:1783–94.
Nikolaou VS, Giannoudis PV. History of osteochondral allograft transplantation. Injury. 2017;48(7):1283–6.
Nitzan DW, Dolwick MF, Martinez GA. Temporomandibular joint arthrocentesis: a simplified treatment for severe, limited mouth opening. J Oral Maxillofac Surg. 1991;49(11):1163–7; discussion 8–70.
Onishi M. Arthroscopy of the temporomandibular joint (author's transl). Kokubyo Gakkai Zasshi. 1975;42(2):207–13.
Perrott DH, Umeda H, Kaban LB. Costochondral graft construction/reconstruction of the ramus/condyle unit: long-term follow-up. Int J Oral Maxillofac Surg. 1994;23(6 Pt 1):321–8.
Plotnikov NA. Methoden der Aufbereitung und Konservierung lyophilisierter Knochen-Homotransplantatezur Substitution bei Unterkieferdefekte. Chir Plast. 1965;2:65.
Pogrel MA, Kaban LB. The role of a temporalis fascia and muscle flap in temporomandibular joint surgery. J Oral Maxillofac Surg. 1990;48(1):14–9.
Popescu V, Vasiliu D. Treatment of temporo-mandibular ankylosis with particular reference to the interposition of full-thickness skin autotransplant. J Maxillofac Surg. 1977;5(1):3–14.
Poswillo D. Experimental reconstruction of the mandibular joint. Int J Oral Surg. 1974;3(6):400–11.
Prein J. Condylar prosthesis for the replacement of the mandibular condyle. Berlin: Springer; 2002. p. 372–6.
Pringle J. Displacement of the mandibular meniscus and its treatment. Br J Surg. 1918;6(23):385–9.
Quinn P. Lorenz prosthesis. Oral Maxillofac Surg Clin North Am. 2000;12(1):93–104.
Ramezanian M, Yavary T. Comparison of gap arthroplasty and interpositional gap arthroplasty on the temporomandibular joint ankylosis. Acta Med Iran. 2006;44(6):391–4.
Raveh J, Stich H, Schawalder P, Sutter F, Straumann F. Conservative and surgical measures to restore temporomandibular joint function and new possibilities and methods for bridging defects in the mandible. SSO Schweiz Monatsschr Zahnheilkd. 1980;90(10):932–48.
Raveh J, Stich H, Sutter F, Greiner R. Use of the titanium-coated hollow screw and reconstruction plate system in bridging of lower jaw defects. J Oral Maxillofac Surg. 1984;42(5):281–94.

Resnick CM, Frid P, Norholt SE, Stoustrup P, Peacock ZS, Kaban LB, et al. An algorithm for management of dentofacial deformity resulting from juvenile idiopathic arthritis: results of a multinational consensus conference. J Oral Maxillofac Surg. 2019;77(6):1152.e1–e33.
Risdon F. Ankylosis of the temporomandibular joint. J Am Dent Assoc. 1933;21:1933–7.
Robinson M. Temporomandibular ankylosis corrected by creating a false stainless steel fossa. J South Calif Dent Assoc. 1960;28:186–9.
Robinson M. Temporomandibular ankylosis corrected by creating a false silastic sponge fossa. J South Calif Dent Assoc. 1968;36(1):14–6.
Rodnan GP, Benedek TG, Panetta WC. The early history of synovia (joint fluid). Ann Intern Med. 1966;65(4):821–42.
Rooney TP, Haug RH, Toor AH, Indresano AT. Rapid condylar degeneration after glenoid fossa prosthesis insertion: report of three cases. J Oral Maxillofac Surg. 1988;46(3):240–6.
Ryba FM, Ali A, Matthews NS. Temporomandibular joint meniscopexy using the Arthrex Corkscrew(R) mini anchor system: technical note. Br J Oral Maxillofac Surg. 2015;53(3):299–300.
Sanders B. Arthroscopic surgery of the temporomandibular joint: treatment of internal derangement with persistent closed lock. Oral Surg Oral Med Oral Pathol. 1986;62(4):361–72.
Sanders B, Buoncristiani R. Diagnostic and surgical arthroscopy of the temporomandibular joint: clinical experience with 137 procedures over a 2-year period. J Craniomandib Disord. 1987;1(3):202–13.
Sanders B, Buoncristiani R. A 5-year experience with arthroscopic lysis and lavage for treatment of painful temporomandibular joint hypomobility. Philadelphia: WB Saunders; 1993. p. 21–4.
Sandler NA, Macmillan C, Buckley MJ, Barnes L. Histologic and histochemical changes in failed auricular cartilage grafts used for a temporomandibular joint disc replacement: a report of three cases and review of the literature. J Oral Maxillofac Surg. 1997;55(9):1014–9.
Schellhas KP, Wilkes CH, el Deeb M, Lagrotteria LB, Omlie MR. Permanent Proplast temporomandibular joint implants: MR imaging of destructive complications. AJR Am J Roentgenol. 1988;151(4):731–5.
Schultz LW. Report of ten years' experience in treating hypermobility of the temporomandibular joints. J Oral Surg (Chic). 1947;5(3):202–7.
Silver CM. Long-term results of meniscectomy of the temporomandibular joint. Cranio. 1984;3(1):46–57.
Silver CM, Motamed M, Carlotti AE Jr. Arthroplasty of the temporomandibular joint with use of a Vitallium condyle prosthesis: report of three cases. J Oral Surg. 1977;35(11):909–14.
Small IA, Brown S, Kobernick SD. Teflon and Silastic for mandibular replacement: experimental studies and reports of cases. J Oral Surg Anesth Hosp Dent Serv. 1964;22:377–90.
Smith AE, Robinson M. A new surgical procedure in bilateral reconstruction of condyles, utilizing iliac bone grafts and creation of new joints by means of non-electrolytic metal; a preliminary report. Plast Reconstr Surg (1946). 1952;9(5):393–409.
Smith AE, Robinson M. A new surgical procedure for the creation of a false temporomandibular joint in cases of ankylosis by means of non-electrolytic metal. Am J Surg. 1957;94(6):837–45.
Snyder CC, Levine GA, Dingman DL. Trial of a sternoclavicular whole joint graft as a substitute for the temporomandibular joint. Plast Reconstr Surg. 1971;48(5):447–52.
Sonnenburg M, Sonnenburg I. Development and clinical application of the total temporomandibular joint (T.M.J.) endoprosthesis. Rev Stomatol Chir Maxillofac. 1990;91(2):165–9.
Sonnenburg I, Fethke K, Sonnenburg M. Pressure load of the temporomandibular joint--an experimental study. Anat Anz. 1984;155(1–5):309–15.
Spagnoli D, Kent JN. Multicenter evaluation of temporomandibular joint Proplast-Teflon disk implant. Oral Surg Oral Med Oral Pathol. 1992;74(4):411–21.
Speculand B, Hensher R, Powell D. Total prosthetic replacement of the TMJ: experience with two systems 1988-1997. Br J Oral Maxillofac Surg. 2000;38(4):360–9.
Spiessl B. First experiences with a temporomandibular-joint prosthesis. Fortschr Kiefer Gesichtschir. 1976;21:119–21.

Swanson AB. Silicone rubber implants for replacement of arthritic or destroyed joints in the hand. 1968. Clin Orthop Relat Res. 1997;(342):4–10.

Szabo G, Barabas J, Matrai J, Gyorgy J, Miklos L. Application of compact aluminum oxide ceramic implants in maxillofacial surgery. J Oral Maxillofac Surg. 1990;48(4):354–61.

Tauras SP, Jordan JE, Keen RR. Temporomandibular joint ankylosis corrected with a gold prosthesis. J Oral Surg. 1972;30:767–73.

TMJ. TMJ device and regulatory history. Milwaukee: The TMJ Association; 2021. Available from: https://tmj.org/living-with-tmj/tmj-implants/tmj-device-and-regulatory-history/.

Tong AC, Tideman H. A comparative study on meniscectomy and autogenous graft replacement of the Rhesus monkey temporomandibular joint articular disc--Part I. Int J Oral Maxillofac Surg. 2000;29(2):140–5.

Topazian RG. Comparison of gap and interposition arthroplasty in the treatment of temporomandibular joint ankylosis. J Oral Surg. 1966;24(5):405–9.

Valentine JD Jr, Reiman BE, Beuttenmuller EA, Donovan MG. Light and electron microscopic evaluation of Proplast II TMJ disc implants. J Oral Maxillofac Surg. 1989;47(7):689–96.

Van Loon JP, Verkerke GJ, de Bont LG, Liem RS. Wear-testing of a temporomandibular joint prosthesis: UHMWPE and PTFE against a metal ball, in water and in serum. Biomaterials. 1999;20(16):1471–8.

van Loon JP, Verkerke GJ, de Vries MP, de Bont LG. Design and wear testing of a temporomandibular joint prosthesis articulation. J Dent Res. 2000;79(2):715–21.

van Loon JP, de Bont LG, Stegenga B, Spijkervet FK, Verkerke GJ. Groningen temporomandibular joint prosthesis. Development and first clinical application. Int J Oral Maxillofac Surg. 2002;31(1):44–52.

Vuillemin T, Raveh J, Sutter F. Mandibular reconstruction with the THORP condylar prosthesis after hemimandibulectomy. J Craniomaxillofac Surg. 1989;17(2):78–87.

Wade M, Gatto D, Florine B. Assessment of Proplast implants in meniscoplasties as temporomandibular joint surgical procedures. 68th annual meeting of the American Association of Oral and Maxillofacial Surgeons New Orleans, LA. 1986.

Wagner JD, Mosby EL. Assessment of Proplast-Teflon disc replacements. J Oral Maxillofac Surg. 1990;48(11):1140–4.

Walker RV, Kalamchi S. A surgical technique for management of internal derangement of the temporomandibular joint. J Oral Maxillofac Surg. 1987;45(4):299–305.

Ward TG. Surgery of the mandibular joint. Ann R Coll Surg Engl. 1961;28:139–52.

Ware WH, Taylor RC. Growth center transplantation to replace damaged mandibular condyles. J Am Dent Assoc. 1966;73(1):128–37.

Watanabe M. Memories of the early days of arthroscopy. Arthroscopy. 1986;2(4):209–14.

Watanabe M, Takeda S. The number 21 arthroscope. J Jpn Orthop Assoc. 1960;34:1041.

Weinberg S, Cousens G. Meniscocondylar plication: a modified operation for surgical repositioning of the ectopic temporomandibular joint meniscus. Rationale and operative technique. Oral Surg Oral Med Oral Pathol. 1987;63(4):393–402.

Westermark A, Koppel D, Leiggener C. Condylar replacement alone is not sufficient for prosthetic reconstruction of the temporomandibular joint. Int J Oral Maxillofac Surg. 2006;35(6):488–92.

Westfall RL, Homsy CA, Kent JN. A comparison of porous composite PTFE/graphite and PTFE/aluminum oxide facial implants in primates. J Oral Maxillofac Surg. 1982;40(12):771–5.

Wilkes CH. Structural and functional alterations of the temporomandibular joint. Northwest Dent. 1978a;57(5):287–94.

Wilkes CH. Arthrography of the temporomandibular joint in patients with the TMJ pain-dysfunction syndrome. Minn Med. 1978b;61(11):645–52.

Wolford LM, Cottrell DA, Henry CH. Temporomandibular joint reconstruction of the complex patient with the Techmedica custom-made total joint prosthesis. J Oral Maxillofac Surg. 1994;52(1):2–10; discussion 1.

Yih WY, Zysset M, Merrill RG. Histologic study of the fate of autogenous auricular cartilage grafts in the human temporomandibular joint. J Oral Maxillofac Surg. 1992;50(9):964–7; discussion 8.

Zhi K, Ren W, Zhou H, Gao L, Zhao L, Hou C, et al. Management of temporomandibular joint ankylosis: 11 years' clinical experience. Oral Surg Oral Med Oral Pathol Oral Radiol Endod. 2009;108(5):687–92.

Distraction Osteogenesis

Dani Stanbouly and Michael Perrino

1 Introduction

Distractions osteogenesis, the biological process of new bone formation between gradually separated bone segments through incremental traction, has very early roots. The renowned Greek physician, Hippocrates, was reported to have mechanically manipulated bone fragments in the repair of fractures. Subsequently, Guy de Chauliac in the fourteenth century first utilized *continuous* traction in the repair of fractures through a pulley system that consisted of a weight attached to the leg by a cord. Years later in the twentieth century, an Italian surgeon named Alessandro Codivilla illustrated one of the earliest instances of external fixation, where he induced limb lengthening of the lower limb through external skeletal traction after an oblique osteotomy of the femur. His device consisted of a traditional plaster cast placed on the leg and cut in half at the level of the osteotomy. While the proximal part of the cast was fastened to a stationary external frame, the distal part of the cast was anchored to the calcaneus via a pin (Samchukov et al. 1998).

Thereafter, distraction osteogenesis quickly increased in popularity across the world and was implemented particularly for the purpose of limb lengthening. Nevertheless, its successes were accompanied with an equal degree of complications, namely, *bone-associated problems* such as delayed healing, non-unions, and deformities and *soft tissue-associated problems* due to overstretching, such as nerve palsy. These significant issues stopped the process of distraction osteogenesis from achieving universal acceptance. While many surgeons responded to the

D. Stanbouly
College of Dental Medicine, Columbia University, New York, NY, USA

M. Perrino (✉)
Riverside Oral Surgery, River Edge, NJ, USA
e-mail: map@riversideoralsurgery.com

E. M. Ferneini et al. (eds.), *The History of Maxillofacial Surgery*,
https://doi.org/10.1007/978-3-030-89563-1_19

complications that erupted with the increasing popularity of distraction osteogenesis overtime, none of them addressed them as effectively as the Russian surgeon, Gavriil Ilizarov. He developed a fixation apparatus that held several advantages over the widely recognized methods at the time. Ilizarov also developed a revolutionary technique called subperiosteal corticotomy for the purpose of limb lengthening. The procedure ensured maximum preservation of the periosteum and endosteum, delivering minimum trauma to the periosteum and to the bone marrow (Samchukov et al. 1998).

It is worth mentioning that in his clinical experience, Ilizarov came to discover a couple of biological principles in distraction osteogenesis: (1) the tension-stress effect on the genesis and growth of tissues and (2) the influence of blood supply and mechanical loading on the shape of bones and joints. On top of his theoretical discoveries, Ilizarov articulated the practical circumstances necessary for their effective implementation through a series of experiments on dogs. His experiments scrutinized several phenomena and illustrated many novel and valid notions. In investigating the effect of the direction of distraction on the orientation of newly formed tissues, Ilizarov discovered that the regenerated bone always formed along the axis/direction of applied traction (Fig. 1). When he explored the influence of the rate and rhythm of distraction on the formation of the bone, his results proved that more frequent rates of distraction led to more favorable regeneration with less soft tissue problems. Despite the innovation that shone through his work, Illizarov remained by and large unknown to the rest of the world until his surgical expertise was requested by the famous Italian alpinist, Carlo Mauri. Carlo Mauri suffered from a foot deformity that could not be treated by the world's leading surgeons, who saw nothing more than a poor prognosis that rested on amputation. Ilizarov's

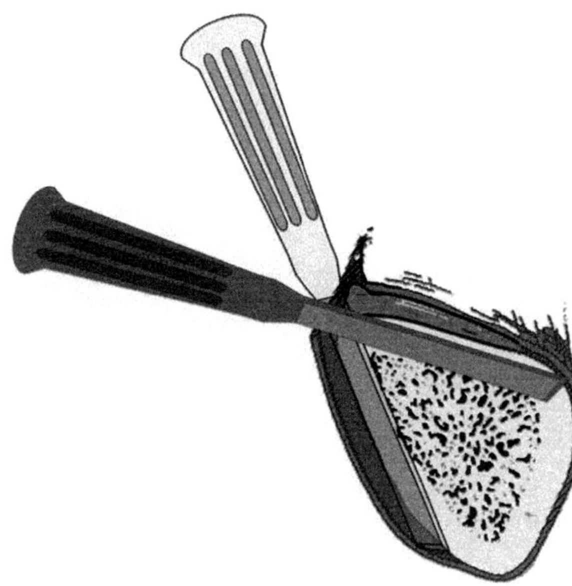

Fig. 1 G.A. Ilizarov's low-energy subperiosteal corticotomy technique. (Reprinted with permission and without alterations from Cope et al. (1999), Original Figure 5)

successful work on Carlo Mauri gained the attention of Italian surgeons, who invited Ilizarov to educate them on his methods. There, the Association for the Study and Application of the Method of Ilizarov (ASAMI) was formed. Subsequently, continental and international districts of ASAMI were formed to foster the exchange of knowledge about different aspects of distraction osteogenesis (Samchukov et al. 1998).

2 Early Applications of Distraction Osteogenesis in Maxillofacial Surgery

The arrival and development of distraction osteogenesis in the field of maxillofacial surgery were possible through the lessons learned from its application on long bones by the surgeons who pioneered the technique, such as Gavriil Ilizarov (Cope et al. 1999). Nevertheless, the time to transfer the knowledge acquired from distraction osteogenesis of the long bones to the maxillofacial region took over 40 years (Erverdi and Motro 2015).

During the early twentieth century and prior, skeletal deformities of the craniofacial complex, such as maxillomandibular hypoplasia, facial asymmetry, and congenital micrognathia, have been addressed in terminally grown patients via osteotomies followed by acute orthopedic movements and skeletal fixation. In order to correct retrognathic mandibles, Brown in 1918 and Bruhn-Linderman in 1921 each performed a vertical osteotomy of the mandibular body followed by acute advancement of the anterior segment, where the consequent gap created would be filled by healing bone regenerate (Limberg 1925). While this paradigm of acute treatment, embodied by orthognathic surgery, has achieved notable success, it has several limitations (Caldwell and Amaral 1960; Converse and Horowitz 1969). One of these limitations is the inability of soft tissues, such as the muscle, to accommodate the abrupt mechanical changes in bone position. Partial or total relapse often results secondary to the acute stretching of the muscle, and/or the forces applied by the myofascial system to the osteotomized segments and intervening bony regenerate. Unless additional surgery accounts for this limitation from large movements or movement vectors that violate the myofascial compartment, stability to the planned reconstruction goal will be compromised (Longaker and Siebert 1996). As a response to the deficits of orthognathic surgery in the correction of the skeletal deformities mentioned earlier, the procedures within this paradigm of gradual treatment, characterized by distraction osteogenesis, were attempted in the maxillofacial region and achieved promising results as compared to traditional orthognathic surgery (Cope et al. 1999).

According to Loboa et al., the daily tension produced by the distraction device causes just enough trauma to the tissues to induce neoformation of mesenchymal tissues without critical damage (Loboa et al. 2004). The triggered bone regeneration comes about through a cascade of biological processes which may include differentiation of pluripotent cells, angiogenesis, osteogenesis, and bone mineralization (Rachmiel and Shilo 2015). The first instance of distraction osteogenesis in the maxillofacial region was performed by Wolfgang Rosenthal in 1927. This "primitive" attempt was followed up by the father of modern plastic surgery, Varaztad H. Kazanjian, who was consulted by a patient with retrusion of the chin that was not correctable through the orthodontics measures taken (Fig. 2). Of note, Kazanjian was an oral surgeon by training. Kazanjian performed L-shaped osteotomies on both sides of the mandible and attached a wire hook directly to the mandibular symphysis. Three days post-operatively, an "over the face" appliance (Fig. 3) was placed and activated with an elastic band that was attached to the wire hook,

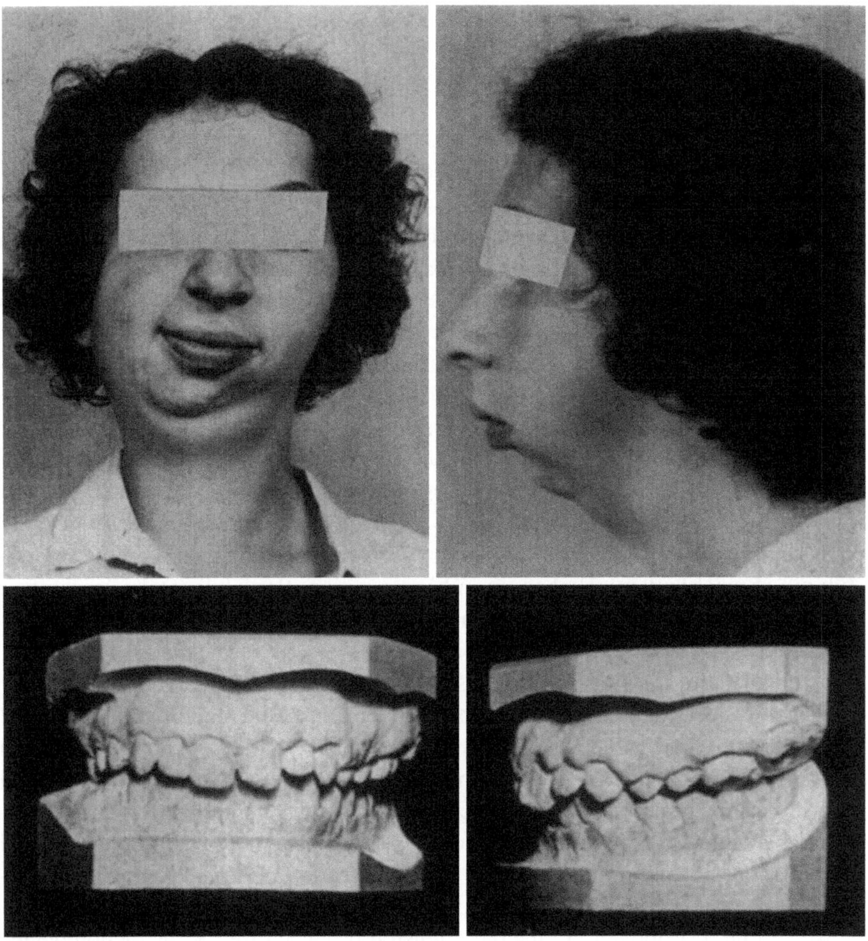

Fig. 2 A photo of the patient who presented to Kazanjian due to a patient with retrusion of the chin. The patient initially presented with severe malocclusion that was corrected through orthodontics as is illustrated here. (Reproduced with permission and without alteration from Kazanjian (1941), Figure 11)

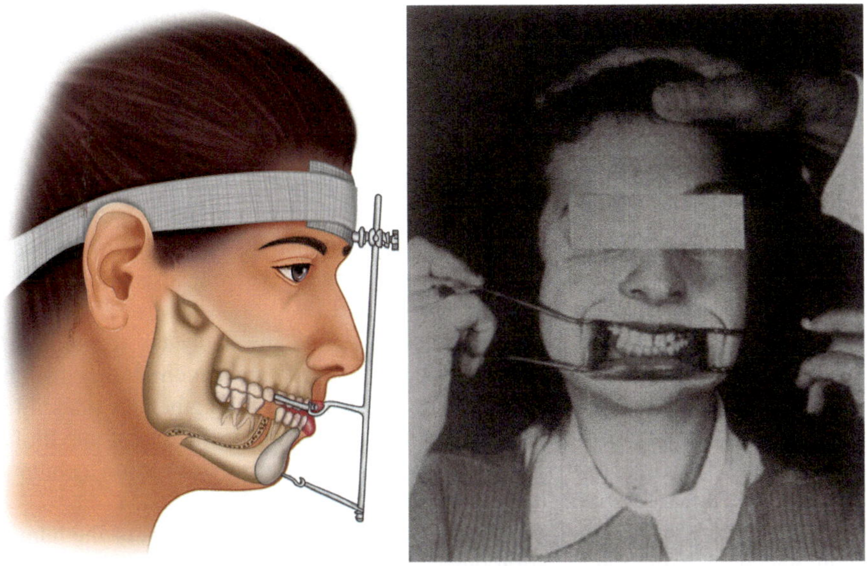

Fig. 3 On the left is an illustration of the "over the face" appliance utilized by Kazanjian. On the right is a picture of the patient post-operation. Her retrusion of the chin, refractory to orthodontics, was fixed through Kazanjian's treatment plan. (Reproduced with permission and without alteration from Kazanjian (1941), Figures 12 and 13)

slowly pulling the mandibular anterior segment forward. Kazanjian additionally placed two pieces of harvested tibial bone directly over the mental protuberance, and the other along the left side of the jaw for cosmetic purposes, which ultimately resulted in an excellent outcome (Fig. 3) (Kazanjian 1941).

Despite the endeavors made by Rosenthal and Kazanjian, distraction osteogenesis was yet to gain widespread acceptance and integration into maxillofacial surgery, namely, due to the inadequacy of distraction appliances and the instability of osseous fixation. A major innovation in mandibular repositioning surgery was conceived and subsequently proven highly versatile with great safety and success shortly thereafter – Trauner and Obwegeser introduced the sagittal split osteotomy, which is considered an indispensable tool in the correction of dentofacial abnormalities to this very day (Cope et al. 1999; Monson 2013).

3 Milestones and Advancements in Maxillofacial Distraction Osteogenesis

As was illustrated in detail in the previous section, premature versions of distraction osteogenesis were made by pioneering surgeons, such as Rosenthal and Kazanjian. The first report demonstrating the application of Ilizarov's principles to the mandible appeared in 1973, when Snyder deliberately excised a unilateral 15-mm bone segment from the mandibular corpus of a dog to simulate a crossbite. Subsequently, he performed an osteotomy on the shortened mandible and placed an extraoral distraction appliance. After a 7-day latency period, the device was activated at a rate of 1 mm per day for 14 days; at the end of which, the original occlusal relationship was successfully achieved. Additionally, the mandibular cortex and medullary canal across the distraction gap were seen after 6 weeks of fixation (consolidation), during which callus maturation and mineralization transpire. Indeed, this was the first application of maxillofacial distraction osteogenesis in a "modern manner" (Cope et al. 1999; Erverdi and Motro 2015).

In 1989, McCarthy was the first surgeon to clinically apply the technique of extraoral osteodistraction on a human mandible, specifically for children with congenital craniofacial anomalies. In the series, he managed to lengthen the mandibles around 18–24 mm. It was this milestone that propelled the technique of maxillofacial distraction osteogenesis in popularity, as an alternative reconstruction technique for the correction of craniofacial deformities (Erverdi and Motro 2015).

Despite these initial reports of success in distraction osteogenesis of the human craniofacial skeleton, the extraoral devices utilized were merely capable of unidirectional (horizontal or vertical) mandibular lengthening only. While the unidirectional vectors generated from the earlier devices were capable of completely correcting mandibular deficiencies located either exclusively in the ramus or the body, they were limited in correcting deficiencies that simultaneously involved multiple regions of the mandible, as is witnessed in congenital syndromes involving mandibular microsomia or micrognathia. It was thought that the restoration of the mandible in such complicated cases can be more effectively addressed using independent distraction in two directions (Cope et al. 1999).

Molina and Ortiz-Monasterio were the first surgeons to perform bidirectional osteodistraction in the mandible. They generated two distraction sites via double-level corticotomies, one horizontal in the ramus and the other vertical one in the corpus, allowing them to lengthen both parts of the mandible simultaneously. They performed their procedure on 87 patients with unilateral hemifacial microsomia and 19 patients with bilateral mandibular hypoplasia, characteristic of Robin sequence and Treacher Collins syndrome. They managed to achieve a mean elongation of 19 mm in the unilateral group and a mean elongation of 7.5 mm vertically and 14 mm horizontally in the bilateral group. They reported successful improvement in the facial asymmetry in all patients (Molina and Ortiz-Monasterio 1995).

Multidirectional extraoral distraction appliances were eventually developed, which enabled manipulation of bone segments in multiple planes of space. Unlike bidirectional distraction appliances, they were capable of correcting severe mandibular deformities in three-dimensional space. Despite the fruitful results brought about by extraoral distraction devices, they come with two major shortcomings: (1) their bulky structure can cause considerable social inconvenience, and (2) their application can lead to permanent facial scars (Cope et al. 1999). These shortcomings instigated the development of intraoral appliances. In 1990, Guerrero was the first surgeon to report the use of intraoral mandibular appliances in the distraction osteogenesis for 11 patients with transverse (horizontal) deficiencies of the mandible. Other designs of the intraoral mandibular appliance were subsequently constructed with improved form and function by McCarthy and Wangerin. The major advantages of intraoral appliances include their inconspicuous nature and the lack of facial scars, exactly countering the disadvantages associated with extraoral appliances.

4 Considerations in Distraction Osteogenesis

There are three phases in the process of distraction osteogenesis which allows for the successful application of this technique to the osteotomized bone. The phases, in order, are latency, activation (or distraction), and consolidation. The latency phase is the time from the completion of the surgical osteotomy gap to the beginning of the lengthening, or separation, of the bone units. The activation phase, otherwise known as distraction, is the period in which the bone is actively separated with the goal to increase its dimension in the desired vector(s). During this phase, immature bone is formed between the bony segments. Consolidation refers to the period of time after the activation is complete, when the immature bone remodels into mature, stable, woven bone, thus creating a single bone unit with the desired increase in dimension.

In order for successful distraction osteogenesis to occur, the phases of treatment must be carefully timed to occur within the physiologic limits of bone regeneration. The newly formed bone is a result of membranous ossification of the regenerate, as there is no cartilaginous intermediate (Saunders and Lee 2008; Gabrick and Runyan 2017). In the early phase of healing, the tissue's response to ischemia and traction are critical factors in angiogenesis and osteoinduction of the newly repaired/forming tissues. It is this sequence of signals that attract mesenchymal stem cells and promotes the proper milieux for bone induction and formation. Though the specifics are beyond the scope of this discussion, it is these interactions between pro-inflammatory cytokines, neo-vascularization and angiogenic factors, transforming growth factor beta superfamily factors including the bone morphogenic proteins (BMPs), and the mechanical stresses placed on the regenerate that promotes bone formation and healing (Saunders and Lee 2008; Gabrick and Runyan 2017).

The latency phase begins after the osteotomy is completed. It is crucial that enough time elapses for the initiation of callus formation across the osteotomy gap, as in typical bone and fracture repair. More specifically, if the latency phase is too short, then there will be insufficient osteoid regenerate deposited between the actively distracted segments, and hence, the result will be a fibrous or non-union of the segments. In contrast, if the latency phase is too long, then consolidation of the segments can occur resulting in inability to actively distract or lengthen the segments or device failure. There is some debate regarding the ideal timing of the latency phase, but it is generally accepted to be between 0 and 7 days. The ideal timing depends upon age, site, blood supply, and any factor that could compromise healing such as radiation, etc. A younger patient requires a shorter latency period for DO. For example, a newborn with Robin sequence undergoing mandibular distraction osteogenesis may have a latency period of 0–2 days versus a teenager with cleft lip and palate undergoing a maxillary LeFort I distraction osteogenesis who may have a latency period of 5–7 days – depending on the surgeon's preference, experience, and patient-specific clinical factors.

The activation phase begins with the purposeful lengthening of the osteotomy gap. Ilizarov described the tenets of successful distraction as being device stability, a latency period, a gradual distraction period, and a sufficient consolidation period (Ilizarov 1988, 1989a, b). Upon completion of the osteotomy, some form of lengthening device, a distractor device, must be fixated to the bone segments. Distraction devices come in many forms including external devices and internal devices, as discussed previously. Though the external devices are bulky and compromise social acceptability, patient comfort, and esthetics – they are more able to manage multiple vectors with the current readily available technology. However, they can be more difficult to manage precise movements. The common internal distractor device typically consists of two foot plates, one each for the proximal and distal bony segment, connected to a rod and screw system that allows the separation of the foot plates as the screw is turned or activated. Each revolution of the screw will lengthen the device in a pre-determined amount, i.e., 0.5 mm per turn. In this way a precise and reliable movement can be obtained eliminating sources of error in the distraction process. Moreover, ratchet systems have been included to the devices to prevent the device from accidentally being manipulated in either direction.

Another concept that Ilizarov introduced was osteotomy with minimal periosteal stripping. The integrity of the periosteum post-osteotomy and application of the stable distractor device allowed for callus formation and an envelope in which the conditions are adequate for lengthening of the regenerate. And because of the gradual lengthening, the surrounding soft tissues including the nerve, muscle, endothelium, etc. are believed to lengthen as well – similar to the effects of a tissue expander. However, debate exists as to the extent of this process and its limitations.

The concept of the rate and rhythm of distraction is also integral to the success of DO. The rate refers to the amount of lengthening per activation of the device, whereas the rhythm refers to the frequency of activation. This is also dependent upon patient-specific factors such as age, site, etc. Again, the pediatric population can be distracted at an increase rate as compared to teenagers or adults. It is common for neonates, infants, and toddlers to undergo distraction to a total of 2 mm per day, with two activations (of 1 mm) occurring daily. In contrast, a teenager or adult undergoing a LeFort I distraction may only undergo a total of 1 mm per day, with 0.5 mm activations occurring twice daily. If the distraction is too rapid, a non-union may result, and if it is too slow, then early consolidation will occur. Surgeon-specific protocols for the rate and rhythm of distraction exist, as a lack of consensus remains as to the optimal protocol. However, complication rates remain low with the aforementioned guidelines (Hollier et al. 2006).

Consolidation is the next phase and is the period during which the osteoid regenerate develops into mature, stable bone. This is again an age-dependent process.

Ilizarov initially described consolidation as a minimal period of 6 weeks or when cortical outlines of the regenerate are visible on radiography. In general, the younger patient will experience consolidation more rapidly. Additional factors include the size of the bone and the length of distraction. Therefore, a small alveolar defect will require less time for consolidation than a 2-cm segment in the body of the mandible. Adults will typically require 3–6 months of consolidation in which the distractor device will act as the fixation device and must remain stable throughout this time. It is this author's experience that infants and neonates can tolerate a 2- to 3-month consolidation period, and older children, teenagers, and adults require a minimum of 3 months. Upon completion of consolidation, the distractor devices are removed. Therefore, it is critical that stable bone healing has occurred.

5 Modern Clinical Implications of Maxillofacial Distraction Osteogenesis

The use of distraction osteogenesis in maxillofacial surgery has increased tremendously over the previous generation, particularly to buttress the maxillofacial skeleton in conditions associated with bone deficiency. Distraction osteogenesis is indicated in deficiency of the maxilla or midface, deficiency of the mandible, and deficiency of the alveolar bone prior to implant placement (Rachmiel and Shilo 2015). Each surgical technique that is available will have certain instances when it will be the preferred or optimal method for obtaining the desired result. Distraction osteogenesis is no exception. At one point, there was a suggestion that distraction was superior and would eliminate the need for traditional orthognathic procedures. However, with time it became clear that though DO has specific indications in which it can provide a superior result to traditional osteotomies and reconstructions, there are limitations.

DO requires that the patient undergoes multiple surgeries including the osteotomy and placement of the distractor device(s), as well as removal of the device(s). The device itself, whether internal or external, is a space-occupying mass which can alter facial form and/or cause discomfort due to the bulk – and will stay in place through the consolidation period. In addition, the device will have a component that will exit and/or be visible through the skin of the neck, face, cranium, or mouth – which is the site where the activation rod is accessed for lengthening or distracting the bone. This provides a point of entry to the underlying tissues with a resulting increased risk of infection. The exit site can also be a source of discomfort. Furthermore, DO is an active process which requires twice-daily activation of the device, which separates the bony segments, and causes a variable amount of discomfort over the period of distraction. This requires a high degree of patient compliance and specifically with pediatric patient's behavioral management can be intensive or prohibitive.

Craniomaxillofacial DO typically occurs with some form of computer simulation and virtual planning after either CT or cone beam CT scan of the facial skeleton. This provides a significant benefit to limit complications by identifying the optimal sites for screw and plate placement with bone density evaluation, ability to avoid vital structures with the osteotomy and screw placement, and vector of distraction for ideal final position of the distracted segment based on the patient-specific morphological defect or condition. This same benefit also exists with computer simulation for traditional surgical procedures. Moreover, as stated earlier, DO can achieve greater lengths of advancement with a lower risk of relapse, as well as eliminate large areas of dead space in large advancements with the gradual movement and no need for bone grafting. However, when considering distraction of dentate segments of the facial skeleton, achieving an ideal dental occlusion is not predictable and can result in additional orthognathic procedures to finalize treatment. In contrast, traditional orthognathic surgery can be performed in a one-stage operation with a predictable occlusal result. Selection of the appropriate treatment, i.e., distraction versus one-stage reconstruction, should be patient specific with the goal being the most predictable result.

DO is optimally performed with the use of computer simulation and virtual surgical planning. As stated earlier, this allows for minimizing damage to important structures while planning for the optimal vectors. Custom surgical guides can be fabricated, and ideal positioning of the distraction device and management of the position and size of the screw fixation will be optimized. In addition, given the success of MDO for Robin sequence, multiple choices of devices are available which can be selected to best fit the individual. Moreover, custom devices will likely be a reality in the near future.

6 Mandibular Distraction Osteogenesis

The primary benefit of distraction osteogenesis is to increase the dimension or length of the selected bone in the desired vector – either for large movements which are less stable or impossible for one-stage reconstructions or for its ability to expand the soft tissue envelope in a gradual manner to decrease dead space or for its effects on the nerve, endothelium, skin and mucosa, and muscle. A primary indication for mandibular distraction osteogenesis (MDO) occurs in individuals born with Robin sequence. Robin sequence is the triad in which a small mandible will lead to glossoptosis and then airway obstruction. Because the retropositioning of the mandible prevents tongue descent from between the palatal shelves, these individuals may have a cleft palate. Neonates or infants who suffer from Robin sequence may require assistance with maintaining a patent airway or with feeding, and the severity presents within a wide spectrum. There are standard algorithms for managing these newborns which includes conservative management with prone positioning, placement of airway devices such as a nasopharyngeal tube, the use of supplemental oxygen devices like CPAP, or tongue-lip adhesion.

Other indications of MDO include hemifacial microsomia (HFM) and Treacher Collins syndrome. It is crucial to note that bilateral mandibular deficiency that characterizes the aforementioned indications can decrease the volume of the pharyngeal airway, potentially resulting in obstructive sleep apnea (OSA) and even tracheostomy dependency (Rachmiel et al. 2005). Mandibular distraction osteogenesis with either an internal or external device following the appropriate osteotomies is indicated for the aforementioned forms of mandibular deficiency (Rachmiel and Shilo 2015).

Severe obstruction, refractory to conservative measures, may require invasive treatment such as intubation, mandibular distraction (MDO), or even tracheostomy until normal growth relieves obstruction. Severe obstruction, refractory to conservative measures, may require invasive treatment such as intubation, mandibular distraction, or even tracheostomy. MDO is proven to be a safe and effective means of predictably relieving upper airway obstruction by creating space for the airway by advancing the tongue base by lengthening the body of the mandible (Breik et al. 2016; Denny et al. 2001; Sidman et al. 2001). There are risk of complications, which include damage to developing tooth buds, injury to the inferior alveolar nerve, injury to the facial nerve, infection, need for additional airway interventions or repeat distraction, and potential growth restriction (Hong et al. 2012; Paes et al. 2016).

Mandibular distraction in an older population including toddlers and young children presents similar anatomical challenges not only due to the developing structures including the dentition but also due to the behavioral management and compliance required for successful treatment. Individuals with distinct craniofacial anomalies, such as Treacher Collins syndrome, may have a deficiency of not only the length of the mandible but also the vertical height of the ramus and an obtuse gonial angle. Vertical distraction of the ramus and condyle remains controversial due to the potential for ankylosis and predictable surgical outcomes.

7 Maxillary and Upper Midface Distraction Osteogenesis

A primary indication for maxillary DO is for large advancements of the maxilla when performing a LeFort I osteotomy. This is more common for individuals born with cleft lip and palate and the resulting restricted anterior-posterior maxillary growth with a Class III malocclusion. Segmental maxillary distraction, or mobilizing a discrete segment of the maxilla, is indicated in the cleft patient with large alveolar defects and has been shown to be successful in closing or reducing the size of the alveolar cleft. In addition, syndromic patients with midface hypoplasia, such as those with Crouzon or Apert, etc., may also benefit from a large advancement with DO at the LeFort I level. In addition, these syndromic persons with significant midface hypoplasia may extend to the LeFort 2 or LeFort 3 level – and DO can be the preferred modality for managing the advancement of the upper midface after the appropriate osteotomy is completed. It is important to remember that the execution of these procedures is more difficult in patients with abnormal anatomy and previous surgeries. Relapse of the desired movement can occur to a higher degree. In addition, obtaining the ideal occlusal result may require a second and definitive reconstruction.

The case of maxillary deficiency is exemplified by an individual born with a cleft palate who underwent the standard algorithm of care with repair to the palate at the ideal time. It is accepted that 25–30% of individuals with a repaired cleft palate will develop a Class III malocclusion that is likely a result of undergoing the initial surgical repair of the cleft palate (Ross 1987).

This can be corrected by a maxillary LeFort 1 osteotomy – however, in certain patients the anterior-posterior desired movement is too great a distance to accomplish with the standard LeFort I procedure. It is in these situations that a LeFort I osteotomy followed by distraction osteogenesis through an internal or external device can improve the ability to achieve the greater desired movement. Similarly, midfacial hypoplasia is a typical feature of syndromic craniosynostosis, such as Crouzon's syndrome, and results in sequelae of exophthalmos, upper airway stenosis, sleep apnea, central face concavity, and dental malocclusion. While this was previously treated through a LeFort 3 osteotomy and subsequent bone grafts to fill the induced bone cuts, distraction osteogenesis following LeFort 3 osteotomy has increased in utility over the recent years. One advantage DO holds over bone grafts is that it is minimally invasive, without the risk of donor site morbidity (Sakamoto et al. 2020).

More recently, the monobloc operation, which consists of advancement of both orbits and the midface in one piece, plus advancement and reshaping of the frontal area, when used in conjunction with distraction osteogenesis has reduced morbidity significantly (Fig. 4). A large retro-frontal space result after acute expansion when the monobloc operation is executed. The subsequent communication between the nasal cavities and the anterior cranial fossa leads to a high (>30%) infection rate due to the dead space created by the advancement that manifests as meningitis, epidural abscess, and/or osteomyelitis of the frontal bones with subsequent bone loss. The gradual expansion of bone when distraction osteogenesis is added into the equation eliminates the formation of a large retro-frontal space. Negligible infectious complications and the evasion of frontal bone loss, meningitis, and epidural abscess have been reported using an internal distraction system (Kumar and Steinbacher 2014).

The final modern indication for DO that will be discussed is alveolar deficiency for the purpose of implant placement. Maxillofacial trauma, periodontal disease, and resection of aggressive large jaw cysts or tumors can all cause a significant reduction in alveolar bone. As was stated earlier in maxillary and midface DO, alveolar DO is advantageous for increasing the dimensions of the jaws due to its minimally invasive nature; there is a decreased need for a bone augmentation surgery with the associated risk of donor site morbidity (Rachmiel and Shilo 2015).

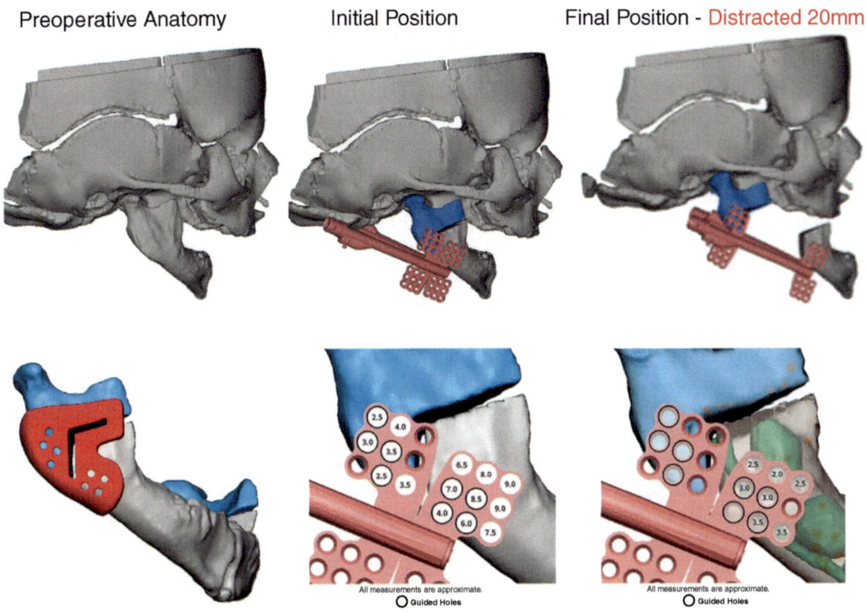

Fig. 4 Virtual surgical planning of distraction osteogenesis

References

Breik O, Tivey D, Umapathysivam K, Anderson P. Mandibular distraction osteogenesis for the management of upper airway obstruction in children with micrognathia: a systematic review. Int J Oral Maxillofac Surg. 2016;45:769.

Caldwell JB, Amaral WJ. Mandibular micrognathia corrected by vertical osteotomy in the rami and iliac bone graft. J Oral Surg. 1960;18:3–15.

Converse JM, Horowitz SL. The surgical-orthodontic approach to the treatment of dentofacial deformities. Am J Orthod Dentofacial Orthop. 1969;55:217–43.

Cope JB, Samchukov ML, Cherkashin AM. Mandibular distraction osteogenesis: a historic perspective and future directions. Am J Orthod Dentofac Orthop. 1999;115(4):448–60.

Denny AD, Talisman R, Hanson PR, Recinos RF. Mandibular distraction osteogenesis in very young patients to correct airway obstruction. Plast Reconstr Surg. 2001;108:302.

Erverdi N, Motro M. Brief history of distraction osteogenesis. In: Alveolar distraction osteogenesis. Cham: Springer; 2015. https://doi-org.ezproxy.cul.columbia.edu/10.1007/978-3-319-07707-9_1.

Gabrick KS, Runyan CM. Biology of bone formation, fracture healing, and distraction osteogenesis. J Craniofac Surg. 2017;28(5):1380–9.

Hollier LH, Higuera S, Stal S, Taylor T. Distraction rate and latency: factors in the outcome of pediatric mandibular distraction. Plast Reconstruct Surg. 2006;117(7):2333–6.

Hong P, Graham E, Belyea J, Taylor SM, Kearns DB, Bezuhly M. The long-term effects of mandibular distraction osteogenesis on developing deciduous molar teeth. Plast Surg Int. 2012;2012:5.

Ilizarov GA. The principles of the Ilizarov method. Bull Hosp Jt Dis Orthop Inst. 1988;48:1–18.

Ilizarov GA. The tension-stress effect on the genesis and growth of tissues: I. The influence of stability of fixation and soft tissue preservation. Clin Orthop. 1989a;238:249–81.

Ilizarov GA. The tension-stress effect on the genesis and growth of tissues: II. The influence of the rate and frequency of distraction. Clin Orthop. 1989b;239:263–85.

Kazanjian VH. The interrelationship of dentistry and surgery in the treatment of deformities of the face and jaws. Am J Orthod Oral Surg. 1941;27(1):C10–30.

Kumar AR, Steinbacher D. Advances in the treatment of syndromic midface hypoplasia using monobloc and facial bipartition distraction osteogenesis. Semin Plast Surg. 2014;28(4):179–83. https://doi.org/10.1055/s-0034-1390170.

Limberg A. Treatment of open bite by means of plastic oblique osteotomy of the ascending rami of the mandible. Dent Cosmos. 1925;67:1191–200.

Loboa EG, Fang TD, Warren SM, et al. Mechanobiology of mandibular distraction osteogenesis: experimental analyses with a rat model. Bone. 2004;34:336.

Longaker MT, Siebert JW. Microsurgical correction of facial contour in congenital craniofacial malformations: the marriage of hard and soft tissue. Plast Reconstr Surg. 1996;98:942–50.

Molina F, Ortiz-Monasterio F. Mandibular elongation and remodeling by distraction: a farewell to major osteotomies. Plast Reconstr Surg. 1995;96:825–40.

Monson LA. Bilateral sagittal split osteotomy. Semin Plast Surg. 2013;27(3):145–8. https://doi.org/10.1055/s-0033-1357111.

Paes EC, Bittermann GK, Bittermann D, Muradin MM, van Hogezand R, Etty E, van der Molen ABM, Kon M, Breugem CC. Long-term results of mandibular distraction osteogenesis with a resorbable device in infants with Robin sequence: effects on developing molars and mandibular growth. Plast Reconstr Surg. 2016;137:375e.

Rachmiel A, Shilo D. The use of distraction osteogenesis in oral and maxillofacial surgery. Ann Maxillofac Surg. 2015;5(2):146–7. https://doi.org/10.4103/2231-0746.175777.

Rachmiel A, Aizenbud D, Pillar G, Srouji S, Peled M. Bilateral mandibular distraction for patients with compromised airway analyzed by three-dimensional CT. Int J Oral Maxillofac Surg. 2005;34:9–18.

Ross RB. Treatment variables affecting facial growth in complete unilateral cleft lip and palate. Part 7: an overview of treatment and facial growth. Cleft Palate J. 1987;24:71–7.

Sakamoto Y, Tamada I, Sakamoto T, Ishii T, Kishi K. Le Fort III distraction osteogenesis without bicoronal incision. J Craniofac Surg. 2020;31(6):1753–5. https://doi.org/10.1097/SCS.0000000000006527.

Samchukov ML, Cherkashin AM, Cope JB. Distraction osteogenesis: origins and evolution. Craniofac Growth Ser. 1998;34:1–36.

Saunders MM, Lee JS. The influence of mechanical environment on bone healing and distraction osteogenesis. Atlas Oral Maxillofac Surg Clin North Am. 2008;16(2):147–58.

Sidman JD, Sampson D, Templeton B. Distraction osteogenesis of the mandible for airway obstruction in children. Laryngoscope. 2001;111:1137.

Craniosynostosis Surgery

Jessica S. Lee and Jason W. Yu

1 Ancient Descriptions of Craniosynostosis

Congenital human deformities, especially of the head and face, have known to be described as early as the time of antiquity. Homer wrote about the warrior, Thersites, who, in the *Iliad*, was described as "…the ugliest man who came before Troy…his head ran up to a point…there was little hair on top of it…" (Homer 1990) (Fig. 1). This was one of the earliest descriptions of a man with craniosynostosis, and the expression *tête à la Thersite* has been used in French literature as a synonym for oxycephaly.

Craniofacial deformities, however, have not always been viewed as sequelae of human malformation; instead, particular head shapes were marks of elitist distinction or divinity in many ancient cultures across the globe (Gaudier et al. 1967). The Taoist God of Longevity, Shouxing, exemplifies this distinction, portrayed with an extremely high cranial vault (Fig. 2). The Japanese, Shinto God of Wisdom, Fukurokuju, has been depicted with a very high forehead (Fig. 3). These marks of distinction have also been found in the Americas (Incas, Mayas, Pueblos, Navajos, and Apaches), Africa (Ethiopians), the Philippines, and France (Montaut and Stricker 1977). In the French regions of Brittany, Normandy, and Toulouse, the practice of skull deformation through bandaging continued until the end of the nineteenth century (Figs. 4 and 5).

J. S. Lee (✉)
Private Practice, Northeast Facial & Oral Surgery Specialists, Florham Park, NJ, USA
e-mail: drlee@nefoss.com

J. W. Yu
Section of Oral & Maxillofacial Surgery, UCLA School of Dentistry, Los Angeles, CA, USA
e-mail: jwyu@mednet.ucla.edu

E. M. Ferneini et al. (eds.), *The History of Maxillofacial Surgery*,
https://doi.org/10.1007/978-3-030-89563-1_20

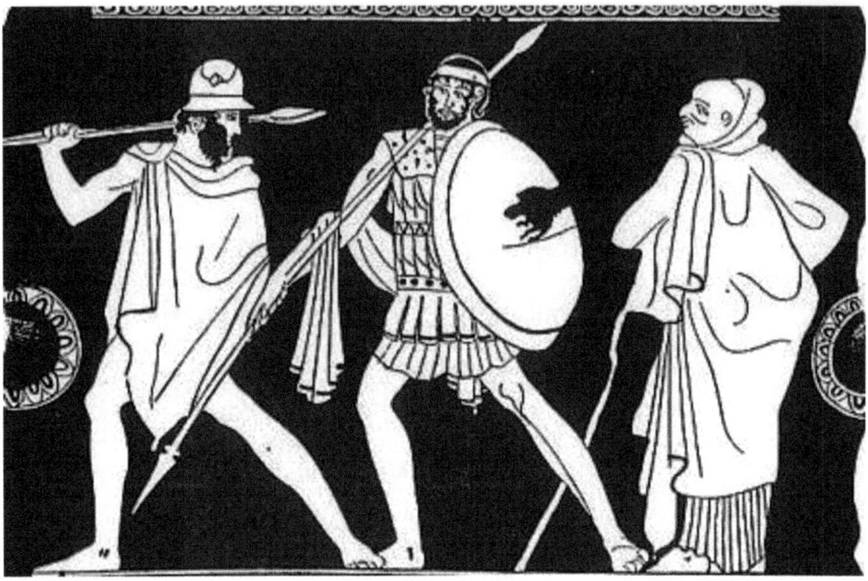

Fig. 1 Odysseus, Agamemnon and Thersites from the *Iliad*

2 Early Scientific Descriptions of Craniosynostosis

By the sixteenth century, anatomists began to document the existence of cranial sutures and broad range of characteristics, including suture patterns and premature suture fusion in a variety of configurations (Hundt 1501), specific abnormal varieties of sagittal and coronal sutures (Dryander 1537), and descriptions of oxycephaly and brachycephaly (della Croce 1583; Vesalius 1543).

In the late 1790s, Samuel Thomas von Sömmerring (Fig. 6), a German physician, was the first to describe abnormal head shapes beyond simple descriptions in the context of abnormal cranial suture development (von Sömmering 1801). His descriptions have laid the foundation for our modern understanding of craniosynostosis and, subsequently, the development of non-surgical and surgical interventions (von Sömmering 1839; Winston 1996).

Several decades later, Adolph Wilhelm Otto, a German anatomist, based on his studies of human and animal anatomy, proposed that a consequence of premature suture fusion was a compensatory cranial expansion along another trajectory in the skull, providing the first explanation of the global cranial abnormalities observed (Otto 1830).

A landmark study published by German physician Rudolf Virchow (Fig. 7) in 1851 described an aberrant growth pattern in which the premature fusion of calvarial bone restricted growth perpendicular to the direction of the involved calvarial suture and promoted compensatory growth, subsequently named Virchow's law (Virchow 1851). He initially described this phenomenon as *craniostenosis*, describing a narrow or structured skull; however, he later more appropriately named it

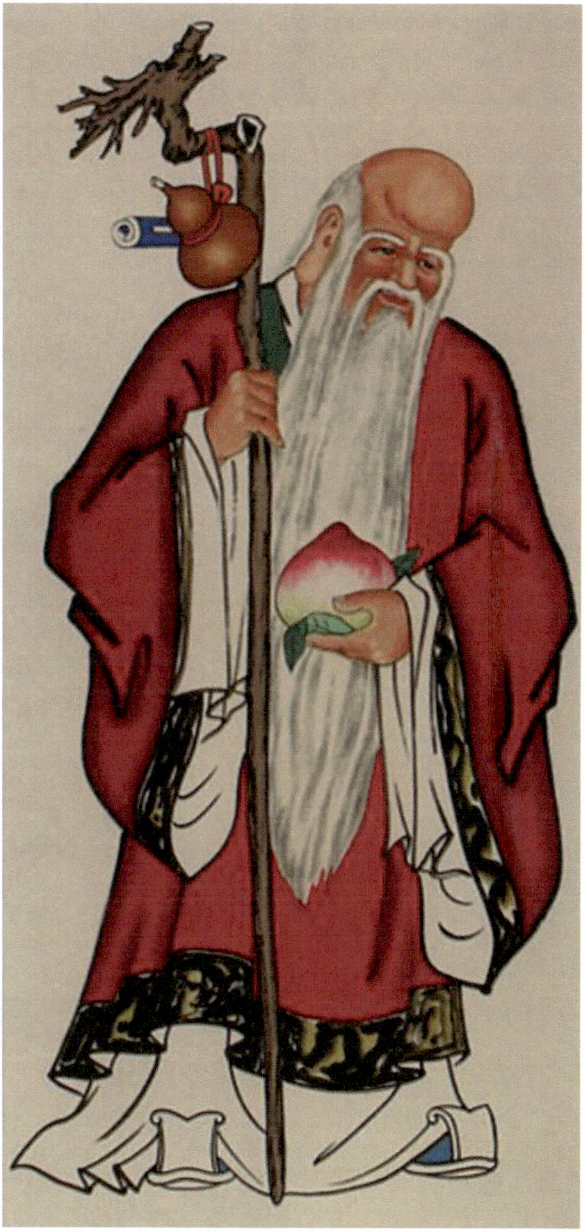

Fig. 2 Shouxing, God of Longevity

craniosynostosis, indicating suture involvement and encompassing all cranial suture anomalies (Virchow 1851; Sear 1937). Virchow's observations and contributions were crucial in the development of surgical interventions for craniosynostosis, and subsequent modifications were based directly on his observations and principles (Mehta et al. 2010).

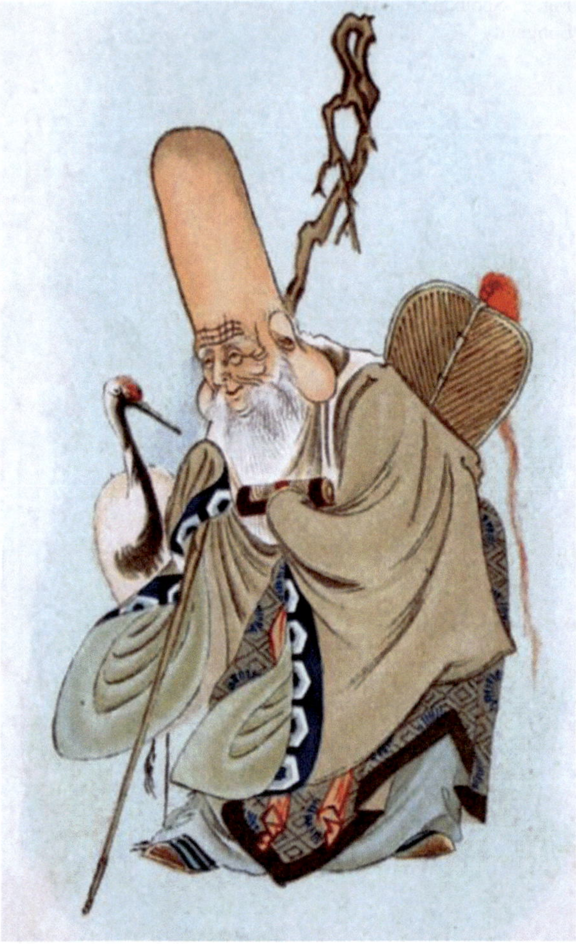

Fig. 3 Shinto, God of Wisdom

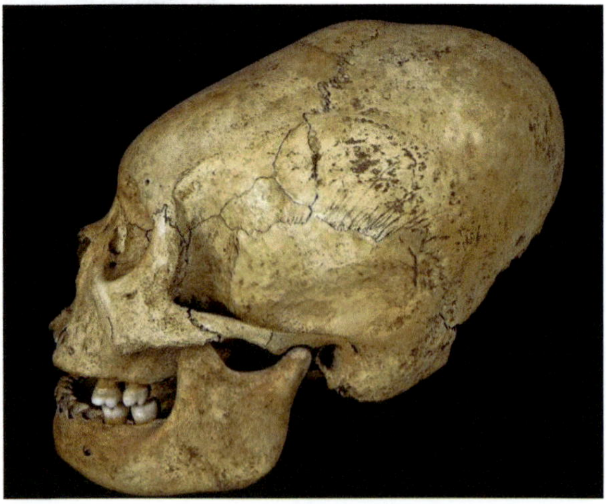

Fig. 4 Ancient Incan Skull

Fig. 5 Man from Toulouse

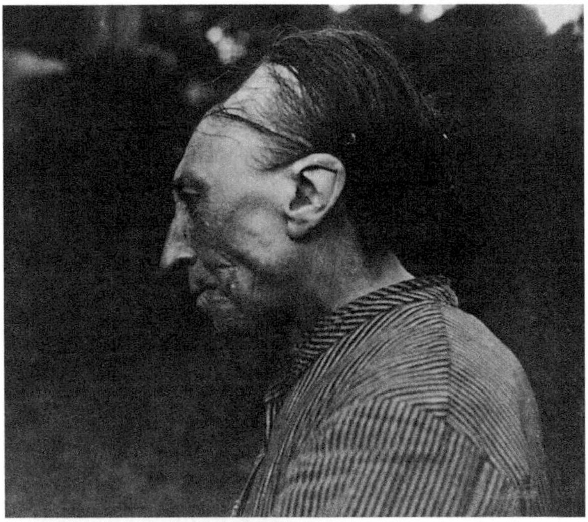

Fig. 6 Samuel Thomas von Sömmerring (1755–1830)

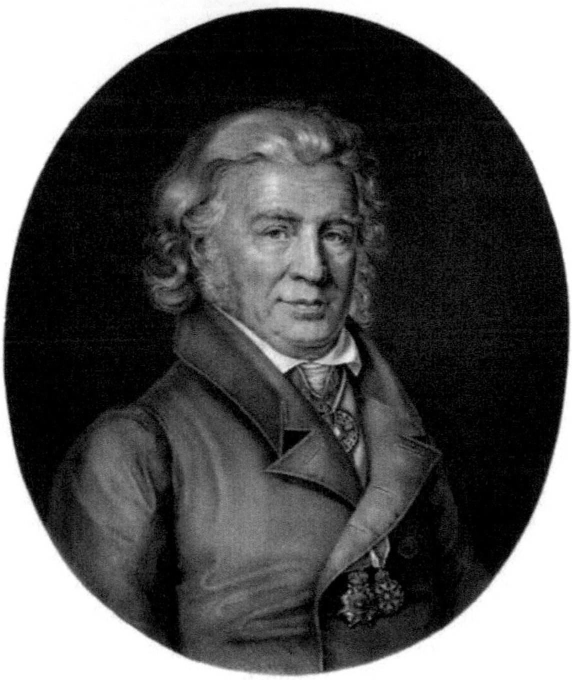

Virchow's hypotheses and contributions on craniosynostosis remained the standard for nearly a century as additional perspectives began to emerge, including the association of craniostenosis with ophthalmological visual loss (von Graefe 1866) and craniosynostosis with optic atrophy (Friedenwald 1893).

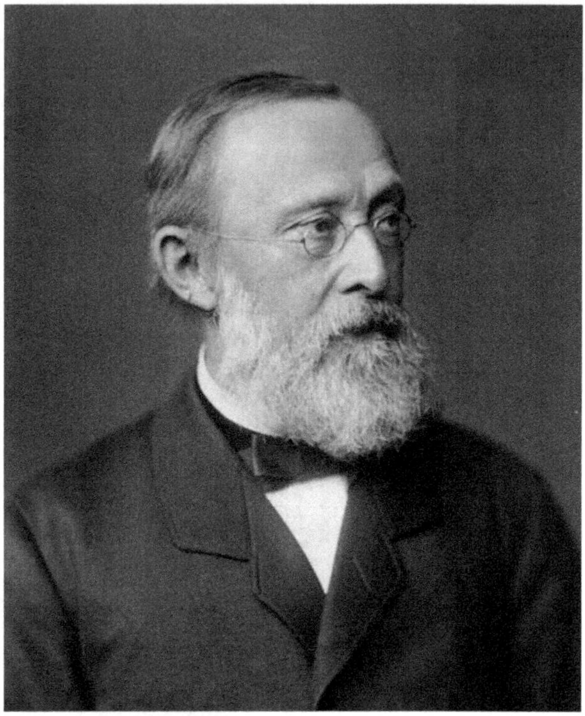

Fig. 7 Rudolf Virchow (1821–1902)

Although more frequently non-syndromic and monosutural, by the early 1900s, craniosynostosis was recognized as a component of more complex, syndromic craniofacial anomalies, most notably by French physician Eugène Charles Apert in 1906 and French neurologist Louis Édouard Octave Crouzon in 1912, after whom two of the most well-known syndromes are named.

In the mid-twentieth century, American anatomist and dentist Melvin Lionel Moss (Fig. 8) proposed that the primary site of abnormality was within the cranial base, which led to the secondary fusion of the cranial sutures (Di Rocco 1995; Moss 1954, 1959). His theory was based on four observations: (1) sutures were often patent at surgery, even when there was a high degree of preoperative suspicion of suture fusion and characteristic skull abnormality; (2) characteristic abnormalities at the cranial base occurred with certain suture patterns; (3) excision of the fused suture did not always improve the cranial shape; and (4) embryologically and developmentally, skull development occurred after cranial base development.

Moss' theory fell out of favor, however, as surgical treatment directed at the prematurely fused suture demonstrated reversal of the deformity and cranial base and facial abnormalities appeared to occur as a result of cranial suture restriction (Persson et al. 1979; Persing et al. 1991). This suggested that craniofacial anomalies were primarily due to the fusion of sutures, not the cranial base. Although Moss' theory on the etiology of craniosynostosis was eventually disproven when it was shown that the suture itself was the primary site of abnormality in craniosynostosis

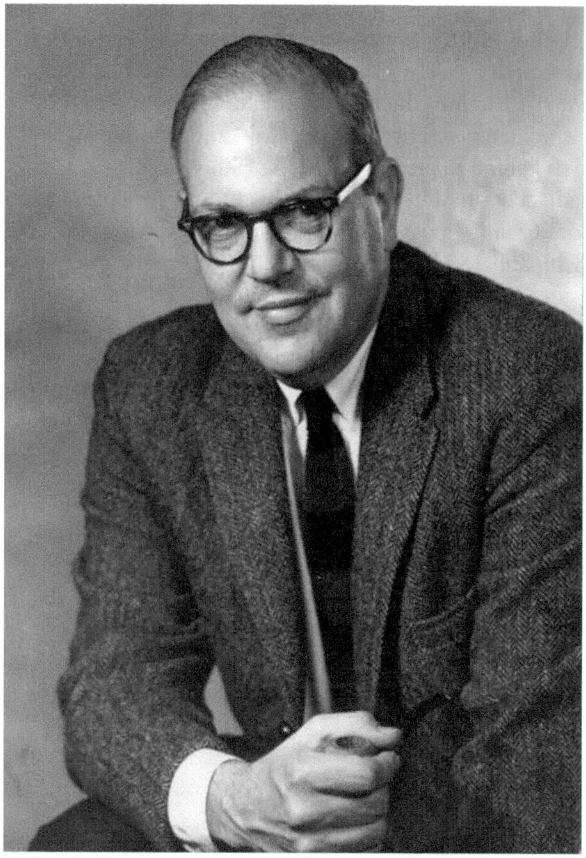

Fig. 8 Melvin Lionel Moss (1923–2006)

as cranial base and facial abnormalities responded when the pathology in the cranial vault was addressed (Marsh and Vannier 1986), his lasting contribution on the functional matrix theory, which proposed that the primary driving force of deposition of bone in cranial sutures was growth of the underlying brain, would later become a part of the basis and justification for the minimally invasive, endoscopic approach for treating craniosynostosis.

3 Early Descriptions of Surgical Intervention

In August of 1888, American surgeon Levi Cooper Lane performed the first strip craniectomy at Cooper Medical College in San Francisco when approached by a mother of a child with sagittal craniosynostosis who pleaded to him, "can you not unlock my poor child's brain and let it grow?" He described the removal of the fused suture with a cross-shaped craniectomy, but due to reported anesthesia complications, the patient died 14 hours postoperatively (Lane 1892).

It was not until year 1890 when the first successful surgical procedure to correct craniosynostosis was performed on a 4-year-old girl with a severe psychomotor deficit in Paris by French surgeon Odilon Marc Lannelongue (Fig. 9) (Lannelongue 1890). He introduced a technique to address sagittal suture synostosis in children, which involved two parallel strip craniectomies lateral to the midline, with a strip of left behind to protect the sagittal sinus. The strip craniectomy continued through the adjacent, unaffected sutures, including the coronal suture anteriorly and the lambdoid suture posteriorly (Fig. 10) (Boulos et al. 2004; Venes and Sayers 1976; Chipault 1894). The main goal of this technique was to alleviate intracranial pressure and decrease mortality but to also correct the abnormal head shape after excising the fused sutures to allow for physiological growth of the cranial vault (Frassanito and Di Rocco 2011). With this technique, Lannelongue completed strip craniectomies on 59 patients, navigating through complications including blindness, cognitive and neurological damage, hydrocephalus leading to irreparable brain damage, and even death of one patient (Alvarez-Garijo et al. 2001; Hunter and Rudd 1976; McCarthy et al. 1995; Speltz et al. 2004). Lane was successful in his second operation in 1892.

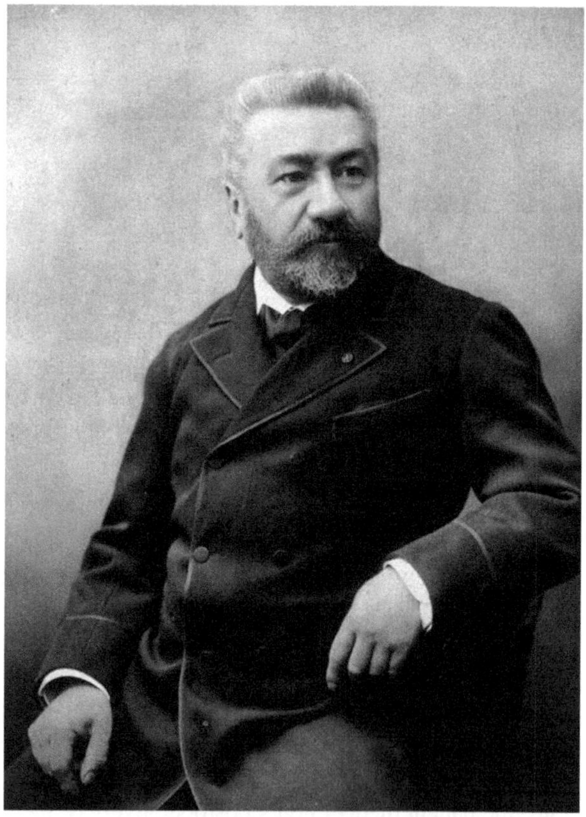

Fig. 9 Odilon Marc Lannelongue (1840–1911)

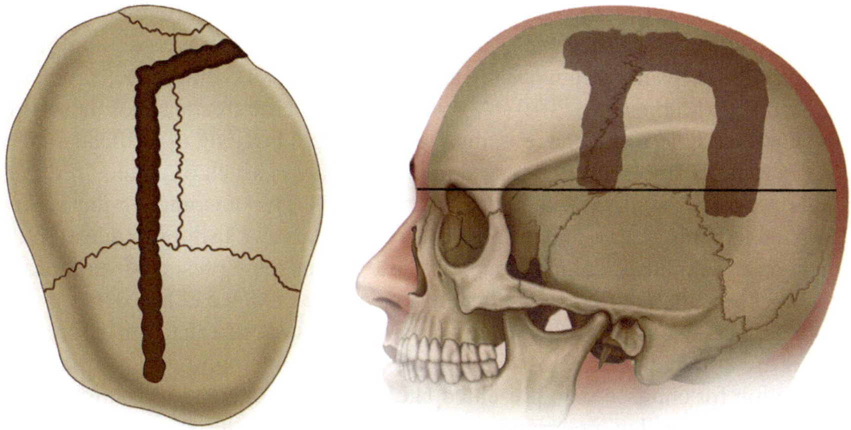

Fig. 10 Early sketches of Lannelongue's linear craniectomy (Chipault 1894)

Despite the quick adoption of surgical technique and use for the treatment of craniosynostosis, German physician Abraham Jacobi, also known as the father of American pediatrics, denounced the practice of open strip craniectomies at an American Academy of Pediatrics meeting after reviewing a series of 33 children surgically treated for presumed craniosynostosis. In his review, he found alarmingly high postoperative mortality rates, with 15 deaths out of 33 children due to major blood loss (Jacobi 1894). Harvey Cushing, one of the most influential neurosurgeons of his time, was also very critical of these early techniques, stating that "the introduction in 1891 of linear craniotomy, which has led to innumerable operations said to have been followed by an improvement in mentality, is a lamentable instance of the furor operandi running away with surgical judgment" (Cushing 1908). With these criticisms, surgical correction of craniosynostosis fell out of favor for nearly three decades.

4 The Revival of Surgical Intervention

Additional controversy around the craniotomy technique delayed further development in the surgical management of craniosynostosis until the early 1920s when German surgeon Arndt Mehner described a successful technique involving simple strip craniectomy, or suturectomy, for complete removal of a fused suture, and the practice of surgical intervention for craniosynostosis was revived (Maher et al. 2010; Mehner 1921). A few years later, American pediatrician Harold Kniest Faber and neurosurgeon Edward Bancroft Towne at Stanford University published a case series, reporting excellent preservation of neurological function with minimal morbidity and mortality (Faber and Towne 1927) and later pioneered the concept of early and prophylactic linear synostectomy for preservation of neurological function and improvement of cosmesis (Faber and Towne 1943).

By the 1940s, strip craniectomies and suturectomies to treat craniosynostosis were once again widely accepted, and the importance of early intervention before 2 months of age resulting in more favorable functional and cosmetic outcomes was demonstrated (Mehta et al. 2010). A new challenge in the treatment of these children, however, emerged when reossification with rapid bridging of artificial sutures was a common complication observed in older children, which often required multiple, extensive cranial vault remodeling procedures. The outcomes in these complex patients with mature and delayed fusion led Harvey Cushing to question the indication of late linear craniectomies in these patients and presented surgeons of the next generation with major challenges to overcome (Mehta et al. 2010).

By the mid-twentieth century, the focus of surgery research, primarily taking place at Boston Children's Hospital, shifted to address the limitations of surgical intervention for children who presented late in the disease course or children who underwent surgery but presented with reossification at the synostectomy site. Donald Darrow Matson and Franc Douglas Ingraham, pediatric neurosurgeons at Boston Children's Hospital, reported the use of polyethylene film on the edges of calvarial bone following strip craniectomy to prevent reossification (Ingraham et al. 1948). Just 1 year prior, neurosurgeons Donald Ray Simmons and William Thomas Peyton at the University of Minnesota reported the use of tantalum foil between the edges of calvarial bone following craniectomy (Fig. 11) (Simmons and Peyton 1947). Both techniques fell out of favor, however, due to reports of reossification and infection (Mehta et al. 2010). Frank Anderson and Forrest Johnson,

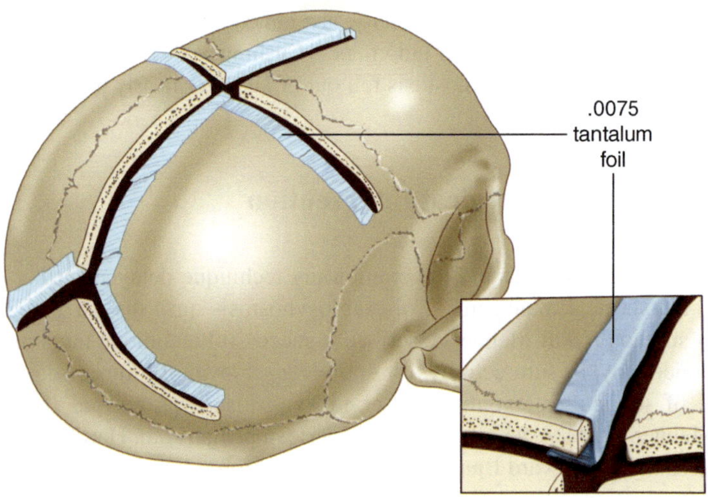

Fig. 11 Tantalum foil adapted to edges of craniectomy to prevent bridging and new bone formation (Simmons and Peyton 1947)

American neurosurgeons, described a technique in 1956 whereby Zenker's solution was applied to the dura to cauterize the ossifying elements within the meninges and promote suture patency but was found to cause seizures (Anderson and Johnson 1956).

Matson and Ingraham's technique of simple craniosynostectomy became a mainstream surgical technique, replaced strip craniectomies as the treatment of choice in most pediatric neurosurgery texts, and became one of the most common approaches during this period (Matson 1969). The craniosynostectomy technique involved removing a strip of bone measuring 1 cm wide at the site of the fused suture and extending the craniectomy across the adjacent, normal sutures and excising the pericranium to prevent reossification.

By the mid-1950s, surgery for craniosynostosis became safer with less morbidity and mortality due to significant advances in anesthesia, blood transfusion, and surgical technique as these procedures were performed at a higher volume at major medical centers such as Boston Children's Hospital. American neurosurgeon John Shillito Jr. and Matson reported only two deaths in a large case series of 519 patients who underwent surgery, demonstrating a mortality rate of 0.39%, refuting Jacobi's observation and results just a few decades ago (Winston 1996; Shillito Jr and Matson 1968). With new reports of safer surgeries for craniosynostosis, the importance of restoring the form of the natural skull early to allow a proper rate of growth for normal brain development was emphasized. As a result, the consideration for aesthetics and cosmesis as one of the primary indications for surgical intervention became generally accepted (Shillito Jr and Matson 1968). Although simple craniosynostectomy and strip craniectomy demonstrated favorable results in young infants, these techniques fell short when treating older children with advanced disease or those who presented with reossification at the site of synostectomy, introducing a new challenge for the next generation of surgeons.

5 Era of Modern Craniofacial Surgery

The early 1960s to 1990s marked a new era in which the innovation of complex calvarial vault remodeling was developed to overcome the limitations of simple craniosynostectomy and strip craniectomy techniques, driven by the need for immediate deformity correction to prevent impending neurological dysfunction in older children and the need to treat secondary compensatory changes at sites away from the diseased suture (Mehta et al. 2010).

The foundation of modern craniofacial surgery was established by Paul Louis Tessier (Fig. 12), a French surgeon, widely regarded as the father of modern craniofacial surgery. Tessier is best known for his work on Crouzon and Apert syndrome craniofacial dysostoses, who, unlike his predecessors, emphasized the importance of aesthetic outcomes to achieve normality (Ghali et al. 2014). Historically, the treatment of craniofacial dysostoses was anchored heavily on the correction of *facial* deformities. Tessier's solution for craniofacial dysostoses included the

Fig. 12 Paul Louis Tessier (1917–2008)

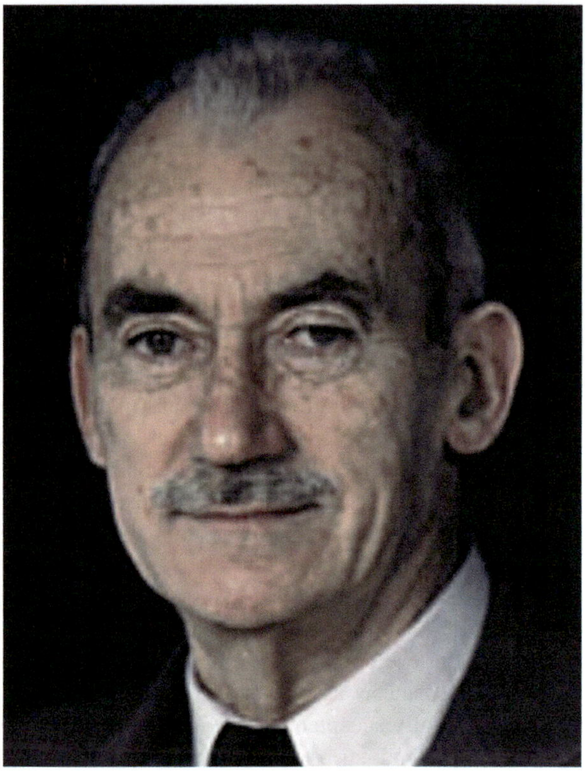

advancement of the forehead of supraorbital rims, which involved creating osteotomies through the entire middle third of the facial skeleton with cuts posterior to the zygoma and orbits along with interpterygomaxillary disjunction to achieve the most optimal aesthetic results (Fig. 13) (Marchac and Renier 1980).

During the late 1960s and into the 1970s, Tessier developed a series of principles and procedures which departed from the limitations of maxillofacial surgery and revolutionized the field of craniofacial surgery by way of transcranial and subcranial correction of orbital dystopias (e.g., orbital hypertelorism), correction of craniofacial dysostoses (e.g., Crouzon, Apert, and Treacher Collins syndrome), and the correction of oro-ocular facial clefts (Ghali et al. 2014). His use of autogenous bone grafts from the rib, iliac crest, or calvarium to prevent relapse in addition to precise osteotomies enhanced the durability and decreased relapse of his reconstructive surgeries (McKinnon 2011). Tessier also developed a collection of surgical techniques and instruments to harvest and secure bone grafts to aid in these procedures, many of which are still in use today by craniofacial surgeons.

Tessier's work gained widespread recognition and praise when he presented a series of Crouzon and Apert patients treated with a surgical technique, on which he collaborated with French neurosurgeon Gérard Guiot, through an intracranial, frontal approach to the upper and midface at the International Congress of Plastic and Reconstructive Surgery in 1967. His successful results were a culmination of Tessier's innovation,

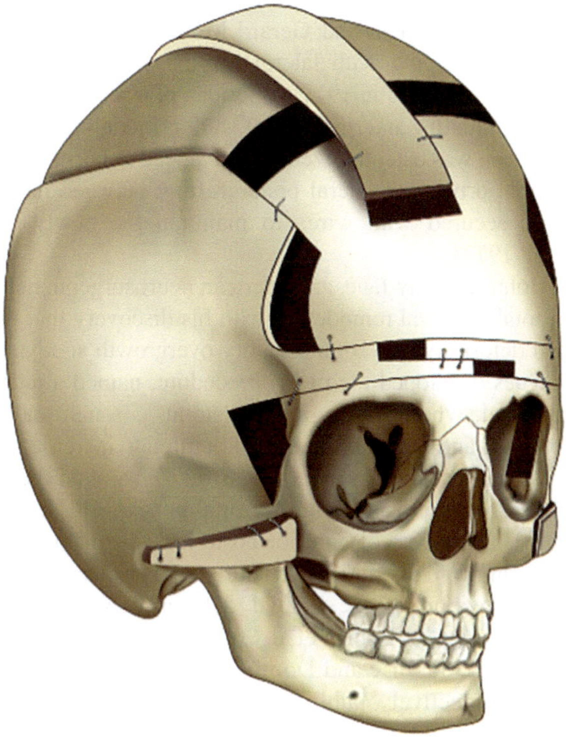

Fig. 13 Monobloc frontofacial advancement developed by Tessier

extensive study of craniofacial anomalies and syndromes including cadaveric dissections of the craniofacial skeleton, and multidisciplinary training by and collaboration with Maurice Virenque (maxillofacial surgery), George Huc (pediatric orthopedics), Sir Harold Gillies and Sir Archibald McIndoe (otorhinolaryngology and plastic surgery, respectively), Pierre Petit (cleft surgery), Gilbert Sourdille (ophthalmology), and Gérard Guiot and Jacques Rougerie (neurosurgery) who were regarded as the world's leaders in each of these fields during this time (Ghali et al. 2014).

Often considered the founding father of craniofacial surgery, Paul Tessier's legacy defined the philosophy of the next generation of craniofacial surgeons. Tessier emphasized the importance of collaboration across multiple disciplines, perhaps honoring his own experiences and training as a young surgeon, and frequently collaborated with physicians and nurses within a multidisciplinary craniofacial team to treat his patients (Ghali et al. 2014).

6 Advanced Cranial Vault Remodeling

Tessier's groundbreaking approaches to the craniofacial skeleton were expanded upon with the development of surgical modifications through the 1970s. French neurosurgeon Jacque Rougerie included remodeling of the anterior cranial vault simultaneously with suture release (Rougerie et al. 1972). Canadian neurosurgeons Harold J. Hoffman and Gerard Mohr described the concept of cranial vault and orbital reshaping with lateral canthal advancement (Hoffman and Mohr 1976). Shortly thereafter in 1977, American plastic surgeon Linton A. Whitaker proposed a technique for anterior cranial vault remodeling where three-fourths of the abnormal orbit was osteotomized and advanced to become the level with the contralateral, normal orbit with lateral bone grafting between the advanced orbit and temporal bone secured with wires to maintain the newly advanced position (Whitaker et al. 1977).

John Anthony Jane, an American neurosurgeon, helped advance the development of total calvarial remodeling with his discovery that the major cause of global cranial deformity was compensatory overgrowth at adjacent sutures. Jane and his colleagues developed the pi (π) procedure, named after the shape of the bone that is removed, where the sagittal, bilateral, coronal, and lambdoid sutures were first removed and parietal bones out fractured to increase skull width. The sagittal suture was then removed and used as a strut to maintain the lateral position of the parietal bones, and the frontal and occipital bones were then secured to the parietal bones with adjustments of anterior-posterior dimension and frontal bossing. This technique allowed the surgeon to address the primary suture fusion and provide immediate correction of the cranial deformity without the need for helmet therapy postoperatively (Boulos et al. 2004; Jane et al. 1978, 2005).

Daniel Marchac and Dominique Renier, French plastic surgeon and neurosurgeon, respectively, published the "floating forehead" technique to manage unilateral or bilateral coronal synostosis, which utilized simultaneous suture release and cranial vault and orbital reshaping where the orbital bandeau segment was loosely attached to the remaining orbits (Marchac and Renier 1979). Marchac and Renier proposed that the growing brain would further advance the "released" orbits and midface forward and allow for natural correction of midface hypoplasia in syndromic patients; however, postoperative evaluation of these patients concluded that their approach failed to support their theory (Marchac et al. 1988). Through the 1980s, Renier further developed a technique to address sagittal synostosis with an "H" pattern, where retrocoronal and prelambdoidal segments were removed together with central segments over the sagittal suture (Di Rocco et al. 2012).

Summarizing the surgical outcomes of this era, American neurosurgeon J. Gordon McComb and his colleagues at Children's Hospital Los Angeles published one of the most significant publications on contemporary surgical management of craniosynostosis in pediatrics, describing their 6-year, institutional experience for 250 patients who underwent surgical treatment of craniosynostosis with relatively low morbidity and mortality rates (6.8% and 0.8%, respectively) (Sloan et al. 1997).

6.1 Distraction Osteogenesis

Distraction osteogenesis, a bone-regenerative process aided first by an osteotomy followed by gradual distraction of the vascularized bone segments with deposition of new bone within the gap, was first pioneered by Italian surgeon Alessandro Codivilla and further developed for use in lower extremities by Russian orthopedic surgeon Gavriil Ilizarov. Distraction osteogenesis was first described with its application for mandibular advancement in the management of craniofacial microsomia by American plastic surgeon Joseph G. McCarthy (Codivilla 2008; Ilizarov et al. 1980; McCarthy et al. 1992). Initially described by McCarthy to improve mandibular asymmetry in patients with craniofacial microsomia, distraction osteogenesis is more commonly applied to the craniofacial skeleton to correct severe functional deficits including upper airway obstruction in neonates born with micrognathia or in adults with severe obstructive sleep apnea. Its application to the midface has become the preferred method over the traditional advancement technique in growing children. Posterior cranial vault distraction is used to delay the need for major cranial remodeling by reducing high intracranial pressure in patients with syndromic craniosynostosis, until a time that major cranial vault remodeling surgery can be more safely performed (Fig. 14) (Runyan et al. 2017).

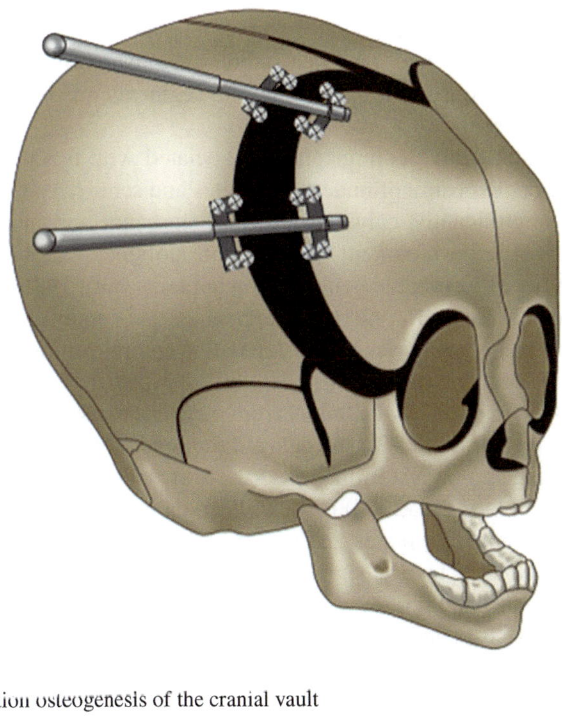

Fig. 14 Distraction osteogenesis of the cranial vault

6.2 Spring-Mediated Cranioplasty (Subsection Under Sect. 6)

The spring-mediated cranioplasty technique, introduced by Swedish surgeon Claes Lauritzen in 1998, was born out of the idea of attempting the results of the surgery to continue to work over a period of time after the incision was closed (Lauritzen et al. 1998, 2008; David 2020). Described as less extensive than the "traditional" cranioplasty techniques, the spring-mediated cranioplasty uses simple linear craniotomies powered by implantable dynamic elements in the form of compressive and/or expansive stainless steel springs, and, therefore, the reshaping of the skull does not rely exclusively on the action of residual brain growth when compared to linear craniectomy techniques alone and does not require cyclic activation of a distractor (Guimarães-Ferreira et al. 2004). Spring placement is most effective if implanted at 3–6 months of age and limits its applications to children who were diagnosed at an early age (David 2020).

7 Technological Advances in Craniosynostosis Surgery

In 1968, German surgeon Hans Luhr was the first to introduce the concept of internal fixation with miniature bone plates and screws in the craniofacial skeleton (Luhr 1968). The use of titanium mini- and microinternal plate and screw fixation evolved into the preferred form of fixation when stability against motion or when complex three-dimensional reconstruction of multiple segments of bone was required (Posnick and Ruiz 2000).

Due to the postoperative complications associated with metallic bone fixation including infection, exposure of underlying plates and screws leading to skin irritation, and, more significantly, calvarial growth disturbance and intracranial migration of hardware, the development of resorbable polymer fixation has led to the clinical availability of resorbable bone fixation implants since 1996 with application to the craniofacial skeleton for the pediatric population (Eppley et al. 2004).

Despite this advancement, risks of postoperative complications related to resorbable hardware failure still remain. A review of 1883 pediatric cranial vault reconstruction surgeries reported device failure from plate fractures, requiring reoperation in the postoperative period (0.3%) and delayed foreign body reactions (0.7%) which resulted in swelling and/or cyst formation (Sanger et al. 2007). Higher complication rates of 15.3% (Eppley et al. 2004) to 17% (Pearson et al. 2008) due to resorbable fixation, including palpable plates and a case in which the resorbable plates were surgically removed due to erythema, have been reported. The development of resorbable mini-plates and screws as a form of stable fixation continues to evolve as a fixation alternative especially for use in growing bones and for immobilization of onlay bone grafts (Posnick 1994).

The continual advancement in extensive cranial vault remodeling during the modern era of craniofacial surgery not only addressed normal neurological development but also achieved excellent aesthetic results even for those patients afflicted with the most complex, multiple-suture synostosis (Vollmer et al. 1984). These procedures, however, were associated with significant operative time, lengthier hospital stay, blood loss frequently requiring transfusion, and postoperative complications, which were considered limitations to extensive cranial vault remodeling and the driving force in the development of minimally invasive, endoscopic techniques.

Three-dimensional computerized tomography (CT) was first applied to the evaluation of craniofacial anomalies in the 1980s (Karatas and Toy 2014; Hemmy et al. 1983). The evaluation of craniosynostosis is enhanced with 3D CT data, and surgical planning can be completed virtually before the patient is brought to the operating room. With the development and advancements in computer-aided design/manufacturing (CAD-CAM), 3D CT data is used to manufacture stereolithographic models of the patient's craniofacial skeleton in addition to osteotomy and positioning guides, which are used intraoperatively (Figs. 15 and 16). This allows the surgeon to transfer the virtually planned surgery to the operating room with improved precision and efficiency of even the most complex, cranial vault remodeling procedure (Fig. 17).

8 Minimally Invasive and Endoscopy-Assisted Craniosynostosis Surgery

Through the 1990s, David F. Jimenez and Constance M. Barone, American neurosurgeon and plastic surgeon, respectively, proposed a novel technique involving a simple suturectomy via an endoscopic approach (Fig. 18) (Jimenez and Barone 1998; Pattisapu et al. 2010). Their technique was based on three basic principles of craniosynostosis: (1) greater success with surgery early in life; (2) based on Moss' functional matrix theory, the rapidly growing brain would cause expansion of the skull into a normal shape if timely intervention occurred; and (3) they employed an adjunct cranial vault remodeling helmet first introduced by American plastic surgeon, John A. Persing, in 1986 into which the brain would help shape the skull (Pattisapu et al. 2010; Persing et al. 1986).

Jimenez and Barone initially published a small case series in 1998 consisting of four patients with sagittal synostosis who underwent early endoscopic strip craniectomy and postoperative cranial molding helmets. They found that when compared to extensive cranial vault remodeling, their procedures demonstrated minimal blood loss, shorter operative times, earlier hospital discharge, and excellent function and cosmetic results (Pattisapu et al. 2010). They subsequently published the results of their technique in 12 patients who were afflicted with various fused suture patterns and, later, studies of up to 185 patient case series with various sutures involved, demonstrating continued, long-term success in the setting of extremely rare postoperative complications of infection, dural sinus tears, cerebrospinal fluid leaks or neurological injury, confirming the safety and efficacy of this approach (Jimenez and Barone 2000, 2010; Jimenez et al. 2002).

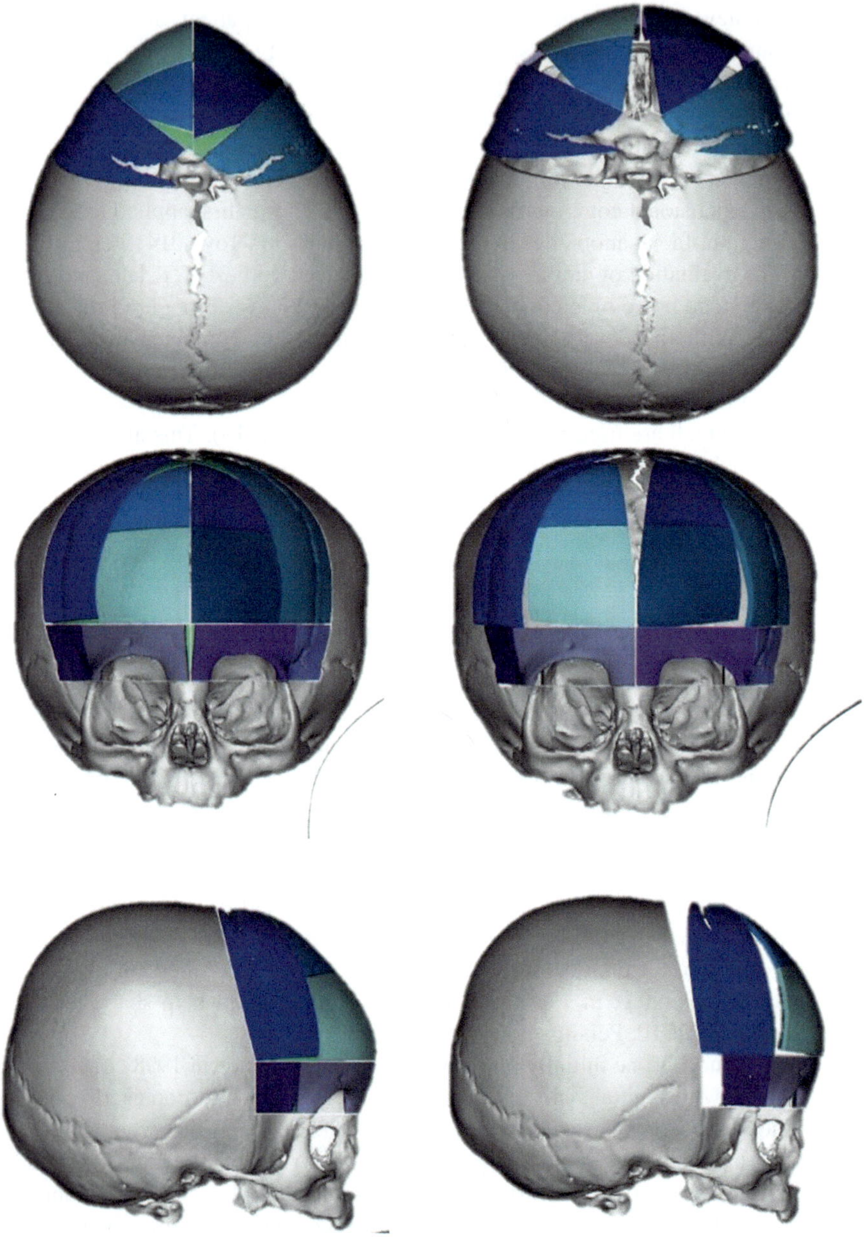

Fig. 15 Virtual surgical planning of anterior cranial vault remodeling for metopic synostosis. An age-matched skull is used to predict the correct cranial morphology

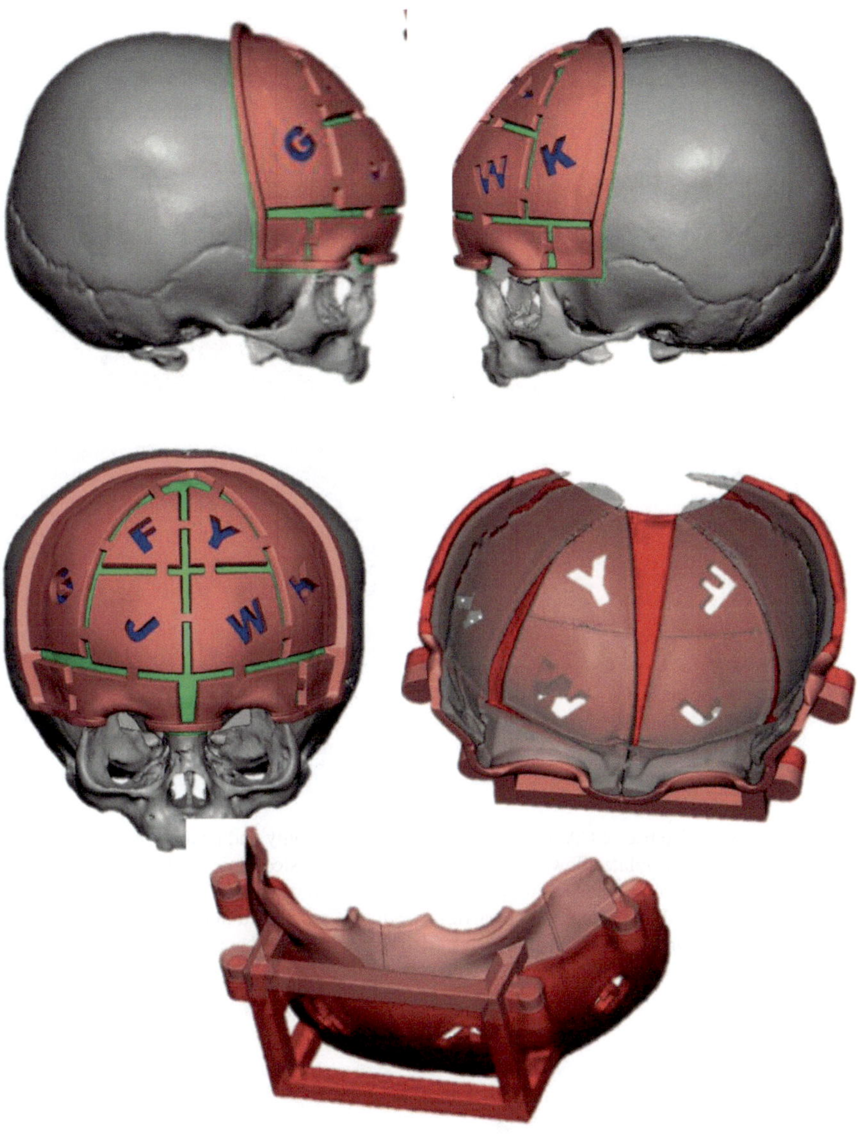

Fig. 16 Patient-specific CAD/CAM manufactured cranial vault osteotomy and positioning guides with labeling of each individual calvarial segment

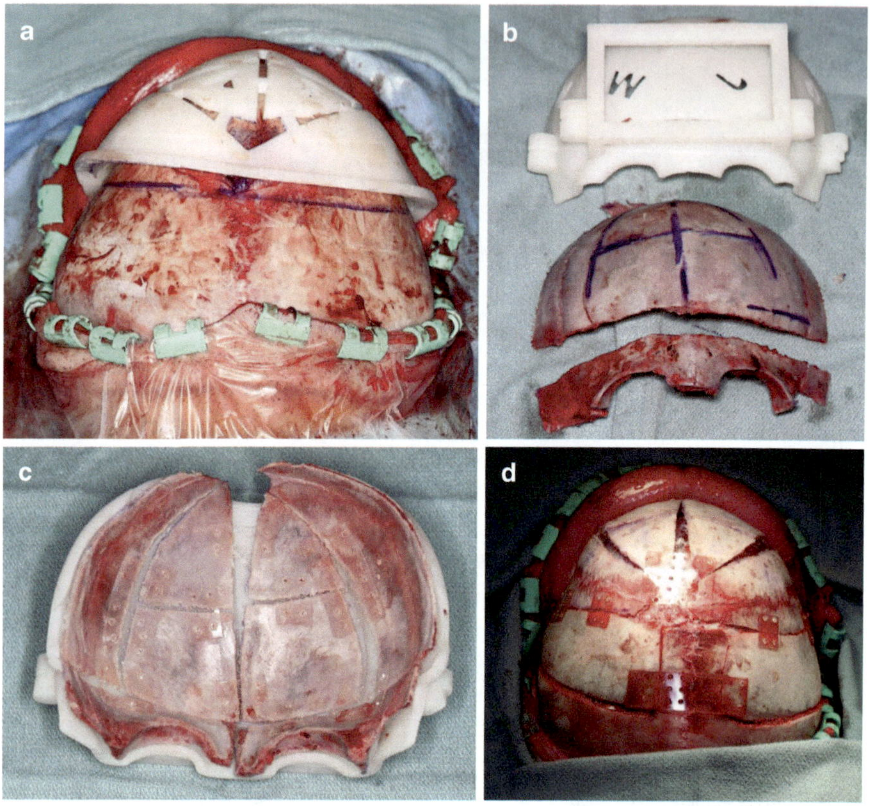

Fig. 17 Intraoperative use of CAD/CAM manufactured osteotomy and positioning guides. (**a**, **b**) Cranial vault cutting template allows for accurate placement of osteotomies and labeling each bone segment. (**c**) A positioning guide allows for accurate placement of individual calvarial segments to achieve normal cranial morphology. The calvarial segments are placed into the internal surface of the template and secured with resorbable plates. (**d**) The reconstructed cranial vault is then returned to the patient's native cranium and secured with resorbable plates

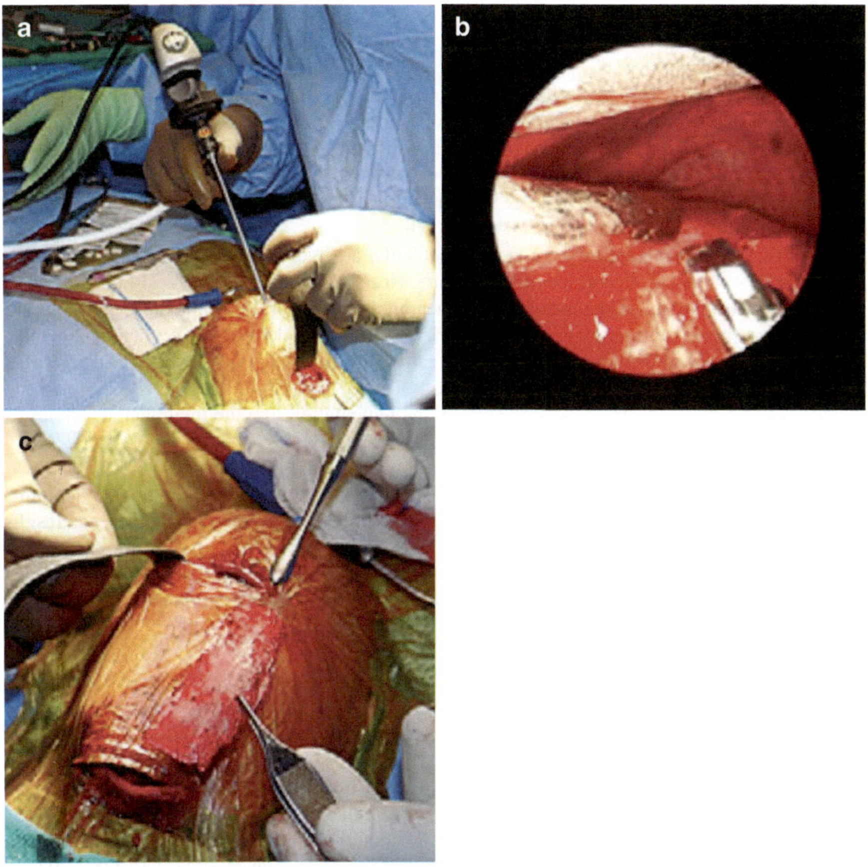

Fig. 18 An endoscope is used to (**a**) visualize and release the fused sagittal suture, (**b**) perform a craniectomy and create barrel staves, and (**c**) remove the entire sagittal suture and adjacent cranial bone

9 Conclusion

The contributions of the pioneers in craniosynostosis surgery allow surgeons today to offer treatment options for their patients that are relatively safe and predictable with excellent functional and cosmetic outcomes. The historical arc of craniosynostosis surgery, first with the development of strip craniotomies in the 1800s, followed by more advanced, open cranial vault surgery and then more recently and, ironically, minimally invasive, endoscopic strip craniectomy, illustrates the creativity, ingenuity, and perseverance of the generations of surgeons who have dedicated their work toward improving surgical outcomes for their patients.

References

Alvarez-Garijo JA, Cavadas PC, Vila MM, Alvarez-Llanas A. Sagittal synostosis: results of surgical treatment in 210 patients. Childs Nerv Syst. 2001;17(1–2):64–8.

Anderson FM, Johnson FL. Craniosynostosis; a modification in surgical treatment. Surgery. 1956;40(5):961–70.

Boulos PT, Lin KY, Jane JA Jr, Jane JA Sr. Correction of sagittal synostosis using a modified Pi method. Clin Plast Surg. 2004;31(3):489–98, vii.

Chipault A. Opérations applicables à la microcéphalie, à l'hydrocéphalie, à l'encéphalocèle. In: Chirurgie opératoire du système nerveux. Paris: Rueff et Cie; 1894. p. 698–734.

Codivilla A. The classic: on the means of lengthening, in the lower limbs, the muscles and tissues which are shortened through deformity. 1905. Clin Orthop Relat Res. 2008;466(12):2903–9.

Cushing H. Surgery of the head. In: Keen WW, editor. Surgery: its principles and practice, vol. 3. Philadelphia: WB Saunders; 1908. p. 17–276.

David L. The history of spring-assisted surgery implementation into the treatment algorithm for craniofacial deformities. J Craniofac Surg. 2020;31(7):2071–3.

della Croce GA. Cirugia Universale e Perfetta. Venetia: Zi- letti; 1583.

Di Rocco C. Surgical management of craniosynostosis and craniofacial deformities. In: Schmidek HH, Sweet WH, editors. Operative neurosurgical techniques: indications, methods, and results, vol. 2. 3rd ed. Philadelphia: Saunders; 1995. p. 135–48.

Di Rocco F, Knoll BI, Arnaud E, Blanot S, Meyer P, Cuttarree H, Sainte-Rose C, Marchac D. Scaphocephaly correction with retrocoronal and prelambdoid craniotomies (Renier's "H" technique). Childs Nerv Syst. 2012 Sep;28(9):1327–32.

Dryander J. Anatomie Capitis Humani. Marburg; 1537.

Eppley BL, Morales L, Wood R, Pensler J, Goldstein J, Havlik RJ, Habal M, Losken A, Williams JK, Burstein F, Rozzelle AA, Sadove AM. Resorbable PLLA-PGA plate and screw fixation in pediatric craniofacial surgery: clinical experience in 1883 patients. Plast Reconstr Surg. 2004;114(4):850–6; discussion 857.

Faber HK, Towne EB. Early craniectomy as a preventive measure in oxycephaly and allied conditions: with special reference to the prevention of blindness. Am J Med Sci. 1927;173:701–11.

Faber HK, Towne EB. Early operation in premature cranial synostosis for the prevention of blindness and other sequelae. Five case reports with follow-up. J Paediatr. 1943;22(5):286–307.

Frassanito P, Di Rocco C. Depicting cranial sutures: a travel into the history. Childs Nerv Syst. 2011;27(8):1181–3.

Friedenwald W. Cranial deformity and optic nerve atrophy. Am J Med Sci. 1893;105:529.

Gaudier B, Laine E, Fontaine G, Castier C, Farriaux JP. Les craniosynostoses (etude de vingt observations). Arch Fr Pediatr. 1967;24:775–92.

Ghali MG, Srinivasan VM, Jea A, Lam S. Craniosynostosis surgery: the legacy of Paul Tessier. Neurosurg Focus. 2014;36(4):E17.

Guimarães-Ferreira J, Miguéns J, Lauritzen C. Advances in craniosynostosis research and management. Adv Tech Stand Neurosurg. 2004;29:23–83.

Hemmy DC, David DJ, Herman GT. Three-dimensional reconstruction of craniofacial deformity using computed tomography. Neurosurgery. 1983;13(5):534–41.

Hoffman HJ, Mohr G. Lateral canthal advancement of the supraorbital margin. A new corrective technique in the treatment of coronal synostosis. J Neurosurg. 1976;45(4):376–81.

Homer. The Iliad. Trans. Robert Fagles. New York: Viking; 1990.

Hundt M. Antrologium de Hominis Dignitate. Leipzig; 1501.

Hunter AG, Rudd NL. Craniosynostosis. I. Sagittal synostosis: its genetics and associated clinical findings in 214 patients who lacked involvement of the coronal suture(s). Teratology. 1976;14(2):185–93.

Ilizarov GA, Devyatov AA, Kamerin VK. Plastic reconstruction of longitudinal bone defects by means of compression and subsequent distraction. Acta Chir Plast. 1980;22(1):32–41.

Ingraham FD, Alexander E Jr, Matson DD. Clinical studies in craniosynostosis analysis of 50 cases and description of a method of surgical treatment. Surgery. 1948;24(3):518–41.

Jacobi A. Non nocere. Med Rec. 1894;45:609–18.

Jane JA, Edgerton MT, Futrell JW, Park TS. Immediate correction of sagittal synostosis. J Neurosurg. 1978;49(5):705–10.

Jane JA, Dumont AS, Lin KYK, Jane JA. Craniosynostosis. In: Moore AJ, Newell DW, editors. Neurosurgery. Springer specialist surgery series. London: Springer; 2005.

Jimenez DF, Barone CM. Endoscopic craniectomy for early surgical correction of sagittal craniosynostosis. J Neurosurg. 1998;88(1):77–81.

Jimenez DF, Barone CM. Endoscopy-assisted wide-vertex craniectomy, "barrel-stave" osteotomies, and postoperative helmet molding therapy in the early management of sagittal suture craniosynostosis. Neurosurg Focus. 2000;9(3):e2.

Jimenez DF, Barone CM. Multiple-suture nonsyndromic craniosynostosis: early and effective management using endoscopic techniques. J Neurosurg Pediatr. 2010;5(3):223–31.

Jimenez DF, Barone CM, Cartwright CC, Baker L. Early management of craniosynostosis using endoscopic-assisted strip craniectomies and cranial orthotic molding therapy. Pediatrics. 2002;110(1 Pt 1):97–104.

Karatas OH, Toy E. Three-dimensional imaging techniques: a literature review. Eur J Dent. 2014;8(1):132–40.

Lane LC. Pioneer craniectomy for relief of mental imbecility due to premature sutural closure and microcephalus. JAMA. 1892;18:49–50.

Lannelongue M. De la craniectomie dans la microcephalie. CR Acad Sci. 1890;110:1382–5.

Lauritzen C, Sugawara Y, Kocabalkan O, Olsson R. Spring mediated dynamic craniofacial reshaping. Case report. Scand J Plast Reconstr Surg Hand Surg. 1998;32(3):331–8.

Lauritzen CGK, Davis C, Ivarsson A, Sanger C, Hewitt TD. The evolving role of springs in craniofacial surgery: the first 100 clinical cases. Plast Reconstr Surg. 2008;121(2):545–54.

Luhr HG. Zur stabilen Osteosynthese bei Unterkieferfrakturen [On the stable osteosynthesis in mandibular fractures]. Dtsch Zahnarztl Z. 1968;23(7):754. German.

Maher CO, Buchman SR, O'Hara E, Cohen-Gadol AA. Harvey Cushing's experience with cranial deformity. Neurosurg Focus. 2010;29(6):E6.

Marchac D, Renier D. "Le front flottant". Traitement précoce des facio-craniosténoses [The "floating forehead". Early treatment of craniofacial stenosis]. Ann Chir Plast. 1979;24(2):121–6. French.

Marchac D, Renier D. Early treatment of facial-craniostenosis (Crouzon-Apert) (author's transl). Chir Pediatr. 1980;21:95–101, (Fr).

Marchac D, Renier D, Jones BM. Experience with the "floating forehead". Br J Plast Surg. 1988;41(1):1–15.

Marsh JL, Vannier MW. Cranial base changes following surgical treatment of craniosynostosis. Cleft Palate J. 1986;23(Suppl 1):9–18.

Matson DD. Craniosynostosis. In: Matson DD, Ingraham FD, editors. Neurosurgery of infancy and childhood. 2nd ed. Springfield: Charles C Thomas; 1969. p. 138–43.

McCarthy JG, Schreiber J, Karp N, Thorne CH, Grayson BH. Lengthening the human mandible by gradual distraction. Plast Reconstr Surg. 1992;89(1):1–8; discussion 9–10.

McCarthy JG, Glasberg SB, Cutting CB, Epstein FJ, Grayson BH, Ruff G, Thorne CH, Wisoff J, Zide BM. Twenty-year experience with early surgery for craniosynostosis: I. Isolated craniofacial synostosis--results and unsolved problems. Plast Reconstr Surg. 1995;96(2):272–83.

McKinnon M. Le refabricant des orbites: a tribute to Paul Tessier. Ann Plast Surg. 2011; 67(6):S36–41.

Mehner A. Beiträ¨ge zu den Augenverä¨nderungen bei der Schä¨deldeformitä¨t des sog: Turmscha ¨dels mit besonderer Beru¨cksichtigung des Ro¨ntgenbildes. Klinische Monatsbl Augenheilk. 1921;61:204.

Mehta VA, Bettegowda C, Jallo GI, Ahn ES. The evolution of surgical management for craniosynostosis. Neurosurg Focus. 2010;29(6):E5.

Montaut J, Stricker M. Les dysmorphies cranio-faciales. Les synostoses prernaturees (craniostenoses et faciostenoses). Neurochirurgie. 1977;23:1–299.

Moss ML. Growth of the calvaria in the rat; the determination of osseous morphology. Am J Anat. 1954;94(3):333–61.
Moss ML. The pathogenesis of premature cranial synostosis in man. Acta Anat (Basel). 1959;37:351–70.
Otto AW. Lehrbuch der Pathologischen Anatomie des Menschen und der Thiere. Berlin: Rücker; 1830.
Pattisapu JV, Gegg CA, Olavarria G, Johnson KK, Ruiz RL, Costello BJ. Craniosynostosis: diagnosis and surgical management. Atlas Oral Maxillofac Surg Clin North Am. 2010;18(2):77–91.
Pearson GD, Havlik RJ, Eppley B, Nykiel M, Sadove AM. Craniosynostosis: a single institution's outcome assessment from surgical reconstruction. J Craniofac Surg. 2008;19(1):65–71.
Persing JA, Nichter LS, Jane JA, Edgerton MT Jr. External cranial vault molding after craniofacial surgery. Ann Plast Surg. 1986;17(4):274–83.
Persing JA, Morgan EP, Cronin AJ, Wolcott WP. Skull base expansion: craniofacial effects. Plast Reconstr Surg. 1991;87(6):1028–33.
Persson KM, Roy WA, Persing JA, Rodeheaver GT, Winn HR. Craniofacial growth following experimental craniosynostosis and craniectomy in rabbits. J Neurosurg. 1979;50(2):187–97.
Posnick JC. The effects of rigid fixation on the craniofacial growth of rhesus monkeys [discussion]. Plast Reconstr Surg. 1994;93:11–3.
Posnick JC, Ruiz RL. The craniofacial dysostosis syndromes: current surgical thinking and future directions. Cleft Palate Craniofac J. 2000;37(5):433.
Rougerie J, Derome P, Anquez L. Craniosténoses et dysmorphies cranio-faciales. Principes d'une nouvelle technique de traitement et ses résultats [Craniostenosis and cranio-facial dysmorphism. Principles of a new method of treatment and its results]. Neurochirurgie. 1972;18(5):429–40. French.
Runyan CM, Flores RL, McCarthy JG. Distraction osteogenesis: biologic and biomechanical principles. In: McCarthy JG, editor. Craniofacial distraction. Cham: Springer International Publishing; 2017. p. 11–43.
Sanger C, Soto A, Mussa F, Sanzo M, Sardo L, Donati PA, Di Pietro G, Spacca B, Giordano F, Genitori L. Maximizing results in craniofacial surgery with bioresorbable fixation devices. J Craniofac Surg. 2007;18(4):926–30.
Sear HR. Some notes on craniosynostosis. Br J Radiol. 1937;10:445.
Shillito J Jr, Matson DD. Craniosynostosis: a review of 519 surgical patients. Pediatrics. 1968;41(4):829–53.
Simmons DR, Peyton WT. Premature closure of the cranial sutures. J Pediatr. 1947;31(5):528–47.
Sloan GM, Wells KC, Raffel C, McComb JG. Surgical treatment of craniosynostosis: outcome analysis of 250 consecutive patients. Pediatrics. 1997;100(1):E2.
Speltz ML, Kapp-Simon KA, Cunningham M, Marsh J, Dawson G. Single-suture craniosynostosis: a review of neurobehavioral research and theory. J Pediatr Psychol. 2004;29(8):651–68.
Venes JL, Sayers MP. Sagittal synostectomy. Technical note. J Neurosurg. 1976;44(3):390–2.
Vesalius A. De Humani Corporis Fabrica. Basel: Oporinis; 1543.
Virchow R. Ueber den Cretinismus, namentlich in Franken: und ueber pathologische Schädelformen. Verh Phys Med Gesamte Wurzburg. 1851;2:230–70.
Vollmer DG, Jane JA, Park TS, Persing JA. Variants of sagittal synostosis: strategies for surgical correction. J Neurosurg. 1984;61(3):557–62.
von Graefe A. Tumor orbitae et cerebri. Graefes Arch Clin Exp Ophthalmol. 1866;12/II:100–14.
von Sömmering ST. Vom Baue des Menschlichen Körpers. Frankfurt am Main: Varrentrapp und Wenner; 1801.
von Sömmering ST. Vom Baue des Menschlichen Körpers. 2nd ed. Frankfurt am Main: Varrentrapp und Wenner; 1839.
Whitaker LA, Schut L, Kerr LP. Early surgery for isolated craniofacial dysostosis. Improvement and possible prevention of increasing deformity. Plast Reconstr Surg. 1977;60(4):575–81.
Winston KR. Craniosynostosis. In: Wilkins RH, Rengachary SS, editors. Neurosurgery, vol. 3. 2nd ed. New York: McGraw-Hill; 1996. p. 3673–92.

Cleft Lip and Palate Surgery

M. Alejandro Fajardo, Derek J. Tow, Christopher Hughes, and Charles Castiglione

1 Origins, Anatomy, and Incidence of Clefts

Orofacial clefts (OFCs) are among the most predominant birth defects worldwide. The prevalence of cleft lip (CL) and cleft palate (CP) varies with ethnicity, population, and gender. Clefts occur due to disturbances in various development processes and can affect the eyes, ears, nose, cheeks, forehead, lips, and palate. There are approximately 15 different forms of facial clefts that have been observed, most of which are rare. Among the different ethnicities, Native Americans and Asians have the highest rates of clefts estimating 2 per 1000 births, Caucasians have a slightly lower rate at approximately 1 per 1000, and African-derived populations have the lowest rates at approximately 1 per 2500 (Marazita 2012).

In general, most OFCs are considered nonsyndromic. Nonsyndromic OFCs account for approximately 70% of CL with or without CP and 50% of CP alone. Currently, with the aid of genetic technology, many of the genetic variations or mutations that give rise to syndromic forms of OFCs have been discovered (Marazita 2012).

During embryogenesis, lip and palate formation begins between 6 and 12 weeks of gestational age. Several tissues are in place by week 4 during normal development: paired maxillary processes, the frontonasal prominence, and paired

M. A. Fajardo
Department of General Surgery, School of Medicine, University of Connecticut, Farmington, CT, USA

D. J. Tow
Division of Oral and Maxillofacial Surgery, University of Connecticut, Farmington, CT, USA

C. Hughes · C. Castiglione (✉)
Division of Plastic Surgery, Hartford Hospital and Connecticut Children's Medical Center/University of Connecticut, Hartford, CT, USA
e-mail: Charles.Castiglione@hhchealth.org

E. M. Ferneini et al. (eds.), *The History of Maxillofacial Surgery*,
https://doi.org/10.1007/978-3-030-89563-1_21

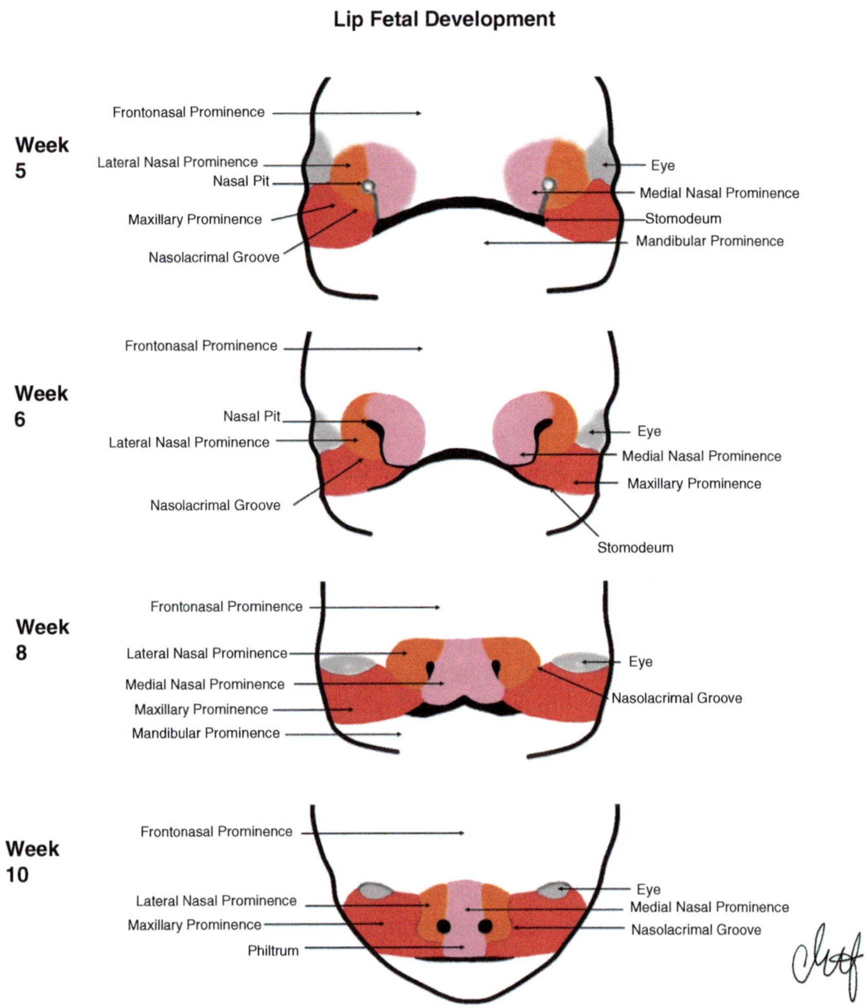

Fig. 1 Lip fetal development. Week 5 consists of paired maxillary and mandibular processes, formed fronto-nasal prominence, and paired medial and lateral nasal processes. Week 6 consists of medial nasal and maxillary processes that make the upper lip and primary palate. From week 6 to week 8, bilateral outgrowths from the maxillary processes start to grow down on either side of the tongue to become the palatal shelves. By week 10 there is culmination of upper lip development with descending of the medial nasal prominence to become the philtrum

mandibular processes surround the oral cavity (Fig. 1). By week 5 the nasal pits make up the paired medial and lateral nasal processes. By the end of week 6, the medial nasal and maxillary processes form the upper lip and primary palate, and by the end of week 10, lip formation is complete (Fig. 1). Bilateral outgrowths from the maxillary processes start to grow down on either side of the tongue to become the palatal shelves during week 6 (Fig. 2). By week 12, the tongue drops down, and the

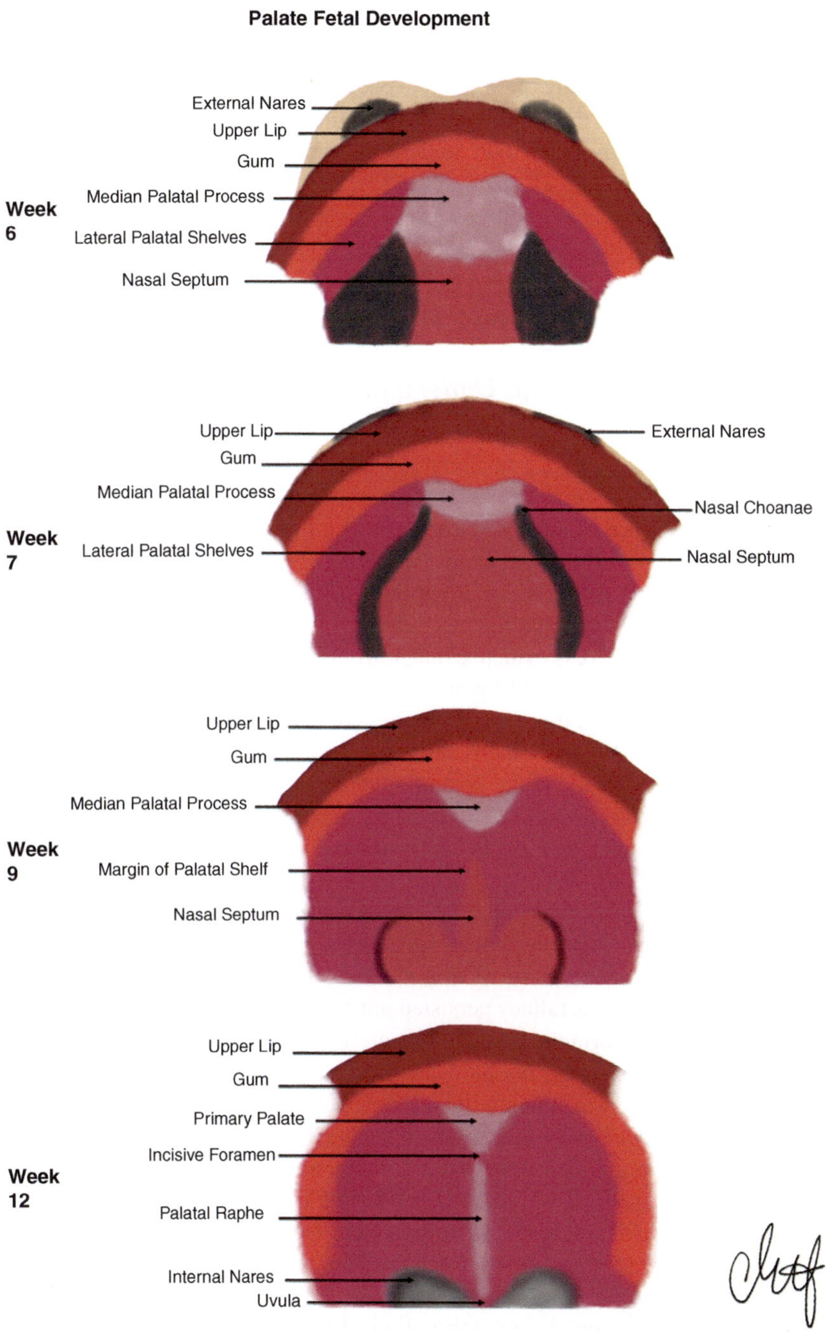

Fig. 2 Palate development. Week 6 consist of bilateral outgrowths from the maxillary processes that start to grow down on either side of the tongue to become the palatal shelves. Week 7 to week 9 consist of continued growth medially by the lateral palatal shelves that undergo fusion in the midline. By week 12 the tongue drops down and the palatal shelves go up and combine to create the palate

palatal shelves rotate up and fuse to create the palate (Fig. 2). The palate and lip are fully formed by 12 weeks. Any disruption in this chain of development can cause an OFC. Studies on the etiology of OFCs date back thousands of years and continue to this day. While much of the ancient studies on OFCs revolve around folklore, modern medicine has advanced our understanding using evidence and science (Marazita 2007).

2 History, Recognition, and Treatment of Clefts

2.1 Cultural History and Understanding of Clefts

Historically, explanations for congenital deformities were focused on a mixture of faith, superstition, invention, and charlatanism. Many deformities were considered to signify the presence of an evil spirit in the child affected, and the affected children would be cast out from their homes, drowned, or thrown off mountains. These events are well documented through various ancient texts on the attitudes toward orofacial clefts (McDowell and Vistnes 1979).

In ancient Sparta, there is evidence that newborn babies with clefts were drowned in the Tiber River or thrown off Mount Tagete (McDowell and Vistnes 1979). In *The Republic*, Plato suggested that discarding these defective children would be considered an action to remove evil omens and preserve the race's goodness. Tord Skoog cited the terracotta statuette in the Potters' Quarter of Corinth found in 1969, which dates from around 700 to 300 BC. The figure portrays a clown in such detail that secondary defects of the premaxilla and nasal alae clearly demonstrate a complete cleft lip model (Millard 1976a).

Olaus Magnus, an archbishop in Uppsala Sweden, proclaimed in 1550 that women may become pregnant by leaping over the heads of a hare and that for this reason these children have a hare mouth, in which the lip permanently separates the mouth from the nose. This fallacy persisted until 1889, when John Keating recorded several congenital abnormalities, including cleft lip, and stated that the mother was causing abnormalities during her pregnancy (Keating 1889).

Interestingly, there was thought to be a lack of facial clefts in ancient Greece, as in *Hippocratic Corpus*, a compendium of medical information of the time, there was no reference to this deformity. Additionally, no mention of OFCs is found in other early Greek medical and anatomical scripts from 124 to 690 BC, a span of over 500 years. This includes writings from famous ancient physicians like Asclepiades, Galen, Oribasius, Caelius Aurelianus, and Paulus Aegineta (Bhattacharya et al. 2009).

The first person to suggest an embryological basis for clefts was the sixteenth-century Italian surgeon Fabrice ab Aquapendente, also known as "The Father of Embryology." He suggested that the upper lip forms in the middle during a late phase of fetal development. Later, eighteenth-century surgeon Meckel theorized that clefts were formed by five distinct processes which eventually merge together to form both the top and bottom lips. The most convincing explanation on the origin of facial clefting was provided by nineteenth-century French surgeon Philippe-Frederick Blandin, who suggested that clefting arose due to the failure of fusion of the palatal bones, the premaxilla, and the maxilla (Bhattacharya et al. 2009). Another theory was presented by nineteenth-century anatomist William His, who suggested that the embryological development of the palate and lips is the result of a fusion of the five processes. Different types of clefts would form depending on which combination of those five processes did not fuse (Bhattacharya et al. 2009). This was also one of the first examples of classifying various types of clefts.

2.2 Evolution of Treatment: Cleft Lip

One of the first documented cases of cleft treatment dates back to 390 BC, China. The first recorded patient was Wey Young-Chi, an 18-year-old male born in Jen City. After the operation, Wey Young-Chi was able to join the imperial army to repress an uprising, eventually becoming the General of the Province of Yee and later the Governor General of six provinces (Millard 1976a).

Early surgical techniques were rudimentary, and detailed accounts date back to the late 900s AD. Tenth-century Arab surgeon Albucasis suggested creating a small cut into the lip, inserting a garlic clove, and leaving it for 15 hours. After the garlic was removed, a bandage moistened with butter was applied to seal the gaps. The Saxon surgeons of pre-Norman Britain, known archaically as "leeches", may very well have been the first to specifically describe the repair of CL in Europe. This was documented in the *Bald's Leechbook*, at the end of the tenth century (McDowell and Vistnes 1979). Turkish surgeons from the fifteenth century carried on traditions from the early descriptions of Albucasis. Cafar ed-Din, a Turkish surgeon of this era, provided depictions in the first Turkish surgical manuscript of cauterization of lip fissure, which is believed the same technique used during cleft lip repair (Fig. 3a) (McDowell and Vistnes 1979).

In the early fourteenth century, Flemish surgeon Yperman named the deformity *sartre moude* which roughly translates to "notched lip." Yperman described both unilateral and bilateral cleft lips and is likely the first to fully document the description of its surgical repair. He proposed that cleft margins be scarified with a bistouri (an early scalpel), sutured with a triangular needle dipped in wax, and reinforced with a long needle passed through the lips to accurately approximate the internal and external wound edges. The needle was then held in place with a wrap-around figure-of-8 suture or thread. Yperman was the first to document important aspects of cleft repair, such as ensuring as little of the lip was cut as possible and minimizing scarring by using the thinnest sutures and needles available (McDowell and Vistnes 1979).

Sixteenth-century surgeon Ambroise Paré, a tutor of Pierre Franco and one of the greatest surgical figures of the renaissance, performed extensive research on the

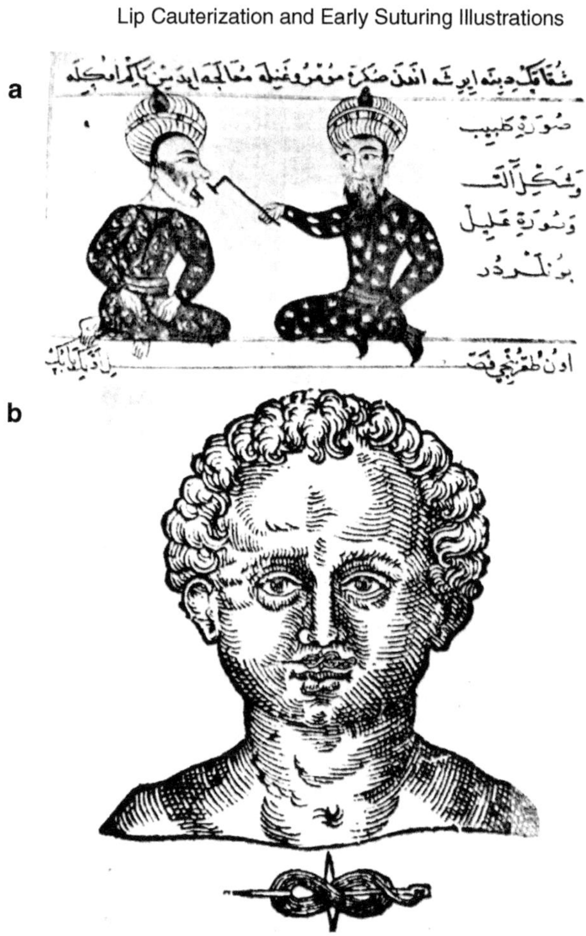

Fig. 3 (**a**) Cauterization of lip fissure, technique believed to be used for repair of cleft lip. (**b**) Copy of Pare's original woodcut suturing techniques. (Taken from "*The Source Book of Plastic Surgery*" by Frank McDowell)

anatomy of lips and palates as well as advanced suturing techniques. Paré is the first surgeon to include illustrations of repaired cleft lips in his surgical texts (Fig. 3b). He described the first example of an operation on a cleft lip and demonstrated impeccable technique. Paré was largely responsible for the gradual abolition of the cauterization methods used by the Arabians. In *Traite des Hernies*, Franco, a pupil of Pare, carefully refined the correction of unilateral and bilateral cleft lips. He recommended that the cleft lip edges be cut either with a knife or scissors or adjusted with a cautery. For double cleft lip, he proposed that superfluous portions of the premaxilla should be cut away with a bone scissors or saw to allow for better closure. He stressed that an accurate repair created a discreet scar, a result as he stated, "particularly desirable when the patient was a female" (McDowell and Vistnes 1979).

The use of adjacent tissue was introduced by Hieronymus Fabricius in the sixteenth century. He suggested the use of buccal mucosa or gingival tissue in closing the cleft lip. For wide clefts, he used bandages to bring the edges of the cleft together which reduced tension at the tissue margins prior to initiating repair. Hendrik van Roonhuysen, a skillful surgeon from Amsterdam in the seventeenth century, was one of the first to recommend repairing CL soon after birth. He suggested operating when the infant was 3–4 months old. However, in 1701, Le Clerc suggested that CL repair should not be done in children, as the constant crying impairs healing and therefore prevents reapproximation of the edges (McDowell and Vistnes 1979).

The French were some of the first to describe bilateral cleft lip repairs. Eighteenth-century surgeon Georges de la Faye from Paris wrote *Observations on Cleft Lip* where he described his first bilateral cleft lip operation. In his text, he describes removing the premaxilla and then bringing the lateral lip edges into the prolabium which was then left to hang free under the nasal tip. The lip was then pinned together with one pin near the nose and the other down the lip. The pins would then be sutured with silk in a figure-of-8 fashion (Faye 1743).

In the early nineteenth century, Joseph-Francois Malgaigne described repair of cleft lip with a different technique. He departed from a straight-line closure and instead created two small flaps to close the defect. In a case report from 1844 of unilateral cleft lip repair, Malgaigne thought that the whistling deformity was an inevitable sequel to a straight-line closure due to the linear contracture of a straight scar (McDowell and Vistnes 1979). In the same year, French surgeon Germanicus Mirault created an innovative method of circumventing this issue by inserting a triangular flap from the lateral side in a gap to create a horizontal incision on the medial side. More than a hundred years later, French surgeon Victor Veau proclaimed “Mirault is the genius of cleft lip surgery” (Bhattacharya et al. 2009).

Delicate and precise surgical technique resulting in decreased scar hypertrophy was discussed by Gustav Simon, a German surgeon who is credited with the preliminary closure of the bilateral cleft lip and whom the term “Simon’s band” is attributed to (Bhattacharya et al. 2009). The term “Simon’s band” or “Simonart’s band” or “Simonart’s band” refers to a small cutaneous or mucosal bridge that spans the lateral and medial components of a cleft lip. Gustav Simon was one of the first to construct labial bands for retrusion of the premaxilla in preparation for a more definite repair of bilateral complete cleft lip. This is rarely used now due to advances in dentofacial orthopedics (Mulliken and Schmidt 2013).

Another modification of cleft lip repair was made by nineteenth-century German surgeon Werner H. Hagedorn, who proposed using a quadrangular rather than triangular flap for the vertical repair. This change gave distinct benefits, particularly for bilateral clefts since a quadrangular flap simplified repair and helped correct its protrusion by exerting pressure on the premaxilla. Later in his career, Hagedorn operated on two children within a week of their birth and became the first to perform a bilateral lip repair in one stage (McDowell and Vistnes 1979).

In 1930 Blair and Brown revived the triangular flap repair, but they used a much larger flap. The triangular flap became the most commonly used technique from 1930 to 1955. In 1938, Victor Veau used a small triangular flap from under the alar base, fitted into a cut in the columella, a feature of Millard’s later operation. By 1940 LeMesurier revived the Hagedorn quadrangular flap, and for quite some time, it was popular (Fig. 4). By 1952, Tennison published a method of marking the

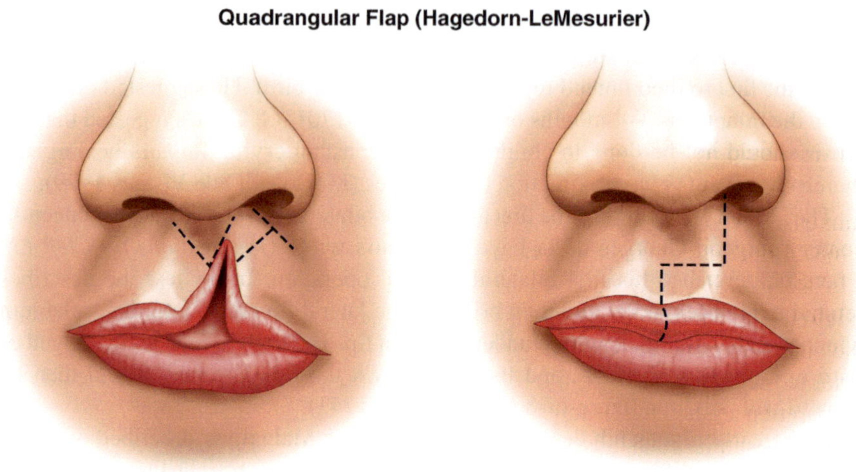

Fig. 4 Quadrangular flap. Quadrangle flap for vertical repair of unilateral cleft defects

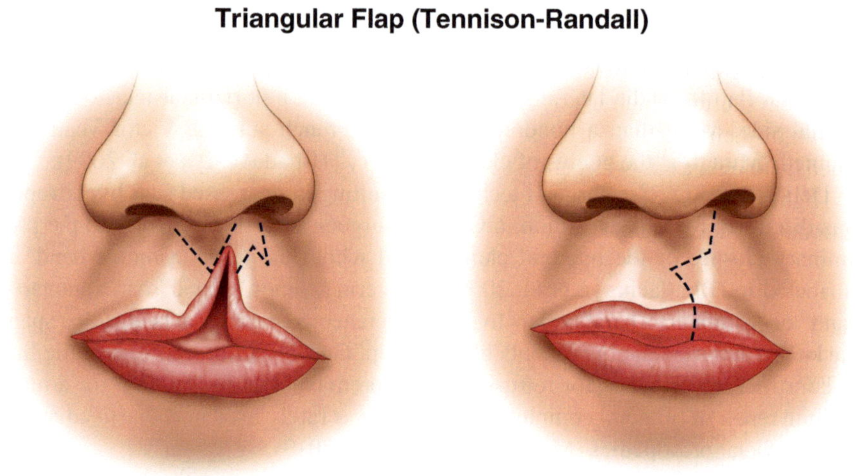

Fig. 5 Triangular flap. Involves lengthening of the medial lip segment by making a back-cut into which a triangular flap on the lateral lip segment is introduced

patient by using a bent wire. In 1959, Randall published a triangular flap method (Fig. 5) in which he created an opening for the flap on the medial side by making an incision similar to that used by Hagedorn and LeMesurier (McDowell and Vistnes 1979).

American surgeon Ralph Millard was introduced to cleft lip repair in 1944 at Boston Children's Hospital while assisting Donald MacCollum. Four years later in England, Millard had the opportunity to perform multiple straight-line lip closures under the supervision of British surgeon William Holdsworth. Dissatisfied with the results, Millard started to experiment with a rectangular flap from the cleft side in an attempt to reproduce a Cupid's bow. Over the next few years, Millard had the opportunity to work with prominent surgeons Brown, McDowell, LeMesurier, Straith, and Gillies to name a few. By 1953, as a Navy volunteer in Korea, Millard had the opportunity to repair multiple cleft lip deformities using the LeMesurier method. However, he continued to be dissatisfied with the results and decided to shift gears by performing his first rotation advancement procedure on a 10-year-old Korean boy. Millard described the first operation where he took a triangular flap from high on the lateral side, under the alar base, and inserted it into an incision on the side of the columella, the first reports of a "rotation advancement flap" (Fig. 6). In 1955, before returning to the United States, Millard presented his rotational advancement method to Gillies. While in London, he was able to present his paper "A Primary Camouflage of the Unilateral Harelip" at the International Congress of Plastic Surgery. Initially there was skepticism, but others adopted his idea and technique. By 1961, a survey of American and Canadian plastic surgeons indicated that the Millard technique was widely accepted and used by about 20% of those surveyed. In the coming years, Millard's rotation advancement method was widely used in Japan, especially Korea given its birth as a technique there, India, the United Kingdom thanks to Gillies, and the United States (Millard 1976a). As described by McDowell, "the best-known technique for the repair of a unilateral cleft lip is the rotation advancement repair, pioneered by Ralph Millard" (McDowell and Vistnes 1979). Over time, many surgeons have created their own modifications based on the rotation advancement flap.

In 1965, surgeon William Manchester from New Zealand stated that treatment of the complete bilateral cleft lip and palate is the most challenging of plastic surgery procedures. Much like Millard, Manchester was familiar with the techniques

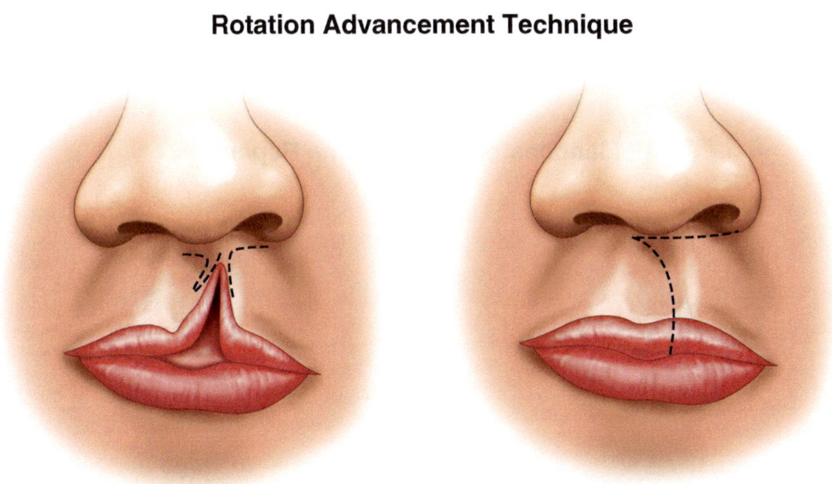

Fig. 6 Rotation advancement flap by Millard. This technique uses an upper lip Z-plasty scar beneath the columella. Described by Millard as the "cut as you go" technique

of LeMesurier but was not satisfied with the results. In the repair of bilateral cleft lip, LeMesurier advocated lengthening of the prolabium which caused the central and lateral portions of the lip to be too long. Even with modifications of the technique, Manchester found the central vermillion border to show too little bulk. He then postulated that the goals moving forward would be to keep the prolabial mucocutaneous ridge at a natural level, allowing the lateral lip to remain short, but add bulk to the central border of the vermillion. Key points of Manchester's technique involved discarding parts of the mucocutaneous ridge, dissecting the prolabial mucosa downward toward the vermillion, and allowing for anterior eversion of the vermillion border. The mucosal dissection is carried to the mucocutaneous ridge without dissecting upward from the premaxilla. This allowed for production of a large surface of the prolabium, allowing flaps of vermillion and mucosa to be made on each side. The flaps were then joined. The resulting eversion of the labial mucosa provided bulk to the midline and a pronounced cupid's bow (Fig. 7) (Manchester 1965).

American surgeon John Mulliken from Boston also described repair of bilateral cleft lip to be more challenging compared to that of unilateral cleft lip. In 1985, Mulliken realized that the residual soft tissue deformities seen with methods of bilateral cleft lip repair could be improved by applying five operative principles: maintaining symmetry, securing primary muscle union, selecting proper prolabial size and configuration, forming the median tubercle and mucocutaneous ridge from lateral lip tissue, and constructing the nasal tip and columella by anatomic placement of the alar cartilages. At that time, the repair was often a two-stage procedure but over the years progressed to a one-stage surgery (Mulliken 1985). By 1995, Mulliken refined his technique and invoked two additional concepts: simultaneous nasolabial repair and columellar modeling from nasal tissue alone (Fig. 8) (Mulliken 1995).

Finally, the timing of surgical repair must be performed at the right time to allow for maximum healing of the cleft. The timing of cleft lip repair has been and is still

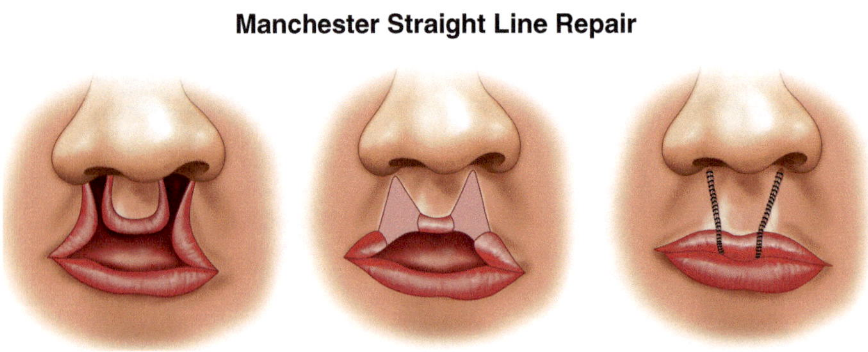

Fig. 7 Manchester straight line repair. Incision across back of the prolabial mucosa, with mucous membrane dissected down from the prolabial skin towards the remaining central mucocutaneous ridge. Flaps are developed from the vermilion of the lateral lip elements

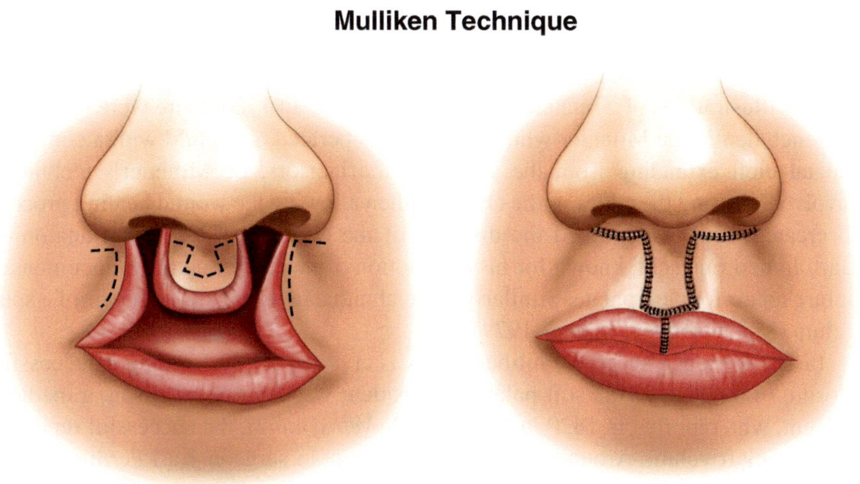

Fig. 8 Mulliken technique for repair of bilateral cleft lip defects. Involves reconstruction of orbicularis oris muscle by advancing bilateral muscle segments

highly debated. Two early voices in this debate in the mid-seventeenth century include Amsterdam surgeons Hendrik van Roonhuysen and Warwick James Cooke. They claimed that surgery should be performed as soon as possible, at an age of only 3 or 4 months, and any younger poses a higher risk of failure. This pacing of the operation continued into the nineteenth century when it was challenged by Italian surgeon Andrea Ranzi. He surmised that while it is possible to correct a simple CL soon after birth, operations for more complicated defects may have to wait until up to 5 years later (Millard 1976a).

The treatment and surgical repair of CL have evolved dramatically over the centuries, and contributions have been made by many trailblazers. Sophisticated techniques are now available for those with cleft lip, and minor modifications are still being suggested.

2.3 *Evolution of Treatment: Cleft Palate*

In the past, cleft palate was believed to be the direct effect of syphilitic infection. Others believed that cleft palate defects were the result of suppurative and/or destructive disorders such as scurvy, tuberculosis, severe dental and alveolar abscesses, or decay. Ideas for correcting this condition did not arise until the sixteenth century, when French surgeon Jacques Houllier proposed suture reconstruction for syphilitic palatal perforations. Pierre Franco was also one of the first to suggest an association between cleft lip and cleft palate, insinuating a congenital origin for defects of the palate (McDowell and Vistnes 1979). By the seventeenth century, Fabrice ab Aquapendente became one of the first to postulate that many newborn infants with cleft palates were unable to suck and frequently died as a result. In 1757, German physician Christopher Jacob Trew published one of the earliest illustrations of a bilateral cleft lip and palate. In 1766, there were reports of a French dentist Le Monnier who successfully operated on a child with a complete palatal cleft extending from the velum to the incisors. Le Monnier's technique involved suturing the edges of the cleft and then allowing the wound healing process to create a scar that bridged the distance of the cleft. In 1776, Italian anatomist Bartolomeo Eustachi, known for his description of inner ear anatomy, documented suture repair for cleft palate. Similarly, his technique involved suture repair of a split velum (McDowell and Vistnes 1979).

In 1819, French surgeon Philibert Roux is credited for performing a successful closure of a defect of the soft palate. The patient was John Stephenson, a medical student, who reported in 1820 in his thesis *De Velosynthesi*, the successful report of his own cleft velum. Around the same time, German surgeon Karl Ferdinand von Graefe reported closure of a soft palate defect. Von Graefe reported applying his surgical repair technique on four patients; however, only one was fully successful. The surgical approach used by von Graefe, which was similar to that used by Roux, consisted of five main steps:

1. Separation of the epidermis from cleft edge, which could be performed in two ways, mechanically or chemically. The mechanical method involved using a "chisel," and the chemical method involved using concentrated hydrochloric acid or sulfuric acid or using a caustic stick. The main goal of both methods was to scarify the edges of the cleft.
2. Insertion of sutures, which consisted of using four or five stitches.
3. Closure, which involved threading both ends of each suture through the cylindrical mother screw of the ligature screws.
4. General support and local care, which involved increasing inflammation and minimizing the production of mucus using clear liquid diets and acidified mouth washes.
5. Keeping the sutures tight, which involved constant readjustment of the slack of the sutures.

Numerous modifications of palatal repair followed von Graefe's original description. In 1826, Johann Friedrich Dieffenbach from Berlin described modifications in suturing and suture material. He continued to acknowledge the fact that cleft palates had congenital associations, and he also pointed out in his report that new techniques were needed to close the hard palate which most often failed. Dieffenbach's contributions also included the introduction of lateral relaxing incisions, the initial concept of repair timing based on palate function, and the modified suture materials, which would become precursors to Veau's wire suture (McDowell and Vistnes 1979).

By 1827, American surgeon Nathan Smith from Massachusetts and Alexander Hodgon Stevens from New York became the first to contribute reports of cleft palate repair in America. Stevens was a successful surgeon who had multiple roles later in his career including professor of surgery at the College of Physicians of New York now Columbia University, founder and president of the New York Academy of Medicine, president of the New York State Medical Society, and president of the American Medical Association (McDowell and Vistnes 1979).

In 1837, British surgeon Robert Liston was the first to illustrate and describe lateral relaxing incisions for repair of the velum. Liston was very skilled and was reported to have other surgical contributions including being the first surgeon to remove a scapula, designing the Liston splint for thigh dislocations, and being the first surgeon to use ether as an anesthetic (McDowell and Vistnes 1979).

In 1843, talented surgeon from Boston, J. Mason Warren, discovered that it was easier to dissect gingiva from the palatine bones than from the nasal mucosa in cleft palate repair. Warren essentially took Liston's contribution and improved upon it to create a more profound extension of the lateral incisions. As a result, Warren was the first to produce loose and relaxed flaps that reached further midline and allowed for tension-free closure of the oral mucosal flaps (McDowell and Vistnes 1979).

By 1845 Scottish surgeon William Ferguson realized wider clefts consistently failed to be fully tension-free despite new techniques like relaxing lateral incisions. Ferguson proposed division of the main components of the palatal musculature: levator palatini, the palatopharyngeus, and the tensor palatini tendon to minimize tension in wide clefts for successful repair (McDowell and Vistnes 1979).

In 1861 Bernhard von Langenbeck from Germany described a different technique for palatal repair using two bipedicled flaps. This became known as the von Langenbeck palatoplasty (Fig. 9). For the next couple of decades, multiple attempts were made by surgeons such as Karl Schoenborn and Theodor Billroth to perform cleft repair with modifications of the von Langenbeck palatoplasty to improve the repair and speech results. In 1925, American surgeon George Morris Dorrance from

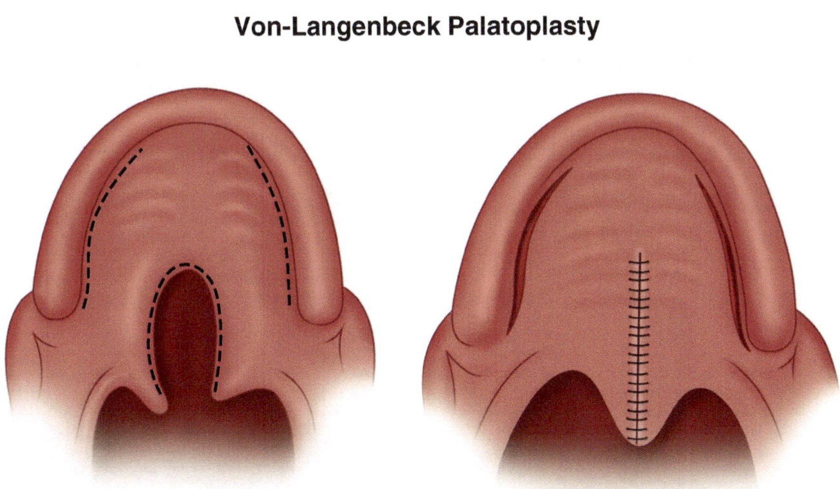

Fig. 9 The Von-Langenbeck palatoplasty involves relaxing lateral incisions with a midline closure of the defect with creation of mucoperiostial flaps

Pennsylvania introduced a palatal pushback and elongation. He also altered the structure and direction of the tensor palatini tendon by fracturing the hamulus (McDowell and Vistnes 1979).

In 1931, German surgeon Victor Veau from Burgundy introduced two innovations: the design of flaps to close the cleft in the hard palate and the direct suture repair for apposition of velar musculature. Veau designed flaps that were detached mesially and were vascularized only by the posteriorly situated greater palatine vessels. The design of the flaps was a major departure from the Langenbeck operation (Marquis 1962). Veau advocated the concept of midline levator palatini muscle reapproximation and emphasized the importance of an encircling suture to pull the levator muscles together, side by side (Leow and Lo 2008). This became the precursor to more sophisticated intravelar veloplasty techniques.

In 1937 British plastic surgeons T. Pomfret Kilner and William Wardill further modified Veau's technique to what became known as the Veau-Wardill-Kilner or V-Y pushback palatoplasty (Fig. 10). This modification allowed more flap advancement than the von Langenbeck technique and enabled posterior lengthening of the palate, thus improving velopharyngeal competence (Millard 1976b).

In 1967 Polish surgeon Janusz Bardach first described the two-flap palatoplasty with intravelar veloplasty. This technique involved creating mucoperiosteal flaps from the oral surface, mucosal flaps from the nasal lining, and muscular retropositioning with intravelar veloplasty (Leow and Lo 2008).

By 1978 American surgeon Leonard T. Furlow from Florida introduced the double opposing Z-palatoplasty at the annual meeting of the Southeastern Society of Plastic Surgeons. This technique involved opposing Z-plasties of the nasal and oral mucosal lining flaps. One side is a myomucosal flap, and the opposite side is a mucosa-only flap. This is reversed for the nasal lining, so that the velar muscles are automatically re- and retropositioned with flap inset. The Furlow repair allows for

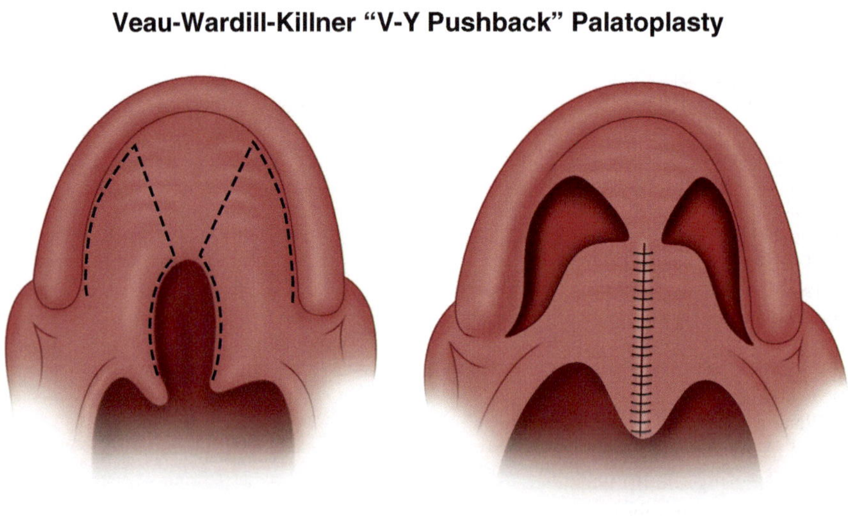

Fig. 10 V–Y pushback palatoplasty. Involves lengthening of the posterior palate by a pushback technique with elevation of muco-periostial flaps

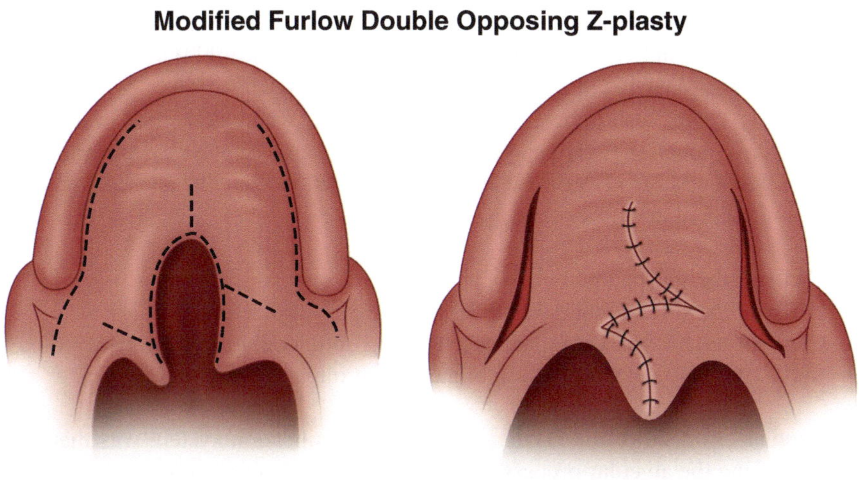

Fig. 11 Modified double opposing Z-plasty. This technique involves Furlow's Z-plasty with the modification by Randall involving bilateral relaxing incisions

soft palate lengthening, and it breaks up a straight-line scar in order to avoid scar-induced palatal shortening (Leow and Lo 2008). During Furlow's presentation, Peter Randall who was one of the moderators at the meeting applauded Furlow's concepts and later in 1986 presented a series of 106 patients using Furlow's technique. Randall employed the use of wide lateral relaxing incisions to maximize tension-free closure (Fig. 11) (Millard 1976a; Leow and Lo 2008).

Most recently, a poll of cleft surgeons in the United States demonstrated that the most frequently used techniques were the Furlow palatoplasty and the two-flap palatoplasty with an intravelar veloplasty (Katzel et al. 2009).

3 Classification of Clefts Through the Years

In addition to an evolution of surgical techniques and treatments, there have also been numerous developments in the classification of clefts. Because clefting occurs in so many ways, creating a classification system that is both simple and inclusive has been a challenge.

In 1922, American plastic surgeons John Staige Davis and Harry P. Ritchie announced that the concept of "harelip" should be abandoned and replaced with the term congenital cleft of the lip (Millard 1976a; Allori et al. 2017). They were among the first to support a standard classification system. The team proposed a three-group classification system allowing a separate definition of the lip, alveolus, and palate using the alveolar process as a dividing line (Burt and Byrd 2000). The first group affecting the lip was termed "prealveolar process clefts" and could be unilateral, bilateral, or median. The second group called "postalveolar process clefts" affected the palate and was further subdivided into soft and hard palate clefts. The third and final group named "alveolar process clefts" was any clefts involving the alveolar process and, similar to group 1, could be unilateral, bilateral, or median (Millard 1976a; Allori et al. 2017; Burt and Byrd 2000).

In 1931, Victor Veau published *Division Palatine*, which described in detail his approach to evaluation and management of cleft palate. Despite respect for his colleagues, Veau was openly critical of prior classification systems, and he developed his simplified and classic system:

1. Clefts of the soft palate
2. Clefts of the soft and hard palate up to the incisive foramen
3. Clefts of the hard and soft palates extending unilaterally through the alveolus
4. Clefts of both palates extending bilaterally through the alveolus

Another criticism of the Davis and Ritchie classification system was that Veau thought using the alveolar process as the dividing line between pre- and postalveolar clefts was set arbitrarily. Danish surgeon Poul Fogh-Andersen was one of many surgeons who considered the incisive foramen rather than alveolar process to be a better dividing line. In *Inheritance of Harelip and Cleft Palate* (1942), Fogh-Andersen proposed an alternative to the Davis and Ritchie classification that was composed of four groups: cleft lip, cleft lip with cleft palate, isolated cleft palate, and rare, atypical clefts (Allori et al. 2017).

Ardent supporters that favored a developmental anatomy-based classification included surgeons Desmond A. Kernahan of Chicago and Richard B. Stark from New York. They supported Fogh-Andersen's classification and added that based on the most recent understanding of facial embryogenesis at the time, the use of the incisive foramen was indeed the embryologically sound division line. The reasoning was that during gestation, the primary palate extends posteriorly with the incisive foramen as the posterior border. From that primary palate, the central upper lip and premaxilla are derived. Should failure of this growth happen, it makes sense that clefting would occur (Millard 1976a).

Detailed knowledge of past cleft palate classifications is important in pushing the boundaries of contemporary cleft treatment. As newer technologies enhance our understanding of human embryology and development, they will also improve our understanding of cleft lip and palate. Perhaps classification systems will be advanced in ways surgeons like Davis, Ritchie, or Veau would have never imagined.

4 Psychological and Cultural Influence on Clefts

Cleft treatment aims to restore the anatomy as well as auditory, speech, and feeding functions of children and enable them to improve physiologically and psychologically. A key component to cleft care is the involvement of a multidisciplinary team in order to provide a comprehensive approach for children throughout the cleft care cycle (Baker et al. 2009). This approach allows for patients to receive the best and most cost-effective results, at the same time allowing professionals such as dentists, orthodontists, speech therapists, audiologists, geneticists, social workers, and psychologists a chance to work with surgeon colleagues to become well trained in all aspects of cleft care (Searle et al. 2017).

That is not to say the results of cleft treatment are perfect. Those born with OFCs have often voiced concerns with respect to fulfillment, alteration to appearance after previous surgery, and issues not addressed within the cleft treatment pathway. Interviews of numerous individuals born with CLP reveal that they did not feel in control of any portion of the decision-making process as child patients. This finding may be due in part to older patients encountering a more paternalistic framework that was pervasive in healthcare when they were adolescents or teens. Unfortunately, younger people overall had not felt that their feelings were adequately considered in their interviews with wellbeing experts. A subjective inquiry of 52 adults born with CLP in the United Kingdom found that many participants questioned the value and necessity of surgical revision. They also felt that treatment decision-making was too influenced by the opinions of those around them and consequently led to further distress (Searle et al. 2017).

While there are many studies that have shown a clear association with CLP and communication difficulties leading to difficulty during school years, there are newer studies that demonstrate a contrary view. In a cross-sectional study performed in the United Kingdom on 103 parents of children and young adults with CLP, there were many negative outcomes including family impact and psychological distress, but these were less significant than the positive growth and adjustment that resulted from their child's condition. The subjects reported higher utilization of social support and less avoidance when it came to coping strategies. The study was careful to say that having these experiences did not necessarily mean it was a net positive on family dynamics but that having these challenges can possibly contribute to developing effective coping mechanisms for both the patient and those around them (Baker et al. 2009).

Families and patients affected by CLP can have a range of experiences in life, and many of these experiences are heavily influenced by numerous factors including severity of physical manifestation, interactions with the treatment team, and cultural coping mechanisms. While it is important to develop new therapeutic modalities and surgical techniques to help correct physical abnormalities, it is equally as important to evaluate and help manage social and psychological concerns.

5 The Present and Beyond

Our understanding and treatment of cleft lip and palate has evolved dramatically over the centuries. Surgeons from all over the world have made great strides to define and reproduce "normal" anatomy with a variety of techniques that continue to improve to this day. Techniques have advanced from simple edge-to-edge suturing to the providing lip length with quadrangular or triangular flaps, to Millard's rotation advancement, to functional muscle repair, and to the addition of primary nasoplasty. This progression of surgical techniques provides a valuable insight into the origins and future directions of cleft care, with a focus on functional repair while maintaining cosmesis.

Further, the classification of clefts has steadily become more accurate over the years to produce an inclusive and descriptive product. Efficient classification systems not only help medical professionals and scientists understand the different types of clefts but also help guide treatment plans and surgical options.

There are large psychological and cultural implications to consider when managing patients with orofacial abnormalities. Even for those with access to care, insecurities associated with poor oral hygiene, communication, and physical attraction can develop. These problems were often not addressed in the past but have now become an integral part of treatment protocols. Common problems that can arise in a child's life include behavioral issues, bullying, seclusion, and insecurities that may persist into adulthood. But evidence has shown that despite these adversities, affected families and patients are often stronger and more able to develop healthy coping mechanisms that permeate beyond issues related to a physical affliction. It then becomes the practitioner's responsibility to approach care with a more holistic approach to optimize not only the surgical outcome but also the overall quality of life of each patient.

References

Allori AC, Mulliken JB, Meara JG, Shusterman S, Marcus JR. Classification of cleft lip/palate: then and now. Cleft Palate-Craniofac J. 2017;54(2):175–88.

Baker SR, Owens J, Stern M, Willmot D. Coping strategies and social support in the family impact of cleft lip and palate and parents' adjustment and psychological distress. Cleft Palate-Craniofac J. 2009;46(3):229–36.

Bhattacharya S, Khanna V, Kohli R. Cleft lip: the historical perspective. Indian J Plast Surg. 2009;42(Suppl):S4–8.

Burt JD, Byrd HS. Cleft lip: unilateral primary deformities. Plast Reconstr Surg. 2000;105(3):1043–55.

Faye G. Observations on the cleft lip. Mem Acad R Chir. 1743.

Katzel E, Basile P, Koltz P, Marcus J, Girotto J. Current surgical practices in cleft care: cleft palate repair and postoperative care. Plast Reconsr Surg. 2009;124(3):899–906.

Keating J. Cyclopaedia of the diseases of children, medical, and surgical. Philadelphia: J.B. Lippincott Publishing; 1889.

Leow A, Lo L. Palatoplasty: evolution and controversies. Chang Gung Med J. 2008;31(4):335–45.

Manchester WM. The repair of bilateral cleft lip and palate. Br J Surg. 1965;52(11):878–82.

Marazita ML. Subclinical features in non-syndromic cleft lip with or without cleft palate (CL/P): review of the evidence that subepithelial orbicularis oris muscle defects are part of an expanded phenotype for CL/P*. Orthod Craniofac Res. 2007;10(2):82–7.

Marazita ML. The evolution of human genetic studies of cleft lip and cleft palate. Annu Rev Genomics Hum Genet. 2012;13(1):263–83.

Marquis J. Victor Veau (1871–1949). Plast Reconstr Surg. 1962;30:225–35.

McDowell F, Vistnes LM. The source book of plastic surgery. Plast Reconstr Surg. 1979;63(1):117.

Millard DR. Cleft craft: the evolution of its surgery, vol. 1. Miami: University of Miami Miller School of Medicine; 1976a.
Millard DR. Cleft craft: the evolution of its surgery, vol. 3. Miami: University of Miami Miller School of Medicine; 1976b.
Mulliken JB. Principles and techniques of bilateral complete cleft lip repair. Plast Reconstr Surg. 1985;75(4):477–87.
Mulliken JB. Bilateral complete cleft lip and nasal deformity: an anthropometric analysis of staged to synchronous repair. Plast Reconstr Surg. 1995;96(1):9–23; discussion 24–6.
Mulliken JB, Schmidt A-G. Gustav Simon's band and the evolution of labial adhesion. J Craniofac Surg. 2013;24(1):108–14.
Searle A, Ali S, Deacon S, Waylen A. Treatment experiences of individuals born with cleft lip and/or palate in the UK. Int J Oral Dent Health. 2017;3:42.

Facial Cosmetic Surgery

Keyur Naik, Pasquale G. Tolomeo, and Elie M. Ferneini

1 Introduction

Cosmetic surgery includes procedures that are intended to improve one's aesthetic appearance. Aging, asymmetries and congenital and acquired deformities are all reasons why patients may pursue cosmetic surgery. A person's self-esteem is frequently tied to their outward appearance. As such, the market for cosmetic procedures has grown dramatically. Facial cosmetic surgery is typically performed by highly skilled surgeons who frequently participate in advanced cosmetic or aesthetic fellowships after residency. Like plastic surgeons and otolaryngologists, oral and maxillofacial surgeons (OMS) can pursue such training. Oral and maxillofacial surgery has a long history in facial cosmetic surgery, and OMS have contributed to the inception and advancement of modern facial cosmetic surgery.

Today's principles of facial cosmetic surgery are rooted in reconstructive surgery. Sir Harold Gillies, a physician originally from New Zealand, is frequently credited as a pioneer in the field of plastic surgery and facial cosmetic surgery. In 1882, Gillies travelled from New Zealand to study at Cambridge University and

K. Naik (✉)
Department of Oral and Maxillofacial Surgery, New York University Langone Medical Center/Bellevue Hospital Center, New York, NY, USA
e-mail: Keyur.Naik@nyulangone.org

P. G. Tolomeo
Tulsa Surgical Arts, Tulsa, OK, USA

E. M. Ferneini
Beau Visage Med Spa and Greater Waterbury OMS, Cheshire, CT, USA

Department of Surgery, Frank H Netter MD School of Medicine, Quinnipiac University, North Haven, CT, USA

Division of Oral and Maxillofacial Surgery, University of Connecticut, Farmington, CT, USA

E. M. Ferneini et al. (eds.), *The History of Maxillofacial Surgery*,
https://doi.org/10.1007/978-3-030-89563-1_22

subsequently to train in otolaryngology at St. Bartholomew's Hospital in London, England (Thomas et al. 2019). At the time, plastic surgery was not an established specialty, and facial cosmetic surgery was not widely practised. During World War I (WWI), Gillies performed reconstructive surgery on soldiers with significant facial injuries. Gillies focused on improving not only on the reconstructive aspect of maxillofacial surgery but also the cosmetic outcome of his patients, which he noted was frequently ignored by other surgeons of his time. His work culminated in a seminal book in the field of plastic surgery titled *Plastic Surgery of the Face* (1920).

Oral and maxillofacial surgeons have performed facial cosmetic surgery since its inception. A French oral surgeon, Dr. Hippolyte Morestin, created a centre for facial reconstruction in Paris and worked alongside Sir Harold Gillies during WWI (Benmoussa et al. 2017). Facial cosmetic surgery has remained a part of oral and maxillofacial surgery since that time. However, facial cosmetic surgery has seen a particular explosion in demand over the past 30 years. As popularity has grown, surgeons from a variety of specialties have begun to incorporate cosmetic procedures into their practices. Oral surgeons have done similarly. The average number of facial cosmetic procedures performed by oral surgery residents has steadily grown as having the number of post-graduate cosmetic fellowship opportunities available to oral surgeons. Facial cosmetic surgery looks to be a rapidly expanding subspecialty within oral and maxillofacial surgery for years to come.

This chapter will explore the premodern and modern history of specific facial cosmetic procedures by citing the literature. It will also explore the advancements in surgical techniques up to the present day. The procedures discussed here are by no means the total sum of facial cosmetic surgeries performed by OMS. Rather, it is a discussion of those most frequently preformed. For the purposes of this chapter, surgeries that fall under the larger umbrella of reconstructive, cleft palate or lip, and orthognathic surgery will not be discussed as they are covered elsewhere. Additionally, minimally invasive cosmetic surgery will be discussed in the following chapter.

2 Rhinoplasty

Rhinoplasty represents one of the most frequently performed facial cosmetic procedures. According to the American Society of Plastic Surgeons (ASPS), approximately 220,000 rhinoplasties are performed annually (Plastic Surgery Statistics n.d.). Rhinoplasty is performed to address cosmetic deformities of the external nose. While rhinoplasty is referred to as a single procedure, the nasal complex is a composite structure, and an intricate understanding of its parts is necessary to obtain the desired result during rhinoplasty. Additionally, the procedure can be combined with septoplasty in order to improve nasal airflow. Two principal techniques of rhinoplasty exist today: open and closed. The open approach is typically taken when a more comprehensive procedure is required such as combined septorhinoplasty or placement of grafts for nasal reconstruction. However, closed rhinoplasty remains an option for those patients requiring only minor modification.

The first known recordings of cosmetic nasal surgery were in the *Ebers Papyrus* written by the Egyptians around 1550 BC. Rhinectomy was a common form of punishment for a variety of crimes in ancient Egypt. Attempts to reconstruct the nose after such mutilation became the first written description of nasal surgery (Whitaker et al. 2007). Rhinoplasty was also documented in ancient Sanskrit texts written on palm leaf named the *Sushruta Samhita*, which dates to 1000 BC. A physician named Sushruta is credited as the author of the text, though parts of the original manuscript have been found throughout India, Nepal, China and Tibet likely signifying a range of contributors. The *Sushruta Samhita* describes a rotational flap from the cheek as a method for reconstruction of traumatic deformities to the nose. Additionally, it describes instrumentation required to perform this early form of rhinoplasty (Singh 2017).

Modern rhinoplasty was first described in the early to mid-1800s. The term *rhinoplasty* was first coined by German surgeon Karl von Graefe in 1818 in his book titled *Rhinoplastik* (Graefe and Hecker 1818). In the text, von Graefe described innovative forms of nasal surgery, including reconstruction of the nose using a free flap from the patient's forearm. However, the surgeon credited as the father of aesthetic rhinoplasty has been debated in the literature. In 1887, an American otolaryngologist, John Orlando Roe, developed intranasal approaches for correction of the nasal tip (Roe 1989). Roe described certain deformities of the nasal tip as a 'pug nose' and developed a closed approach to correct it. In his first publication, Roe was able to demonstrate his post-operative outcomes through illustrations. In 1891, Roe published a second article titled *The Correction of Angular Deformities of the Nose by a Submucous Operation*, which included endonasal approaches to the dorsal hump and management of saddle nose deformities as well as pre- and post-operative photographs of his patients (Fig. 1) (Roe 1981). Others credit Jacques Joseph, a German orthopaedic surgeon, as the father of modern rhinoplasty. In 1898, Joseph pioneered rhinoplasty using external incisions and presented his technique as a case report to the Berlin Medical Society (Bhattacharya 2008). Included in this case report was a unique theory for the time. Joseph stated that aesthetic surgery can better the psychological health of his patients. This theory was considered radical by his fellow physicians who viewed medicine as a curative practice for physical ailments. In 1931, Joseph published a book of surgical techniques, entitled *Rhinoplasty and Other Facial Plastic Surgeries* (Joseph 1931). A number of prominent American surgeons travelled to Germany to learn Joseph's techniques and brought rhinoplasty to the United States by the mid-1900s. Two American surgeons, Irving Goldman and Maurice Cottle, became leaders of rhinoplasty in the United States. Goldman became the first president of the American Academy of Facial Plastic and Reconstructive Surgery (AAFPRS) in 1964, while Cottle established the American Rhinologic Society in 1954 (Stucker 2003).

The nasal surgery pioneered by Roe and Joseph is termed 'reduction rhinoplasty' and was performed with a closed approach. Endonasal rhinoplasty remained the standard approach until the early 1970s. A Croatian surgeon, Ivo Padovan,

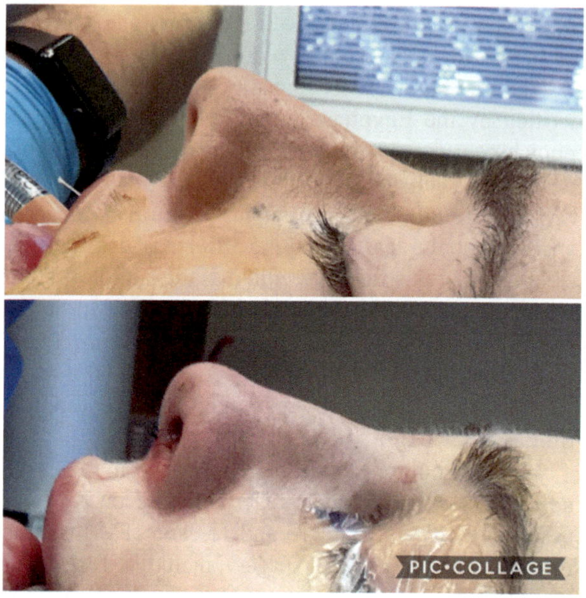

Fig. 1 Dorsal hump reduction. (Courtesy of Dr. Angel Cuzalina)

presented an external approach to rhinoplasty performed on a series of 400 patients at the first meeting of the AAFPRS (American Academy of Facial Plastic and Reconstructive Surgery 1972). The technique was quickly adopted by American surgeons, namely, Wilfred Goodman and Jack Gunter. In 1978, Goodman published a paper in the Canadian *Journal of Otolaryngology* entitled *Technique of external rhinoplasty*, which described advancements that he had made to Padovan's methods (Fig. 2) (Goodman 1973). In 1987, Gunter presented a secondary rhinoplasty via an open approach in his article *External Approach for Secondary Rhinoplasty* (Gunter and Rohrich 1987). Additionally, the 'reduction-only' methods that were demonstrated by Joseph were replaced by techniques that included both reduction and grafting. In 1978, Jack Sheen, a plastic surgeon from the University of California at Los Angeles, published a text *Aesthetic Rhinoplasty* which included techniques that advocated preservation of nasal cartilage and its use to shape other aspects of the nose (Sheen and Sheen 1978). The open approach and 'preservation' techniques are based on the work of these surgeons and their contemporaries. Advances in rhinoplasty have continued throughout the early twenty-first century. As a greater understanding of nasal anatomy is appreciated, the transition from a reductive to a structural approach remains the driving ideology behind rhinoplasty today. The greater understanding of nasal anatomy and multiple approaches to rhinoplasty now allows for individualized treatment for each patient. The cosmetic surgeon must understand that the nose is the centrepiece of the face and must focus on improving one's surgical skill in addition to one's knowledge. The nose is a framework that involves various skin types, cartilaginous and bony infrastructures. Each patient must be addressed individually being that one nose is unlike the other; a standardized treatment plan for all patients will result in a sub-aesthetic outcome.

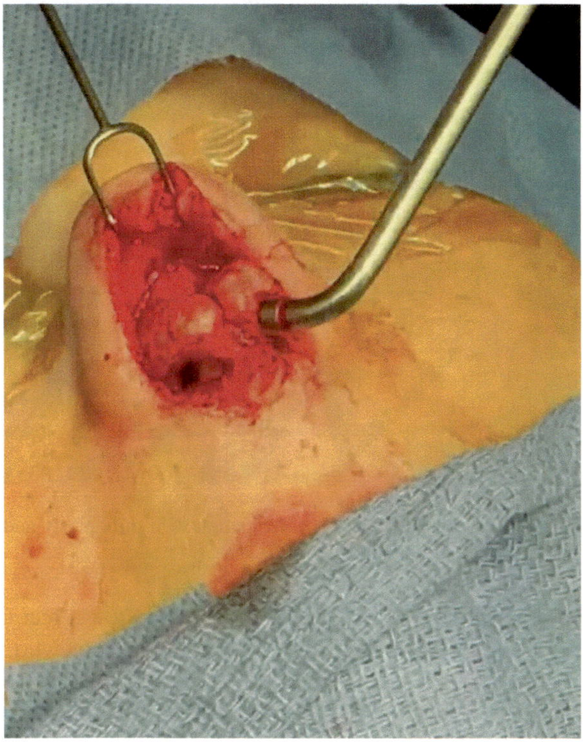

Fig. 2 Open rhinoplasty. (Courtesy of Dr. Angelo Cuzalina)

3 Forehead and Browlifting

The upper facial third contributes to the youthful and aesthetic face as well as non-verbal communication. As such, forehead or browlifting has become an increasingly requested procedures, primarily by older female patients. Typical candidates for browlifts are patients between the ages of 40 and 65. Ptosis of the brows progresses as we age. The purpose of a browlift is to reverse drooping and to produce a more youthful appearance to the upper facial third. As gravity affects the forehead and brow, the lateral canthal lines, or crow's feet, and upper eyelid dermatochalasia, or baggy upper eyelids, become more pronounced. The inclination may be to pursue eyelid surgery, but brow ptosis may be the true culprit. The surgeon must be able to identify the true cause of disruption to the upper eyelid complex and address the issue, i.e. lateral hooding may present as excessive tissue of the upper eyelids. A number of browlift techniques exist, both open and endoscopic. In this section, we will discuss the history of open approaches to browlifting.

Forehead and browlifting have been described in the medical literature for over 100 years. The first description was published by French surgeon, Raymond Passot, in 1919 in an article titled *La chirurgie esthetique des ridges du visage* (which roughly translates to 'Aesthetic surgery of face wrinkles') (Fig. 3). In the article, Passot describes the elliptical excisions anterior to the hairline and lateral to the eye

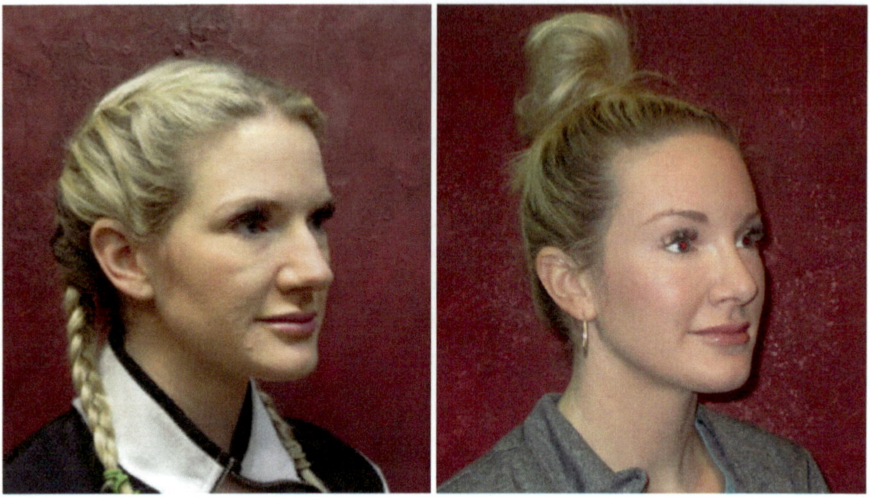

Fig. 3 Brow-/forehead lift in combination with rhinoplasty and lower blepharoplasty. (Courtesy of Dr. Angelo Cuzalina)

in order to lift the forehead and decrease crow's feet (Passot 1919). Passot's technique was followed by that of H. Lyons Hunt who proposed coronal excisions within the hair-bearing scalp in his 1926 book *Plastic Surgery for the Head, Face and Neck* (Hunt 1926). A number of surgeons followed the work of Passot and Hunt in the 1930s. Advancements in technique included undermining of the pericranium and resection of the corrugators as described by Fomon in 1939 (Fomon 1939). Others recommended rhytidectomy in conjunction with the previously described techniques.

Despite early advances, the procedure remained largely unchanged for the following 20 years. In the 1950s, the browlift techniques previously described were derided in the literature due to the inability to maintain long-lasting change. New approaches involved modifications to the frontalis. Chemical destruction of the temporal branch of the facial nerve was attempted to decrease innervation to the frontalis, but a number of unfavourable side effects were encountered including brow ptosis (Marino and Gandolfo 1964). In 1964, Marino and Gandolfo introduced the pretrichial incision design which remains popular for open browlifts to this day. In 1965, Vinas proposed excision of a strip of the deep aponeurosis-muscle layer formed by the frontalis, extending out to the lateral brow. Vinas differentiated wrinkles that appear during action from those that are permanent. He determined that correcting permanent wrinkles would require dermal abrasion and could not be corrected by browlifting alone. He also showed that elevation of the lateral brow was necessary to accomplish a long-lasting correction (Vinas 1965). In 1972, Regnault published the first description of the 'biplanar' approach to the temporal region as a way of performing traction on crow's feet. She advocated a subgaleal dissection to the eyebrows and upper margin of the crow's feet with relaxing incisions in the galea for traction (Regnault 1972). The work of Vinas was further developed by a surgeon named Kaye in 1977. While Kaye added to the surgical techniques of the time, he also contributed to the understanding of forehead aging and the necessary preoperative exam required for improved surgical planning. Kaye recognized that sagging upper eyelid skin may not be reversed by blepharoplasty alone. The correct treatment for many patients may in fact be browlifting. In order to determine the need for forehead lifting, Kaye recommended elevating the forehead and eyebrows preoperatively and assessing the effect on eyelid ptosis. By doing so, a surgeon can more accurately determine which procedure is more appropriate for a patient (Kaye 1977). This assessment is now a routine in the workup of patients presenting with eyelid ptosis. In 1991, Flowers published an article entitled *Periorbital Aesthetic Surgery for Men: Eyelid and Related Structures* (Flowers 1991). In the article, he further develops the ideas of Kaye and describes the importance of proper brow positioning prior to blepharoplasty. Since the early 1990s, the approach to the browlift has remained largely unchanged. The introduction of endoscopic forehead lifting has provided surgeons with minimally invasive ways of achieving the results requested by patients. Despite this advancement, open browlifting remains a mainstay of treatment.

4 Facelift

Like other cosmetic surgery procedures, facelift has become increasingly popular. While browlift was intended to reverse the signs of aging of the upper face, the goal of facelift is to rejuvenate the lower face and neck. The term 'facelift' does not describe one but a number of procedures that can be used to enhance the appearance of the lower face, including neck lifts liquid facelifts, nonsurgical lifts via radiofrequency and plasma energy, minitucks as well as thread lifts. This group of procedures aims to address gradually increasing skin laxity and changes in the subcutaneous soft tissues of the face and neck. With aging, there is a loss of elasticity and decreased skin thickness along with the development of wrinkles. Preoperative evaluation of the skin remains one of the most important aspects of facelift treatment planning. The surgeon can not only determine the type and extent of procedure required but also advise the patient on the potential for relapse based on dermal thickness. Correction of the changes to the subcutaneous soft tissues is equally important. Laxity of the platysma and superficial musculoaponeurotic system (SMAS) accentuates the nasolabial folds, facial wrinkles, jowls and the appearance of a droopy chin. An understanding of the changes in the superficial and deep fat planes of the face is also crucial for sculpting the lower face during a lift. With age, the superficial plane increases in total volume, while the deep layer descends and atrophies. Adjusting the superficial fat plane sometimes with adjunctive procedures helps maximize the cosmetic outcome of a facelift. As technology has progressed, a number of nonsurgical modalities have been developed in an attempt to achieve similar results. Despite that, facelift surgery remains a cornerstone of facial cosmetic surgery. This section will explore the development of the procedure and how an increasing understanding of the multiple layers of the lower face and neck has influenced facelift surgery over the years.

Tord Skoog, a Swedish plastic surgeon, is commonly credited as the pioneer of modern facelift surgery. Prior to Skoog's demonstration of a deeper dissection to manipulate the appearance of the face, a number of surgeons described elevation and excision of the skin alone or skin and underlying superficial fat. These types of lifts were first described in the 1920s and 1930s by Dutch and German surgeons. However, the effects of such facelifts were limited in their ability to produce any long-lasting change. Only including the skin and subcutaneous fat without involving the underlying muscle caused significant tension on the skin, which resulted in frequent and rapid relapse. In 1974, Skoog described a thick cervicofacial flap developed by raising the skin, the subcutaneous fat and the SMAS together (Skoog 1974). By repositioning these planes in a superior and posterior direction, he was able to produce reliable tightening of the lower face and neck. While the flap was robust, dissection occurred in a dangerous plane with a great risk for facial nerve injury. Additionally, the tissues could only move in one plane, resulting in limited improvement particularly in the anterior face. As a greater understanding of the subcutaneous layers of the face and neck was developed and described in the literature, facelift became a more nuanced procedure. Mitz and Peyronie were the first to describe the SMAS in *Plastic and Reconstructive Surgery* in 1976 (Fig. 4) (Mitz

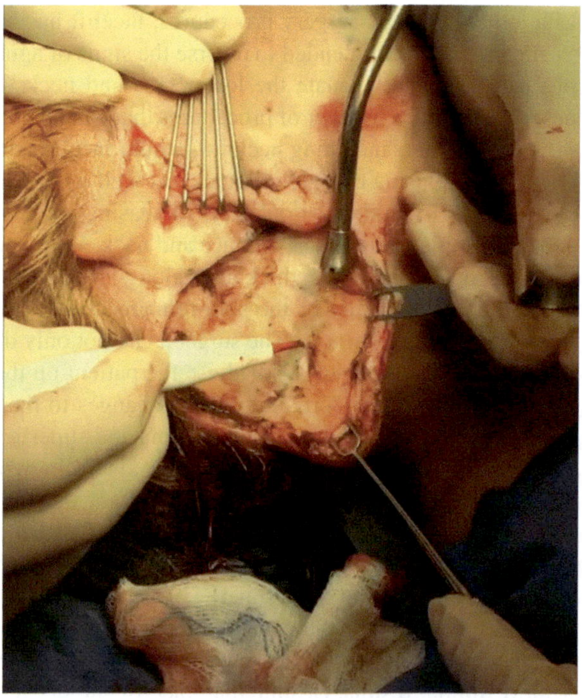

Fig. 4 Facelift. (Courtesy of Dr. Angelo Cuzalina)

and Peyronie 1976). Subsequent studies demonstrated how the SMAS serves as an investing layer of the muscles of the upper lip and a safe dissection plane for avoiding injury to the facial nerve. Surgeons had begun to develop various techniques to address longevity and obtain even greater results including SMAS plication and imbrication as well as a combination of platysma transection with medial plication and lateral pull. Additionally, retaining ligaments were first described by Bosse and Papillon in 1987 (Bosse and Papillon 1987). These ligaments suspend the SMAS to the underlying muscle and bone. Laxity of the retaining ligaments results in mid-cheek grooves and facial jowls. Repositioning of the SMAS can help eliminate these signs of aging.

In the early 1980s, Owsley, Connell and Aston separately furthered the work of their predecessors by describing a biplanar or lamellar lift by separating the skin from the underlying SMAS (Owsley 1983; Connell and Marten 1995; Aston 1983). While this approach allowed for greater vector control in sculpting of the lower face, the risks were considerable. Loss of blood supply to the skin or SMAS and tearing of the SMAS flap were feared complications. In order to avoid these risks, Hamra furthered the initial technique put forth by Skoog and described the deep plane facelift in 1990. In an article titled *The Deep Plane Rhytidectomy* published in *Plastic and Reconstructive Surgery*, Hamra demonstrated the composite facelift in which the orbicularis, malar fat and platysma are raised together with the overlying skin. In this technique, the SMAS is elevated off the parotid capsule and superficial to the branches of the facial nerve anteriorly in order to avoid motor nerve damage (Hamra 1990). In 1995, Ramirez described the subperiosteal approach to the facelift. The purpose of this approach was to release the retaining ligaments of the face and to allow for greater passive repositioning of the soft tissues (Ramirez 1995).

The facelifts described by Owsley, Connell, Aston and Hamra, amongst others, were significantly more invasive than the early lift proposed by Skoog. However, over the past 20 years, the development of adjunctive procedures has lessened the need for extensive facelifts. Fat grafting or lipofilling is the most common procedure done in conjunction with a facelift that addresses facial fat atrophy and allows for restoration of the facial volume. Approximately 85% of cosmetic surgeons utilize fat grafting to enhance the outcomes of the facelifts they perform (Sinno et al. 2015). The deep medial cheek is a particularly important area to fat graft as significant volume is lost in the compartment with aging. By performing lipofilling at the end of a lift procedure, a surgeon can accentuate the mandibular line angle, restore malar projection and improve tear trough deformities without more invasive surgery. An equally important adjunct procedure is skin resurfacing. Unlike fat grafting, skin resurfacing procedures are completed at the conclusion of a facelift after the quality of the skin and flap thickness are visually confirmed. Erbium and CO_2 lasers and trichloroacetic acid peel are commonly used, though the utility is limited to fair-skinned patients (Fitzpatrick I to III) (Wright and Struck 2015). The advent of new technology has allowed surgeons today to perform less extensive surgery, leading to shorter operating times and lower rates of serious complications.

5 Blepharoplasty

Blepharoplasty encompasses a wide range of surgical procedures performed on the upper or lower eyelid to improve appearance. Changes in eyelid appearance are most commonly secondary to aging though environmental factors such as sun damage and aging can also contribute to unaesthetic eyelids. Blepharoplasty focuses on the removal of excess eyelid skin, modification of herniated fat pads and creation of a more aesthetic eyelid crease in order to reverse the effects of aging and long-term environmental exposures. Simply, blepharoplasty can be divided into cosmetic procedures performed on the upper eyelid and those performed on the lower eyelid. The indications for surgery differ. Upper eyelid blepharoplasty is typically performed to improve dermatochalasis, asymmetry and muscle laxity. Certain upper eyelid conditions can be accentuated by brow ptosis. Cosmetic surgeons should evaluate brow ptosis and counsel on the need for a browlift in order to maximize the results of upper lid surgery. Lower eyelid blepharoplasty can improve dermatochalasis, steatoblepharon and herniated fat but also ectropion or entropion.

Though the first eyelid surgeries are hard to date, the first recordings of eyelid diseases can be found in ancient Egyptians' texts. Dated to 1550 BC, the Ebers Papyrus describes ectropion, entropion and trichiasis and medical treatments for each condition (Johnson 2005). The ancient Greeks expanded on the ocular and periocular diseases described by the Egyptians. The Hippocratic treatises document cases of eyelid ptosis, blepharitis and epiphora in addition to a litany of other conditions that effect the eye and eyelids. Despite the number of conditions described in ancient Greek texts, descriptions of surgical correction are limited. It is not until the development of Roman medicine do surgical procedures of the eyelids become more commonplace. In 30 AD, Aulus Cornelius Celsus compiled an encyclopaedia of diseases along with medical and surgical treatments into a text called *De Medicina* (Lazzeri et al. 2012). In this textbook, surgical treatments for a number of periorbital diseases including eyelid tumours, dacryocystitis and lagophthalmos in addition to those conditions were previously described by the Greeks. The medical traditions of the ancient Greeks and Romans were furthered by the Arabs who invaded the Roman Empire in 600 AD. The early Arabic conquests resulted in an Islamic Empire that stretched from Central Asia to Northern Africa and present-day Spain and Portugal. The strong tradition of written text in the Arabic culture resulted in over 30 textbooks on ophthalmology that were written over the course of the following 500 years. The most notable of these texts named Tadhkirat al-Kahhalin was written by Ali ibn Isa, a surgeon from Iraq. Isa documented the first upper lid blepharoplasty. In the text, Isa described sustained compression and subsequent necrosis of excess upper lid skin (Haq and Khatib 2012). Another physician of the time, Albucasis, wrote about cauterization of excess eyelid skin in order to correct eyelid ptosis (Al-Benna 2012).

A greater understanding of eyelid anatomy resulted in the modernization of the procedure by European surgeon in the mid-1800s (Fig. 5). In 1844, Jules Sichel, a French surgeon, published an article describing the role of herniated orbital fat in

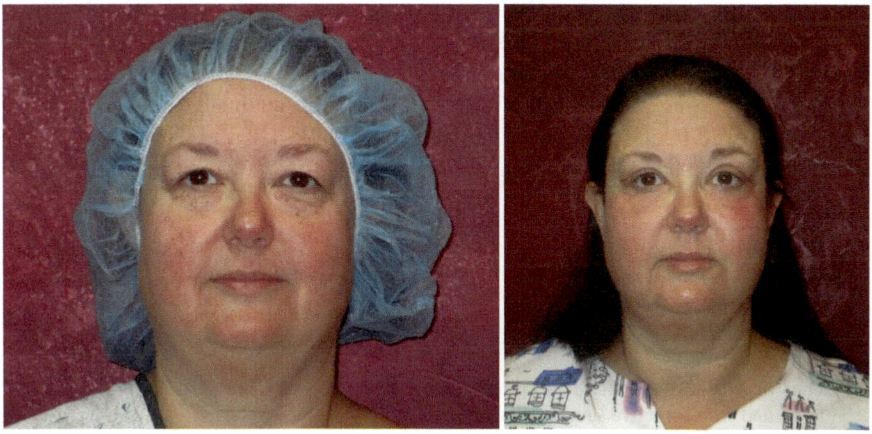

Fig. 5 Pre- and post-op upper and lower blepharoplasty. (Courtesy of Dr. Angelo Cuzalina)

the appearance of excess upper eyelid skin (Sichel 1844). This idea was furthered by Ernst Fuchs who demonstrated that laxity of fascial attachments between the upper eyelid skin and the underlying levator palpebrae resulted in a pronounced eyelid skin fold. Drawing on his findings, Fuchs described a surgical technique that not only called for removal of excess upper lid skin but also modification of these attachments to the levator and tarsus (Fuchs 1896). American surgeon Charles Conrad Miller made significant contributions by publishing the one of the first textbooks dedicated to facial cosmetic surgery in 1907. In his text titled *Cosmetic Surgery: The Correction of Featural Imperfections*, Miller was the first to describe lower lid blepharoplasty through a subciliary incision (Miller 1907). Another French surgeon, Julien Bourguet, advanced lower eyelid surgery by describing transconjunctival approach to blepharoplasty. He used this approach to remove herniated fat in order to tighten the lower eyelid (Bourget 1924). These facial cosmetic surgeons of the nineteenth and early twentieth century laid the groundwork for the subsequent advances in eyelid surgery which occurred after World War I.

World War I and II saw an increased need for facial reconstructive surgery, which led to improved understanding of facial anatomy and rapid advancement of surgical techniques. Facial cosmetic surgeons, including those who perform blepharoplasty, drew on the lessons learnt during the two world wars. In 1951, Salvador Castanares published a comprehensive article describing the orbital fat compartments (Castanares 1951). He drew on his own work to present novel techniques for treating herniation of periorbital fat, brow ptosis and lower eyelid bags over the following 15 years. Castanares' methods were largely reductive in nature. He advocated removal of orbital fat and excess skin in order to make cosmetic enhancements. As other surgeons have built on his work, there has been shift away from a reductive approach towards preservation of and addition to the periocular soft tissues. In his 1981 article entitled *Fat Pad Sliding and Fat Grafting for Leveling Lid Depressions*, Loeb was one of the first to describe utilizing and repositioning the herniated orbital fat in order to sculpt the periorbital area and soften the tear trough (Loeb 1981). Like other facial cosmetic surgeries, adjunct procedures have reduced the extent of surgical correction required during blepharoplasty. In 1997, Coleman described additive fat grafting to the periorbital areas in order to augment the appearance of the lower eyelid (Coleman 1997). The advent of new technology and preservative techniques has shortened surgical time, reduced operative complications and enhanced patient outcomes.

References

Al-Benna S. Albucasis, a tenth-century scholar, physician and surgeon: his role in the history of plastic and reconstructive surgery. Eur J Plast Surg. 2012;35:379–87.

American Academy of Facial Plastic and Reconstructive Surgery, editor. Proceedings of the first international symposium of the AAFPRS. New York: Grune & Stratton; 1972.

Aston SJ. Plastysma-SMAS cervicofacial rhytidoplasty. Clin Plast Surg. 1983;10:507–20.

Benmoussa N, Hansen K, Charlier P. Use of fat grafts in facial reconstruction on the wounded soldiers from the first World War (WWI) by Hippolyte Morestin (1869–1919). Ann Plast Surg. 2017;79(5):420–2. https://doi.org/10.1097/SAP.0000000000001221.

Bhattacharya S. Jacques Joseph: father of modern aesthetic surgery. Indian J Plast Surg. 2008;41(Suppl):S3–8.

Bosse JP, Papillon J. Surgical anatomy of the SMAS at the malar region. In: Transactions of the 9th international congress of plastic and reconstructive surgery. New York; 1987.

Bourget J. Les hernies graissueses de l'orbite: Notre: traitement chirurgical. Bull Acad Nat Med. 1924;92.

Castanares S. Blepharoplasty for herniated intraorbital fat; anatomical basis for a new approach. Plast Reconstr Surg. 1951;8:46–58.

Coleman SR. Facial recontouring with lipostructure. Clin Plast Surg. 1997;24:347–67.

Connell BF, Marten TJ. The trifurcated SMAS flap: three-part segmentation of the conventional flap for improved results of the midface, cheek and neck. Aesthet Plast Surg. 1995;19:415–20.

Flowers RS. Periorbital aesthetic surgery for men: eyelids and related structures. Clin Plast Surg. 1991;18:689–729.

Fomon F. The surgery of injury and plastic repair. Baltimore: The Williams & Wilkins Company; 1939.

Fuchs E. Uber Blepharochalasis (Erschlaffung der Lidhaut). Wien Klin Wochenschr. 1896;9:109.

Gillies HD. Plastic Surgery of the Face Based on Selected Cases of War Injuries of the Face, Including Burns. With Original Illustrations. JAMA. 1920;75(25):1738. https://doi.org/10.1001/jama.1920.02620510052037.

Goodman WS. External approach to rhinoplasty. Can J Otolaryngol. 1973;2(3):207–10.

Graefe CF, Hecker GF. De Rhinoplastice sive arte curtum nasum ad vivum restituendi commentatio. Berolini; 1818.

Gunter JP, Rohrich RJ. External approach for secondary rhinoplasty. Plast Reconstr Surg. 1987;80(2):161–74. https://doi.org/10.1097/00006534-198708000-00001.

Hamra ST. The deep-plane rhytidectomy. Plast Reconstr Surg. 1990;86(1):53–63.

Haq I, Khatib HA. Light through the dark ages: the Arabist contribution to Western ophthalmology. Oman J Ophthalmol. 2012;5(2):75–8. https://doi.org/10.4103/0974-620X.99367.

Hunt HL. Plastic surgery for the head, face and neck. Philadelphia: Lea & Febiger; 1926.

Johnson HA. Fish bile and cautery: trachoma treatment in art. J R Soc Med. 2005;98(1):30–2.

Joseph J. Nasenplastik und sonstige Gesichtsplastik nebst einem Anhang. Leipzig: Kabitzsch; 1931.

Kaye BL. The forehead lift: a useful adjunct to face lift and blepharoplasty. Plast Reconstr Surg. 1977;60:161–71.

Lazzeri D, Agostini T, Figus M, Nardi M, Spinelli G, Pantaloni M, Lazzeri S. The contribution of Aulus Cornelius Celsus (25 B.C.–50 A.D.) to eyelid surgery. Orbit (Amsterdam, Netherlands). 2012;31(3):162–7.

Loeb R. Fat pad sliding and fat grafting for leveling lid depressions. Clin Plast Surg. 1981;8:757–76.

Marino H, Gandolfo E. Treatment of forehead wrinkles. Prensa Med Argent. 1964;51:1368–71.

Miller CC. Cosmetic surgery: the correction of featural imperfections. Philadelphia: Davis; 1907.

Mitz V, Peyronie M. The superficial musculo-aponeurotic system (SMAS) in the parotid and cheek area. Plast Reconstr Surg. 1976;58(1):80–8.

Owsley JQ. SMAS-platysma face lift. Plast Reconstr Surg. 1983;71:573–6.

Passot R. La Chirurgie esthetique des rides du visage. Presse Med. 1919;27:258.

Plastic Surgery Statistics. n.d. Retrieved January 20, 2021, from https://www.plasticsurgery.org/news/plastic-surgery-statistics.

Ramirez OM. Endoscopic subperiosteal browlift and facelift. Clin Plast Surg. 1995;22(4):639–60.

Regnault P. Complete face and forehead lifting, with double traction on "crow's feet". Plast Reconstr Surg. 1972;49:123–9.

Roe JO. The correction of angular deformities of the nose by a subcutaneous operation. Med Rec. 1981;40:57.

Roe JO. The deformity termed 'pug nose' and its correction by a simple operation. By John Orlando Roe, 1887. Arch Otolaryngol Head Neck Surg. 1989;115(2):156–7. https://doi.org/10.1001/archotol.1989.01860260030010.

Sheen AP, Sheen JH. Aesthetic rhinoplasty. Saint Louis: Mosby; 1978.

Sichel A. Aphorismes pratiques sur divers points d'opthalmologie. Ann Ocul. 1844;12:185.

Singh V. Sushruta: the father of surgery. Natl J Maxillofac Surg. 2017;8(1):1–3.

Sinno S, Mehta K, Reavey PL, Simmons C, Stuzin JM. Current trends in facial rejuvenation. Plast Reconstr Surg. 2015;136:20e–30e.

Skoog T. New methods and refinements. In: Plastic surgery. Stokholm: Almgrist and Wicksell International; 1974.

Stucker FJ. Rhinoplasty from the Goldman/Cottle schools to the present: a survey of 7447 personal cases. Am J Rhinol. 2003;17(1):23–6.

Thomas RL, Fries A, Hodgkinson D. Plastic surgery pioneers of the central powers in the great war. Craniomaxillofac Trauma Reconstr. 2019;12(1):1–7.

Vinas JC. Plan general de la ritidoplastia y zona tabu. Transactions of the 4th Brazilian congress on plastic surgery. 1965.

Whitaker IS, Karoo RO, Spyrou G, Fenton OM. The birth of plastic surgery: the story of nasal reconstruction from the Edwin Smith Papyrus to the twenty-first century. Plast Reconstr Surg. 2007;120(1):327–36.

Wright EJ, Struck SK. Facelift combined with simultaneous fractional laser resurfacing: outcomes and complications. J Plast Reconstr Aesthet Surg. 2015;68:1332–7.

Minimally Invasive Cosmetic Procedures

Elizabeth M. Will, Brian M. Will, Michael J. Will, and Alia Koch

1 Introduction

To understand where we are going, it is important to understand where we have been. For as long as history has been documented, the human race has attempted to alter appearance through jewelry and costumes, tattooing, and body painting. The desire for eternal youth is pervasive throughout all cultures. In ancient Egypt, women would attempt to soften their skin and treat wrinkles by applying ointments made of mixtures of incense, wax, freshly squeezed olive oil, cypress, and fresh milk (Parish and Crissey 1988). The word *cosmetic* originated in the seventeenth century and comes from the Greek word *kosmos* which means order or adornment (Oumeish 2001). Taken literally, cosmetics assist in maintaining order. The order that most cosmetic patients desire is the restoration of youthful appearance. As we age, the amount of collagen in our skin's extracellular matrix decreases, the dermis and epidermis thin, and there is facial volume loss through lipoatrophy. This results in skin laxity, wrinkles, and increased skin transparency. These changes are seen in all humans but affect each individual at varying rates depending on genetic and environmental factors.

E. M. Will
Department of Obstetrics & Gynecology, New York University Langone Medical Center/Bellevue Hospital Center, New York, NY, USA

B. M. Will · A. Koch (✉)
Division of Oral and Maxillofacial Surgery, NewYork-Presbyterian/Columbia University Irving Medical Center, New York, NY, USA
e-mail: ak2045@cumc.columbia.edu

M. J. Will
Will Surgical Arts, Urbana, MD, USA

E. M. Ferneini et al. (eds.), *The History of Maxillofacial Surgery*,
https://doi.org/10.1007/978-3-030-89563-1_23

The emphasis on aesthetics seems to only increase as time passes, and the revolution in cosmeceutical science has reflected that. For the human race, the face is the focal point in the evaluation of appearance, and the ideals of what constitutes an aesthetically pleasing facial structure have changed over time. The face constitutes the foundation for most nonverbal messages including the emotional state of a person, as it is best stated in the ancient proverb, "the face is an index of the mind" (Kattimani et al. 2019).

The explosion of social media has had an enormous impact on influencing what we as a society consider beauty. Makeup, air-brushing, and digital engineering have created an almost unattainable ideal of beauty. This has resulted in an insatiable demand for facial cosmetic procedures to enhance perceived inadequacies or to defy the inevitable effects of aging. Many patients are willing to undergo general anesthesia and surgical cosmetic procedures, but an even greater patient population elects for regular treatments of minimally invasive cosmetic therapy. In 2019, there were 18.1 million cosmetic procedures performed in the United States, 16.3 million of which were minimally invasive (an increase of 2% from 2018) (American Society of Plastic Surgeons Plastic Surgery Statistics Report 2019). This chapter will focus on the most popular and frequent in-office injectable treatments.

2 Needle and Syringe

The use of injectables would not have been possible without the advent of the needle and syringe as there would be no means of delivering therapeutic substances to the dermis and subcutaneous soft tissues. The hollow needle was invented by physician Francis Rynd in Dublin, Ireland, in 1844 (Kravetz 2005). He manufactured the needle by annealing the edges of a flat strip of steel to make a hollow tube. Rynd first used the needle to inject sedatives for the treatment of neuralgias (Rynd 1861). The hypodermic needle and syringe were developed independently in 1853 by French orthopedic surgeon Charles Pravaz and Scottish physician Alexander Wood. The first syringe involved a screw-type piston allowing subcutaneous delivery of small amounts of fluid. Pravaz used the needle and syringe to administer coagulant to sheep, and Wood used them to inject morphine into humans (Feldmann 2000; Ellis 2017). Wood generally receives credit for the discovery of the hypodermic needle as he was the first to use it to deliver medications to humans. Sadly, Pravaz's wife died of opioid overdose after self-administration of morphine injections. The basic functional design of the hypodermic needle and syringe has remained unchanged since the initial discovery. Advancements such as interchangeable and disposable plastic parts in the 1950s have resulted in the universal use of these essential medical devices.

3 Neurotoxins

A chapter on the history of minimally invasive cosmetics would not be complete without talking about the most popular in-office cosmetic procedure in the United States, botulinum toxin type A (Botox™) (American Society of Plastic Surgeons 2018). Botox™ is not the only neurotoxin treatment currently available, but it was the first to be approved by the Food and Drug Administration (FDA) in the United States and is so commonly used that the word is part of the vernacular of both medical and non-medical individuals. This neurotoxin offers successful outcomes with a very limited side effect profile (Jandhyala 2013). In fact, botulinum toxin has such a low-risk profile that its injections can be used in almost any patient population. The only absolute contraindications are infection at the site of injection or known hypersensitivity to a component of the product. Relative contraindications include pregnancy, breastfeeding, neuromuscular junction disorders (myasthenia gravis or Lambert-Eaton syndrome), and amyotrophic lateralizing sclerosis (Zhou et al. 2017).

Botulinum toxin is an infamous neurotoxic protein that is the main virulence factor produced by the bacterium *Clostridium botulinum*. The toxin is a protease that is composed of one heavy chain and one light chain (Giordano et al. 2017). It cleaves the SNAP-25 protein in the presynaptic nerve terminal of the neuromuscular junction, preventing the fusion and exocytosis of vesicles containing the excitatory neurotransmitter acetylcholine and resulting in a flaccid paralysis (Fig. 1) (Giordano et al. 2017).

Ingestion of this toxin can cause botulism, with its trademark symptom of descending flaccid paralysis that begins in the muscles of the face and oropharynx. Classically, this occurs in adults when they ingest preformed toxin from improperly canned foods and in infants when they ingest *Clostridium* spores in honey. Botulinum toxin is so potent that Lamanna et al. described it as "most poisonous of all poisons" in their publication in *Science* in 1959 (Lamanna 1959).

Food-borne botulism has existed for as long as humans have attempted to preserve and store food. Several ancient methods of food storage became a perfect environment for the growth of *Clostridium botulinum* and subsequent production of botulinum toxin. Examples include placing ham in barrels of brine in France, hanging liver sausages from rafters in Austria, and fermenting trout in willow baskets in Scandinavia (Erbguth 2004). These processes all provide the ideal anaerobic environment for *Clostridium* to thrive and sporulate.

Seven serotypes of botulinum toxin (A, B, C1, D, E, F, and G) produced by different strains of the bacterium have been discovered. Types A and B are the isoforms that are capable of causing diseases in humans and are also the serotypes utilized in medical therapy. It is fascinating to note that the very same neurotoxin that has the ability to cause fatal disease in both adults and young children can be purified and used in a wide variety of medical and cosmetic treatments. Botulinum toxin type A is the most common isoform used in aesthetic clinical practice.

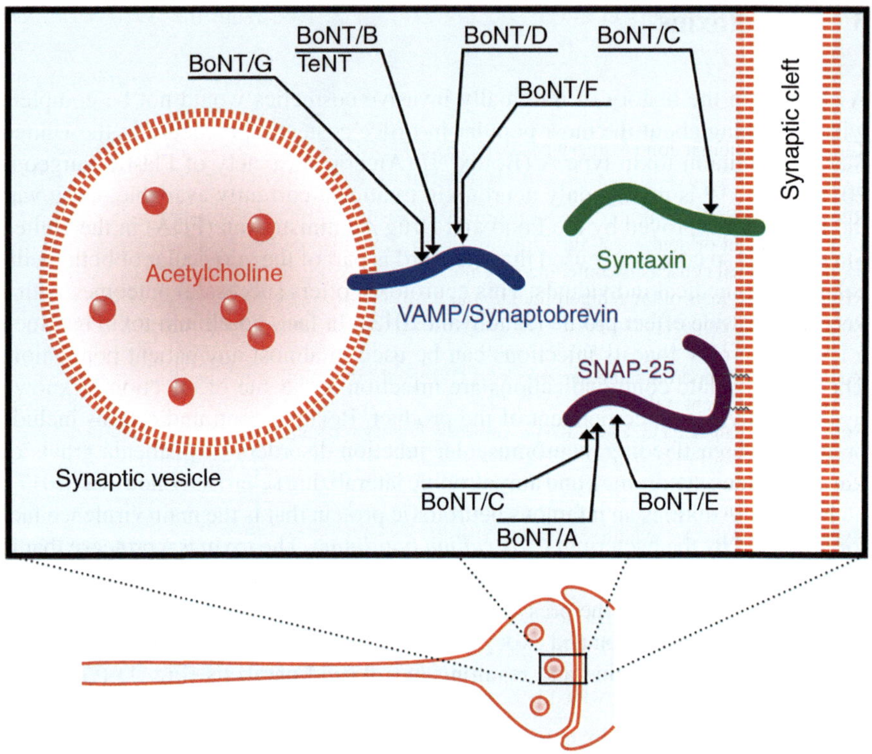

Fig. 1 Mechanism of action of the various known botulinum toxin subtypes. All forms of botulinum toxin interfere with components involved in the exocytosis of ACh at the neuromuscular junction. Botulinum toxin A is the most well-known, illustrated interfering with the SNAP-25 protein. (GNU head Permission is granted to copy, distribute, and/or modify this document under the terms of the GNU Free Documentation License, Version 1.2, or any later version published by the Free Software Foundation; with no Invariant Sections, no Front-Cover Texts, and no Back-Cover Texts. A copy of the license is included in the section entitled GNU Free Documentation License. "https://commons.wikimedia.org/wiki/Commons:GNU_Free_Documentation_License,_version_1.2" (Barr et al. 2005))

Similar to other landmark medical discoveries, botulinum toxin was discovered by serendipity. Botulism or "sausage poisoning" as it was originally described was discovered by a small-town German health officer and romantic poet in 1817 named Justinus Kerner. The study of the toxin was prompted by a 1793 outbreak in Wildbad, Germany, that originated from locally produced blood sausage (Kerner 1817). The outbreak involved 13 victims, 6 of whom succumbed to the illness. Before long, more than 200 cases of the food-borne intoxication were known in this region of Germany, prompting Kerner to publish the first paper on the disease in 1820 based on a extensive clinical observation of 76 patients afflicted by what he called "sausage poisoning" (Kerner 1820; Jaspers et al. 2011). In his paper, he describes symptoms of mydriasis, diplopia, gastrointestinal upset, and progressive muscle paralysis

(Kerner 1820; Jaspers et al. 2011). Botulism is derived from the word "botulus," sausage in Latin (Erbguth 2004; Torrens 1998).

Kerner went on to conduct experiments on animals and himself with botulinum toxin. He concluded that the toxin worked by interrupting signal transmission in somatic and autonomic motor systems while sparing sensory systems and mentation (Kerner 1820; Erbguth 1998). He noted that the toxin forms under anaerobic conditions and possesses lethality at very low doses (Erbguth 2004; Erbguth 1998). These descriptions of the effects of botulinum toxin earned Kerner recognition as the pioneer and father of botulinum toxin therapy.

The discovery of botulism propagated across the globe. In 1895 in Berlin, Emile van Ermengem, a bacteriologist and student of the infamous Robert Koch, isolated extract from a raw, partially salted ham that poisoned 34 people attending a funeral in Ellezelles, Belgium (Devriese 1999). The afflicted experienced symptoms of mydriasis, dysphagia, dysarthria, and descending muscle paralysis (Erbguth 2004). Ermengem successfully grew the same bacterium from the ham extract and autopsy specimens (Van Ermengem 1897; Ting and Freiman 2004). Ermengem also correctly established that botulism was an intoxication produced by *Clostridium botulinum*, not an infection (Van Ermengem 1897). He noted that the toxin only caused clinical disease in certain animal species and quickly lost its virulence when heated. As the canned food industry boomed over the next few decades, botulism became known in popular culture as a public health hazard. Botulinum toxin was even investigated as a potential biochemical warfare agent during World War II at Fort Detrick in Maryland. However, the toxin was never utilized in chemical warfare as it reportedly could not be aerosolized (Lamanna et al. 1946).

The US government first allowed academic investigation of *Clostridium* bacterium in the 1940s. The first indication that botulinum toxin may have medicinal uses was in the field of ophthalmology. Ophthalmologists specializing in eye muscle disorders were seeking non-surgical injection treatment options for the correction of strabismus. Various agents were utilized with limited success including local anesthetics, alcohols, enzymes, enzyme blockers, and snake venom.

In 1973, the ophthalmologist Alan B. Scott published a paper reporting that injecting botulinum toxin into the extraocular muscles of monkeys provided long-term, non-surgical treatment of strabismus without significant side effects (Scott et al. 1973). Scott and colleagues developed techniques for freeze-drying and buffering the toxin with albumin while maintaining potency, sterility, and safety and applied for investigational drug use approval from the US FDA. In 1978, the FDA granted Scott approval to begin testing small amounts of botulinum toxin type A in human volunteers. His team injected 56 doses of toxin into 16 patients with strabismus, utilizing an electromyographic needle to record muscle activity and thereby ensure that the injections were placed into the appropriate extraocular muscle belly. Scott and colleagues reported that the toxin was able to correct gaze misalignment without significant local or systemic side effects in his landmark paper, published in 1980 (Scott 1980). Scott trained hundreds of other colleagues to perform these injections with the novel agent which he called the Latin term for "eye aligner,"

Oculinum™. In 1989, the FDA approved the use of Oculinum™ for the non-surgical correction of strabismus, blepharospasm, hemifacial spasm, Meige syndrome, and the treatment of cervical dystonia and spasmodic torticollis (Walton et al. 1999). In 1989, the pharmaceutical company Allergan purchased Scott's company and renamed the toxin Botox™, a name that is synonymous with the toxin today.

In the late 1980s, the oculoplastic surgeon Jean Carruthers in Vancouver, British Columbia, incidentally discovered the use of botulinum toxin for facial cosmetic purposes. Jean was first introduced to botulinum toxin type A after spending 3 months with Alan Scott in 1982 as one of the early investigators in the studies that eventually led to FDA approval of botulinum toxin (Carruthers 2003). Carruthers began utilizing botulinum toxin type A injections for the treatment of blepharospasm in her patients. In 1987, she reported that injections to the medial brow of a patient resulted in an "unworried, un-troubled appearance," first noticed by the patient's family (Carruthers 2003). Jean Carruthers shared this observation with her husband, Alastair Carruthers, an accomplished dermatologist. Alastair experimentally injected isolated botulinum toxin type A into the glabellar regions of his receptionist the very next day. After 2–3 days, he observed that the receptionist's glabellar wrinkles had disappeared.

The Carruthers, desiring further characterization of this new use for botulinum toxin, recruited subjects from their respective practices into a small prospective study. Jean and Alastair published the first paper reporting the cosmetic appeal of botulinum toxin in 1992, demonstrating minimized glabellar wrinkles in 18 patients with intramuscular injections of botulinum toxin A with minimal side effects (Carruthers and Carruthers 1992). The Carruthers demonstrated that botulinum toxin was more effective and possessed a favorable side effect profile in the treatment of glabellar wrinkles when compared to other soft tissue augmentation practices of the time, such as injectable filler and fat grafting (Fig. 1). Of note, the Carruthers were not the only ones to note the potential use of botulinum toxin in facial cosmetics. A group at Columbia University observed similar clinical manifestations, but chose not to pursue these findings due to interests in other potential neurologic uses of botulinum toxin (Blitzer et al. 1993).

The doctors Carruthers had the perfect ingredients to launch a robust botulinum toxin practice, with Alastair's dermatologic patient population and Jean's access to purified botulinum toxin (Fig. 2). At first, many patients were hesitant to allow injection of a potentially fatal toxin into their bodies. However, as the doctors Carruthers conducted additional trials and presented their findings at dermatology meetings, their practice gained traction. Their treatment of forehead and ocular wrinkles with botulinum toxin injections became so popular that Jean completed training in cosmetic surgery and stopped treating ophthalmological patients altogether, and Alastair stopped performing dermatologic cancer surgery, limiting his practice to head and neck cosmetic procedures.

Since the Carruthers' landmark paper in 1992, many different formulations of botulinum toxin have become available and approved for use worldwide. In 2009, the FDA recommended the use of specific names rather than serotypes when

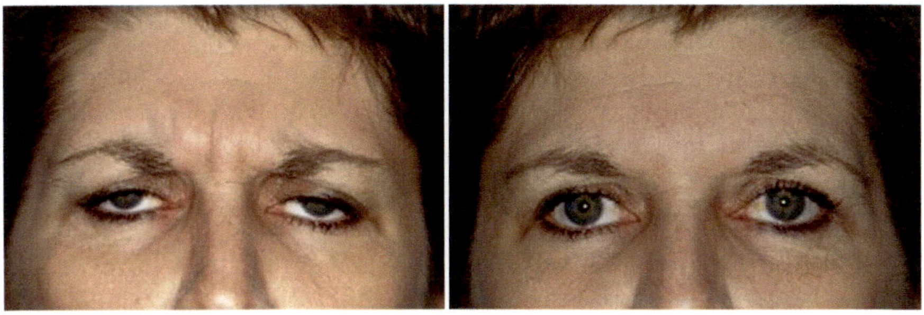

Fig. 2 Illustrates the effectiveness of botulinum toxin A injections in elimination glabellar wrinkles. The image on the left is prior to neurotoxin injection, and the right image was after 25 units of botulinum toxin A to the glabella. (Picture used with permission. Courtesy of Michael J. Will MD, DDS, FACS)

referring to the available formulations of botulinum toxin in order to prevent confusion. The formulations available in North America include on abotulinum toxin A, abobotulinum toxin A, incobotulinum toxin A, and prabotulinum toxin A. There have been numerous large randomized control trials proving the effectiveness of various individual formulations of botulinum toxin for the treatment of dynamic rhytids, glabellar lines, and crow's feet (Carruthers et al. 2002; Grimes and Shabazz 2009; Carruthers et al. 2006). Few randomized trials have directly compared the efficacy of the different formulations of botulinum toxin. Studies have suggested, however, that there is not much difference in overall efficacy of the various formulations, although they differ in onset of action, pain with injection, and duration of action (Sattler et al. 2010; Flynn 2010).

The popularity of botulinum toxin injections has increased dramatically since its first use in facial cosmetics. From 2000 to 2008, minimally invasive cosmetic treatment with botulinum toxin increased by 537% to an estimated five million treatments per year (American Society of Plastic Surgeons 2010). Over the same time period, surgical cosmetic procedures such as facelift and blepharoplasty decreased by 16% and 32%, respectively (American Society of Plastic Surgeons 2010). In 2019, 7.7 million Botox™ procedures were documented, an increase of 4% from 2018, making it again the most popular minimally invasive cosmetic procedure in the United States (American Society of Plastic Surgeons Plastic Surgery Statistics Report 2019). Botulinum toxin is now utilized for multiple facial cosmetic concerns that can be improved with regional muscle relaxation, including dynamic rhytids on the upper face and skin lines located on the lower face and neck.

Botulinum toxin is also used to treat a variety of non-cosmetic conditions in the head and neck region, including oromandibular dystonia, cervical dystonia, tension headaches, migraine headaches, post-herpetic neuralgia and myofascial temporomandibular dysfunction. Botulinum toxin was first used in oral and maxillofacial surgery in 1992 when Dr. Alistair Smyth published the remarkable effects it had on patients with "square jaws" or masseteric hypertrophy (Smyth 1994). In 1999, Dr.

Brian Freund was the first oral surgeon to report the effective use of the toxin in treatment of TMD with injections into the masseter and temporalis under electromyographic (EMG) guidance (Freund and Schwartz 1999). Today, botulinum toxin is used throughout medicine and dentistry, and its indications for use will likely continue to broaden.

4 Dermal Fillers

Over the past two decades, most medical and dental practices that offer cosmeceuticals have embraced the art and science of facial fillers. Soft tissue fillers are the second most common cosmetic procedure performed worldwide after injection of botulinum toxin (Ballin et al. 2015). In 2019, 2.7 million soft tissue filler procedures were performed in the United States, a 1% increase from 2018 (American Society of Plastic Surgeons Plastic Surgery Statistics Report 2019). Middle-aged women comprise the majority of injectable filler patients, but it is becoming more and more common for facial cosmetic practices to treat both younger and older patients of both sexes (American Society of Plastic Surgeons Plastic Surgery Statistics Report 2019).

As we age, there is decreased thickness and elasticity of the skin, lipoatrophy, and resorption of the craniofacial skeleton, all of which lead to facial volume loss (Ballin et al. 2015). It has been long appreciated that facial volume loss is one of the primary factors contributing to an aged look. Clinical signs of age-related facial volume loss include decreased facial contours, sagging skin, flatter cheeks, depression of the oral commissures, and hollowing of the eyes. A 2007 study utilizing facial dissection of cadavers demonstrated that subcutaneous fat in the face is highly compartmentalized and changes in the volume and positioning of these compartments contribute to the aging facial appearance (Rohrich and Pessa 2007). The administration of fillers can be used to restore a semblance of youth by replacing the lost tissue volume and inducing effacement of overlying skin wrinkles. The cosmetic applications of dermal filler are vast, including softening of glabellar and horizontal forehead lines, replacing periorbital fat, elevating the brow, correcting temporal fossa wasting, adding fullness to the cheeks, decreasing depth of the nasolabial and nasojugal folds, treating melomental (marionette lines) and oral folds, and even chin, lip, and mandibular augmentation. Soft tissue fillers can also be used to correct or repair cosmetic contour defects that are unrelated to the aging process such as HIV-associated lipoatrophy, atrophic scarring, and acquired or congenital facial asymmetry secondary to bony or soft tissue abnormalities.

There are over 100 filler products at the disposal of the facial cosmetic practitioner. There are currently five main materials that make up the majority of fillers available on the market. The available absorbable filler materials are collagen, hyaluronic acid, calcium hydroxyapatite, and poly-L-lactic acid. The only non-absorbable or permanent material available is composed of polymethylmethacrylate (PMMA) beads, a popular compound used in ophthalmology and restorative dentistry. This chapter cannot possibly cover all of the available formulations. Instead, the discussion will focus on the key historical discoveries and broad categories of facial fillers that helped shape today's facial cosmetic rejuvenation opportunities.

From a historical perspective, it is helpful to be aware of the original filler products, their discovery, and their shortcomings to gain an appreciation and understanding of the fillers available for use today. History has taught us that novel technologies and agents must be used with extreme caution as serious complications can arise, sometimes many years after the initial treatment.

The first technique utilized for injectable filler was fat grafting. The first documented fat grafting procedure occurred in 1893 when the German surgeon Gustav Neuber filled out facial defects resulting from osteomyelitis scars by transplanting dermal fat from the upper extremity to the orbital region (Klein 2006). Neuber did this by performing a lipectomy from the upper arm and transferring the gross harvest to the dermis of the atrophic site; however, this technique resulted in significant resorption over time. In 2020, a similar technique of fat grafting is still being used by many cosmetic surgeons and was recently repopularized with the advent of suction-assisted lipectomy with blunt cannulas for fat harvest.

The first reports of injections of a foreign substance for use as a filler can be traced back to 1899, when the Austrian surgeon Robert Gersuny injected petrolatum mineral oil to replace a missing testicle following castration caused by tuberculous epididymitis (Glicenstein 2007). The immediate success of this treatment encouraged Dr. Gersuny to utilize petrolatum as a filler for soft tissue defects. However, petrolatum has a melting temperature similar to body temperature and became quickly liquified when injected subcutaneously, and so the search for the material for an injectable filler continued.

The German chemist Baron Karl Ludwig von Reichenbach discovered paraffin in 1830 by isolating it through the dry distillation of beech-wood tar (Goldwyn 1980). He observed the substance to be inert and unreactive and aptly named it paraffin from the Latin word parum (barely) and affinis (affinity). Soon, surgeons began experimenting with using the material as a cosmetic filler as it had a melting temperature of 65 degrees Celsius, well above body temperature. However, paraffin injections were associated with severe secondary late complications including embolization, migration into the surrounding tissue causing nodules, paraffinomas, and granuloma formation (Glicenstein 2007; Ridenour and Kontis 2009). By 1901, literature emerged outlining the potential life-threatening complications of injectable paraffin, including a report of a 39-year-old woman who underwent paraffin injection for urinary incontinence and went on to develop pulmonary and cerebral emboli (Goldwyn 1980). The most infamous paraffin filler complication causing disfigurement was seen in the Duchess of Marlborough, Gladys Spencer-Churchill (Fig. 3). The Duchess underwent paraffin injection in 1901 to the nasal dorsum that subsequently migrated to her chin, producing paraffinomas throughout her face and causing severe disfigurement (Ridenour and Kontis 2009). Even with the reports of these severe and even life-threatening complications, paraffin fillers remained popular for the first 20 years of the twentieth century. They were used primarily for

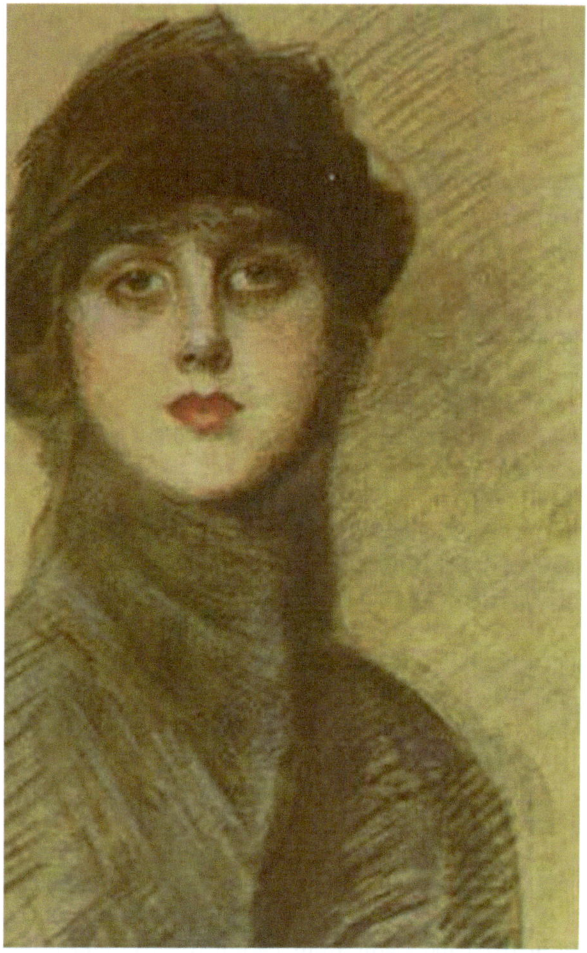

Fig. 3 The Duchess of Marlborough Gladys Spencer-Churchill (1881–1977), the second wife of the ninth Duke of Marlborough. She was well-known for her beauty before undergoing injections with paraffin filler complicated by migratory "paraffinomas" that caused severe facial disfigurement "https://creativecommons.org/publicdomain/mark/1.0/deed.en"

cosmetic indications such as filling of face wrinkles, adding volume to the cheeks, and augmenting nasal defects.

The next foreign body substance utilized as a filler was silicone. Like paraffin, silicone is an inert, clear, oily substance that can be easily injected. Since its initial use, there has been debate over its safety. The literature is inundated with examples of disastrous complications associated with silicone injections, and these cases have received worldwide media attention. However, proponents of the use of silicone as an injectable agent assert that the complications can be explained by the use of impure silicone in improper amounts. Proponents of silicone assert that pure medical-grade silicone can be an excellent filler agent when delivered by an experienced provider.

The Swedish chemist Johann Berzelius is credited as the first to isolate elemental silicon in 1824 (Chasan 2007). Silicone was originally produced in mass quantities by the Dow Corning Corporation for use in the aerospace, electronics, and defense industries (Chasan 2007). John Holter, a toolmaker, was the first to bring attention to the potential of silicone's medical use. After having a baby affected by hydrocephalus, Holter was motivated to develop a silicone-based hydrocephalic shunt that was placed in the first patient in 1955 (Chasan 2007). In Japan following World War II, silicone was used for the first time in cosmetics. Silicone was injected into the breasts and buttocks of prostitutes in an attempt to achieve a more "westernized" appearance (Chasan 2007). This practice spread to the United States, becoming especially popular in the entertainment capitals of California and Nevada.

The plastic surgeon James Barrett Brown was among the first to recognize the potential use of silicone for soft tissue supplementation to the face, publishing his findings in 1953 (Brown et al. 1953). Simultaneously, JT Scales published a list of criteria for the ideal soft tissue substitute which included a substance not modified by soft tissue, chemically inert, lack of inflammation or foreign body reaction, non-carcinogenic, non-allergic, sterilizable, able to be fabricated in the desired form, and capable of resisting mechanical strain (Scales 1953). Brown believed silicone would fit Scales criteria, and although his initial interest was the use of silicone in burn victims, he reasoned that silicone injections would offer a safe treatment for small contour deficiencies like scars and wrinkles. However, by the 1960s, Barrett Brown and others noted that silicone had many complications similar to those seen with paraffin injectables including migration, fistulation, and even several reported cases of death. It was particularly concerning that the severe inflammatory complications could be seen many years after silicone injections.

In 1965, Dow Corning Corporation developed a purified medical-grade silicone to be tested as an injectable, referred to as MDX4-4011. In a 1977 study, the Canadian plastic surgeon Theodore Wilkie published a study on the treatment of 92 patients with a total of 230 treatments with MDX 4-4011 over a 10-year period showing 13 granuloma formations, most occurring in the glabella (Wilkie 1977). The consensus at that time was that because of this complication, silicone injectables were not safe for use. In 1989, a group of dermatologists reviewed the safety of silicone and concluded that the previously reported problems with silicone soft tissue augmentation were associated with impure products, excess volumes, or inappropriate locations (Swanson 1989). In 2013, a team that included the Carruthers published a study where they evaluated the safety and efficacy of highly purified medical-grade 1000-cst liquid injectable silicone to treat HIV-associated facial lipoatrophy. They utilized the "micro-droplet" technique, whereby small amounts of silicone were deposited deep into the dermis and subcutaneous tissue over the course of months. Twenty patients with HIV-associated lipoatrophy were treated with injectable silicone over the course of a maximum of six sessions with 2.0 cc injected each session. The results showed that at 18 months, there were no adverse effects and all patients achieved complete correction of lipoatrophy (Chen et al. 2013). This study suggested that liquid injectable silicone could be safe when used in the hands of an experienced provider.

The use of injectable silicone for facial cosmetics remains a hotly debated topic today. The US FDA considers injectable silicone an investigational device and has yet to approve silicone for widespread cosmetic use. Cosmetic surgeons and emergency rooms throughout the United States continue to see the complications of silicone filler treatments, most performed in other countries with silicone of unknown purity.

In many ways, the quest for the perfect filler still continues today, although new innovations are constantly being made. The universally agreed-upon characteristics of the perfect filler are still in line with Scales criteria from the 1940s with a few additional desirable features including the following: the volume injected is the volume of correction, long-lasting, a natural feel and look, inexpensive, and fully reversible. Currently, there are no fillers on the market that meet all criteria, but there are many formulations that come close.

Animal collagen-based products were the first to be FDA-approved for use as cosmetic injectables and laid the foundation for the many filler products that succeeded it. After several years of study, development, and testing, collagen gained FDA approval in 1981 (Knapp et al. 1977). The first of these bovine-derived collagen fillers to hit the market were Zyderm™ and Zyplast™. The use of collagen filler for lip enhancement became popularized in American culture by actress Barbara Hershey in the 1988 movie *Beaches* (Klein 2006).

While successful, the bovine collagen fillers did have several notable side effects, most significantly a foreign body reaction. Bovine collagen requires a sensitivity test before use to ensure that the patient's immune system will tolerate the foreign substance. Classically, patients had to be inoculated with the material in the forearm, and if no local allergic response was seen at 30 days, the material was assumed safe for further dissemination. Some providers advocated for two consecutive monthly negative allergy tests prior to cosmetic injections to the face. The need for allergy testing was a major drawback to its use, as cosmetics patients were reluctant to wait 30–60 days to achieve their desired effect. Bovine collagen is also associated with severe swelling at the site of injection, likely due to local immune response to the foreign material. Furthermore, the bovine collagen products did not have the long-lasting effects that patients were seeking, lasting only several months. Finally, outbreaks of avian flu, swine flu, and prion diseases made animal-based collagen fillers less attractive to patients. Despite these drawbacks, the bovine collagen product Bellafill™ remains available on the market and is approved for use as a filler for nasolabial folds and moderate to severe facial acne scars.

While the bovine collagen products were successful and safe compared to prior available injectables, there was a demand for a substance that lasted longer and did not require sensitivity testing prior to injection. This resulted in the development of hyaluronic acid (HA) products. HA was first discovered in the vitreous humor of cow's eyes in 1934 (Meyer and Palmer 1934). It was used overseas as a filler decades before receiving FDA approval for cosmetic use in the United States in 2003 after many studies found it to be safe and effective (Duranti et al. 1998). HA is by far the most popular and commonly used filler today.

HA is a naturally occurring glycosaminoglycan that is found ubiquitously throughout the extracellular matrix of human connective tissue. It is responsible for stabilizing intercellular structures, producing a viscoelastic framework for collagen and elastin to bind. It is extremely hydrophilic, capable of binding 1000 times its weight in water (Olenius 1998). HA-based filler has a much longer duration of effect compared to collagen fillers (Narins et al. 2003). The extended longevity of HA fillers is due in large part to the process of isovolumetric degradation. Collagen fillers are continually metabolized through phagocytization and degradation, whereas HA fillers are degraded as water is drawn into the hydrophilic glycosaminoglycan molecule.

HA is harvested in large quantities for use in filler by two methods: bacterial fermentation and extraction from rooster combs. The rooster-derived products have a shorter duration effect compared to their bacterial-derived counterparts (Ridenour and Kontis 2009). There has been some hesitation from patients to have animal products injected, prompting innovation of non-animal HA fillers. The first non-animal HA filler to receive FDA approval for use in the United States, and credited for the explosion in popularity of HA fillers, was Restylane™ in 2003 (Fig. 4). There was an enormous marketing campaign targeting baby boomers associated with the introduction of Restylane™ in the United States, securing a significant market share for the product (Niamtu 2011). In 2005, the FDA-approved popular competitor Juvederm™. Other animal-based HA fillers introduced in the early 2000s include Hyalaform™ and Captique™. However, these products were produced via the rooster comb technique, received with hesitation by patients, and did not last long as the non-animal-based HA fillers. For these reasons, the non-animal options Restylane™ and Juvederm™ have remained the most popular HA fillers since their introduction.

Since the introduction of the non-animal HA fillers, there have been minor enhancements to the products. For example, Juvederm Ultra XC™ was released in 2010 and included local anesthetic with the injectable although many clinicians do not see significant utility in this advancement. The noxious stimulus of the needle and fluid bolus would have already occurred by the time the local anesthetic took effect, providing minimal increased comfort during the treatment. However, many

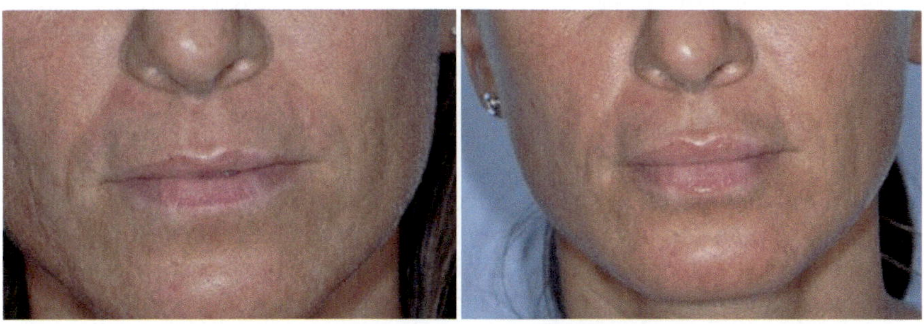

Fig. 4 Illustrates the effectiveness of Restylane™ (HA filler) at treating deep nasolabial folds and atrophic lips. The image on the left was prior to volume enhancement, and the image on the left was taken 1 week following Restylane™ injections to the nasolabial fold (2 cc) and upper and lower lips (1 cc). (Image used with permission, courtesy of Michael J Will MD, DDS, FACS)

patients come in demanding the formulations that have a combined local anesthetic due to successful marketing campaigns conducted by the filler companies.

While HA products remain most popular, newer technologies such as the injectable implant poly-L-lactic acid from the alpha hydroxy acid family have been introduced. Sculptra™ was the first of these products to become FDA approved for the treatment of HIV-associated facial lipoatrophy in 2004. The poly-L-lactic acid particles initiate an inflammatory reaction causing local tissue fibroblasts to produce collagen. Sculptra™ treatments typically require multiple sessions as the full clinical effect of the injections may not be apparent for 1–2 weeks. This product is used by some clinicians for the off-label filling of lines and wrinkles (Niamtu 2011).

Injectable calcium hydroxyapatite, marketed as Radiesse™, is another new technology, receiving FDA approval in 2006 for the correction of facial lipoatrophy and moderate to severe wrinkles (Ridenour and Kontis 2009). Radiesse™ is composed of 30% calcium hydroxyapatite suspended in a sodium carboxymethylcellulose, glycerin, and high-purity water gel carrier (Ahn 2007). The calcium hydroxyapatite microspheres are similar to the inorganic components of bone and teeth. Radiesse™ is injected deep into the subdermal plane, where the gel carrier is degraded over a period of 1–3 months, and the calcium hydroxyapatite particles serve as a scaffold for new collagen deposition, inducing local collagen production from fibroblasts. Radiesse™ filler provides immediate correction, and clinical effect can last 1–2 years (Ahn 2007).

The only permanent filler on the market contains PMMA beads, originally marketed as ArteFill™. ArteFill™ was rebranded in 2014 as Bellafill™, a suspension of PMMA beads in a bovine collagen delivery vehicle. The PMMA beads are not absorbed by the body, inducing fibroplasia and becoming encapsulated by endogenous collagen (Ballin et al. 2015). A major drawback to Bellafill™ is that a sensitivity test is necessary before use to ensure there is no allergy to the bovine collagen. The major concern with the use of permanent filler is the possibility of late-onset complications such as migration of the material, as was seen in prior permanent filler materials like paraffin and silicone (Funt and Pavicic 2013). Despite this concern, Bellafill™ was FDA approved for correction of nasolabial fold in 2006 and the treatment of acne scars in 2015.

5 Conclusion

The demand for products to fight the effects of facial aging and enhance appearance will likely continue to increase. History has shown us that the human race has an insatiable need to alter perceived defects in appearance with cosmeceuticals of various kinds. This high demand provides lucrative opportunities for both drug companies and practitioners and will likely continue to drive the development of new products and expand the utility of existing products.

References

Ahn MS. Calcium Hydroxylapatite: radiesse. Facial Plast Surg Clin North Am. 2007;15:85–90.

American Society of Plastic Surgeons 2010 Report of the 2009 Statistics.

American Society of Plastic Surgeons 2018 Plastic Surgery Statistics Report.

American Society of Plastic Surgeons Plastic Surgery Statistics Report 2019: ASPS National Clearinghouse of Plastic Surgery Procedural Statistics.

Ballin AC, Brandt FS, Cazzaniga A. Dermal fillers: an update. Am J Clin Dermatol. 2015;16:271–83.

Barr JR, Moura H, Boyer AE, Woolfitt AR, Kalb SR, Pavlopoulos A, McWilliams LG, Schmidt JG, Martinez RA, Ashley DL. Botulinum neurotoxin detection and differentiation by mass spectrometry. Emerg Infect Dis. 2005;11:1578–83.

Blitzer A, Brin M, Keen M. Botulinum toxin for the treatment of hyperfunctional lines of the face. Arch Otolaryngol Head Neck Surg. 1993;119:1018–22.

Brown JB, Fryer MP, Randall P, Lu M. Silicones in plastic surgery: laboratory and clinical investigations, a preliminary report. Plast Reconstr Surg. 1953;12:374–6.

Carruthers A. History of the clinical use of botulinum toxin A and B. Clin Dermatol. 2003;21:469–72.

Carruthers JDA, Carruthers JA. Treatment of glabellar frown lines with C. botulinum-A exotoxin. J Dermatol Surg Oncol. 1992;18:17–21.

Carruthers J, Lowe N, Menter M. A multicenter, double-blind, randomized, placebo-controlled study of the efficacy and safety of botulinum toxin type A in the treatment of glabellar lines. J Am Acad Dermatol. 2002;46:840–9.

Carruthers A, Carruthers J, Said S. Dose-ranging study of botulinum toxin type a in the treatment of glabellar rhytids in females. Dermatol Surg. 2006;31:414–22.

Chasan PE. The history of injectable silicone fluids for soft-tissue augmentation. Plast Reconstr Surg. 2007;120:2034–40.

Chen F, Carruthers A, Humphrey S, Carruthers J. HIV-associated facial lipoatrophy treated with injectable silicone oil: a pilot study. J Am Acad Dermatol. 2013;69:431–7.

Devriese PP. On the discovery of clostridium botulinum. J Hist Neurosci. 1999;8:43–50.

Duranti F, Salti G, Bovani B, Calandra M, Rosati ML. Injectable hyaluronic acid gel for soft tissue augmentation: a clinical and histological study. Dermatol Surg. 1998;24:1317–25.

Ellis H. Alexander wood: inventor of the hypodermic syringe and needle. Br J Hosp Med (Lond). 2017;78:647.

Erbguth FJ. Botulinum toxin, a historical note [18]. Lancet. 1998;351:1820.

Erbguth FJ. Historical notes on botulism, clostridium botulinum, botulinum toxin, and the idea of the therapeutic use of the toxin. Mov Disord. 2004; https://doi.org/10.1002/mds.20003.

Feldmann H. Die geschichte der injektionen. Bilder aus der geschichte der hals- nasen-ohren-heilkunde, dargestelt an instrumenten aus der sammlung im Deutschen medizinhistorischen museum in ingolstadt. Laryngorhinootologie. 2000;79:239–46.

Flynn TC. Botulinum toxin: examining duration of effect in facial aesthetic applications. Am J Clin Dermatol. 2010;11:183–99.

Freund B, Schwartz M. The use of botulinum toxin for the treatment of temporomandibular disorders: preliminary findings. 1999.

Funt D, Pavicic T. Dermal fillers in aesthetics: an overview of adverse events and treatment approaches. Clin Cosmet Investig Dermatol. 2013;6:295–316.

Giordano CN, Matarasso SL, Ozog DM. Injectable and topical neurotoxins in dermatology: basic science, anatomy, and therapeutic agents. J Am Acad Dermatol. 2017;76:1013–24.

Glicenstein J. The first "fillers," Vaseline and paraffin: from miracle to disaster [in French]. Ann Chir Plast Esthet. 2007;52:157–61.

Goldwyn RM. The paraffin story. Plast Reconstr Surg. 1980;65:517–24.

Grimes PE, Shabazz D. A four-month randomized, double-blind evaluation of the efficacy of botulinum toxin type a for the treatment of glabellar lines in women with skin types v and VI. Dermatol Surg. 2009;35:429–36.

Jandhyala R. Impact of botulinum toxin a on the quality of life of subjects following treatment of facial lines. J Clin Aesthet Dermatol. 2013;6:41–5.

Jaspers GWC, Pijpe J, Jansma J. The use of botulinum toxin type A in cosmetic facial procedures. Int J Oral Maxillofac Surg. 2011;40:127–33.

Kattimani V, Tiwari RVC, Gufran K, Wasan B, Shilpa PH, Khader AA. Botulinum toxin application in facial esthetics and recent treatment indications (2013–2018). J Int Soc Prev Commun Dent. 2019;9:99–105.

Kerner J. Vergiftung durch verdorbene Würste. Tübinger Blätter für Naturwissenschaften und Arzneykd. 1817;3:25.

Kerner J. Neue Beobachtungen über die in Würtemberg so häufig vorfallenden tödtlichen Vergiftungen durch den Genuß geräucherter Würste. 1820.

Klein AW. Techniques for soft tissue augmentation: An "A to Z". Am J Clin Dermatol. 2006;7:107–20.

Knapp TR, Kaplan EN, Daniels JR. Injectable collagen for soft tissue augmentation. Plast Reconstr Surg. 1977;60:398–405.

Kravetz RE. Hypodermic syringe. Am J Gastroenterol. 2005;100:2614.

Lamanna C. The most poisonous poison: what do we know about the toxin of botulism? What are the problems to be solved? Science (80-). 1959;130:763–72.

Lamanna C, Mcelroy OE, Eklund HW. The purification and crystallization of clostridium botulinum type a toxin. Science (80-). 1946;103:613–4.

Meyer K, Palmer JW. The polysaccharide of the vitreous humor. J Biol Chem. 1934;107:629–34.

Narins RS, Brandt F, Leyden J, Lorenc ZP, Rubin M, Smith S. A randomized, double-blind, multicenter comparison of the efficacy and tolerability of restylane versus zyplast for the correction of nasolabial folds. Dermatol Surg. 2003;29:588–95.

Niamtu J. Cosmetic facial surgery. St Louis: Elsevier; 2011.

Olenius M. The first clinical study using a new biodegradable implant for the treatment of lips, wrinkles, and folds. Aesthet Plast Surg. 1998;22:97–101.

Oumeish OY. The cultural and philosophical concepts of cosmetics in beauty and art through the medical history of mankind. Clin Dermatol. 2001;19:375–86.

Parish LC, Crissey JT. Cosmetics: a historical review. Clin Dermatol. 1988;6:1–4.

Ridenour B, Kontis TC. Injectable calcium hydroxylapatite microspheres (Radiesse). Facial Plast Surg. 2009;25:100–5.

Rohrich RJ, Pessa JE. The fat compartments of the face: anatomy and clinical implications for cosmetic surgery. Plast Reconstr Surg. 2007;119:2219–27.

Rynd F. Description of an instrument for the subcutaneous introduction of fluids in affections of the nerves. Dublin Q J Med Sci. 1861;32:13.

Sattler G, Callander MJ, Grablowitz D, Walker T, Bee EK, Rzany B, Flynn TC, Carruthers A. Noninferiority of incobotulinumtoxinA, free from complexing proteins, compared with another botulinum toxin type A in the treatment of glabellar frown lines. Dermatol Surg. 2010;36:2146–54.

Scales J. Discussion on metals and synthetic materials in relation to tissues. Proc R Soc Med. 1953;46:641–562.

Scott AB. Botulinum toxin injection into extraocular muscles as an alternative to strabismus surgery. Ophthalmology. 1980;87(10):1044–9. healio.com.

Scott AB, Rosenbaum A, Collins CC. Pharmacologic weakening of extraocular muscles. Investig Ophthalmol Vis Sci. 1973;12:924–7.

Smyth A. Botulinum toxin treatment of bilateral masseteric hypertrophy. Br J Oral Maxillofac Surg. 1994;32:29–33.

Swanson NA. Dermal implants: safety of products injected for soft tissue augmentation. J Am Acad Dermatol. 1989;21:992–8.

Ting PT, Freiman A. The story of clostridium botulinum: from food poisoning to Botox. Clin Med J R Coll Phys London. 2004;4:258–61.

Torrens JK. Clostridium botulinum was named because of association with "sausage poisoning". BMJ. 1998;316:151.

Van Ermengem E. Ueber einen neuen anaeroben Bacillus und seine Beziehungen zum Rotulismus. 1897.

Walton M, Otrr, Dctda, Goldenthal K. Division of Clinical Trial Design and Analysis HFM-576 Medical Officer Review. 1999.

Wilkie TF. Late development of granuloma after liquid silicone injections. Plast Reconstr Surg. 1977;60:179–88.

Zhou R, Pan B, Wang C, Wang D. Mandibular rim trilogy with botulinum toxin injection: reduction, projection, and lift. Facial Plast Surg. 2017;33:102–8.

Index

E. M. Ferneini et al. (eds.), *The History of Maxillofacial Surgery*,
https://doi.org/10.1007/978-3-030-89563-1

N

O

S

T

GPSR Compliance

The European Union's (EU) General Product Safety Regulation (GPSR) is a set of rules that requires consumer products to be safe and our obligations to ensure this.

If you have any concerns about our products, you can contact us on ProductSafety@springernature.com

In case Publisher is established outside the EU, the EU authorized representative is:

Springer Nature Customer Service Center GmbH
Europaplatz 3
69115 Heidelberg, Germany

Batch number: 10732076

Printed by Printforce, the Netherlands